8週穩糖減重密技

降三高、消脂甩肉，健檢不再秀紅字

余宜叡醫師◎著

目錄

PART 1 糖尿病與血糖的親密關係

PART 3 拒絕糖胖的關鍵秘訣

Ch3 藥物與體重管理 ……244

PART 4 專業團隊讓減重&穩糖更有成效

Ch1 好團隊很重要 ……260

Ch2 案例分享 ……276

附錄 成人肥胖治療流程與藥物重點重要圖表 ……290

推薦序 1 |

從穩糖減重開始，打造自我的全方位健康

欣聞余宜叡主任即將出書，將其費心整理的許多臨床案例編集成冊，造福更多糖尿病及肥胖症患者，深化病患對自我健康照護的意識與知識，並提升健康管理的能力，裨益社會整體健康的發展。對於宜叡主任的用心與努力，深表肯定與敬佩！

宜叡在本體系員榮醫院、員生醫院擔任社區醫學部主任，是一位具專業又充滿活力的醫師。不只用智慧與熱誠帶領社區護理師、衛教師、個管師等團隊；還對臨床服務有專業投入，也經常在報章媒體發表淺顯易懂的衛教文章，呼籲國人重視自我健康照護，讓患者與家屬理解與因應糖尿病與肥胖症在生活中的各種困境，以營造生理、心理與社會的全方位健康。

本人身為心臟科醫師，深知糖尿病對全身大小血管的危害，也瞭解對病患衛教的重要性。在心臟科經常遇到與死神拔河搶救的心血管病患，卻有不少患者對於已罹患糖尿病渾然不知或未有良好控制，日積月累終演變為糖尿病的嚴重後果「心肌梗塞」；有些病患甚至因而猝死，令人十分遺憾與難過。

另外，肥胖症也是現今社會盛行率相當高的重要課題，肥胖症常伴隨高血壓、高血糖、高血脂等三高症狀和相關疾病，若長期忽

略未加控制，同樣會衍生為心肌梗塞、腦中風等心血管疾病，嚴重威脅民眾健康。

員榮醫療體系正在籌設「員榮總醫院」，未來將網羅更多優質專業人才。除了持續落實急重症醫療，也將深耕社區，大力推動預防保健與健康管理，以預防疾病發生及提升民眾自我健康識能為目標，並用心呵護更多糖尿病與肥胖症患者，達到延緩或避免產生嚴重併發症的效果。深切期盼宜叡主任持續發揮其專長，帶領團隊服務鄉親，做到全人全家全程的優質醫療服務。

本書分為前後兩部分，前半部主要是糖尿病照護，後半部則是減重照護；

每個臨床個案的分析都深入淺出，點出在臨床上穩糖減重過程中患者常遇到的各種疑問，同時也提供深具參考價值的因應之道。

相信藉由本書的出版，將散播正確衛教的種子，幫助更多需要的人，讓患者的病情更容易獲得控制，一般民眾也能夠因而維持健康避免產生疾病；如此，我們的社會將更健康美好，這是身為醫者的我最衷心的期待。

（員榮醫療體系總院長）

張克士

推薦序 2 ｜

見解獨到、實用有效的祛糖胖、穩血糖完全手冊

在台灣，糖尿患者口已經逼近 250 萬人，而且以每年近 16 萬人的速度增加。如何妥善管理血糖？不但是糖友關注的重要議題，也是你我應該了解的健康議題。很高興看到余宜叡醫師出了這本書，提供大家關於糖尿病血糖與體重管理的全面知識，也能幫助糖友們穩定血糖並且達到理想的體重。

余醫師在台北醫學大學醫學系畢業之後，就接受完整的家庭醫學科訓練，並且曾經擔任過彰化基督教醫院的主治醫師與鹿東分院的家庭醫學科主任，目前是員榮醫院社區醫學部主任，對於糖尿病的治療與體重管理，有豐富的臨床經驗與獨到的見解，由他來分享相關的知識，是再適合也不過了。

本書分為 4 個部分，每一部分都涵蓋了重要的主題，包括糖尿病的基礎知識，以及實務上的血糖監測、用藥原則、飲食策略，以及減重和專業團隊的重要性，內容豐富而完整。特別的是，本書的章節編排頗費心思，針對讀者可能想知道的問題來組織，每個主題都用精要的文字加以說明，這樣的編排有助於快速的查到心中想知道的問題。

在本書的第一部分，介紹了糖尿病的分類、主要症狀和診斷標

準，以及糖尿病的併發症、血糖監測與胰島素治療。第二部分則針對藥物、飲食與運動等生活習慣，進行詳細的說明。在第三部分，分享了減重的重要性，以及減重的關鍵秘訣，包括飲食策略、運動與藥物治療。最後，在第四部分中，則強調專業團隊在糖尿病管理和減重方面的重要性，並分享一些案例和工作坊學員的寶貴經驗。

這些內容，無論是已經被診斷為糖尿病的糖友，還是想要更了解血糖和體重的調節與管理，都會覺得很實用。此外，這本書提供了實際的建議和解決方案，讓大家能夠更了解自己的健康，並讓糖友透過血糖與體重控制，減少併發症的風險，並增加生活品質。

不過，由於每個人的狀況都不同，因此要提醒大家的是，本書主要是提供一個架構，讓大家能有整體的觀念與知識，實際上的狀況還是要跟你的醫師討論後再進行。

最後，恭喜余醫師順利的出版這本書，希望這本書能讓更多的人認識糖尿病，了解血糖控制與減重的關鍵，也能對糖友們的血糖與體重管理有所助益！

（臺大醫院內科臨床教授、中華民國糖尿病學會理事、糖尿病關懷基金會執行長）

李弘元

推薦序3 |

案例最多、
糖友最想擁有的穩糖減重全書

一位認真的好醫師，一本架構清晰寫作完整的好書，連結了糖尿病和血糖的親密關係。糖尿病的可怕在全世界及台灣都是無庸置疑的，有關糖尿病的科普書籍也非常的多，但是文筆清晰、邏輯完整的相關書籍卻非常有限。然而，我在余宜叡醫師的這本大作當中，同時看到了這兩個特徵。他把最新的概念，融入教育患者的科普書籍中，讓我們閱讀起來平易近人、如沐春風。

余醫師是一位非常認真的醫師，平日不但需要幫患者做教育，也花了很多時間來跟同儕討論，以及提攜下一代的年輕醫師，這本書不僅僅適合讓患者完整了解穩糖與減重，還能幫助資淺的醫護人員能夠清楚看到糖尿病的相關特徵以及併發症。所以，當余醫師希望我幫他寫序言，除了感到非常榮幸之外，心中更是感動。因為願意看患者的醫師很多，但是願意用文字留下記錄，而且展望未來者的反而很少。

本書當中舉出了非常多的案例，可以讓讀者好好來學習如何面對血糖，這比教科書中硬梆梆的知識好太多了，因為我們面對的是患者，而不是課本，在這本書中，充分的展現以患者為師的風範，讓我們能夠在病患的生活型態，以及併發症上，學習真正跟患者溝通的知識。

同時，本書也展望未來糖尿病的重點──體重的管理。相信從社區醫學、減重及家庭醫學等余醫師的專長出發，可以帶領我們的病患，遠離對糖尿病的恐懼，學習跟慢性病為友，身體健康就自然可以天長地久。

恭喜余醫師完成這本大作，除了推薦給糖尿病病友之外，我也非常推薦本書給年輕的醫護人員作為臨床看病患入門的參考。期待在醫師、糖尿病衛教師等歌專業人員的通力合作的努力下，幫助每位糖友都能獲得健康幸福。

（台大醫學院內科教授、中華民國糖尿病衛教學會理事長）

王治元

推薦序 4 ｜

最親切、詳盡的余式穩糖減重好書

余宜叡醫師是我在彰化基督教醫院的前同事，他具有做事非常認真的人格特質，而且不只擁有非常到位的專業精神，更永遠都帶著熱情和執著在服務人群。因此，當我看到他竟然能夠在自由時報寫醫學專欄，以幾乎每個禮拜有一篇短文刊登的頻率的時候，我的內心不僅僅非常佩服他的毅力之外，更由衷讚嘆他愛護糖友及家屬的這種大愛。也更由此，他總能由蒐集到的諸多案例當中，導入正確的衛教知識，不只教導糖友和家屬，甚至連參加其所舉辦推廣增進穩糖減重的工作坊的醫藥專業人員，都獲益非淺。此舉絕對堪稱「仁心仁術」，我要大大為他按無數個讚！

本書雖然是余醫師的首本大眾保健養生著作，但讀來毫無生澀感，反而充滿濃濃的愛護糖友的愛心。其最大特色就是，完全都是以案例解說病情和解決方案的「余氏風格」和大家說話——也就是從認識糖尿病，到穩糖的關鍵秘技，再到拒絕糖胖的關鍵秘訣，最後以專業團隊讓減重和穩糖更有成效做結尾，形成本書的 4 大部分。

每篇文章讀來無不令人覺得異常親切之外，更從他舉出的諸多的故事案例當中，讀者很容易都可以對號入座地對應到自己的狀況，從中掌握關鍵的糖尿病知識，汲取做為己用，讓自己邁向更健康的正途。就算是讀者是家屬，也都根本無礙於傳達給糖友和患者當事人，因為易讀、易懂、好操作，一讀就懂、一看就會，自然能夠馬上協助糖友和患者進行實作。

所以，我們完全可以說這是一本既淺顯易懂，又正確傳遞糖尿病防治和減重穩糖知識的好書，破除網路社群媒體常見似是而非的片段經驗以及不當藥物宣傳等眾多迷思，推薦給你一起研讀，和余醫師一起創造更健康美好的人生。

（糖尿病衛教學會前理事長）

杜思德

推薦序 5 ｜

能真正穩糖減重者，才是真富貴

糖尿病是台灣最重要的公共衛生問題之一，多年來一直是十大死因的第五位；目前台灣成年人 1/8 罹患糖尿病，而糖尿病前期患者更高達 1/4，也在走向糖尿病的路上，意即 1/3 的台灣人身體泡在糖水裡。糖尿病對病患造成的健康危害很廣，從急性到慢性、從輕微疲憊到洗腎、失明、截肢，都與糖尿病有關，一年也用掉健保約 1/8 的費用，真是令人憂心的富貴病。

糖尿病的治療在西醫次專科分類上屬於新陳代謝疾病，所以內分泌專科醫師是醫療院所治療糖尿病的專家，但全台高達 200 萬以上的用藥病患，散落在各科醫師門診中。我本身是胃腸肝膽專科醫師，專研在肝臟疾病的診治，但脂肪肝患者的研究發現「肥胖的脂肪肝患者在體重下降後不僅肝臟改善，連血糖都變好了！」所以個人臨床上雖然以處理肝臟疾病為主，但會注重肥胖症對健康的危害，特別是血糖、血壓、血脂等三高問題，也會在醫學研討會上讓更多臨床醫師瞭解。

欣聞余宜叡醫師要出版新書《八周穩糖減重密技：降三高，消脂甩肉，健檢不再秀紅字》非常開心，樂於為之序。還記得在肥胖研究學會課程與研討會上余醫師認真的提問與互動，顯然有把肥胖醫學的精髓吸收並運用在臨床診治患者之上。

本書第一、二部分為傳統必須了解的糖尿病相關知識，而第三、四部分則著重在體重控制的好處與秘技，這些知識由新陳代謝科專科醫師來寫更有說服力，建議讀者要好好拜讀。傳統的糖尿病用藥只能控制，無法逆轉糖尿病，但糖尿病患者若積極控制體重卻有機會在不用藥的情況下逆轉糖尿病。最後以唐朝藥王孫思邈在《備急千金要方》中所言與大家共勉

古人善為醫者 上醫醫未病之病
中醫醫欲病之病 下醫醫已病之病

恭喜有機會讀到此書的讀者，因為余醫師是上醫，能運用肥胖醫學知識做醫療健康傳播，達到預防醫學的理想。最後也祝宜叡新書大賣，造福更多讀者。

（中華民國肥胖研究學會榮譽理事長）

蕭敦仁

用熱情與誠懇，跟大家一起打擊糖尿病

認識余宜叡醫師，是參與林瑞祥教授和陳宏麟院長在埔里所舉辦的臨床帶教活動，算起來也已經不少年。最初的印象就是一位笑起來有點靦腆的大男孩，好學不倦的出現在北中南各式各樣的進修課程中，他像海綿一樣不停吸收大量知識，拓展深度與廣度。這些年看著他日益成長茁壯，勤於把所學運用在工作上，用無比的熱情和執著持續精進自己的醫術，真的很令人感動，也為他的病患感到慶幸，能遇見一位用生命在燃燒衛教魂的好醫師。

這本書的內容就跟他本人一樣，充滿熱情與誠懇。不僅深入淺出的將糖尿病的知識以清晰易懂的圖文呈現，更搭配案例的實戰經驗幫助讀者理解。在這個全球都在對抗著肥胖與糖尿病的時代，面對無孔不入的健康威脅，我們需要更全方位的了解糖尿病對人體的影響。除此之外，如何將知識付諸於實際行動，才是真正扭轉疾病進程的關鍵因素。

市面上有許多相關書籍，為什麼還需要這麼一本書呢？翻開這本書處處可見余宜叡醫師的風格，身為家庭醫學科，他對不同領域也多有涉獵，不光是血糖，許多居家照護相關的問題也貼心的為讀者解惑。加上長期教學的經驗，他特別擅長將複雜的論述解釋，變成簡短精要易於記憶的短句，佐以精心挑選的圖片。句句單刀直入，毫不拖泥帶水，說是秘笈再不為過。

有趣的是，當翻到後面居然看見拙作《幸福瘦》一書被放進內文時不禁失笑，余醫師推廣書籍比我這個作者還認真呢！真可謂長江後浪推前浪，身為前浪的我希望有更多後浪急起直追，因為我們正迎向高齡化社會的銀髮海嘯，糖尿病與肥胖衍生的問題正在風口浪尖上，眼看就要吞噬你我的健康！

總之，誠摯推薦這本充滿熱誠的作品給想要認識糖尿病與肥胖治療的一般民眾和醫療從業人員，跟著余宜叡醫師一起打擊糖尿病吧！

（天主教耕莘醫院內分泌科主任暨衛教諮詢中心主任）
馬文雅

短文推薦

血糖穩，牙齒才會好

非常感謝余宜叡主任在本書中對糖尿病精闢的解說，讓因生活愈來愈好的社會大眾能有機會預防、控制日趨嚴重的血糖問題。

身為看診多年的牙醫師，臨床上常發現病患罹患牙周病且治療效果不佳，請病患一併確認身體健康狀況後，往往都會發現伴隨血糖過高的情況，需要進一步的轉診治療。

研究顯示，牙周炎與糖尿病有雙向高關聯性，一方的存在會導致另一方發生，而一方得到治療也可改善另一方的病情。

余主任書上所提的跨科合作來改善目前牙周炎及糖尿病相互影響也是我們牙醫師相當重視的病因之一。而有效的控制糖尿病，也會有較佳的口腔治療效果。

身為牙醫師的我們，相當推崇余主任以淺顯易懂條理分明的方式提升民眾們對口腔健康的照顧，及對糖尿病衛教的重視。在此特別推薦本書給大家。

（員榮醫療體系員生醫院醫療副院長）

沈紋瑩

控糖瘦身祕笈，帶領大家走出糖尿病大觀園

就像進入冒險遊戲需要勇氣、智慧和堅持不懈一樣，當你走進糖尿病的大觀園，就將面對各種挑戰，但請以積極正向的心態來克

服困難，與糖尿病和平共處。透過獲取和理解相關知識，我們能夠增加勇氣和自信面對困難和挑戰。

這本書以深入淺出、生動有趣的方式描述糖尿病的成因、症狀和診斷標準。作者的洞察力和筆觸令人驚嘆。他提醒讀者，糖尿病患者也要特別小心牙周病、肺炎和泌尿道感染等風險。此外，書中還介紹了各種降血糖藥物和胰島素的使用方式，以及如何自行測量血糖和積極監測血糖的重要性。作者還分享了適合的運動、生活習慣調整和疫苗接種對糖尿病管理的影響。另外他也提供了許多穩定血糖並減少併發症的寶貴建議。

這本書以生動易懂的方式呈現複雜的醫學知識。無論你是糖尿病患者還是關心糖尿病的人，都將成為寶貴的健康指南，幫助你更好地理解和應對糖尿病。別猶豫了，一起加入這場糖尿病大冒險吧！

（彰基新陳代謝科前主任）

王舒儀

糖友要看，
醫護人員更要看的控糖瘦身示範手冊

宜叡是我在彰化基督教醫院擔任家庭醫學科主任期間的主治醫師，對於糖尿病的衛教以及治療特別有興趣。他持續舉辦了許多次的糖尿病工作坊與衛教班，不遺餘力在傳授及推廣穩糖控糖，以及減重相關的專業知識和相關技能，讓不論是專業的醫護人員或糖有都受益良多。

此次更將相關的專業知識以及其臨床經驗寫成書籍，將可為大眾提供糖尿病以及減重更多深入淺出的知識，透過書籍傳播健康，這個理念令人激賞，在此要特別推薦給大家。

（亞洲大學附屬醫院預防暨社區醫學中心主任）

林益卿

最能幫助糖友的穩糖減重模式

剛剛從美國參加美國糖尿病協會年會（簡稱「ADA」）回來，就收到余宜叡醫師的關於穩糖減重的新書書稿。而今年 ADA 的熱門議題就是強調體重管理和糖尿病之間的關係。

余醫師和我一樣是家醫科醫師，而他透過自己的模式幫助了許多糖尿病病友和肥胖的患者達成健康目標，而今他將這些經驗透過深入淺出的文字編輯成書，分享給大家，希望能幫助更多有需要的人，特此推薦。

（西園醫院家醫科主任）

馬世明

健康控糖、快樂生活

糖尿病是國人常見的慢性病。許多民眾對糖尿病的成因或治療不甚清楚或有所誤解，甚至誤信偏方，延誤治療先機。也有糖友雖認真積極抗糖，但成效有限，感到挫折。

本書藉由淺顯易懂的文字敘述，讓民眾了解糖尿病的成因及治療方式；文中多處運用案例說明，讓讀者更能感同身受。閱讀此書，有助於糖友或是重視健康，想維持健康生活型態的您，學習如何健康控糖、快樂生活！特此為文推薦。

(中國附醫社區暨家庭醫學部主治醫師)

楊鈺雯

品質最好的糖尿病自我照護專書

余宜叡醫師不只長期致力於照護與陪伴糖尿病友，進行穩糖與減重兩大工作；更擅長培訓後進醫師，一起加入穩糖、減重的行列。此次余醫師編寫的糖尿病自我照護專書，品質讓人非常放心，特此推薦給大家。

(蔡醫師線上瘦身課程創辦人、內分泌新陳代謝專科)

蔡明劼

絕不藏私，教你與糖共舞的好書

很高興收到余醫師的邀約，跟余醫師認識大約是十年前，他親自送了營養師一個推廣健康飲食的桌遊，他說他自己買了玩了，覺得透過遊戲推廣健康飲食方式，能增加民眾的對健康飲食認識及朝正向改變，也鼓勵營養師發揮衛教創意，增加患者對飲食衛教的認知及遵循。從此發現他是個非常喜歡教學、喜歡跟病患交談，透過交談中加入衛教元素促使患者達成目標的醫師，也非常樂於分享他的經驗。

這次他將他的經驗透過這本書，傳遞全方位的糖尿病管理經驗，還有藥物、飲食、運動等多個面向，也很實用的教大家如何尋找一個好的醫療團隊，可以清楚知道如何去開始管理糖尿病。如此好書當然要推薦給所有想要了解糖尿病和正在與糖共舞的諸多糖友一起來閱讀。

（彰化基督教醫院營養師）

游欣亭

與糖的距離好近好近！

糖尿病就醫人口數逐年增加，根據衛福部健保署的最新統計 111 年罹患人數有 256 萬 8409 人，同時醫療費用的支出多年來在健保都是第三名，如此龐大的醫療負擔，是我們全體國民不懂得如何照顧嗎？在我們的健保照顧之下有相當多的糖尿病照護團隊等等，同時在坊間也有相當多的糖尿病照護書籍可以自我學習，如將出刊的「8 週穩糖減重密技」，作者用平易近人的文筆呈現出大家容易懂的糖尿病照顧方式，書中是先讓閱讀者了解糖尿病，再說明醫療端會有哪些治療模式，進而我們該如何做個聰明的有智慧的健康照護者，是一本非常實用並值得您參與學習的書籍。

（中國附醫糖尿病衛教師、護理師）

葉桂梅

穩糖武功秘笈

糖尿病是最常見的生活習慣相關疾病之一，控糖瘦身說起來容易，控制起來卻是充滿挑戰。

余宜叡醫師常常在報章雜誌發表文章，這一次能將過去的著作重新整理集結成穩糖武功秘笈，用案例的解說，個案的觀點，從糖尿病的成因，到穩糖的關鍵秘技；從飲食對策，運動生活習慣以及監測，也談到穩定體重的重要性以及和醫療團隊協同合作等等。運用平鋪直述的方式，讓民眾能夠很快就掌握健康穩糖的方法，這是一本容易入手學習的糖尿病寶典，推薦大家一起來輕鬆學習，快樂控糖。

（陳宏麟診所主治醫師）

陳宏麟

學會自我控糖、調整體重，就能人生精彩

第一次見到余宜叡醫師是在 2017 年 6 月聖地牙哥參加美國糖尿病協會年會的時候，幾日相處下來，了解余醫師是位積極學習糖尿病照護的醫師。往後這幾年來，他除了積極參與國內外糖尿病相關會議外，在臉書上更是常發表最新糖尿病藥物和照護新知。此外，為了推廣糖尿病相關知識，他更是不辭辛勞辦理各種課程，以滿足大家學習的渴望。

糖尿病是一個和生活習慣極度相關的慢性病。統計顯示，全球糖尿病流行率一直持續升爬中，此現象和肥胖有著密切的關聯。只要認識糖尿病，學習自我照護能力，從藥物、飲食和運動三方面著手，就可以將糖尿病控制好，擁有精彩人生。

本書中余醫師說明糖尿病的原因、糖尿病和胰島素的關係之外，更提供了穩糖密技和如何拒絕糖胖，只要確實執行這些方法，並持之以恆，一定能夠成功。如此好書，很高興推薦給您！

（陳敏玲內科診所院長、台灣基層糖尿病協會秘書長）

陳敏玲

戰勝糖胖必看的攻略寶典

根據國民健康署統計，全國糖尿病及肥胖的「會員」皆達上百萬人，分布在每個年齡層，不分性別共同關心著這不退流行的話題，因此坊間陸續分別出現非常多相關的書籍，但是，將這兩大流行結合在一起的專業書籍卻是少見，當多月前得知余宜叡醫師著手進行催生這本書，當下即非常期待此書的出版。

這本書以淺顯易懂的文字，將艱深的專業用深入淺出的方式敘述出來，從認識糖尿病、成因、藥物、併發症到如何與糖共舞的穩糖關鍵密技，以及飲食藥物之於體重管理的迷思、成效、成癮等，最後也提到了如何選擇及搭配專業團隊來達到必勝方程式，如此一層一層鉅細靡遺的搭配實際案例，每看完一個單元總會發出「哇！原來如此！」的讚嘆聲。

本書細心蒐集並整理相關專業資料及案例，不但適合一般民眾，也是一本適合醫師、營養師、藥師、護理師等專業人士參考的工具書，身為營養師，我認為此書相當值得仔細閱讀並收藏。

（員榮醫院營養師）
童雅惠

自序｜

十年磨一劍，惟願糖友血糖穩、幸福瘦，足矣

臨床經驗超過十年，看了不少糖尿病與減重患者，也開辦多梯的糖尿病與減重的工作坊與衛教講座，發現許多患者家屬有許多糖尿病與減重的誤解與迷思。整體來說，糖尿病的治療，原則是簡單，但是持續地做對做足，實務上是有許多考驗的，因為，大家必須補足很多正確觀念：

- 與血糖藥相比，高血糖更傷害身體。
- 糖尿病併發症一旦產生就回不去了。
- 補充胰島素，可以讓胰臟適度休養。
- 胰島素能有效穩糖不傷身、可以很有生活品質地與糖共舞。
- 糖尿病藥不一定要用一輩子。

因此，本書會從以下幾個方面深入淺出地跟大家說明，協助大家掌握穩糖減重密技，最終達成「與糖共舞」的雙贏局面。

降低低血糖風險

低血糖是許多糖尿病患者家屬的夢魘。每每聽到糖尿病患者因至親或朋友使用胰島素或糖尿病藥物的不良經驗，除了同理患者難過與恐懼的心之外，更堅定早期介入治療與有效衛教的決心。

隨著超長效胰島素，與許多難低血糖的優質血糖藥問世，輔以持續在臨床進修交流的醫療團隊，溝通討論出難低血糖的治療計劃，是可以大幅減少低血糖不良事件發生。

掌握糖尿病前期，逆轉情勢，恢復健康

長期以來，糖尿病前期是許多醫療人員與民眾忽視的一塊。許多患者執行成人健康檢查後，空腹血糖偏高，但是醫療人員的衛教卻是「血糖還在正常值，不是糖尿病」「目前血糖穩定，請不用擔心」如此會造成民眾對血糖掉以輕心。殊不知絕大部分的糖尿病，都是經由糖尿病前期，漸漸演變成糖尿病。

很多確診糖尿病的患者，檢視先前的成人健檢、員工體檢或自費健檢的血糖值，往往都已達到糖尿病前期的標準。願此書的問世，可讓醫療人員與患者家屬在糖尿病前期就可以管理血糖，不需等到糖尿病確診再開始介入。

「前面麻煩，後面就不麻煩；前面怕麻煩，後面就麻煩」是治療糖尿病多年的重要心得。許多在糖尿病前期或初期就診斷，同時做飲食、運動或藥物上的治療，都能將血糖控制得相當穩定，同時藥物不用使用太多太重，甚至有機會逆轉血糖至與正常人一樣；反而是將血糖不當一回事的人，常常需要使用多種口服與針劑藥物，才能將血糖控制下來，若是產生糖尿病的併發症，只能求不再惡化，很難治癒。

胰島素迷思 & 妙用

實務上醫療端，很多人對胰島素，還停留在過去易低血糖、不好使用、腎功能不好的最後用藥等諸多陳舊觀念，加上民眾以為用

了胰島素就會洗腎、使用胰島素還要抽取、很困難與麻煩、使用胰島素會很痛等等錯誤迷思，造成目前胰島素的使用率偏低。

然而，臨床個案印證，越早使用胰島素治療的患者，後續常如研究結果一樣，減藥的機率越高！即使是無法減藥的胰島素使用患者們，常跟醫師分享「我吃得和親友（正常人）一樣，他們都不知道我有糖尿病」「為什麼我飲食和之前一樣，沒改變太多，但血糖為什麼如此穩定」其實他們共同的秘訣就是「治療計劃中有搭配胰島素」而已。

別讓血糖併發症出現！

在有效控糖顧腎的衛教講座裡，詢問民眾「糖尿病併發症不可逆的情況下，你最想要哆啦 A 夢的那一種道具來幫忙？」結果大部分的民眾回答是「時光機」回到從前。但是千金難買早知道。因此收集多年門診常遇到的臨床問題與迷思，補充因應之道與衛教內容，集結成此書。

願此書能幫忙醫療人員瞭解到更多臨床控糖上遇到的問題與因應之道；幫忙更多患者家屬早知道高血糖的危害，做好預防措施，遠離血糖的危害。

遠離復胖，幸福瘦

曾遇到為肥胖所苦的大姐，她光是搬個東西就氣喘呼呼，過度進食的原因是不為人知的家庭問題；遇到減重手術後復胖的患者，一直認為減重手術不是一勞永逸的，怎麼會復胖？遇過在學校被霸凌或親子關係出現問題的重度肥胖青少年；遇過使用蘋果減重法、168 減重法、不知澱粉減重法……等，卻一直體重減不下來，或是減了很快就復胖回去，甚至更胖！

因此，在本書加入減重的臨床重點，期待讀者找到減重的盲點，打破減重的迷思，幸福瘦又不復胖。

感謝師長

十年磨一劍，學習糖尿病的治療超過十年，中間遇到許多師長們的分享與教導。

彰化基督教醫院新陳代謝科的老師們：廖培湧醫師、林世鐸醫師、杜思德醫師、王舒儀醫師、許上人醫師、蔡東華醫師、謝芳傑醫師、糖尿病衛教師的啟蒙老師謝明家醫師、指導糖尿病研究論文的李弘元教授、減重工作坊合作的馬文雅醫師、同糖尿病治療上精進的陳宏麟醫師、陳敏鈴醫師與馬世明醫師等。還有許多家庭醫學科、新陳代謝科、心臟內科、腎臟內科與神經內科老師們的教導，讓我可以吸收到不同科對糖尿病治療的觀點，與糖尿病併發症的預防處置。

也謝謝員榮醫院張克士總院長、沈紋瑩副院長，以及其他長官師長們，在糖尿與病與減重精準醫療上的協助與幫忙。願這本書讓更多人在糖尿病與肥胖預防與因應上，有一本臨床實務個案的參考書，達到糖尿病負成長，延緩發生，糖尿病併發症不出現，越來越多開心減重不復胖的人。

最後特別感謝，辛苦家務還要幫忙潤稿的愛妻，以及幫忙協助出書的原水文化團隊。感謝再感謝。

PART 1

糖尿病與血糖的親密關係

CHAPTER 01 認識糖尿病

糖尿病的形成主因

正常人平常的血糖，主要集中在 80 ～ 200mg/dl。但是，如果胰島素分泌不夠或作用不佳，造成血糖在體內超標，並且持續一段長期的時間，就會形成糖尿病。

一般會有以下三種成因。

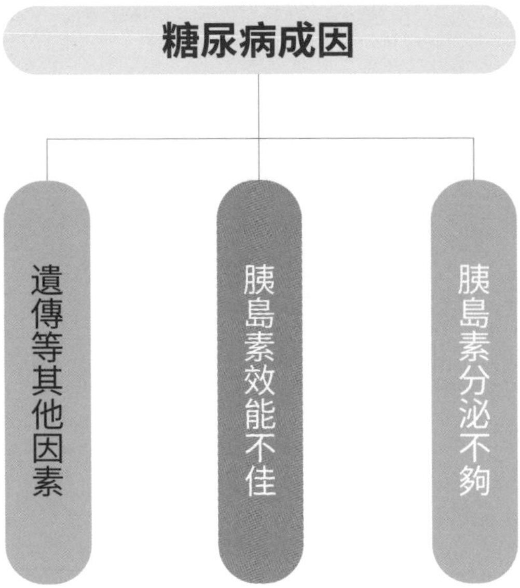

胰島素分泌不夠

不管是第一型糖尿病或者第二型糖尿病，只要分泌的胰島素低於身體需求，就會導致血糖降不下來。因為，第一型糖尿病是完全不分泌胰島素，需要利用胰島素來治療；第二型糖尿病則是可選擇胰島素或口服藥，來提升胰島素，滿足身體的需求。

胰島素效能不佳

另一種說法是胰島素阻抗性變高，造成胰島素的效能不佳，導致身體需要更多胰島素才能降低血糖。例如一般人 10 單位的胰島素，就可將血糖穩定下來，但如果胰島素的效能不佳，就需要 15 ～ 20 單位才能達成同樣的血糖穩定，這問題常見於過重與肥胖的糖友。此時若能好好減輕體重，胰島素效能就可能重新恢復或讓阻抗性變低，是有機會讓糖尿病病情不用藥物逆轉血糖值。

遺傳等其他危險因素

這部分分為不可控制與可控制的危險因子。

不可控制的危險因子主要有家族遺傳（父母都有糖尿病，更是高風險群）與器官退化（年紀增長、胰臟漸漸退化）；可控制的危險因子則是飲食沒控制（飯麵、飲料……等醣類攝取太多）、運動不足（沒有規律的習慣）、體重過重（增加胰島素的阻抗性，胰島素的效率變差，需要更多的胰島素……）

同時根據 2019 年的糖尿病年鑑顯示，台灣糖友除了一直增加中，罹病年齡也一直下修中，可見問題之嚴重。

糖尿病常見症狀與診斷標準

常見症狀

一般來說，糖尿病的症狀包括：

- 多尿（頻尿）：尿頻增加，可能需要在夜間起床排尿。
- 異常口渴：口渴感增加，尤其在夜間。
- 食慾增加：食慾不斷增加，但體重可能下降。
- 疲倦和乏力：經常感到疲倦，缺乏精力。
- 模糊視力：視力模糊，可能出現眼前物體的清晰度降低。
- 更頻繁的皮膚發病：可能出現搔癢或感染。
- 傷口癒合困難：傷口癒合時間延長。

註：但最常見的症狀就是「沒有症狀」。

診斷標準

糖尿病的診斷通常是通過測量血糖水平來確定的。以下是根據美國糖尿病學（協）會（American Diabetes Association）的診斷標準：

1. **空腹血糖測試**（Fasting Plasma Glucose，FPG）：在空腹狀態下，即至少 8 小時沒有進食，測量血糖水平。如果空腹血糖水平等於或高於 126mg/dL，則兩次以上可以確定為糖尿病。

2. **口服葡萄糖耐量試驗**（Oral Glucose Tolerance Test，OGTT）：此測試需要在空腹狀態下測量血糖水平，然後給予一定量的葡萄糖溶液，再於兩小時後再次測量血糖水平。如果兩小時後的血糖水平等於或高於 200mg/dL，則兩次以上可以確定為糖尿病。

3. **隨機血糖測試**（Random Plasma Glucose）：無論進食與否，隨機測量血糖水平。如果隨機血糖水平大於或等於 200mg/dL，並伴隨糖尿病相關症狀，如多尿、口渴和體重下降，則可以確定為糖尿病。

此外，有時還可以使用**糖化血色素**（HbA1c）測試來診斷糖尿病。糖化血色素是血紅蛋白上的一個血糖指標，可以反映近期血糖情況。根據美國糖尿病協會的建議，如果糖化血色素水平等於或高於 6.5%，則可以確定為糖尿病。

請注意，這些診斷標準僅供參考，最終的診斷應由醫師根據個人情況和多種評估因素來確定。如果您懷疑自己可能患有糖尿病，建議您立即諮詢醫師進行進一步的診斷和確診。只有醫師可以根據您的症狀、身體檢查和相關的血糖測試結果來做出準確的診斷。

糖尿病的分類

糖尿病根據其病因和特點，可以分為多種不同類型。主要會分成第一型糖尿病、第二型糖尿病和妊娠糖尿病三種：

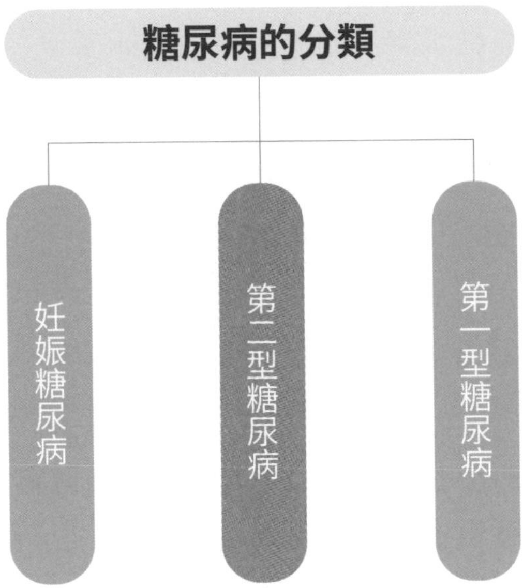

第一型糖尿病

第一型糖尿病，又稱**為胰島素依賴型糖尿病**或**少年型糖尿病**，主要是由於自體免疫攻擊導致胰島細胞受損，無法產生足夠的胰島素。這種類型的糖尿病通常在年輕時期發生，患者需要定期注射胰島素來控制血糖水平。

第二型糖尿病

第二型糖尿病是最常見的糖尿病類型，占所有糖尿病患者的大多數。它主要由兩個因素引起：胰島素分泌不足和身體對胰島素的抵抗。這種糖尿病通常與生活方式和遺傳風險因素密切相關，例如肥胖、缺乏運動和不良的飲食習慣。

妊娠糖尿病

妊娠期間發生的糖尿病被稱為妊娠糖尿病。它主要是由於懷孕期間荷爾蒙變化導致胰島素分泌不足或胰島素作用不佳。妊娠糖尿病通常在懷孕晚期（妊娠第 24 周以後）開始發展，並在分娩後自行消失。妊娠糖尿病是由於懷孕期間體內產生的荷爾蒙變化和胰島素的作用降低所引起。

此外，正常人要罹患糖尿病前，大部分都會經過糖尿病前期。下表列出正常人、糖尿病前期和糖尿病三個階段的葡萄糖和糖化血色的標準，讓大家在看健檢報告時可以有所依據。

	正常	前期	糖尿病
葡萄糖（AC glucose mg/dl）	<100	100 ～ 125	126
糖化血色素（HbA1c%）	<5.7	5.7 ～ 6.4	6.5

糖尿病前期

糖尿病前期（Prediabetes）是指，人體的血糖水平高於正常範圍，但尚未達到糖尿病的確診標準的一種狀態。它被視為糖尿病發展的早期階段，通常是在實際發病之前的幾年產生。這是一個警示信號，顯示罹患糖尿病的風險較高。

糖尿病前期是一個重要的健康狀態，它提醒人們需要採取積極的措施來預防糖尿病的發展。人們患有糖尿病前期時，胰島細胞功能可能已經受損，而身體對胰島素的敏感性也可能降低。這意味著需要更加關注自己的生活方式和飲食習慣，以降低糖尿病發生的風險。

以下再將這四種情形列表說明，讓大家一目了然。

	第一型糖尿病	第二型糖尿病	妊娠糖尿病	糖尿病前期
胰臟功能	胰臟功能完全喪失	胰臟功能已經部分受損>50%	懷孕中才血糖偏高	胰臟功能開始受損
所占族群	少數	最主要族群	少數	加上隱藏，比第二型還多
是否可逆		可	可	可
飲食療法	○	○	○	○
運動療法	○	○	○	○
口服藥治療	○（排糖藥小心使用）	○	○（特定口服藥）	○
胰島素治療	○	○	○	○

吃太多、動太少，糖友愈來愈多

想想自己最近曾經持續運動至少 20 分鐘是在什麼時候？如果一週內都沒有的話，那至少有從事 10 分鐘的運動吧？如果還是沒有，大家就應該能正視，我們的確身處在一個運動量變少的不愛運動的環境裡，不論是搭捷運或公車、坐火車、騎機車、開車、搭電梯或升降梯、送貨、食物外送等行為都不算運動，而這些在 20 ～ 30 年前根本不是那麼普及，可見我們運動量因為生活模式的改變，也大大減少了運動的機會！

再想想自己什麼時候，以享用宵夜、零食、甜點、水果……等等理由，吃了任何想吃的食物？是不是就發生在剛才或昨天！

由此可知，現代的文明生活，食物取得很方便，同時間身體活動減少，形成身體易攝取到過多醣類，但卻缺乏活動消耗掉。如此日積月累下來，胰臟就容易過度勞累，造成胰島素分泌量開始下降變少；雪上加霜的是，處在吃多動少的生活下，很容易形成過重、肥胖，此時胰島素效能就更差，需要更多胰島素作用。如此雙重作用的惡性循環下，糖尿病就漸漸產生。也因此，越來越多 40 歲不到，甚至才 20 多歲的年輕人被確診為糖尿病。

幸運的是，大部分糖友都會經過糖尿病前期這個階段，只要在平常或糖尿病前期就介入調整生活習慣，血糖還是有機會回復到正常人的程度。

關於糖尿病的治療，飲食療法與運動療法都有一定的成效。藥物治療也有多種選擇。

飲食主要是管理醣類的攝取；運動主要是增加血糖的消耗，以及提高胰島素的敏感性。

藥物療法方面，口服藥與胰島素都是不錯的選擇。若是想保存胰臟內分泌胰島素β細胞的功能，可以提早使用胰島素（胰臟可適當休息，不用繼續過勞），或者早期使用兩種以上的複方藥物，一次讓血糖達標（減少高血糖對β細胞的傷害）。除非是早期診斷的糖尿病，否則一延誤糖尿病治療時間，通常要使用到第二、第三，甚至第四種藥物。

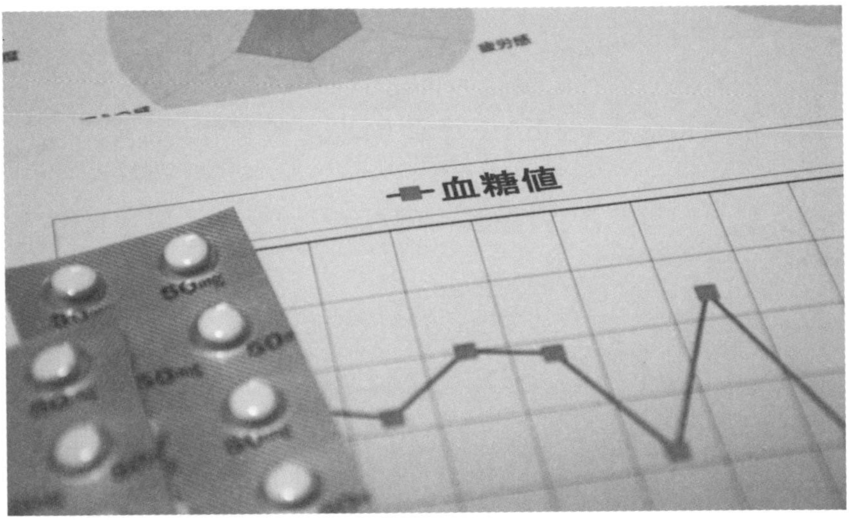

▲血糖數值可輔助判斷是否身處糖尿病前期或糖尿病（照片提供／余宜叡）

糖尿病前期或糖尿病積極治療可逆轉病情

案例 1

白先生，38 歲，因長期疲倦不適求診，發現隨機血糖高達 300mg/dL，糖化血色素為 8.0%。醫療團隊建議他優先使用胰島素控糖，並進行衛教。白先生同意口服藥搭配胰島素治療，一週後血糖數值正常化，三個月後糖化血色素降至 6%，六個月後停止胰島素使用，只用口服藥控糖，糖化血色素仍維持在 6.0%。

案例 2

林小姐，40 多歲，家族有糖尿病病史，健檢發現 BMI 為 31，空腹血糖超過 150mg/dL，糖化血色素為 7.6%。由於屬於肥胖體型，醫生建議使用腸泌素或排糖藥物。林小姐選擇排糖藥物治療，三個月後糖化血色素 HbA1c 降至 6.2%，體重減少了近 3 公斤。

案例 3

王先生，40 多歲，在糖尿病前期就開始定期追蹤。由於生活忙碌，飲食和運動難以改變，因此他選擇自費使用藥物控糖。8 年後，他仍然保持在糖尿病前期，糖化血色素維持在 5.7 ～ 6.0%。王先生對這樣的結果感到滿意，他的目標是比父母晚確診糖尿病，希望能在 60 多歲後不發展成糖尿病。

案例 4

吳女士，60 歲，在健檢中發現空腹血糖為 116mg/dL，糖化血色素為6.2%。由於不想自費用藥，她接受了飲食和運動的衛教。半年後，糖化血色素 HbA1c 升至 6.8%，空腹血糖為 138mg/dL，確診為糖尿病。

吳女士意識到糖尿病前期若沒有適當處置，會進展成糖尿病。她也明白自己需要更加調整飲食和增加運動量來控制血糖。她更了解到即使處於糖尿病初期，也有可以獲得給付的用藥選項，不必自費。因此，她主動積極地致力於改變生活方式並遵從醫療團隊的建議，以便更好地管理糖尿病，降低併發症風險。

案例 5

李先生，60 多歲，在健檢中發現血糖偏高，糖化血色素 HbA1c 為 7.5%，確診糖尿病。他開始使用含有兩種口服藥的複方藥物治療，不到兩週的時間，血糖數值已達標，三個月後的糖化血色素 HbA1c 降至 6.5%。

如上述 5 個不同年紀、性別和狀況各異的例子來說，可以非常明顯看出，糖尿病前期族群，不論因何而發現患有糖尿病，都要正向看待、提高警覺，因為這都已經顯示是需要改變生活方式，並使用藥物來穩定血糖的時候了，當然更好的時候是從「現在」開始

一般來說，在糖尿病病史不長的情況下（1 年內），胰臟通常仍具有一定的功能。若能積極地早期治療，並融合飲食調整、運動以及藥物治療，有極高的機會能夠達到理想的血糖控制同時兼顧生活品質。

早期糖尿病一般會有以下三種治療方法：

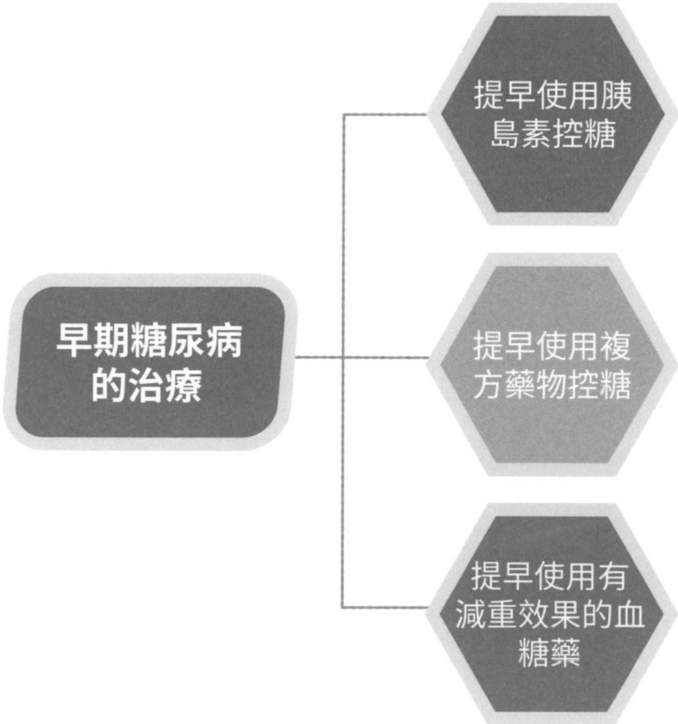

提早使用胰島素控糖

研究顯示，與先使用口服藥物的族群相比，先使用胰島素的糖友在之後減藥或停藥的比例更高。這也得到臨床實踐的驗證，一開始就使用胰島素的糖友有更大的機會最終能夠減少藥物劑量並穩定血糖。無論是不需要使用口服藥物，只需每天注射一次胰島素；或者不需要使用胰島素而只使用 1～2 種口服藥物就能維持血糖穩定。

提早使用複方藥物控糖

根據權威醫學期刊《刺胳針》上的研究指出，與單一藥物治療相比，早期使用兩種藥物的糖友能夠有效延緩加藥的機會，減少至少 2 年以上才需要開始使用胰島素。

提早使用兼具減重效果的血糖藥物

這個方法適用於過重或肥胖的糖友。根據糖尿病學會的糖尿病照護指引，體重減少 5%以上就能明顯改善血糖控制，例如 60 公斤的糖友，只需減少 3 公斤體重就能有明顯的改善。

然而，考慮到藥物給付限制，排糖藥物相對容易獲得給付。對於預算有限的族群而言，可以優先考慮使用排糖藥物，但需要注意這些藥物可能帶來的副作用，主要包括泌尿生殖道感染。對於經濟能力較強的族群，可以考慮使用排糖藥物並結合腸泌素來穩定血糖同時達到減重的效果。

重要的是，早期治療對於控制糖尿病的發展至關重要。無論選擇哪種治療方法，與醫生密切合作，遵從醫療建議，並持續監測血糖水平，這將有助於確保糖尿病的良好管理和提高生活品質。

除了藥物治療外，飲食調整和適度的運動也是管理糖尿病不可或缺的重要因素。請尋求營養師或專業醫療團隊的指導，制定適合個人狀況的飲食計畫和運動方案。

糖尿病確實存在遺傳風險

案例 提醒親人做身體檢查，有時竟然就意外發現糖尿病前期或糖尿病。

67 歲的林女士，糖尿病控制穩定三年多了。這次門診剛好 40 多歲的兒子與女兒陪同就醫。醫療團隊鼓勵他們執行成人健檢，結果意外兒子也確診糖尿病，女兒則確定為糖尿病前期，他們都不可置信地說：「怎麼會這樣？根本沒有任何症狀或不適！」再確認後才發現林女士的先生也罹患糖尿病，因此大幅度提高了兒女罹患糖尿的風險。

有遺傳關係，但不一定會發病

遺傳與糖尿病的關係一直是受到關注的問題。研究顯示，若是父母任一有糖尿病，會增加 30%糖尿病罹病機率；若是父母都有糖尿病，則會增加 70%糖尿病罹病機率。

然而，即使存在遺傳風險，也不意味著一定會罹患糖尿病。重要的是針對遺傳風險採取適當的預防措施，以降低罹患糖尿病的機率。

臨床上有些糖友可能會自我放棄，認為父母或雙親都罹患糖尿病，那自己也一定會得糖尿病，因此就在生活型態上放任自己。

然而，根據研究結果，即使存在 30%或 70%的增加機率，如果提前採取適當的處置和預防措施，糖尿病的罹患機率可以控制在 1%左右。相反地，如果不採取行動並無所作為，原本的 5%罹患機率可能會增加到 40 %，再加上無法改變的先天遺傳因素，罹患糖尿病的機率可能會達到 52%或 68%。

因此，對於有糖尿病家族史的人來說，重要的是明白這只是一個風險增加的指標，而不代表一定會罹患糖尿病。我們無法選擇自己的先天基因，但我們可以在後天的生活中採取積極的措施來降低罹患糖尿病的風險。

良好生活習慣可大幅降低風險

從小就培養良好的生活習慣是關鍵。

在飲食方面，建議攝取大量蔬菜，每餐都應該有一碗青菜，並每天飲用 1500 毫升以上的白開水。

在運動方面，每週至少需要運動 5 天，每天至少累積 20 分鐘以上的運動時間。當身體適應後，可以逐漸提高運動的強度，例如將走路變成快走，或將原地小步走變成原地高抬腿。

此外，**進行定期的體檢也是重要的**。成人、員工或自費體檢都是合適的選擇。自費體檢可以選擇與成人健檢項目相同的小額健檢，價格約在 3000 ～ 5000 元左右，建議包含糖化血色素的檢測項目。對於已經使用血糖機並進行血糖監測的人群，建議進行隨機、飯前或飯後的血糖檢測。如果檢測出血糖偏高，請多次進行檢測，或直接進行糖化血色素的檢測。

如果血糖數值正常，請維持良好的生活方式；如果血糖數值偏高，除了保持良好的生活方式外，還應定期追蹤並適時進行藥物治療，以延緩糖尿病的確診。如果已經確診為糖尿病，則務必早期介入進行穩定的血糖控制，以減少長期高血糖對器官的損害，同時適度調整藥物使用的速度。

總結來看，雖然糖尿病具有遺傳風險，但這並不意味著一定會罹患糖尿病。我們可以通過培養良好的生活習慣，包括健康的飲食、適度的運動和定期的體檢，來降低罹患糖尿病的風險。即使有糖尿病家族史，只要能夠延後罹患糖尿病的時間，就能夠取得重要的進步。因此，讓我們把握後天的努力，努力採取預防措施，以延緩或避免糖尿病的發生。

主要併發症：下肢循環疾病

案例 1 李先生是一位糖尿病患者，他常常在走路一段時間後感到下肢疼痛，但稍作休息後症狀會稍有緩解。ABI 檢查顯示他存在下肢血管硬化的跡象。醫生提醒李先生，下肢循環併發症的嚴重性，並敦促他控制好血糖和血壓，以避免併發症進一步惡化。

糖尿病主要有六大併發症，分別有三項大血管併發症：腦中風、心肌梗塞與下肢循環疾病，以及三項小血管併發症：糖尿病視網膜病變、腎病變與糖尿病神經病變。依目前的的醫療技術，上述六大併發症，一旦發生是很難治癒或回復的，糖尿病患者能做的，就是好好穩定血糖至標準值內，持續糖化血色素小於 7%。

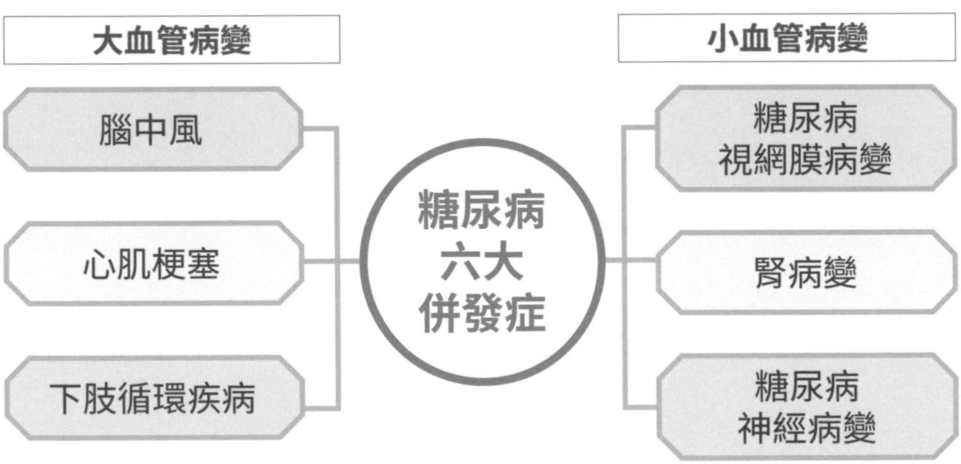

糖尿病患者在面對下肢循環疾病時需要格外留意。

下肢循環不良可能導致傷口難以癒合，進而引發感染，嚴重時甚至需要截肢。患者常常出現走路跛行的症狀，走一段路後下肢感到疲痛，但休息後症狀可能會暫時緩解。這對需要長時間走路或奔跑的工作，如農耕、巡視或警察工作等，會造成極大的影響。

為了治療下肢循環疾病，可以採取多種方式。藥物治療方面，可以使用一些通血管的抗血小板藥物或抗凝血藥物。嚴重情況下，可能需要像通心導管這樣的手術來疏通已堵塞的血管。在極端情況下，可能需要考慮截肢等措施。

除了糖尿病，其他因素如缺乏運動、高血脂和高血壓也可能導致血管硬化，進一步影響下肢循環。避免產生週邊血管性疾病也是一個重要的考量。因此，除了控制血糖和血壓外，這些風險因素也需要被注意和管理。

此外，適當的運動也可以促進下肢循環，但需要在痛覺和循環之間取得平衡，否則可能會導致惡性循環。同時，保持適度的運動也是提升下肢循環的關鍵。

通過適合的運動，可以促進血液循環，改善下肢的供血狀況。然而，病患應留意在運動時的舒適度，避免過度劇烈的活動，以免引發疼痛或造成更嚴重的循環問題。最好在醫生或專業體育教練的指導下進行運動，制定適合個人情況的運動計畫。

總而言之，與醫療團隊密切合作，制定適合自身狀況的綜合治療方案，以降低下肢循環併發症的風險，維護健康和生活品質。

其他高風險疾病 1：牙周病

糖尿病易造成齒齦的發炎，長久下來會造成牙齒的地基受損不穩定，當地基都壞掉後，形成所謂的牙周病，此時牙齒容易脫落，原本可以用到 80 歲的牙齒，很可能在 50 歲不到，就會成為沒有可用牙齒的「無齒之徒」。牙周病可能伴隨的症狀包括牙齦脹痛、牙齦容易流血、口臭或口腔出現異味。

牙周病是糖友常會發生的身體疾患之一，其他還有泌尿道感染以及肺炎兩大問題，這三種「特定疾病與糖尿病」。

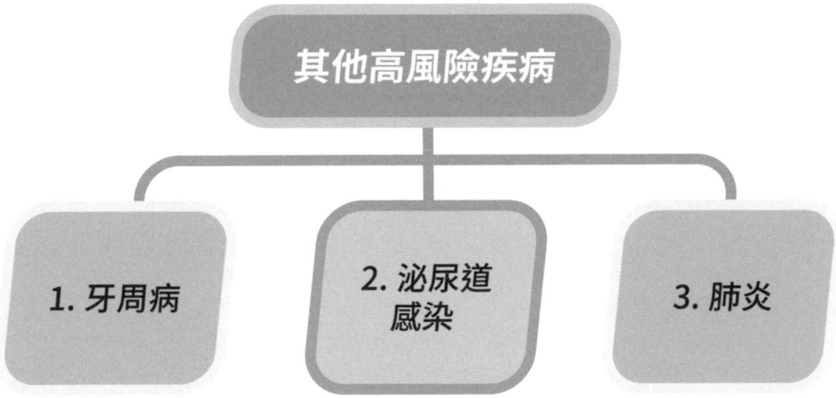

糖尿病與牙周病的關係密切

高血糖的環境有助於口腔內牙周病致病菌的生長。因此，糖友相較於一般人，罹患牙周病的風險增加了 2 ～ 3 倍。此外，糖尿病患者容易口乾舌燥，唾液的分泌量會減少，不利於口腔的自我清潔。

由於牙周病初期症狀常被忽視，糖友往往等到牙齦經常出血或口臭嚴重時才就醫，此時可能已經造成了牙齒根基被破壞，需要格外謹慎對待。

定期護牙很重要

定期洗牙是保持口腔健康的重要步驟之一。除了日常的餐後清潔牙齒外，每半年找牙醫師洗牙也至關重要。然而，有些糖友可能認為每天自己清潔牙齒就可以了，但省略了牙醫專業的洗牙程序，使得牙垢不斷累積，形成牙結石，增加牙周病的風險。一旦牙周病產生，需要花費更多心力治療。

在照護牙齒方面，血糖的穩定達標是至關重要的。有些人可能認為只要進行植牙就可以解決「無齒」問題，但植牙不僅費用不便宜，而且如果牙齦基礎不良，植牙的持久性也會受到影響。因此，保持血糖的穩定達標，降低牙周病的發生，是保持牙齒健康的根本。

臨床上，牙醫師若要手術，都會事先評估患者是否罹患糖尿病，以及其血糖情況。如果血糖超標過多，會建議病人先尋求醫療團隊的協助，血糖達標，才會做後續的牙齒處置，減少潛在的抱怨和爭議。

糖尿病患者需要特別注意口腔健康，並定期回診牙科進行追蹤。糖尿病患者的牙周病控制需要與牙醫合作，如果能夠同時改善口腔健康和糖尿病狀況，絕對是雙贏局面。

其他高風險疾病 2：泌尿道感染

案例　60 多歲的李女士，已患糖尿病超過十年由於口渴才喝水，每天的水分攝取常常不到 1000cc。

最近，她因為吃了親友贈送的餅乾而感到尿意不適，並頻繁去小便。為了減少小便的次數，她甚至進一步減少了水分攝取量。然而，這樣的行為卻導致了她晚上

開始感到身體不適，整個人虛弱無力。家人立即為她測量體溫，發現她的體溫高達攝氏 38.5 度。

家人立刻將她送往急診室進行治療。血糖檢測顯示血糖為 348mg/dl，在排除其他疾病後，確診為泌尿道感染。醫師建議她住院控制血糖，同時使用抗生素治療泌尿道感染。

泌尿道感染比肺炎更常見，雖然其危害沒有肺炎大，常常表現為無症狀或僅在小便時感到不適或疼痛。然而，如果不妥善治療，嚴重感染仍有可能導致敗血症，死亡率也會大幅上升。

患者長時間憋尿或忍尿的工作習慣會增加泌尿道感染的機會。此外，使用最近問世的降血糖藥物「排糖藥」也可能增加泌尿道感染的風險。臨床上，女性比男性更容易患上泌尿道感染。

在這種情況下，幾個因素可能導致泌尿道感染的增加，包括：平時飲水量偏低、血糖控制不達標（免疫力下降）、長時間使用導

尿管以及使用降血糖藥物時缺乏衛教等。

因此，我們強烈建議加強以下幾個方面的注意：

定期更換導尿管

對於需要使用導尿管的患者，每月定期更換導尿管非常重要。長時間使用同一支導尿管容易滋生細菌，增加泌尿道感染的風險。因此，定期更換導尿管可以有效降低感染的機會。

勤飲水

保持足夠的水分攝取，對於預防泌尿道感染至關重要。糖尿病患者由於尿糖排出較多，容易導致口渴和脫水。因此，每天飲水量應該達到充足的水平，通過多喝水來稀釋尿液，減少細菌在泌尿道滋生的機會。

不憋尿

盡量避免長時間憋尿或忍尿的情況。憋尿會增加尿液在泌尿道停留的時間，使細菌有更多機會滋生和繁殖。因此，定時排尿並遵從身體的自然需求是預防泌尿道感染的重要措施。

加強泌尿生殖道清潔

保持良好的個人衛生習慣，特別是在進行排尿和排便後要進行適當的清潔。使用溫和的清潔產品，從前向後擦拭，以防止細菌從肛門區域進入泌尿道。

除了上述注意事項外，對於糖尿病患者使用降血糖藥物「排糖藥」的情況，醫療團隊應加強對患者的衛教，使其充分了解該類藥物的副作用和風險，以及可能引起泌尿道感染的潛在危害，並在使用這些藥物時採取相應的預防措施。

綜上所述，對於糖尿病患者，特別是長期患病且年齡較大的患者，泌尿道感染是一個需要特別關注的問題。通過加強上述注意事項的執行，我們可以降低泌尿道感染的風險。

其他高風險族群 3：肺炎

案例 1 石女士患有糖尿病已超過 15 年，在中風後變得臥床不起，需要另一半照料日常生活。在家訪時，建議石女士接種肺炎疫苗，以降低患肺炎的風險。然而，在等待接種肺炎疫苗的期間，石女士卻感染了肺炎住院。她住院了將近 10 天才出院，但身體功能卻明顯下降。原本在訪視時可以與醫療團隊隨意交談，而現在只能說出幾個單詞。

案例 2 這個案例來自天下雜誌，涉及前花旗銀行董事長管國霖的父親。管國霖表示：「我父親在成大退休後，本來身體很健朗，但在 5 年前因患肺炎住院後，逐漸失去行動能力，臥床不起。」這一年來，他的父親已經無法開口說話了，狀態逐漸惡化。

肺炎對於糖尿病患者來說，是一個相當危險的疾病。根據統計資料，肺炎已連續四年成為國人十大死因中的第三名，其中一些潛在原因包括抗生素抗藥性的增加、病毒的進化以及人口老化等。因此，對於糖尿病患者來說，預防肺炎至關重要。

抗生素治療

對於糖尿病患者而言，血糖控制並不一定能夠始終穩定。如果血糖長時間保持在較高的水平，免疫力就可能下降，容易受到病毒或細菌的侵害，進而引發肺炎。其中，細菌性肺炎最常見的病原菌之一是肺炎鏈球菌。事實上，肺炎鏈球菌本身就存在於人體的鼻腔內，在免疫力不足的情況下，就有可能侵入人體並引發感染。

在肺炎的治療方面，對於輕度的細菌性肺炎，醫師可能會門診開立抗生素供病人回家服用。而對於嚴重的細菌性肺炎，則需要住院注射抗生素，通常至少需要 5 天。然而，許多人可能錯誤地認為只需要住院治療和注射抗生素就可以解決問題，卻忽略了這樣的治療方式可能帶來的負面影響。每次住院都會導致身體功能下降和免疫力下降，增加下次發生肺炎的機率，這樣的惡性循環可能最終導致死亡的後果。

應該戴口罩、注射疫苗

有效的肺炎預防措施包括佩戴口罩、勤洗手、保持營養均衡、進行足夠的運動、減少到公共場所的頻率、接種肺炎疫苗以及戒菸等。這些措施的執行程度越高，降低感染風險的效果就越好。其中，最簡單且不需要依賴記憶力和意志力的方式就是接種肺炎疫苗。一旦接種完成，對於肺炎的保護力就會提高。

因此，接種肺炎疫苗成為非常重要的防護手段。目前台灣提供的肺炎疫苗有 13 價和 23 價可供選擇。23 價疫苗可以在滿 65 或 75 歲時（視各地主管機關規定）時公費接種，而 13 價疫苗則需要自費。值得一提的是，13 價疫苗具有細胞免疫的效果，根據家庭醫學會的建議，建議終身接種一劑。

除了糖尿病患者外，還有一些高風險族群也應該接種肺炎疫苗。這些高風險族群包括脾功能缺損或切除者、免疫功能不全者（包括愛滋病感染者）、人工耳植入者、腦脊髓液滲漏者、免疫抑制劑或放射治療的惡性腫瘤患者或器官移植者、患有慢性疾病的糖尿病患者（如慢性腎病變、慢性心臟病、慢性肺臟病、高血壓、慢性肝病與肝硬化）、酗酒者和菸癮者。此外，除了肺炎疫苗，也不要忘記接種每年一劑的流感疫苗，以及目前正在接種的COVID-19疫苗。

最後，根據研究，接種13價肺炎疫苗對於COVID-19的差異具有顯著效果。它可以降低住院致死率約三分之一。這一點特別重要，特別是對於糖尿病患者來說，因為他們可能面臨更高的感染風險和併發症風險。糖尿病患者由於免疫功能可能受損，且血糖控制不佳時容易引發病毒或細菌感染，增加罹患肺炎的風險。而接種肺炎疫苗可以提高對肺炎的防護力，減少感染的機會，進而降低併發症和死亡的風險。

因此，對於糖尿病患者和其他高風險人群來說，接種肺炎疫苗是非常重要的防護措施。除了接種疫苗外，也應該遵循預防肺炎的措施，如保持良好的個人衛生、避免接觸有感染風險的場所和人群、保持適當的血糖控制、均衡飲食、定期運動等。

總結來說，通過接種疫苗，可以降低罹患肺炎的風險，減少併發症和死亡的可能性。因此，我們強烈建議糖尿病患者儘早接種肺炎疫苗，以保護自己的健康。同時，也提醒其他高風險人群注意肺炎的預防措施，並在醫生的指導下接種相應的疫苗，以確保身體的健康和安全。

提供疫苗相關訊息如下表給大家參考。

	流感疫苗	COVID ~ 19 疫苗	肺炎疫苗
致病源	病毒（流感病毒）	病毒（COVID ~ 19 病毒）	細菌（肺炎細菌）
每年接種	○	可能	
減少病毒肺炎	○	○	
減少細菌肺炎			○
減少病毒引發細菌肺炎。	○	○	○
減少細菌引發病毒肺炎	○	○	○
費用	公費與自費	公費	公費與自費

可能的併發症：腎病變

案例 1 王先生從年輕時就是一個美食家，雖然他盡情享受美食，但卻忽視了自己的身體狀況。結果不到 50 歲的時候，他患上了糖尿病、高血壓、高血脂和高尿酸等現代生活中常見的富貴疾病。儘管如此，除了定期就醫治療痛風發作外，王先生仍然自認沒有任何不適症狀，繼續正常地大吃大喝。然而，即使他使用胰島素注射和口服藥物，他仍然無法有效控制血糖水準。

醫療團隊對王先生進行了健康教育，告訴他控制血糖、血壓、血脂和尿酸的重要性，特別是對心血管疾病和腎臟病變的影響。然而，每次王先生回診時都聽而不聞，沒有做出任何生活方式的改變。

五年後，王先生的腎功能開始惡化，微量白蛋白尿也被檢測出來，確診為糖尿病引起的腎病變。此時，除了控制碳水化合物的攝入外，他還需要開始限制蛋白質的攝入，選擇優質蛋白質，如豆類、魚類和肉類。不幸的是，即使他在飲食上有很多限制，服藥的依從性也很高，但在過去的三年裡，王先生的腎功能逐漸衰退，最終不得不接受洗腎治療。

王先生悔恨不已，如果他從一開始就重視血糖、血壓、血脂和尿酸的控制，也許就不會陷入到連很多食物都不能吃的困境中。

案例 2

沈先生已經超過 60 歲了，這次因為感冒不適來門診就醫。沈先生患有糖尿病已經超過 20 年，已經接受洗腎治療 6 年了。他在門診中分享，如果當時有人好好向他宣傳血糖對腎臟的危害，他一定會遵循醫囑服藥，並尋求營養師的幫助來進行飲食調整。目前，他只能抓住當下，穩定血糖水準，延緩其他糖尿病併發症的發生。

然而，沈先生也非常感激目前能夠接受洗腎治療並獲得給付。如果這發生在沒有給付的年代，他可能無法承擔治療費用，只能任由疾病發展而去世。

案例 3

50 多歲的白女士患有糖尿病、高血壓和高血脂已達 5 年之久。在門診時，她向醫生詢問：「醫生，我知道若糖尿病控制不好，會影響腎功能，請問我目前的控制情況如何？除了控制血糖達到標準，還有哪些顧腎的措施可以請教醫生？」

醫生仔細檢視了她的血壓記錄和血脂數值後，建議她在控制血糖的同時，也需要注意控制血壓和血脂。

案例 4

60 多歲的戴先生已經患有糖尿病近 10 年，雖然最近的血糖控制接近達標，但他的腎功能卻正在緩慢下降。醫生建議戴先生可以在戒菸門診的協助下，戒除持續了近 20 年的抽菸習慣。此外，醫生還鼓勵他增加每天運動次數至 5 次以上，每次運動時間至少 30 分鐘。

同時，醫生建議他加上排糖藥物來輔助血糖控制。並根據最新的 KDIGO 指南，來顧腎。

當腎病變與糖尿病共存時，蛋白質的攝入需要開始進行限制，無法像以前那樣隨意地食用大量的魚肉。相對於沒有糖尿病的人群，糖尿病患者在飲食方面需要更多的限制。因此，建議那些注重美食或熱衷於美食的人努力避免患上糖尿病。

如果不幸確診為糖尿病，目標應該是穩定長期地控制血糖，這樣可以有效減少糖尿病腎病變的發生，並且在控制血糖的過程中仍然可以享受美食。

腎病變分期與洗腎

腎病變的分期主要通過兩個指標來判斷：尿液中的微量白蛋白尿和抽血檢查的肌酐水準，通過這兩個指標可以估算出腎小球濾過率（eGFR）。不過要提醒的是，肌酐水準容易受到許多因素的影響而波動，例如脫水、發燒等，因此建議多次檢查以確定結果。腎病變分期如下表：

期別	腎小球濾過率（eGFR）	說明
G1	≧ 90	正常或高
G2	60-89	輕微下降
G3a	45-59	輕微至中度下降
G3b	30-44	中度至嚴重下降
G4	15-29	嚴重下降
G5	＜ 15	腎衰竭

根據 2020 年臺灣腎病年報，接受透析治療（洗腎）的糖尿病患者占糖尿病患者的比例為 46.2%如下表。由此可見，糖尿病併發症之一的腎病變的危害程度。

新發透析患者主診斷為糖尿病比率(%)

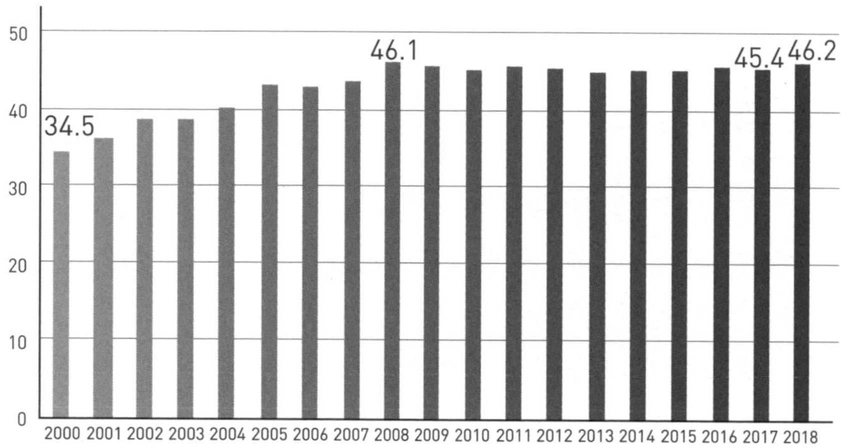

早期介入和達到血糖目標已經成為糖尿病患者的當務之急。目前糖尿病治療指南建議，患有腎病變的糖尿病患者優先使用排糖藥物，這可以有效延緩腎病變的進展，甚至有研究顯示可以延緩透析的時間達 11 年。

只要能夠延緩進入透析階段，除了可以節省大量的醫療費用，還可以改善糖尿病患者的生活品質。糖尿病患者可以主動向醫療團隊諮詢是否適合使用排糖藥物來穩定血糖。

糖尿病腎病變的預防措施如下：

預防 1：控制血糖

將血糖控制在目標範圍內（糖化血色素小於 7%），這是最重要的預防措施。根據目前最新的研究指出，排糖藥可以有效延緩腎病變的發生，甚至在腎功能很差的情況下仍然具有相同的效果，有助於延緩進入洗腎階段。

另外，腸泌素是一種在排糖藥之後可以考慮使用的藥物選擇。相較於其他藥物，許多腸泌素在腎功能不佳的糖友身上不需要調整劑量。然而，腸泌素可能會影響糖友的食慾，進而影響到糖友攝取足夠的熱量或蛋白質。

預防 2：控制血壓和血脂

血糖達標之外，糖尿病共病中的高血脂與高血壓，也要一併達標。這是許多糖友易忽略的地方。一旦長期高血脂與高血壓，日積月累的情況下，腎臟的血管就會開始硬化受損，之後腎功能會跟著慢慢下降。

因此，建議要好好地穩壓降脂。高血脂可優先選用 statin 類用藥降脂，同時減少加工食品的使用；高血壓部分優先使用 RAS 降血壓用藥，同時減少過量鹽份的攝取。

預防 3：充足的水分攝入

每天攝入足夠的水分（建議 1000 ～ 1500 毫升），保持良好的水分平衡，有助於腎臟的正常功能。

預防 4：處理尿酸問題

對於有高尿酸的病人，需要治療尿酸或尿酸結石問題，避免尿酸沉積引起的腎臟損害。

預防 5：避免長期使用止痛藥物

長期或過量使用止痛藥物，特別是非類固醇抗發炎藥，可能對腎臟產生負面影響。在使用止痛藥物時要謹慎，最好在醫生的指導下進行使用。

預防 6：控制體重和運動

如果存在超重或肥胖問題，建議減輕體重，以減輕腎臟的負擔，從而延緩腎功能的下降。規律足量的運動，可以保持腎臟血管的良好循環，正常有效地工作，此外也可以輔助降低血脂與血壓，一舉數得。

預防 7：戒菸

戒菸是一項具有挑戰性的過程，但幸運的是，有許多輔助方式可供選擇。單靠意志力戒菸的成功率只有不到 5%，然而，若配合使用藥物進行戒菸，成功率可以提升至 20 ～ 30%。此外，每年國家健康署提供兩次 8 週的戒菸療程補助，詳細資訊可參考「抽菸族群」相關資料。

儘管戒菸是具有挑戰性的過程，但藉助藥物輔助和戒菸療程，可以大幅提升成功戒菸的機會。除此之外，還有其他輔助方法，例如心理諮詢、支持團體和替代行為培養等，都可以協助減少戒菸的困難度。

大魚醫師小叮嚀：四高指數要穩定

血糖、血壓、血脂和高尿酸一樣重要，努力使其保持在標準範圍內。

合理使用止痛藥物，對於感冒、頭痛、經痛等需要使用止痛藥的情況，只在有需要時短期適量使用，實際上不會影響腎功能。

--CHAPTER-- 02 認識胰島素與血糖的關係

胰島素的重要性

胰島素的發現

在胰島素發明之前，糖友必須節制或禁止攝取任何碳水化合物，也就是現在所謂的低碳水化合物或生酮飲食維持血糖的穩定。尤其是第一型糖友完全缺乏胰島素，無法將血糖有效轉化為身體所需的能量，血糖持續升高，有時甚至可能導致昏迷或死亡，預期壽命不會太長。當時無可用的藥物治療，唯一的希望是嚴格控制碳水化合物攝取（生酮飲食），以延長存活時間。然而，這種飲食方式會長期導致體重減輕、身體衰弱，無法持續很久。直到胰島素的發現，情況才有所改觀。

1921 年，班廷及貝斯特發現胰島素，並在隔年在麥克勞德（John MacLeod）、柯立普（James Collip）的協助下製成可使用的藥物，拯救了當時無藥可治的糖友。隨後，這個由加拿大多倫多大學團隊發現的成果贏得了 1923 年的諾貝爾醫學獎。

起初，胰島素的供應量有限，直到 George Clowes（後來成為 Lilly 禮來公司）和 August Krogh（後來成為 Novo Nordisk 諾和諾得公司）獲得了加拿大多倫多大學的授權，在加拿大境外生產胰島素，才能夠讓更多的糖友受益。班廷和貝斯特以僅 1 美元的價格出讓專利，表達出「胰島素屬於全球」的理念。（本段文字來源出自糖尿病衛教學會會訊《如是我聞之胰島素發現史》）

大魚醫師醫學小教室：胰島素的發現

班廷（Frederick Banting，1891 ～ 1941）是加拿大的一位外科醫生。他在一戰期間擔任過醫療人員，對於戰爭中的傷病治療積累了豐富的經驗。戰後，他進入了多倫多大學醫學院攻讀醫學專業，並在那裡成為一名教師和研究員。

貝斯特（Charles Best，1899 ～ 1978）是加拿大的一位生理學家和研究員。他在多倫多大學攻讀生理學學位，並在那裡遇到了班廷。班廷注意到貝斯特對生理學和內分泌學有著深厚的興趣，並邀請他參與研究，進而就發現了胰島素。

為什麼需要胰島素？

從出生開始，人體就會分泌胰島素。平時，人體會分泌基礎胰島素，維持基本的生理功能。在進行用餐時，人體會再分泌速效胰島素，以穩定血糖水平。

但是，對於完全失去胰臟功能的第一型糖友或糖尿病長期患者來說，如果要模擬人體正常的胰島素分泌，建議使用一天一次的長效基礎胰島素，並根據用餐次數施打相應的速效胰島素。例如，如果每天吃三餐，則需要使用三次速效胰島素；如果每天吃兩餐，則使用兩次速效胰島素，以此類推。

《幸福瘦：不節食、不復胖，從心開始的 23 堂療癒減重對話》一書的作者馬文雅醫師就說「胰島素就像金錢一樣」。當我們購買物品時，必須付出金錢，同樣的情況，在我們進食時，也需要支付胰島素（分泌胰島素），以維持血糖的穩定。

同時，胰臟更像一個會分泌汽油（胰島素）的油箱，它在正常運作下維持著人體的運作。一旦分泌的汽油（胰島素）不足或油箱（胰臟）失去功能，該怎麼辦呢？只能外加汽油（胰島素）來讓車輛（人體）繼續運作！

胰島素可控制血糖，減少肝腎負擔

胰島素對於肝腎功能不良的糖友來說是穩定血糖的最後一道防線。

由於肝腎功能不良的糖友已經無法使用許多口服降血糖藥物，因此胰島素成為他們穩定血糖的最佳的選擇之一。此外，對於腎功能不良或腎病變末期的糖友來說，由於只能使用胰島素，再加上這些患者可能需要進行血液透析（洗腎）治療，造成了許多人對「使用胰島素後很快就需要洗腎」的誤解。事實上，快要進行血液透析的患者往往只剩下胰島素作為穩定血糖的選擇，這並不表示使用胰島素會加速進入洗腎狀態。相反地，胰島素可以有效地幫助控制血糖，減少糖尿病對肝腎的負擔。

因此，對於肝腎功能不良的糖友而言，胰島素可能是他們唯一的選擇。

總之，使用胰島素需要在醫生的指導下進行，以確保劑量和使用方式符合個人的需要。胰島素的使用可以根據血糖控制目標和個人情況進行調整，以達到最佳的血糖管理效果。

大魚醫師醫學小教室：胰島素和血糖的真實關係

糖尿病是一種由於胰島素分泌不足或細胞對胰島素反應不佳而導致的慢性高血糖狀態。在糖尿病患者中，胰島素的功能受到損害，血糖無法有效地進入細胞，導致血糖濃度升高。

因此，糖尿病的治療中，胰島素的補充或增加胰島素的敏感性成為重要的治療手段，如此才能維持正常的血糖水平。

胰島素的分類

胰島素是糖尿病治療中常用的藥物之一，根據作用時間的不同，胰島素可分為速效、短效、中效、長效和超長效五種基本類型，此外還可另外區分出預混型、混和型等兩類。以下分別介紹之。

目前推薦一天施打一次的超長效胰島素搭配隨餐施打的速效胰島素，這種治療方案最符合人體生理機制，對於完全缺乏胰島素的糖友特別適用。

除了第一型糖友需要使用胰島素外，對於第二型糖友來說，隨著更多研究結果的出爐，早期使用胰島素有助於讓胰臟休息，並使血糖控制更長久和穩定。

然而，一些對胰島素的誤解以及胰島素仍需使用微小針頭的問題，使得一些人對胰島素治療的接受度較低，相對而言，口服降血糖藥物的接受度更高。

速效、短效、中效胰島素等 7 種

速效胰島素

這類胰島素通常在進食前或飯後立即注射，以迅速降低血糖水平。它們的作用開始迅速，作用時間短暫，通常可持續約 2 到 4 小時。常見有胰島素膠體和胰島素噴霧劑。

短效型胰島素

這類胰島素通常在進食前注射，以在飯前降低血糖水平。它們的作用開始較快，作用時間較快速作用型胰島素稍長，通常可持續約 4 到 6 小時。例子包括常規人胰島素和胰島素注射液。

中效型胰島素

這類胰島素通常在早上或晚上注射，以提供較長時間的血糖控制。它們的作用開始較慢，作用時間較長，通常可持續約 12 到 18 小時。例子包括中效型胰島素和胰島素混合物。

相關資料以下列表給大家參考。

胰島素種類	商品名	中文名	持續作用
速效胰島素			
Novorapid Apidra	Novorapid Apidra	諾和瑞 愛胰達	3-5 小時
Insulin glulisine			
短效胰島素			
Regular	Humulin R	優泌林常規型	4-6 小時
中效胰島素			
NPH		因速來達	10-16 小時

預混胰島素

針對血糖很高的族群，預混胰島素內含速效胰島素可降血糖，另外又含中效胰島素來穩定血糖。不過缺點就是，針對非定時定量的族群使用，常會發生低血糖的情況。可惜的是，屬於定時定量的糖友比例不高。

相關資料以下列表給大家參考。

胰島素種類	商品名	中文名	持續作用
預混型胰島素			
70/30 human insulin	Humulin 70/30	優泌林 混合型 70/30	10-16 小時
70/30 aspart insulin	NovoMix 30	諾和密斯 30	
50/50 aspart insulin	NovoMix 50	諾和密斯 50	
75/25 lispro insulin	Humalog Mix25	優泌樂筆混合型 25	
50/50 lispro insulin	Humalog Mix50	優泌樂筆混合型 50	

長效胰島素

長效胰島素是一種類似人體胰島素分泌模式的胰島素藥物，可以提供長時間的血糖控制效果。目前市面上有幾種不同的長效胰島素可供選擇，包括 Lantus（蘭德仕）和 Levemir（瑞和密爾）。

長效胰島素的作用持續時間較長，可以提供持續的胰島素釋放，幫助糖友控制血糖。這些胰島素藥物的作用機制是透過改變胰島素分子結構，使其釋放速度減慢，從而延長作用時間。

使用長效胰島素的好處是可以減少胰島素的施打次數，尤其適用於不便於多次施打胰島素的糖友。此外，長效胰島素還有助於穩定血糖，減少血糖波動，提高血糖控制的穩定性。

特別適合長效胰島素的人群包括：

第二型糖友

對於第二型糖友，長效胰島素可以提供穩定的胰島素供應，幫助控制血糖水平。這些患者通常需要每天施打胰島素，長效胰島素可以減少施打次數，提高用藥依從性。

第一型糖友

第一型糖友通常需要每天多次施打胰島素以控制血糖。長效胰島素可以作為基礎胰島素使用，提供 24 小時的胰島素覆蓋，減少胰島素施打次數。

不便於多次施打胰島素的人群

一些人可能因為工作、生活方式或身體狀況的原因，不便於多次施打胰島素。長效胰島素可以提供持續的胰島素供應，減少施打次數，增加便利性和依從性。

特殊族群

例如懷孕婦女或有特殊狀況的糖友，長效胰島素被廣泛應用。這是因為長效胰島素的安全性研究相對完善，可以在這些情況下提供有效的血糖控制。

超長效胰島素

超長效胰島素相比之前的長效胰島素更貼近人體生理，能夠減少血糖波動並具有更長效的穩定血糖作用。目前市面上有幾種不同的超長效胰島素可供選擇，包括 Toujeo（糖德仕）和 Tresiba（諾胰保）。

其中，Toujeo（糖德仕）屬於濃縮型胰島素，需要使用專用的裝置來調整劑量，裝置已經設計好換算，刻度顯示的單位即為胰島素單位數，。濃縮型胰島素容積相同但含有更多胰島素，適用於需要大量補充胰島素的糖友，可裝在一支筆型裝置內，減少每月所需的胰島素筆型裝置數量。

濃縮型胰島素不能像非濃縮型胰島素一樣直接抽取使用，否則容易導致低血糖等血糖不穩定情況的發生。超長效胰島素還有以下兩種混合劑型可運用：

超長效胰島素＋速效胰島素

在不影響某餐的攝取下，可以有效降低餐後血糖，同時也可以有效低血餐前血糖。對於腸泌素有不良反應、特定餐吃較多或想要吃得盡興點的糖友，會是比較好的選擇。

超長效胰島素＋短效腸泌素

可以有效降低餐前血糖外，也可讓減少某餐的攝取，達到血糖控制的問題。對於食慾較高的糖友，會是較好的選擇。使用前不需要搖動混合。

預混型胰島素

預混型胰島素是一種結合了不同種類胰島素的藥物，用於糖尿病患者的胰島素治療。它由快速作用胰島素和中等或長效作用胰島素混合而成。

混和型胰島素的配製可以根據不同的需要和病情進行調整，以滿足患者對胰島素的需求。一般而言，預混型胰島素分為以下兩種類型：

快速作用胰島素＋中等作用胰島素

這種混合型胰島素通常由一種快速作用的胰島素（例如胰島素葡萄糖注射液）和一種中等作用的胰島素（例如胰島素 NPH）混合而成。這種組合可以提供即時的血糖控制和較長效的血糖穩定，適合需要多次進食和胰島素注射的患者。

快速作用胰島素＋長效作用胰島素

這種混合型胰島素由一種快速作用的胰島素和一種長效作用的胰島素（例如胰島素葡萄糖注射液和胰島素葡萄糖混合注射液）混

合而成。這種組合提供了即時的血糖控制和持續的胰島素覆蓋，可以模擬身體自然胰島素的分泌模式。

相關資料以下列表給大家參考。

胰島素種類	商品名	中文名	持續作用
長效胰島素			
Insulin glargine (U－100)	Lantus	蘭德仕	20-24 小時
Insulin detemir (U－100)	Levemir	瑞和密爾	
超長效胰島素			
Insulin glargine (U－300)	Toujeo	糖德仕	36 小時穩定要 5 天
Insulin degludec (U-100)	Tresiba	諾胰保	42 小時穩定要 3-4 天
混和型胰島素			
Glargine 100+ Lixisenatide	SOLIQUA	爽胰達	
Degludec + Aspart	RYZODEG	諾胰得	

胰島素的施打方式

隨著醫學技術的進步，要正確施打胰島素已經變得容易，以下有兩種方式，方便、簡單，糖友和家屬趕快學起來，就不會想要拒打了。

筆型胰島素注射，輕鬆上手

以前傳統的胰島素需要從瓶裝胰島素中抽取，但現在主流的是筆型胰島素，就像使用自動筆一樣方便。建議糖友仔細聆聽糖尿病衛教師的指導，學習如何使用筆型胰島素，這樣就可以輕鬆上手，自行施打。

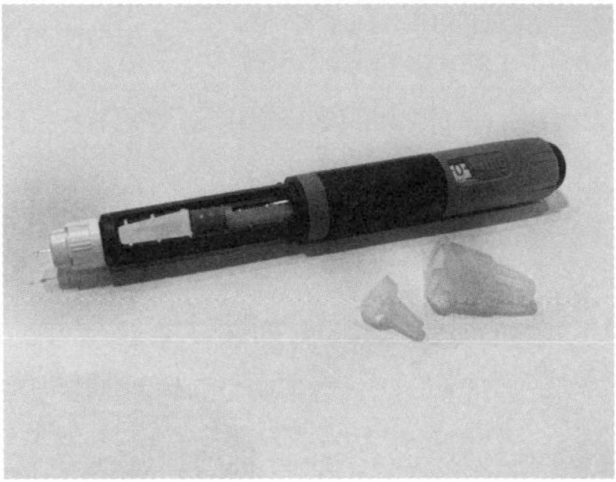

小針頭，幾乎不會痛

目前使用的針頭如圖是最常見的有 4mm 和 8mm 兩種尺寸。如果劑量不大，優先選擇 4mm 的針頭，幾乎不會感到疼痛。此外，如果使用冷藏的胰島素，記得在注射前先回溫，這也可以減少注射時的不適感。

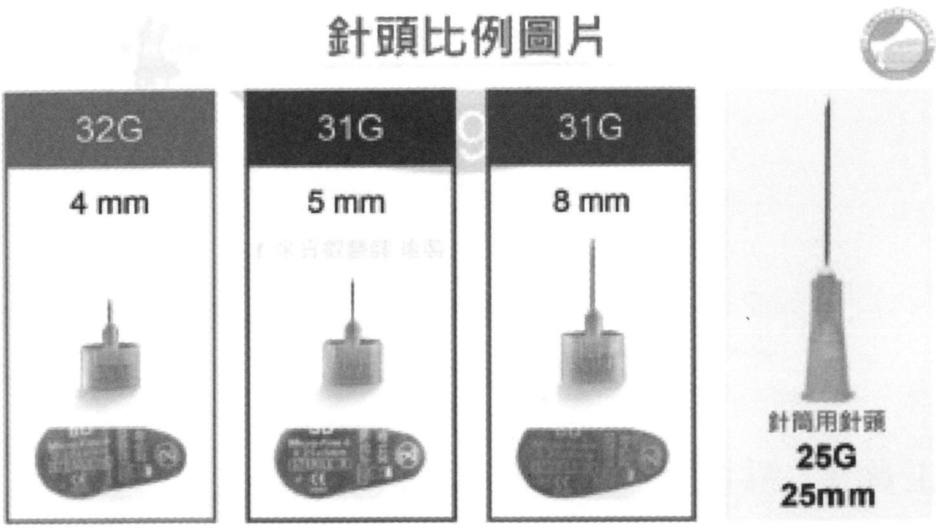

如何自我量測血糖？

量測血糖目前一般可以分成三種方法，一是抽血檢測，二是扎手指測血糖，三是利用連續血糖監測儀。

這三種方式當中以抽血測血糖和扎手指測血糖最常見。抽血檢測一般都要去醫療機構，本文則介紹扎手指測血糖方式，也是大家最常用的自我量測血糖方法。同時順帶簡介連續血糖監測儀。

方式 1：扎手指測血糖

扎手指測血糖需要使用採血筆、血糖試紙和血糖機。建議對於從未量測過血糖的糖友或家屬，接受衛教師的指導，學習如何正確量測血糖。如果可能的話，學習完後可以在衛教師面前進行現場測量一次。

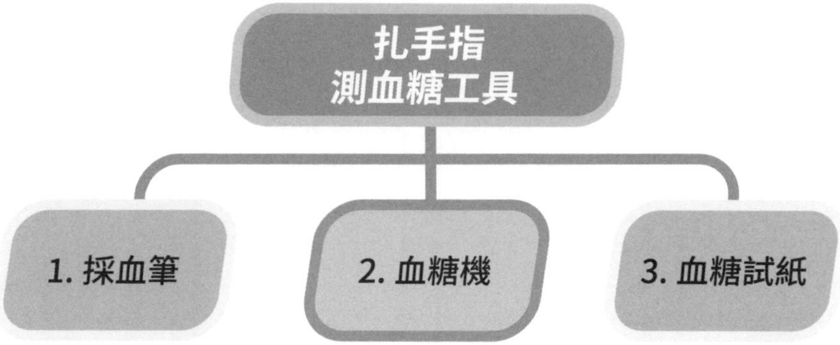

工具 1：採血筆

採血筆上有刻度，通常用數字表示，可調整採血的深度。調得越淺，測量時越不痛，但如果設定太淺，可能會出現血液流不出來或採血量不足，需要再次採血，也只能扎兩次手指了。建議調整適當的刻度，平衡痛感和採血量之間，一次採血足夠，確保測量成功。

此外，有一些方法可以減少血糖測量時的不適，例如採血時選擇手指側邊而非中央、使用專利微針等。不論使用何種方式，都應確保足夠的採血量，以提高血糖監測的準確性。

工具 2：血糖機

選擇和購買血糖機時，可以向衛教師、醫生、藥師等醫療團隊成員詢問意見。目前的血糖機功能越來越多，例如放大字體、台語發音、記憶量測數據、藍牙上傳、提醒量測等。建議在購買前列出需要的功能，以便選擇合適的血糖機。

工具 3：血糖試紙

不同品牌的血糖機通常配有相對應的血糖試紙，建議購買廠商推薦的血糖試紙，通常是同廠牌的配套使用。此外，血糖試紙有一定的有效期限，建議不要一次購買太多。如果買得太多，可能無法在有效期內使用完畢，過期的試紙可能會導致血糖測量結果不準確。

為了確保血糖監測的正確性，請留意血糖試紙的有效期，並適量購買以確保能在有效期內使用完畢。

方式 2：連續血糖監測儀

如果您想更加精確地掌握血糖數值的變化，可以考慮使用連續血糖監測儀。這種儀器可以實時監測血糖的波動情況，讓您更好地了解自己的血糖控制狀況。然而，需要注意的是，目前的連續血糖監測儀仍有些需要使用血糖機進行校正，以確保監測數值的準確性。

其他提醒

如果只是偶爾測量一兩次血糖，想要知道自己的血糖水平，除了可以借用親友的血糖機，也可以前往附近的醫療機構付費進行測量。只有進行血糖測量，才能了解自己的血糖情況。

如果使用他人的血糖機，請注意確認血糖試紙是否過期或受潮。如果需要頻繁測量血糖，建議擁有自己專屬的血糖機，甚至在工作場所和家中都準備有一台專屬的血糖機。

血糖量測方式比較

以下列表分享扎手指、連續血糖監測儀和抽血這三種類型的量測血糖方式和大家分享，大家可根據需求和條件參考。

量測血糖方式	扎手指	連續血糖監測儀	抽血
比喻	手機拍照	攝影機	單眼相機
精確度	++	++	+++
方便性	隨時想測就測	隨時掌握血糖	限醫療人員執行
侵入性	++	+	+++
痛	+	+	++
給付	院所回診時可幫忙檢測；在家檢測則需自費；第一型與妊娠糖尿病有給付血糖試紙	無（除非第一型糖尿病，有重大傷病，限一年使用兩次）	有（但一定的次數限制）
意義	當下血糖	一段時間內的血糖值	當下血糖或糖化血色素
糖化血色素	× 大部分血糖機不行	可估算	可確認
血糖試紙使用	要	要（校正用）	不用
餐前餐後血糖	餐前餐後測兩次（配對測）	抓時間點，即可得到數值	餐前餐後抽血兩次
臨床應用	飲食、運動與藥物對血糖影響	飲食、運動與藥物對血糖影響 夜間低血糖 可估算糖化血色素	飲食、運動與藥物對血糖影響，以及過去三個月的整體情況

大魚醫師醫學小叮嚀：血糖測量的準確性

扎手指測血糖或連續血糖監測機與抽血測血糖相比，都存在一定的時間誤差和量測誤差（在正負 20%的範圍內仍屬正常）。儘管如此，扎手指測血糖或連續血糖監測機仍然具有很高的參考價值，可以在日常生活中幫助您了解血糖的控制情況。

血糖測量結果可能會因抽血和血糖機量測之間存在一定誤差。抽血測血糖直接從血管中抽取血液進行測量，而血糖機則是使用組織液體進行測量後換算為血糖值，因此會有一定的誤差。例如，以正負 20%的誤差為例，如果抽血測得的血糖數值為 100mg/dL，那麼血糖機測量的結果在 80 ～ 120mg/dL 都可以接受。

目前市面上有正負 10 ～ 15%誤差的血糖機可供選擇，精準度越高的血糖機可能價格較高。除了採血方式，血糖測量結果還受到其他許多因素的影響，例如空腹狀態、採血量、消毒後手指上是否有酒精殘留等。為了提高血糖測量的準確性，請避免上述的干擾因素。

為何要積極監測血糖？

案例 林先生和白先生都是 40 多歲的糖友，初始時他們的糖化血色素分別為 9.5%和 9.3%。醫生為他們制定了相同的治療方案，包括口服藥物和胰島素。三個月後的追蹤結果顯示，林先生的糖化血色素下降到了 7.8%，而白先生的糖化血色素僅有些微改善，仍然有進步的空間。

為什麼兩人相同的治療方案卻有不同的結果？深入瞭解後發現，林先生非常勤勞地監測自己的血糖，他快速發現了自己高醣飲食習慣導致的餐後高血糖。他遵從營養師建議的飲食方式，有效地穩定了血糖。此外，他每天花約 20 分鐘散步，成功降低了血糖水平。醫療團隊根據他的血糖數據快速調整了藥物劑量，讓林先生對治療計畫充滿信心，形成了一個正向循環。經過三個月的努力，他的血糖穩定在正常範圍。

相比之下，白先生的血糖監測不夠勤勞，無法產生像林先生那樣的正向循環。雖然他的血糖有些改善，但仍有進步的空間。

以上兩個案例告訴我們，積極監測血糖的重要性。現在讓我們再來看看幾個關於血糖監測的重要事項。

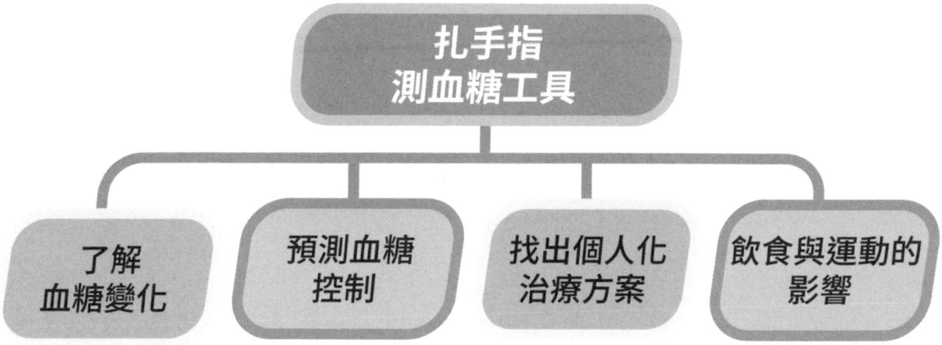

檢討飲食內容與運動方式對血糖的影響

了解不同食物、飲料和運動對血糖的影響是監測血糖的第一步。例如，儘管芭樂是被推薦的水果之一，但飲食後食用過多芭樂會使血糖數值升高。同樣地，糖尿病專用飲品被設計為低 GI（血糖指數）飲品，但如果在用餐後再飲用一罐糖尿病專用飲品，血糖數值可能會增加。食用肉粽、泡麵搭配餅乾等高碳水化合物食物也可能導致血糖升高。因此，了解飲食內容對血糖的影響，能幫助你做出更好的飲食選擇。

找出個人化治療方案

每個人對於藥物、飲食和運動的反應都不盡相同。因此，個人化的糖尿病治療是關鍵。監測血糖可以幫助醫療團隊了解你的血糖變化情況，並根據數據調整治療方案和藥物劑量，以確保血糖控制得到最佳效果。

可以預測血糖控制

監測血糖可以作為預測糖化血色素（HbA1c）的指標。HbA1c 是血液中紅血球上血糖平均水平的指示器，常用於評估長期血糖控制情況。通過經常監測血糖，你可以預測自己的 HbA1c 是否會達到目標範圍。

有助了解血糖變化

監測血糖可以幫助你了解血糖的變化情況。不同人的胰島素作用效率不同，即使進食相同的食物，血糖反應也可能不同。透過監測，你可以更清楚地了解自己的血糖變化模式，並針對性地進行調整。

綜上所述，監測血糖對於糖尿病管理至關重要。它可以幫助你了解飲食、運動和治療對血糖的影響，並預測長期血糖控制的情況。透過持續監測，你可以更好地調整生活方式和治療方案。

正確認知 1：監測血糖有 4 大好處

案例 王先生的餐後血糖為 320mg/dl，相較於餐前血糖 100mg/dl，表示他在該餐中攝取了過多的醣類，導致血糖大幅上升 220mg/dl。這顯示餐後血糖的增加問題主要出在飲食中攝取過多的碳水化合物。

然而，若餐前血糖已經高達 270mg/dl，但血糖僅上升 50mg/dl，此時過多的醣類攝取就不是主要問題，反而需要尋找造成餐前血糖升高的原因。可能的原因包括上一餐進食過多或在餐與餐間進食了其他食物等。因此，透過配對血糖值，我們能更有效地找出飲食中的問題點。

總而言之，通過監測血糖並進行配對分析，可以更好地了解飲食對血糖的影響。在第一種情況下，王先生的餐後血糖升高主要是由於醣類攝取過多，而在第二種情況下，需要進一步探究造成餐前血糖升高的原因。這樣的分析有助於個人調整飲食習慣，以實現更好的血糖控制。

另外，有些糖友可能認為只有血糖高或使用胰島素的人才需要監測血糖。 實際上，不論是第一型糖尿病的糖友或每天使用胰島素 1 ～ 4 次的糖友，都建議頻繁地監測血糖。即使是使用口服藥物治療的糖友，也應該監測血糖，因為無論是口服藥物還是注射藥物，都存在引起高低血糖的風險。監測血糖有助於早期發現血糖異常並做出相應的調整。

此外，正常人或糖尿病前期的糖友也可以進行血糖監測，以更好地了解飲食和運動對血糖的影響，進而調整生活方式以維持健康和穩定的血糖水平。

有些人可能覺得監測血糖很難，但只要認真聆聽衛教師的指導，並進行幾次現場示範，大多數人都可以學會如何監測血糖。此外，還有連續血糖測量儀可以供選擇，更加方便和準確。

另外，有些人擔心監測血糖會導致貧血。實際上，在進行血糖監測時，只需要採集一小滴血液，即使一天多次測量，也不會流失太多血液，不會導致貧血的情況。

最後，還有人認為監測血糖不準確，因此不願意進行監測。雖然與抽血比較起來，血糖監測可能存在 10 ～ 15%的誤差，但仍具有很高的學習價值。通過監測血糖，我可以更好地了解自己的血糖控制狀況，並根據監測結果調整飲食、運動和藥物治療等方面的措施，以達到良好的血糖管理。

血糖監測可以提供以下幾個好處：

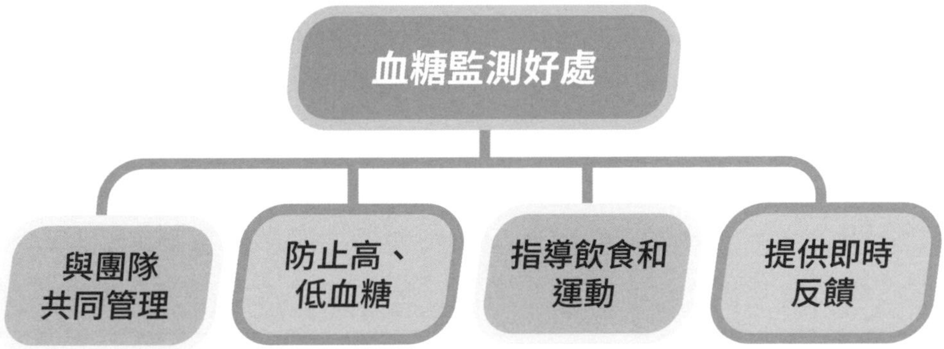

提供即時反饋

血糖監測可以幫助你了解自己每天不同時間段的血糖變化情況。這對於調整飲食和藥物劑量以達到理想的血糖控制非常重要。

指導飲食和運動

通過監測血糖，你可以確定哪些食物和運動方式對你的血糖水平有影響。這樣你就可以調整飲食組成和運動計畫，以達到更穩定的血糖控制。

防止低血糖和高血糖

血糖監測可以幫助你及時發現低血糖或高血糖的情況，從而及時採取措施調整血糖水平。這對於預防低血糖和高血糖的併發症非常重要。

與醫療團隊共同管理

通過監測血糖，你可以提供有價值的數據給醫療團隊，幫助他們評估你的糖尿病管理情況並作出相應的建議。這樣可以實現更有效的共同管理，以達到更好的血糖控制效果。

總之，血糖監測對於糖尿病管理非常重要，無論是使用傳統的血糖測量儀器還是連續血糖測量儀，它都可以提供有價值的信息，幫助你更好地掌握自己的血糖控制狀況，從而改善生活質量並減少併發症的風險。記得與你的醫療團隊密切合作，他們可以為你提供指導和支持。

正確認知 2：不用一輩子監測血糖

案例 60 歲的楊媽媽曾一度血糖高達 502mg/dl，但經過 3 個月的血糖監測和糖尿病相關知識的學習後，他成功地將血糖數值控制在標準範圍內。醫療團隊提醒他，在回診前 2 週內進行血糖監測即可，或者在感覺血糖偏高或偏低時進行監測。

很多都人誤解以為一旦開始監測血糖，就必須一輩子持續下去，但實際上這並非必需。

監測血糖並不一定是終身負擔，只要能夠掌握不同飲食、運動、藥物和心理狀態對血糖的影響，並將血糖保持在標準範圍內，就可以逐漸減少血糖監測的次數，甚至最終不再需要監測血糖。當然，如果發現血糖不穩定，增加監測頻率是必要的。

由多次逐漸減少

建議的做法是從多到少逐漸減少血糖監測的次數。例如，從每天一餐測量，可以減少到每隔 2 天一餐，或者專注於血糖不穩定的早上或睡前時段，或者在早、午、晚餐中的某一餐測量。此外，如果身體感到不適，或者有高低血糖的症狀，或者進食了一些特別的食物等，建議隨機進行血糖監測，以確定血糖是否穩定。

數值穩定是先決條件

增加或減少血糖監測的次數取決於血糖穩定的持續程度。就像學生在大考表現出色後可以逐漸減少小考的次數一樣，因為他們已經知道如何應對大考一樣。小考可以類比為血糖監測（使用血糖試紙或連續血糖機），而大考可以類比為糖化血色素檢測（需要抽血）。糖友就像是一個學生，如果使用連續血糖監測，每天只需校正血糖 1 至 3 次，就能了解各個時間點的血糖情況，這對於那些積極想要掌握血糖狀況的人來說非常適合。

當然，減少血糖監測的情況要特別注意試紙是否已過期，請記得購買適量的血糖試紙以免出現供應不足的情況。

總而言之，血糖監測並不需要一輩子持續下去。通過掌握不同飲食、運動、藥物和心理狀態對血糖的影響，並將血糖保持在標準範圍內，可以逐漸減少血糖監測的次數，甚至最終不再需要監測血糖。但是，對於血糖不穩定的情況，增加監測的頻率是必要的。

記住，血糖監測是維持良好糖尿病管理的重要工具之一，而減少監測次數應基於個人情況和醫療專業人士的建議。

認識糖化血色素

案例 1

李女士是一位 40 多歲的教職員工。在員工體檢中，她的空腹血糖值為 243mg/dl，糖化血色素值為 9.8%。面對這些數據，她感到有些困惑，因此在門診時提出了一系列問題：「糖化血色素代表什麼意思？」、「為什麼我的糖化血色素是 9.8%時醫師就建議使用胰島素？」、「糖化血色素數值需要達到多少才算血糖控制達標？」這些都是糖友關心的重要問題。

案例 2

馬先生是一位 50 多歲的男性。三年前他進行成人健康檢查時，空腹血糖值為 106mg/dl，糖化血色素值為 5.9%。最近，他感到頭暈和疲倦，因此在進行血液檢查時，也同時追蹤了糖化血色素的數值。結果顯示，糖化血色素值為 6.9%，空腹兩小時血糖值為 225mg/dl，這證實了他患有糖尿病。馬先生問道：「從 5.9%升到 6.9%，僅增加了 1%，這需要接受治療嗎？」

我們從以下幾個糖化血色素的定義和功能來回答以上兩個案例的問題。

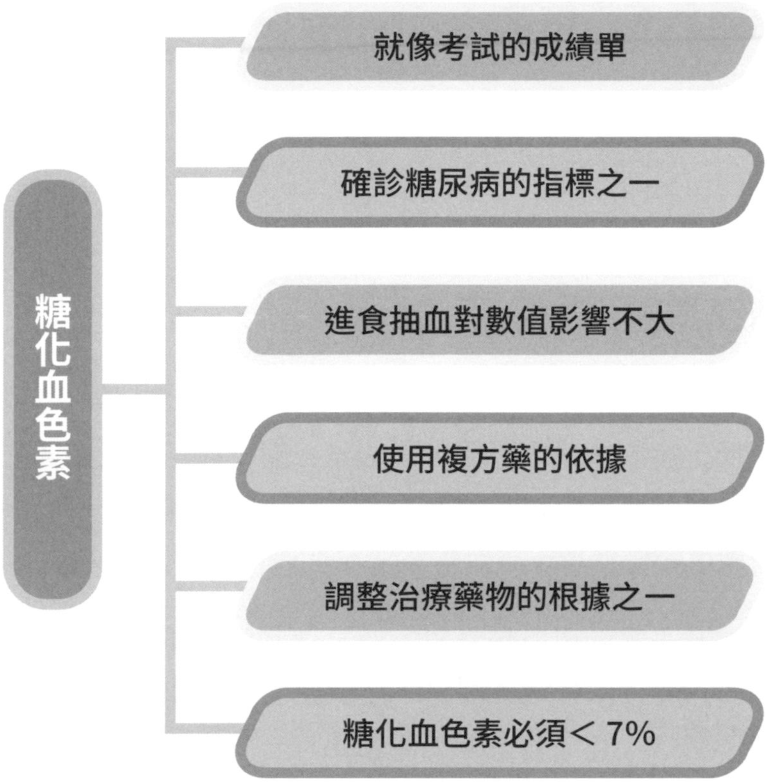
糖化血色素
就像考試的成績單
確診糖尿病的指標之一
進食抽血對數值影響不大
使用複方藥的依據
調整治療藥物的根據之一
糖化血色素必須＜ 7%

就像考試的成績單

糖化血色素是一個重要的指標，用來衡量過去三個月的血糖控制情況。它可以有效確認是否患有糖尿病或處於糖尿病前期。糖化血色素的數值可以配合餐前和餐後的自我血糖監測，協助了解血糖在這些時段的情況。現在的連續血糖儀器也具備計算功能，可以提早預測糖友的糖尿病血糖控制情況。簡單來說，糖化血色素就像是一份過去三個月血糖的成績單，提供了評估血糖控制的重要依據。

確診糖尿病的指標之一

確診糖尿病的指標中，其中有一項為糖化血色素≧ 6.5%為糖尿病，5.7 ～ 6.4%為糖尿病前期。因此，這是確診糖尿病的重要指標之一。

進食抽血對數值影響不大

「醫師不是要空腹才能抽血？」這是一個常見的疑問。實際上，單純檢測糖化血色素並不需要空腹抽血。糖化血色素是過去三個月的平均血糖值，與最近幾餐的攝取量無關。因此，是否空腹對糖化血色素的數值影響很小，可以直接進行抽血檢測。

然而，在平常的血液檢查中，通常會同時檢測空腹血糖和血脂肪等指標。對於這兩個檢查項目，建議空腹進行檢測，因為飲食攝取會直接影響這些數值的正確性。因此，一般會建議在空腹狀態下進行一次抽血，同時檢測這些指標。

需要注意的是，糖化血色素並不包含在一般成人健康檢查的項目中，除非自行選擇或進行特定的自費體檢，才會包含這項指標的檢測。

使用複方藥的依據

複方藥和胰島素是根據糖化血色素數值來判斷治療方案的依據。根據糖尿病學會的建議，當糖化血色素≧ 7.5%時，可以考慮使用複方藥來控制血糖；而當糖化血色素≧ 9%時，可以考慮使用胰島素進行治療。因此，血糖控制的嚴格程度或寬鬆程度也是以糖化血色素數值作為標準。

醫師調整治療藥物的根據之一

糖化血色素的檢測通常每隔 3 至 6 個月進行一次。透過檢測糖化血色素，醫師可以評估過去三個月的血糖控制情況。如果糖化血色素超過標準範圍，這意味著目前的飲食、運動或藥物治療可能不足以達到穩定的血糖控制，因此需要調整治療計畫。只有在下次檢測時糖化血色素達到正常範圍，才能確保血糖控制的有效性。

需要注意的是，糖化血色素代表過去三個月的成績，並不代表之後或將來的血糖控制狀況。

糖化血色素必須＜ 7%

研究結果顯示，建議糖化血色素（HbA1c）保持在小於 7%的水平，有以下原因支持這一標準。許多糖友對於這個標準的由來感到好奇。根據英國糖尿病研究（UKPDS）的研究發現，糖化血色素小於 7%的人群，相較於高於 7%的人群，其糖尿病相關併發症的風險顯著降低。這意味著在達到小於 7%的糖化血色素水平時，器官受到的損害相對較輕微。（正常人的糖化血色素水平為小於等於 5.6%）

此外，許多研究也證實，維持小於 7%的糖化血色素有助於減緩藥物劑量的增加速度。相反地，高於 7%的糖化血色素水平會增加增加藥物劑量的需求。這意味著達到小於 7%的糖化血色素目標，可以減少藥物劑量的調整頻率。

此外，在高血糖情況下，胰臟中分泌胰島素的胰島細胞會持續受到損害。這導致身體需要依靠藥物來促進胰島細胞分泌胰島素或增強胰島素的效果。然而，長期以來，胰島細胞可能會過勞而失去功能，這對於口服藥物的療效產生負面影響，口服藥無法穩定血糖，最終只能依靠補充的胰島素或腸泌素來穩定血糖。

大魚醫師的小叮嚀：糖化血色素轉算成血糖公式

糖化血色素與平均血糖值之間有一個基本的換算公式，即：
(糖化血色素值 - 2) × 30 = 平均血糖值

例如，以糖化血色素 7%為例，(7 - 2) × 30 = 150，平均血糖值為 150 mg/dL。以糖化血色素 9%為例，(9 - 2) × 30 = 210，平均血糖值為 210 mg/dL。以糖化血色素 12%為例，(12 - 2) × 30 = 300，平均血糖值為 300 mg/dL。因此，每增加 1%的糖化血色素，相當於平均血糖值增加 30 mg/dL。

需要注意的是，糖化血色素小於 7%是一個基本目標，但同時也要兼顧生活品質和穩定血糖。達到這一目標，讓糖尿病與糖共舞更加順暢。

輕忽低血糖也可能致命

案例 1

2018 年的新聞報導中提到一起交通事故，一輛計程車載著三名男女乘客，在行經北市西寧南路要上忠孝橋時突然撞上橋墩，造成車輛翻覆 180 度。初步警方調查顯示，這起事故是因為駕駛人在駕駛過程中由於沒有進食，導致低血糖發作並且意識不清，最終導致直接撞上橋墩。事故發生時，路口的監視器也拍下了這一驚險的一刻，畫面中可以看到計程車並沒有減速，直接撞向橋墩。

案例 2

2020 年的新聞報導中提到知名導演楊冠玉因血糖過低在自家休克過世，享年57歲。楊冠玉是一位曾執導過《我的秘密花園》、《我要變成硬柿子》等戲劇，並捧紅了林依晨、楊謹華等藝人的知名導演。這起事件發生在 7 月 4 日，楊冠玉因血糖過低而陷入休克狀態，在自家中不幸過世。

案例 3

我曾問過一位 50 多歲的女性計程車司機，是否常常感到肚子餓並需要進食。她對於我如何知道她的生活情況感到驚訝，並承認自己經常因為肚子餓而感到不適，並且經常依賴車上準備的餅乾或糖果來應對這種情況。長期以來，她一直認為這樣的情況在控制糖尿病時是正常的。

案例 4 類似的情況也發生在 60 多歲的務農者李先生身上。他經常在田地中從事粗重的工作，工作進行到一半時，常常感到肚子餓和無力。這時，他會迅速喝些飲料來消除這種感覺。

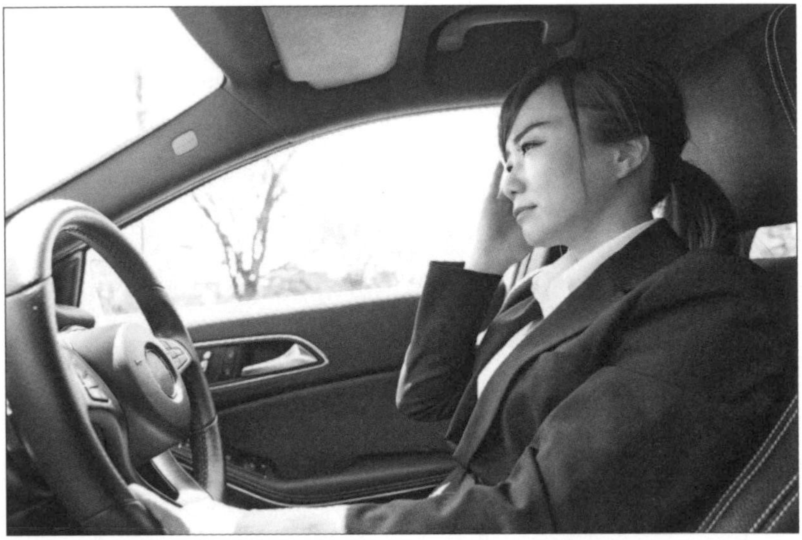

▲駕駛或勞力密集等行業，更要減少低血糖頻率；圖為情境照，圖中人物與本文無關。（照片提供／余宜叡）

從以上 4 個例子可以明顯看出，相較於高血糖逐漸引發併發症，低血糖的症狀更加即時和致命。糖友在血糖過低時常常會發生低血糖事件，例如肚子餓、發抖、情緒不穩或身體感覺異常等症狀。嚴重情況下，低血糖可能導致昏迷和死亡，之前常聽說糖友因低血糖而陷入昏迷無法醒來。

低血糖症狀實際上也可能發生在一般人身上，只要不進食足夠長時間，就可能出現低血糖。然而，正常人體內的血糖調節功能比糖友更好，加上沒有使用藥物，不太可能導致嚴重的低血糖。

在過去的 10 年中，出現了許多難以引發低血糖的藥物，並且新型的超長效胰島素的發明顯著減少了低血糖的發生率。然而，即使如此，只要使用血糖藥物，仍然有可能出現低血糖症狀，這一點不可掉以輕心。

即使使用難以引發低血糖的藥物，仍然可能發生低血糖，更不用說使用易引發低血糖的藥物。如果糖友在治療過程中使用易引發低血糖的藥物，並且經常出現低血糖症狀（見下文），且血糖監測值確實低於 70mg/dl，請務必記錄下來，主動告知醫療團隊，檢視可能造成這次低血糖的問題所在，並檢查是否需要調整飲食、運動和藥物。在更新治療計畫時，需要頻繁測量血糖，以確認血糖值的狀況。

低血糖可能出現的症狀

根據糖尿病衛教學會出版的《糖尿病照護核心教材》顯示，低血糖可能會引發以下症狀：

自主神經方面	包含發抖、顫動、冒汗、心悸、脈搏加速、體溫變化、四肢刺感、呼吸困難等。
中樞神經方面	包含思考緩慢、視力模糊、口齒不清、動作不協調、麻木感覺、無法集中、暈眩、疲倦嗜睡等。

情緒方面	包含焦慮、挫折感、緊張、憤怒、壓力感、憂傷、惱怒、悲觀、輕浮、興奮、情緒波動等。
其他方面	包含飢餓感、噁心、四肢無力、頭痛、感覺不對勁、爭吵、哭泣、拒抗治療、暴力行為、不洽當的社交（性）行為。

總而言之，許多症狀都可能是低血糖發生的表現。

這些症狀提醒糖友在血糖過低時要格外留意，並及時處理。如果您有糖尿病，且出現上述症狀，應立即檢測血糖值，如果確認低於正常範圍，應儘快攝取含糖食物或飲料以提升血糖水平。若症狀嚴重或無法自行處理，應尋求醫療專業人士的幫助。

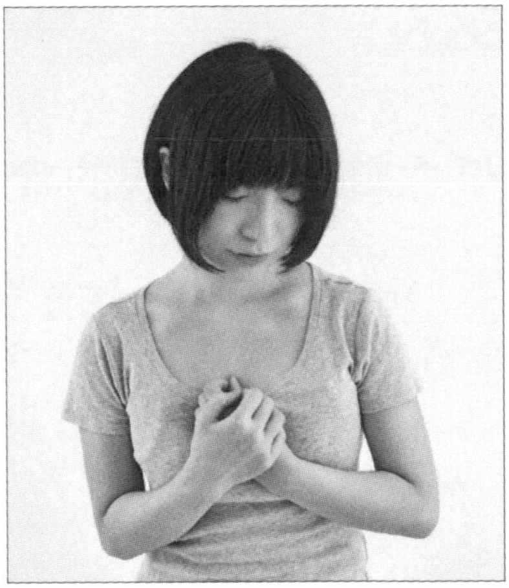

▲如果經常發生心悸、冒冷汗等症狀，絕非正常。（照片提供／余宜叡）

此外，糖友和其家屬應該接受相關的教育和培訓，以了解低血糖的症狀和處理方法，並掌握相關應急措施。定期檢查血糖、遵從醫療團隊的建議和治療計畫也是重要的，以確保血糖控制在安全範圍內，減少低血糖發生的風險。

低血糖當下處置

根據「社團法人中華民國糖尿病衛教學會」所出版的《糖尿病核心教材》當中的指示，在出現低血糖或不適症狀時，以下是低血糖的當下處置步驟：

1. 測血糖

若有可能，立即測量血糖濃度，確認是否為血糖過低。如果無法立即進行血糖測量，應當視為低血糖並進行處理。

2. 意識清楚時

立即服用含有 15 克糖分的食物或飲料，例如果汁、糖水、3 至 5 顆方糖、一湯匙蜂蜜或一湯匙糖漿。等待 15 分鐘後，檢查血糖是否有改善。如果血糖未回升，重複上述的處理方式，並立即尋求醫療協助。

3. 昏迷狀態時

將病人的頭部側放，然後輕輕將一湯匙蜂蜜或糖漿擠入病患口中。可以輕輕按摩病患的臉頰，以幫助促進糖分的吸收。請勿給予固體食物，以免嗆到或阻塞呼吸道，並立即送醫。如果有升糖素（升血糖濃度的藥物）可用，可在急救過程中自行注射。

此外，無論是何種原因造成的低血糖，事後都應進行檢討，找出引起低血糖的原因，並採取相應的因應措施，以避免再次發生低血糖情況。

藥物減量或換不易低血糖藥物

根據糖尿病學會 2020 年的臨床指引，每種血糖藥物都有降低血糖的效果，同時也存在發生低血糖的風險。根據指引，這些藥物可以分為易造成低血糖和較不易低血糖兩類。在檢視這位上述案例 3 的女司機和案例 4 的李先生的用藥情況後，我減少了易造成低血糖的藥物劑量，或將其替換為較不易引起低血糖的藥物。此外，我建議糖友減少攝取西點類或含糖飲料等容易引起血糖波動過大的精緻飲食。

結果，這位女司機回診時分享了自己目前挨餓不適狀況已經改善，可以更順心地開車。而李先生的後續回診顯示，血糖穩定且達到目標，低血糖症狀也有所改善，發生頻率從原本的每週 3 至 5 次降至每 1 至 3 個月 3 至 5 次。

這些結果表明，通過調整用藥方案並改善飲食習慣，可以有效控制低血糖的發生，提升糖友的生活品質和血糖管理狀況。重要的是，在治療過程中緊密與醫療團隊合作，定期追蹤血糖，並進行必要的調整，以確保血糖穩定且符合目標範圍。

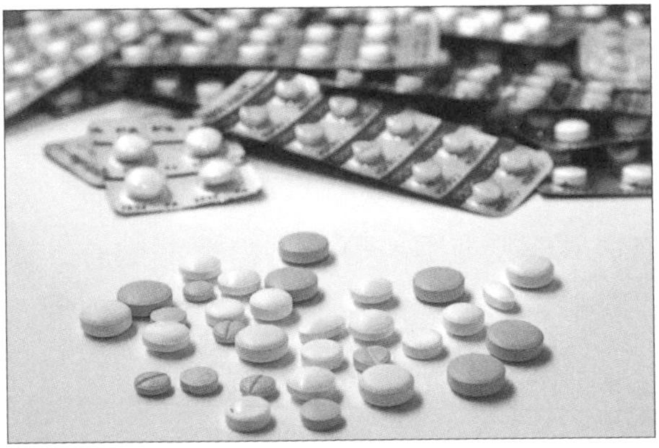

◀血糖藥能降低血糖，同時也有低血糖的風險。（照片提供／余宜叡）

大魚醫師的小叮嚀：如何知道自己低血糖？

要正確了解血糖的數值，最好的方法是進行自我監測血糖或使用連續血糖監測機。這些工具可以提供實時的血糖數值，讓你更準確地了解自己的血糖狀況。

依據進食量、糖尿病藥物的劑量和症狀來判斷是否低血糖只能帶來高度懷疑，並不能確定低血糖的存在。症狀可能與其他因素相關，而進食量和藥物劑量也可能受到其他因素的影響。因此，為了確切知道自己的血糖水平，建議進行正確的血糖監測。

不測血糖如何穩糖？

案例 1

孔先生是一位 50 多歲的糖友，最近剛確診。他面臨經濟上的困難，無法購買血糖機來監測血糖情況。在醫療團隊的建議下，他被囑咐按時服藥，並好好聆聽衛教師和營養師的指導，進行飲食的調整和藥物的使用。雖然他無法監測血糖，但透過正確的用藥和飲食管理，他仍然可以控制血糖，以維持良好的血糖水平。

案例 2

劉女士是一位 60 多歲已有 5 年多糖尿病史的患者，雖然她使用胰島素和口服藥物，但血糖一直難以控制，糖化血色素的數值也未能達標。她拒絕監測血糖的原因是因為測量手指頭會感到疼痛並且心跳加速。醫生了解她的情況後，調整了治療計畫，降低了胰島素的劑量，同時搭配了難低血糖的口服藥物。半年後，她的血糖值接近達標。

「醫師，我還可以做什麼讓我的血糖可以達標？」劉女士對於改善血糖控制提出了問題，衛教師告知她可以加強監測餐後血糖，以更好地了解飲食對血糖的影響。她也了解了傳統血糖機和連續血糖監測儀的差異後，選擇了不需要每次從手指取血的連續血糖監測儀。

雖然她仍需要使用一天 1 ～ 2 次的校正血糖儀，但這讓她能隨時了解血糖情況，包括三餐前後的血糖、睡前和半夜的血糖狀況。這使得她和醫療團隊能更全面地了解她的血糖狀況，並找出更多可以進一步調整的問題點。

不測血糖的常見原因

不測血糖常見原因包括以下幾點：怕痛、血糖機和試紙費用昂貴、需要頻繁監測、無醫療人員檢視血糖記錄、不知道如何測量血糖、缺乏時間（工作繁忙）、不希望他人發現有血糖問題等。然而，這些常見原因可能導致不了解測量血糖的重要性以及為何需要進行血糖監測。

測量血糖是穩定血糖的基本技巧。在臨床實踐中，我們經常遇到一些患者無論如何都不願意測量血糖，或者願意讓血糖保持較高水平的情況。然而，若不測量血糖，這些患者很難學習到飲食對血糖的波動有何影響，因為飲食和運動的控制需要嚴格遵守，無法隨意進食和運動。為了減少血糖的波動，我們需要做到定時定量的飲食和運動控制。當患者不願配合測量血糖時，醫療人員只能優先考慮減少低血糖的發生，並使用難低血糖的藥物組合。

對於糖尿病前期或初次診斷的患者，以及病程較短且胰臟調節功能尚好的患者，血糖波動可能較小，因此在這些族群中可以少量甚至不進行血糖測量。然而，對於病程較長的患者，血糖波動較大。如果您害怕進行血糖監測，請在正常或糖尿病前期時，始終做好預防工作，並保持良好的生活習慣。

定時飲食、運動等生活作息，對糖尿病患者的穩定非常重要，但不易做到

不測血糖必須遵守事項

對於血糖容易出現高低起伏的糖友，在沒有進行血糖測量的情況下，建議採取以下幾點措施：

定時定量

按照固定的時間進食或進行運動，並且在不同時間點保持飲食和運動內容的一致性，避免劇烈差異。雖然定時飲食、運動等生活作息，對許多糖友來說，不易做到，但仍應該堅持下去，直到成功為止。

按時用藥

按照指示按時使用藥物，確保體內藥物能夠有效發揮作用並維持穩定的藥物濃度，以達到持續穩定血糖的效果。

選擇難低血糖的藥物組合

對於血糖極高的糖友，可能需要使用多種藥物來穩定血糖，但需要減少使用 SU 類或 glinides 類藥物，以及高劑量的胰島素，以確保血糖能夠得到有效控制。

定期回診測量餐前或餐後血糖

通過定期回診並測量餐前或餐後血糖，可以大致了解血糖的情況。然而，需要記住的是，測量時應該按照日常的飲食、運動和用藥情況進行，而不是刻意調整以獲得更好的血糖值。這樣才能真實反映平時的血糖控制狀況，自己與醫療團隊才能精準介入穩糖。

透過這些措施，即使沒有進行血糖測量，血糖容易高低起伏的糖友仍然可以努力穩定血糖，減少血糖波動對身體造成的負面影響。然而，測量血糖仍然是更準確了解血糖控制狀況的重要手段，建議糖友在醫療團隊的指導下進行定期血糖監測，以達到更好的管理效果。

連續血糖儀是好幫手

若是糖化血色素小於 7%，連續兩次以上且無身體不適，可以考慮減少或不必頻繁測量血糖。然而，若是糖化血色素超過標準範圍，但又不希望每天都進行血糖測量，可以考慮使用連續血糖監測儀。

連續血糖監測儀分為即時型和盲目型兩種。即時型監測儀可以即時顯示血糖情況，而盲目型則需要拆機後才能獲得血糖數值，每種都有其優點和缺點。根據個人需求，可以與醫療團隊討論並選擇合適的監測儀器。

原則上，容易緊張焦慮的糖友不建議使用即時型連續血糖監測儀，以免增加生活上的焦慮和不安感。配合飲食和運動的記錄，可以借助連續血糖監測的輔助，更加了解飲食和運動對血糖的影響，進一步調整飲食和運動習慣。

對於怕痛的糖友，可以考慮購買具有特殊專利的血糖機，這些血糖機在取樣時較不痛感。

這些行為或原因會導致血糖無法達標

案例 曾先生是一位年過30的糖友，已經罹患這個疾病超過10年。他是透過他的母親介紹來到醫師這裡，而在這位醫師的指導下，他的血糖終於達到了標準範圍。母親之所以轉介他兒子給這位醫師，是因為儘管她已經年紀比較大，但她的血糖一直能夠控制在正常範圍內，為什麼她兒子就無法做到呢？

檢視曾先生過去五年來的藥物使用情況，發現他只使用了一種血糖藥物，而他的糖化血色素一直保持在超過8.5%的高水平。每次回診時，處方總是不變，加上他原本的醫療團隊只能與他短暫接觸，並沒有足夠的時間對他進行飲食和運動的強調與調整。然而，曾先生卻不知道應該從哪裡著手，加上每三個月才回診一次。

檢視曾先生的飲食內容，發現他的飲食與一位30多歲的人的飲食內容和份量並無不同。營養師為曾先生提供了基本而實用的飲食建議，醫師將他的血糖藥物調整為三種不會影響他工作的藥物，而衛教師則提供了幾個增加運動量的方案，讓曾先生回去實際試行。一個月後，曾先生的血糖水平大多數低於250mg/dl，餐前甚至多次低於130mg/dl；六個月後，曾先生終於糖化血色素降至小於7%，這是他確診糖尿病以來的第一次。

臨床上糖友血糖一直沒辦法達標的原因，不外是飲食、運動，與藥物方面。以下是常見的的幾個原因：

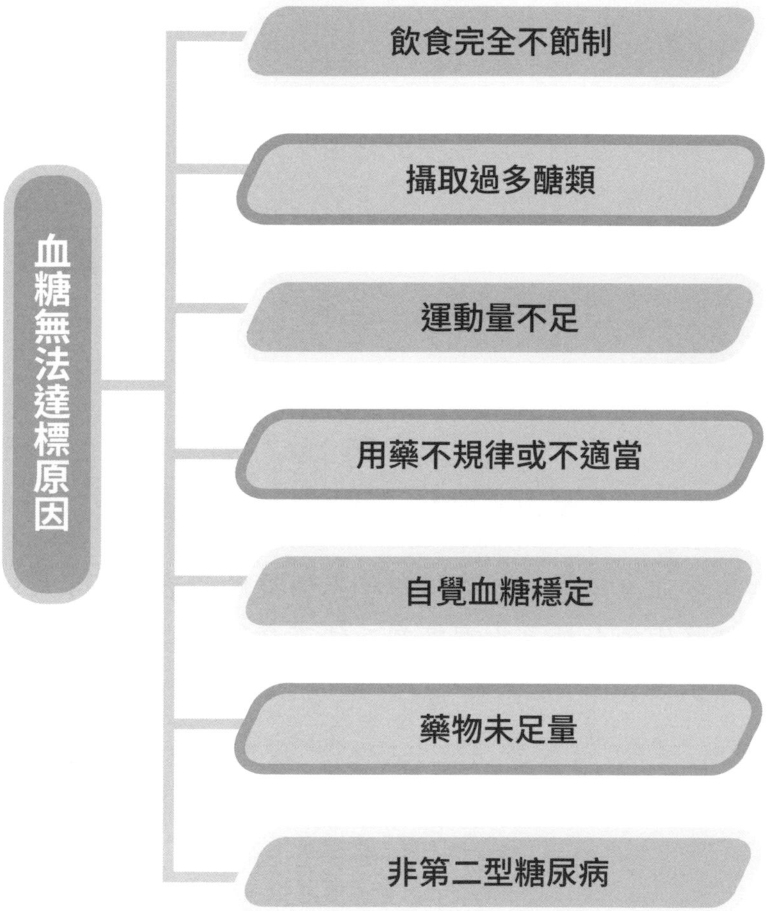
血糖無法達標原因
飲食完全不節制
攝取過多醣類
運動量不足
用藥不規律或不適當
自覺血糖穩定
藥物未足量
非第二型糖尿病

飲食完全不節制

糖友飲食攝取量太多，但減少份量時遇到的飢餓感、工作應酬的必要性以及藉由飲食抒壓等原因，都可能成為飲食調整的障礙。

攝取過多醣類

糖友的飲食習慣通常包含大量的米飯、麵食和含糖飲料，例如一到兩份便當或盛滿肉醬的飯，再加上一杯奶茶。另一個問題是攝取過多自以為是蔬菜的醣類，例如玉米、山藥、豌豆和毛豆等。

運動量不足

糖友認為只要稍微活動一下就算是運動，但實際上運動量遠遠不足。可能每週只在爬山上花上一個小時，或者每天只在家裡走路五分鐘，就以為已經足夠運動了。

用藥不規律或不適當

糖友害怕用藥過量會導致低血糖、成癮或傷害器官等身體問題，因此要求醫師不要再增加藥物劑量，或自行減少藥物的使用頻率，結果造成血糖藥物的療效不夠。

自覺血糖穩定

糖友認為只要使用血糖藥物就可以讓血糖保持穩定，且沒有出現任何身體不適。他們要求醫師繼續開立連續處方箋，卻不知道只有糖化血色素小於 7%才算達到治療目標。

藥物未足量

醫師開立的藥物和劑量並未考慮到糖友目前的飲食和運動狀況。口服藥物通常只能對糖化血色素降低 0.5 ～ 1%，而胰島素則可以達到超過 1%的降幅。如果糖友的糖化血色素距離 7%的目標還有一段距離，他們可能需要使用兩種以上的血糖降低藥物。

非第二型糖尿病

糖友有可能是缺乏胰島素的糖友，例如第一型糖尿病或 LADA 族群（潛伏性成人自體免疫糖尿病，Latent autoimmune diabetes in adults，簡稱 LADA，同時具有第一型糖尿病和第二型糖尿病的特徵，因此稱為「1.5 型糖尿病」）。換句話說，口服藥物對他們並無療效，需要直接使用胰島素進行治療。

這 3 招有助穩定血糖並減少併發症

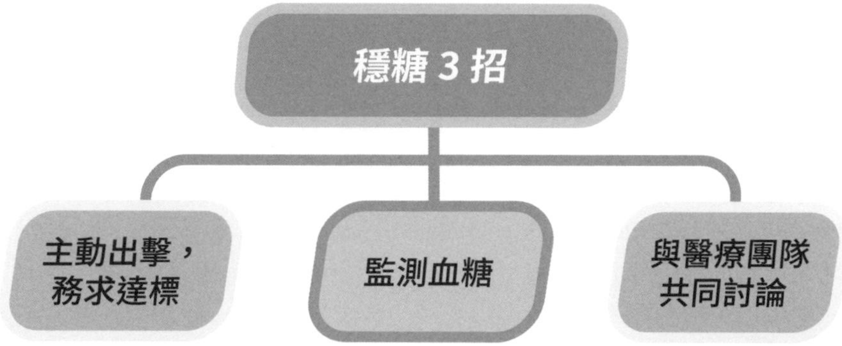

主動出擊，務求達標

這是最重要的應對方法。如果您是糖友，請努力使血糖達到目標範圍，並詢問醫生是否需要調整治療方案。如果血糖未達標，請醫生不要開立連續處方箋。

如果您是糖友的親友，請陪同就醫，提供醫療團隊有關糖尿病血糖控制的相關資訊，例如運動頻率、藥物使用等。

監測血糖

定期測量血糖並進行配對，或者考慮使用連續血糖監測儀。這樣可以瞭解飲食、運動和藥物對血糖的影響，了解三餐或一整天的血糖波動是否在標準範圍內，確保配對血糖值保持在 90 ～ 180mg/

dL 之間，連續血糖監測儀的標準範圍內時間（time in range）是否超過 70%。

與醫療團隊共同討論

如果每次就診等待時間超過 3 個小時，但醫生只花了不到 3 分鐘的時間看診，衛教內容常常草率或者過於制式化，同時糖化血色素持續高於 7%，建議尋找一個能夠與您進行良好溝通和共同討論的醫療團隊。一起找出飲食、運動和藥物方面的問題，定期調整治療方案，甚至可以尋求第二個專業意見，作為溝通討論的參考依據。

遵循上述三點將有助於提早穩定血糖並減少糖尿病併發症的風險。

PART 2

穩糖的關鍵密技

--CHAPTER-- 01 正確用藥

原則 1：好，可以再好！

糖友有時候會感到缺少某些飲食享受，或者只能以限制頻率或份量的方式品嚐，這常常讓他們感到遺憾。然而，他們也必須考慮到放縱可能帶來的血糖上升風險。然而，好消息是，當血糖達標時，我們仍然可以維持生活品質。以下是一些建議，可以幫助我們在血糖控制良好的同時享受生活。

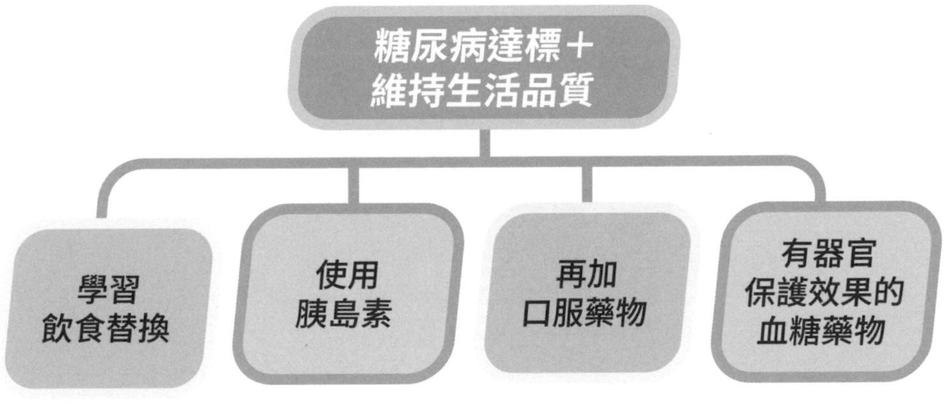

學習飲食替換

向營養師學習飲食替換的技巧，這樣我們可以吃到想吃的東西，同時保持血糖在標準範圍內。舉例來說，如果我們想多吃一點水果（或其他食物），就需要減少大約 1/3 碗的米飯份量。在學習和實踐這些替換技巧時，建議進行自我血糖監測或使用連續血糖監測儀，以了解血糖的波動和數值，以及飲食替換的效果和血糖控制情況。

使用胰島素

身體本身就會持續穩定地分泌胰島素，但糖友的胰島素作用效果較差。在這種情況下，補充類似的基礎胰島素可以使我們的體內產生足夠的胰島素，減少血糖的波動。如果再配合口服藥物使用，效果更好，可以讓我們在享用高血糖食物後仍維持良好的血糖數值。

再加口服藥物

我們可以選擇增加一種藥物，或者調高現有藥物的劑量，這樣可以提高飲食的容錯度。然而，需要特別注意是否會發生低血糖的情況。

選擇有器官保護效果的血糖藥物

在血糖達標的情況下，選擇具有器官保護效果的血糖藥物是非常重要的。這些藥物可以幫助保護我們的器官，減少併發症的風險。以下是幾種具有器官保護效果的血糖藥物：

排糖藥

這些藥物可以顧腎護心，特別適用於有心血管疾病和腎病變的糖友。

腸泌素

腸泌素藥物可以減少蛋白尿和心血管疾病的發生，同樣適用於有心血管疾病和腎病變的糖友。

DPP-4 抑制劑

有些 DPP-4 抑制劑藥物可以減少蛋白尿的發生。

需要注意的是，隨著更多重要研究的問世，血糖藥物的額外器官保護效果和適用族群一直在不斷更新。因此，我們應該定期與醫療團隊溝通和討論，以確定自己是否適合使用這些藥物，並且符合醫療保險的給付規定。

原則 2：適當用藥的重要性

關於適當用藥的原則，本文提供以下 7 個方面給大家參考。

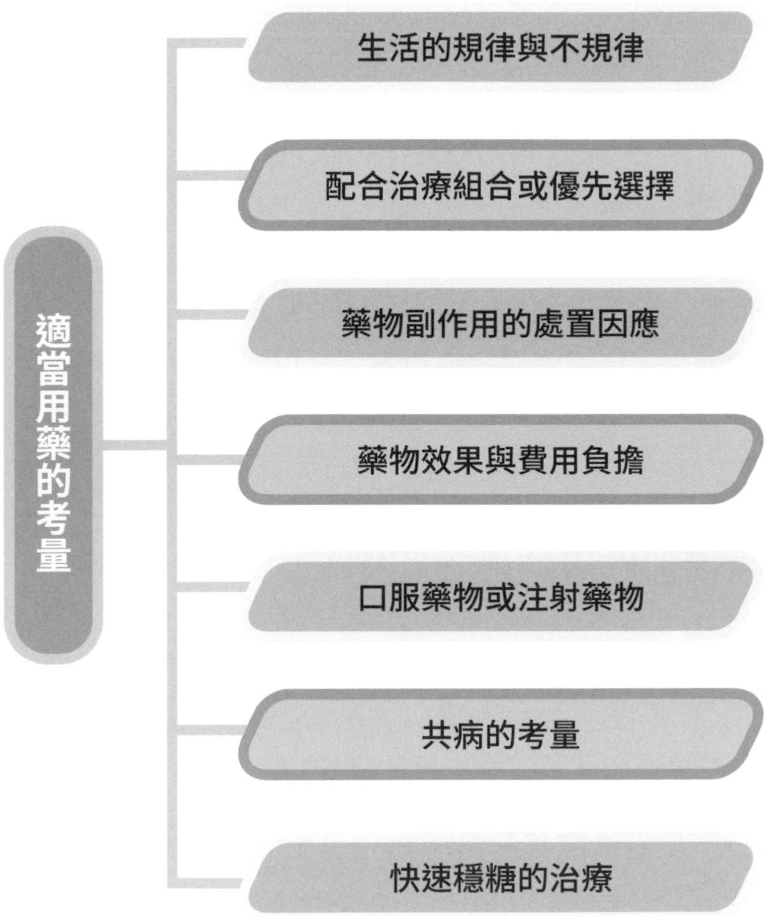
適當用藥的考量
生活的規律與不規律
配合治療組合或優先選擇
藥物副作用的處置因應
藥物效果與費用負擔
口服藥物或注射藥物
共病的考量
快速穩糖的治療

生活的規律與不規律

在穩定血糖的過程中，生活的規律性對於用藥的頻率有很大的影響。如果生活作息不規律，最好選擇使用一天一次或一週一次的治療方法。然而，對於有規律生活的糖友來說，可以使用更多種類的藥物，或以較少的花費達到血糖控制的目標。

配合糖友需求的治療組合或優先選擇

根據糖友的需求，在治療組合中做出適合的選擇和調配是非常重要的。這可能包括讓胰臟休息、只使用口服藥物、選擇小顆藥物、選擇顆數較少的治療方式、優先選擇原廠藥、選擇顧心組合或護腎組合、方便家人照護的藥物使用方式、以及適合減輕體重或增加體重的治療方案。這些選擇應該基於所在的醫療機構所提供的治療選項。

針對藥物副作用的處置因應

不同的藥物可能會產生不同的副作用，我們需要針對這些副作用做出相應的因應。舉例來說，使用舊型的預混型胰島素時，如果能夠按時按量使用，可以減少低血糖的發生。

另外，使用排糖藥時需要補充足夠的水分並注意上廁所的頻率。對於使用腸泌素的糖友，可能會出現食慾抑制的情況，影響正常的日常生活，因此建議在一開始使用時不要過量使用。

考量藥物的效果與費用負擔

在選擇藥物治療方案時，費用是需要考慮的一個因素。如果負擔增加，我們需要考慮藥物的花費。藥物花費越高，造成的負擔就越大。因此，找到自己的治療方案中的CP值高的治療方式非常重要。這意味著要找到費用與療效之間達到平衡的治療。

有時候，便宜的藥物並不一定是最佳的選擇，因為它們可能無法提供足夠的糖尿病控制效果。因此，在選擇治療方案時，需要綜合考慮藥物的療效和花費，找到最適合自己的選擇。

配合糖友建議口服藥物或學習注射藥物

藥物的操作和服用方式也是需要考慮的因素之一。口服藥物相對於注射藥物更容易使用，對於學習或自主能力有問題的糖友來說，建議優先考慮口服藥物。另外，針對需要注射藥物的糖友，可以根據家庭的支持程度提供一週一次的針劑藥物，由定期返家探視的家屬協助施打。無論是口服藥物還是針劑藥物，都建議聆聽糖尿病衛教師的指導，如果可能的話，實際操作給衛教師看，以確保正確的使用方法。

聆聽糖尿病衛教師的指導，這一步驟非常重要，因為糖友以為自己會使用藥物，但實際執行時才會知道是否真的掌握了技巧，有沒有真的學會。

糖友有共病的考量

有些糖友可能還伴隨著其他疾病，如腎功能不全、中風、心肌梗塞等。在制定治療計畫時，需要考慮這些共病的存在。目前的指引中已經提供了對於共病相關的治療建議，可以與醫療團隊充分討論，找到最適合自己的治療方式。

快速穩糖的治療控制

根據治療指引，如果需要快速有效地將血糖降至標準範圍內，優先考慮使用胰島素治療。雖然有些糖友可以僅使用口服藥物將血糖控制在正常範圍內，但通常需要使用 2 至 4 種口服藥物，並配合飲食和運動的調整才能取得良好的降糖效果。

原則 3：能使用針劑最好，否則也有多種選擇

臨床上我們常會遇到對針劑藥有莫名恐懼感的糖友。醫師也知道，每個人小時候都有注射疫苗的經驗，都害怕打針，連我自己也不例外。因此，也可以配合以下方式做調整。

針劑用藥沒您想像的疼痛

還記得當時去學習胰島素的時候，護理師問我是否要試打胰島素，我內心稍有抗拒，但同時也想體驗一下那根細小的針頭穿刺肚皮的感覺。於是我詢問護理師是否已經打過了，她回答說：「早就打好了。」令我意外的是，我完全沒有感到任何不適或疼痛！只有在親自體驗過後才發現，其實打針並不會痛！相比起用手指測血糖時的刺痛感，使用胰島素或其他注射藥物時，可以說是無痛或幾乎沒有感覺。

這樣的體驗讓我明白，對於需要使用胰島素或腸泌素等針劑藥物的人來說，注射並不是一件可怕或痛苦的事情。現代的注射器和針頭設計越來越細小，使得注射過程變得更加舒適。此外，醫護人員的專業技巧和細心操作也能夠確保注射的舒適性。

因此，若你有需求使用這些藥物，不用過度擔心注射的疼痛，相信你也會像我一樣驚訝地發現，打針其實並不可怕，甚至可以說是無痛或幾乎沒有感覺。與其因為擔心疼痛而拒絕必要的治療，不

如嘗試一次，親自體驗這個過程，你可能會發現，注射藥物是一個相對輕鬆且無痛的過程，可以讓你更好地管理糖尿病。

口服藥物需服用較多種，且對肝腎較有負擔

儘管我們花費了很多心力進行糖尿病衛教，但仍有許多糖友希望嘗試單純口服藥物來穩定血糖。對於初次診斷且血糖不高的糖友來說，可能僅需使用一至三種口服藥物就能使血糖達到標準範圍。

然而，對於血糖水平較高的糖友（血糖超過 200 以上），除非在飲食和運動方面有很大的進步空間，換句話說，就是飲食和運動存在嚴重問題，例如飲用含糖飲料、習慣性吃完餐點、完全沒有運動等，否則在不使用注射藥物的情況下，通常需要使用四至六種口服藥物來穩定血糖。但是，這樣的藥物組合會增加對肝臟和腎臟的負擔，對於肝腎功能不佳的糖友來說，口服藥物幾乎成為禁忌，無法使用的選項。

這也是為什麼對於某些糖友來說，注射藥物成為穩定血糖的少數選擇之一。相較於口服藥物，注射藥物在這方面較少有顧慮，對於肝臟和腎臟的負擔也較小。當口服藥物幾乎成為禁忌症，無法使用時，注射藥物提供了一種穩定血糖的選項。

使用注射藥物是長期抗戰的首選

穩定血糖需要長期的努力和抗戰。

對於那些僅使用口服藥物來穩定血糖的糖友來說，臨床上常常

遇到在穩定期持續 1 至 5 年後，需要調整血糖藥物的劑量或新增另一種機制的血糖藥物，才能繼續保持穩定的血糖水平。然而，使用注射藥物的糖友卻能減少這種情況發生的機會，有些人超過 5 年都沒有再次調整過藥物，甚至可以逐漸減少口服藥物，血糖仍然能夠保持穩定。

其中最主要的原因是，口服藥物的主要作用機制是刺激胰臟與身體各器官產生降糖相關物質，而注射藥物則是直接補充胰島素進入體內，使得身體各器官能夠得到充分的休息。想像一下每天都需要工作而無法休息的工人和每天都能得到適度休息的工人，哪一位工人能夠持續工作更久呢？

然而，值得注意的是，每位糖友的情況不同，治療方式應該根據個體化的需求進行調整。無論是口服藥物還是注射藥物，都應該在醫療團隊的指導下進行治療，並密切關注血糖控制的效果以及任何需要調整的情況。此外，適當的飲食控制、適量的運動和定期的體檢也是維持穩定血糖的重要因素。

選擇口服藥物，需配合調整飲食與加強運動

對於拒絕使用針劑藥物的糖友來說，與使用針劑藥物的糖友相比，口服藥物的劑量和種類通常會更多，而且血糖達標且穩定的持久度也會較差。如果想要減少口服藥物相對於針劑藥物的劣勢，需要加強飲食和運動方面的調整。這樣才能像針劑藥物一樣，讓胰臟的「工人」做更少的工作，或者做得更有效率。

針劑藥物對特殊族群較便利

對於那些不喜歡或不方便調整飲食和運動的糖友來說，例如中風後長期臥床、運動受傷或行動不便的人、以及對於美食有很高要求的人，可以優先考慮使用針劑藥物來穩定血糖，同時在生活品質和血糖管理之間取得平衡。

對於行動不便的糖友，如中風後長期臥床的病患或肢體障礙的人，進行常規的運動可能存在困難。在這種情況下，使用針劑藥物可以提供一種便利的方式來控制血糖，減少依賴口服藥物的需求。這樣可以簡化治療方案，同時保持血糖穩定。

原則 4：了解自費用藥的目的是提供更好的照護

案例 1

唐先生是 40 多歲的病患，因長期感到身體疲倦而前往門診求助。檢測結果顯示他的血糖極高，達到 410mg/dl，糖化血色素則為 12%。醫生與唐先生討論後，決定採用胰島素和兩種口服藥物的治療方案來穩定血糖水平。

由於這是唐先生第一次就診，他還不符合加入糖尿病照護網的資格，因此無法享受糖尿病照護網提供的衛教資源。為了學習如何注射胰島素和血糖監測等重要的穩糖技能，唐先生需要支付糖尿病衛教費用，接受糖尿病衛教師的指導。

一週後的回診中，唐先生的血糖記錄大多數都在 250mg/dl 以下。第二次回診時，他同意並符合加入糖尿病照護網的條件，從此可以接受糖尿病照護網提供的衛教服務，無需再支付額外費用。

案例 2

50 多歲的李女士已患糖尿病三年多，她一直努力使血糖接近標準範圍，糖化血色素也一直維持在小於 7% 的水平。然而，在某次回診中，她意識到自己的飲食仍有許多需要改進的地方。為此，李女士決定支付營養諮詢費用，與營養師進行一對一的討論，針對一週的飲食情況找出問題所在。

在兩次營養諮詢後，她增加了蔬菜攝取量，減少了宵夜的頻率。令人驚喜的是，在未調整藥物的情況下，李女士的糖化血色素首次降至小於 7%，達到了標準範圍。對於她來說，支付營養諮詢費是非常物超所值的！透過與營養師的專業討論，李女士了解到她的飲食中存在的問題，並得到了有針對性的建議和指導。

基本上，醫師跟糖友講自費用藥、檢查、檢驗或諮詢，是為了讓在此給付規定下，給予糖友更好品質的糖尿病照護。以下是一些與自費用藥相關的注意事項：

排糖藥與 DPP-4 抑制劑

排糖藥與 DPP-4 抑制劑在健保給付上有不同的規定。

基於健保財務狀況，目前的給付規定是選擇排糖藥與 DPP-4 抑制劑之一，或選擇排糖藥與腸泌素之一。然而，根據國際糖尿病照護指引，排糖藥與 DPP-4 抑制劑、或排糖藥與腸泌素可以相互輔助使用，因為它們具有不同的作用機制。

建議在符合給付規定的情況下，可以考慮同時使用排糖藥與 DPP-4 抑制劑的複方藥物，只要糖化血色素超過 7.5%且使用一種藥物已超過半年以上，即可獲得給付。

腸泌素

如果不符合給付條件，腸泌素的使用需自費。目前的給付條件根據不同的腸泌素而有所不同，例如 SOLIQA 限定半年以上，糖化血色素達到 8%；其他腸泌素如 TRULICITY、OZEMPIC、

VICTOZA 限定半年以上，糖化血色素達到 8.5%。只要不符合這些規定，糖友需要自行支付腸泌素的費用。

血脂藥

若不符合給付條件，血脂藥的使用需自費。一般來說，只要低密度膽固醇（LDL）超過 100mg/dl，就可以使用血脂藥，因此大部分情況下，血脂藥的費用不需要自行負擔。

血壓藥

只要在家量測血壓，並符合高血壓診斷標準，就可以獲得高血壓用藥的給付。這意味著糖友只需自費購買血壓計並進行血壓測量，而高血壓用藥的費用通常不需要自行負擔。

神經病變用藥

若下肢神經檢查未出現多重神經病變，或未經神經內科醫師診斷，則糖尿病神經病變用藥（如：Lyrica 和 Cymbalta 等藥物）需自費。

減重藥物

用於減重的藥物一律需要自費，不論是否已獲得減重適應症。

疫苗

除了流行性感冒疫苗和肺炎鏈球菌 23 價疫苗符合公費的族群外，其他許多疫苗都需要自費。例如肺炎鏈球菌 13 價和 23 價疫苗、帶狀皰疹疫苗、A 型和 B 型肝炎疫苗等，糖友需要自行支付疫苗的費用。

糖尿病前期用藥

目前糖尿病前期用藥不符合給付條件，糖友需要自費。根據美國糖尿病學會的建議，目前已經證實有效的糖尿病前期用藥還沒有獲得健保給付。

糖尿病衛教師與營養衛教

未加入照護網的糖友，需要自費支付糖尿病衛教、營養衛教或諮詢的費用。具體收費方式因醫院或診所而異，一些機構也提供免費的服務。然而，在沒有照護網給付的情況下，支付合理的費用是對專業服務的尊重和肯定。

總之，糖友在面對自費費用時，可以依據醫師的建議、個人經濟能力和疾病狀況做出適合的選擇，並確保獲得適切的糖尿病照護。

原則 5：可幫助糖友減藥的 5 大重點

案例

55 歲的曾女士因為身體持續減輕，擔心罹患癌症，所以前往家醫科門診求診。在進行血液檢查後，意外發現她的血糖高達 500mg/dl。醫療團隊立即與曾女士討論治療方案，她同意使用胰島素和口服藥物來穩定血糖水平。

同時，醫療團隊詢問了曾女士的飲食情況。曾女士因為以前常感到口渴，所以經常飲用鳳梨汁。此外，由於黑糖有益健康的關係，她也習慣在鳳梨汁中加入黑糖。醫療團隊建議曾女士改喝白開水，因為這樣會更有益於她的健康。

一週後，曾女士的血糖已降至 200mg/dl，且體重不再減輕。隨後，曾女士接受了營養諮詢，學習了如何測量血糖，並定期回診與醫療團隊討論治療方案。當曾女士的血糖穩定後，醫生開始逐漸減少她的胰島素劑量，最終不再需要使用胰島素，只需口服藥物。

隨著曾女士養成運動習慣，她也開始逐漸減少口服藥物的劑量，最終達到不需要口服藥物的程度。目前，她定期回診追蹤血糖是否穩定，並成功實現無藥一身輕的狀態。

根據醫生的臨床經驗，如果希望幫助糖有控制血糖並能夠減少糖尿病藥物的使用，請努力配合以下事項：

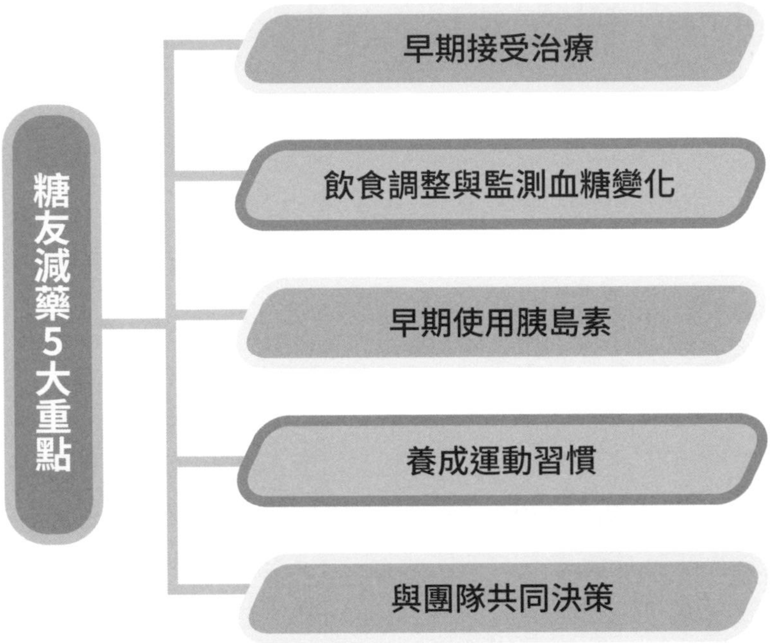

糖友減藥5大重點
早期接受治療
飲食調整與監測血糖變化
早期使用胰島素
養成運動習慣
與團隊共同決策

早期接受治療

確診後立即開始治療，而不是拖延數年才就醫。

飲食調整與監測血糖變化

記錄飲食並與營養師討論如何調整飲食，兼顧生活品質；同時也透過監測血糖，學習飲食對血糖的影響，並掌握適當的食物份量控制。

早期使用胰島素

在血糖過高的情況下，及早使用胰島素補充，減少高血糖引起的發炎反應，同時讓胰臟得到休息。這不僅可以快速穩定血糖，還有可能逐漸減少胰島素劑量，甚至停止使用。

養成運動習慣

逐漸養成運動習慣，每週至少運動 5 天以上，總計達到 150 分鐘以上。

與醫療團隊共同決策

每次回診時與醫療團隊詳細討論治療現況，並根據需要調整治療計畫。

如果您希望幫助親友控制血糖並減少藥物使用，請努力培養這幾個重點，都是成功減藥的重要因素。

常用藥物 1：不易低血糖的 DPP-4 抑制劑

案例 1 范先生，73 歲，被診斷患有糖尿病已經 3 年。在門診期間，他的餐後血糖值達到了 224mg/dL，糖化血色素則為 8.1%。一開始，醫生就給他開立了二甲雙胍和 DPP-4 抑制劑的治療方案。令人驚訝的是，在不到一個月的時間內，只使用了這兩種藥物，范先生的餐前和餐後血糖就非常穩定。如今已經過去了近 3 年，藥物的劑量沒有變動，他的糖化血色素一直保持在達標水平以下，小於 7%。

案例 2 李女士，66 歲，已經罹患糖尿病 5 年。這次她因血糖偏高而前往門診尋求幫助。醫生為她開立了胰島素、二甲雙胍和 DPP-4 抑制劑的治療方案，主要目的是減少高血糖情況下引發酮酸中毒的風險。經過一週的治療，她的血糖值已經有九成恢復到正常範圍內。最重要的是，她可以繼續享用自己喜歡的食物，且生活品質沒有受到太大的影響。李女士和她的家人對目前的治療計畫都非常滿意。

日本首選用藥

DPP-4 抑制劑在日本是首選用藥，穩糖效果不錯且不易引起腸胃不適症狀，但在台灣目前的給付條件下，只有在特殊情況下才能直接開立使用 DPP-4 抑制劑，例如對 metformin 過敏或有嚴重腸胃不適，或是高齡 80 以上的長者。

台灣給付規定

在使用 DPP-4 抑制劑之前，台灣的給付規定要求先使用 metformin，單方的排糖藥不能與單方的 DPP-4 抑制劑一同給付。然而，根據治療指引的建議，同時使用 metformin 和 DPP-4 抑制劑可以增加穩定血糖的效果。使用 DPP-4 抑制劑與排糖藥的複方需要滿足一定條件才能給付，例如使用其中一種藥物至少 6 個月以上且糖化血色素≧ 7.5%。

DPP-4 抑制劑的優點

DPP-4 抑制劑的優點之一是副作用很少且發生率低，主要常見副作用是感冒症狀。臨床上，在開立藥物處方時，通常只需提供簡單的衛教，除了用藥不適和感冒症狀外，再提醒糖友按時用藥即可。

DPP-4 抑制劑的有效性和適用性

需注意的是，除了 linagliptin 外，其他 DPP-4 抑制劑在使用時需要根據腎功能來調整劑量，而對於肝功能不佳的糖友，建議停用除 linagliptin 外的其他藥物。目前對於心血管或腎臟的保護效果，DPP-4 抑制劑並沒有額外的證據支持。其中，saxagliptin 可能增加心衰風險，其他 DPP-4 抑制劑的副作用相對較少見，主要是一些罕見的不良反應，可能會被誤認為其他疾病所引起。

有一項研究發現，DPP-4 抑制劑的一種成分 galvusmet，在早期使用 metformin 和 DPP-4 抑制劑的介入治療中具有潛在價值。該研究發現，如果在糖尿病初期同時使用這兩種藥物並達到血糖控制目標，可以減緩糖尿病的加藥速率，這從長遠的角度來看，可以減少加藥和併發症的風險，達到一舉兩得的效果。在門診時，糖友可以主動詢問醫生，是否可以同時使用這兩種藥物（尤其是對於已有臨床實證支持的 DPP-4 抑制劑治療）。

此外，糖友血糖控制達標仍然非常重要，因為這可以減少後續併發症的發生風險。

最後值得注意的是，有研究收集相關論文進行整合分析後發現，在住院的 COVID-19 患者中，使用 DPP-4 抑制劑可以降低 COVID-19 重症死亡的機率。

下表列出目前台灣有的 DPP-4 抑制劑表格，給大家參考。

學名	商品名	中文	複方名	注意事項
Vildagliptin	Galvus	高糖優適	高糖優美	
Linagliptin	Trajenta	糖漸平	糖倍平	肝腎不佳不需調整劑量
Sitagliptin	Januvia	佳糖維	捷糖穩	
Saxagliptin	Onglyza	昂格莎	康併莎	康併莎已退出台灣市場

附註：5mg 康併莎已退出台灣市場，目前只剩 2.5mg。

常用藥物 2：降糖效果優異的 SU 與 glinide 類藥物

案例 1 白女士是一位 60 多歲的糖友，她已經使用糖尿病藥物超過 10 年了，但最近血糖數值呈現逐漸上升的趨勢。儘管她一直遵循正常的飲食和運動習慣，她開始擔心為什麼血糖控制變得困難。

在與醫療團隊的討論中，他們注意到她目前的處方包括 SU（磺脲類）藥物以及其他藥物。衛教人員向她解釋了血糖上升的可能原因，可能是由於她的胰島素分泌功能退化，需要進一步補充胰島素，或者添加其他類型的降糖藥物。

案例 2 石先生是一位 50 多歲的糖友，已經患有糖尿病三年多。最近，他的血糖數值有些偏高，為了控制血糖，他的醫生增加了第四種藥物的劑量。然而，他開始經常出現低血糖的症狀。回診時，醫生判斷這可能是由於他目前正在使用的 SU 藥物引起的。為了解決這個問題，醫生將 SU 藥物的劑量減半使用。調整後，石先生的低血糖症狀明顯減少了。

SU 與 glinide 類藥物，長期使用可能造成胰臟功能過勞，降低降糖效果。還有，此類藥物屬於易低血糖藥物，一旦攝取的醣類減少，或延後用餐時間，就有發生低血糖的風險。

藥物療效

SU 是一種廣泛使用的血糖藥物，具有優異的降糖效果，與二甲雙胍相當。它是被廣泛使用的血糖藥物之一，歷史悠久且價格便宜。

SU 與 glinide 類藥物具有相似的作用機制，都能刺激胰臟分泌胰島素。然而，長期使用這些藥物可能導致胰臟功能過勞衰退，使降糖效果不如一開始好。

Glinides 類藥物與 SU 類似，但屬於速效藥物，需要隨餐使用。它們的優勢在於可以根據進食情況進行劑量調節，若進食量較大，可以額外降糖。相較於 SU，隨餐使用的 glinide 類藥物低血糖風險較低。

藥物使用

長效的 SU 建議每天使用 1 ～ 2 次。短效的 glinide 類藥物則根據用餐次數而定，可能需要每天使用 1 ～ 4 次不等。

藥物副作用

SU 與 glinide 類藥物的作用機制是刺激胰臟分泌胰島素以降低血糖。優點是具有良好的降糖效果，不亞於二甲雙胍。然而，這些藥物的缺點是易引起低血糖。

糖友若忘記進食或延遲用餐，可能會發生低血糖。

糖友須知

在臨床上，當醫師加入第三種藥物時，會增加低血糖的風險。然而有趣的是，許多糖友會誤以為是新加入的第三種藥物導致低血糖的發生。事實上，真正引起低血糖的元兇是長期使用易引起低血糖的藥物，如 SU 或 glinide 類藥物，而不是後續加入的藥物。

大魚醫師小提醒：預防使用 SU 或 glinide 類藥物的低血糖

使用 SU 或 glinide 類藥物時，要特別注意低血糖的發生。低血糖症狀多樣化，除了常見的冒冷汗和飢餓感外，還可能出現身體的不適感或情緒波動等症狀。建議量測血糖以確認低血糖的情況。

若使用 SU 或 glinide 類藥物後出現低血糖，可以嘗試調整用藥劑量或在用餐前增加碳水化合物的攝取量，以避免低血糖的發生。

若糖友有忘記進食或飲食延誤的情況，應立即補充碳水化合物，例如飲用含糖飲料或進食點心，以預防低血糖的發生。但以上的低血糖處置可能造成血糖超標，因此，減少低血糖的發生才是根本之道。

常用藥物 3：把握 2 不 3 要，二甲雙胍安心吃

案例 1

李先生是一位 40 多歲的病患，最近被診斷出患有糖尿病，其糖化血色素值高達 7.9%。為了更有效地控制血糖達到目標，醫生開立了二甲雙胍和 DPP-4 抑制劑的處方。然而，當李先生回診時，他對自己的血糖記錄感到不滿意，並懷疑是藥物或飲食的問題。進一步詢問，他透露他每天只服用一次較大劑量的二甲雙胍，因為擔心可能引起低血糖。

經過醫療團隊的解釋和衛教後，他瞭解到正確使用二甲雙胍的重要性和療效。從此以後，他開始規律地按時服藥，結果血糖也得到了穩定。

案例 2

錢女士是一位 50 多歲的病患，她在使用二甲雙胍藥物時提前回診。她常常出現腸胃不適和腹瀉的症狀。排除其他可能原因後，發現這些副作用可能與她換用不同廠牌的二甲雙胍有關。當她使用 A 廠牌的二甲雙胍時，她並未出現腸胃道副作用，然而，一旦換成 B 廠牌的產品，這些問題就再度出現。

這個案例提醒我們，在轉換藥廠或品牌時需要留意可能的影響，並與醫生討論。

案例 3

顧先生已經罹患糖尿病超過 10 年，過去他成功將糖化血色素控制在 7% 以下。然而，在最近的半年內，他兩次的檢查結果卻顯

示「超標」，原來醫生要他一天服用兩次二甲雙胍類的降血糖藥物「Metformin」。但顧先生常常忘記服用第二次，因為他沒有感覺到身體有異狀，所以自行改為一天只服用一次。

在接受醫療團隊的衛教後，顧先生瞭解到 Metformin 的控糖療效和重要性。他決定遵照醫囑，每天按時服用兩次藥物。經過三個月的治療後，他的血糖再次達到標準範圍。這次經驗讓他深刻明白，減少一半的 Metformin 劑量對血糖控制的影響是如此重大。

考量到二甲雙胍是療效很好且價格不高貴的藥物，因此是各國糖尿病照護指引的第一線建議用藥。然而，使用二甲雙胍時常常會有糖友覺得藥丸很大顆或要一次吃兩次以上的困擾，因此減藥或停藥，但這樣會影響血糖的控制成效，可能需要再加上其他種類的藥物。除非是藥物過敏、腸胃不適的症狀太嚴重或腎功能嚴重不好，才會建議不要使用二甲雙胍。

二甲雙胍的常見副作用主要是腸胃道不適，例如便秘、腹瀉、脹氣等。然而，使用一段時間後，有些糖友會對這些副作用產生耐受性，副作用的程度也會減輕。在上面顧先生案例的實際應用中，如果院所更換了 Metformin 的藥廠，副作用的程度可能會有所增加或減少，因此在臨床使用時需要特別留意。

二甲雙胍是一種百搭藥物，可以與任何血糖藥物併用。正因如此，有許多包含二甲雙胍和其他類血糖藥物的複方藥物可供選擇，例如加上 DPP-4 抑制劑、排糖藥或 TZD 等。

值得注意的是，之前有爆發二甲雙胍製藥的原物料內含致癌風險的情況。因此，建議大家留意食藥署的報告或新聞，選擇有信譽的藥廠製造的二甲雙胍產品。

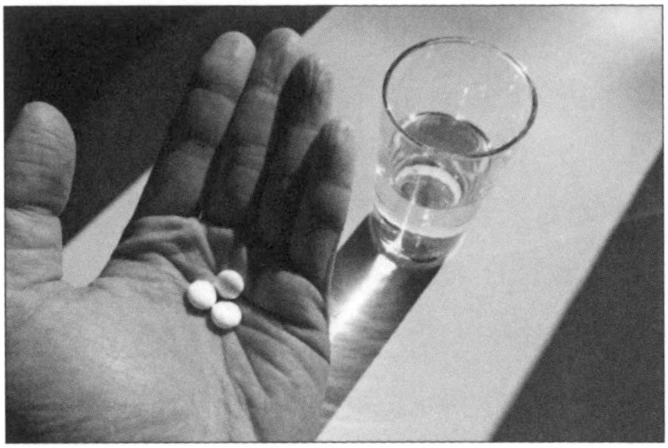
▲ Metformin 是很常用的降血糖藥。（照片提供／余宜叡）

總結起來，建議糖友們做好以下「二不三要」，以降低風險：

二不

「不」擅自減藥或停藥

Metformin 是糖尿病治療的首選用藥，具有良好的降糖效果和臨床實證支持。減藥或停藥會導致血糖升高，增加糖尿病併發症的機率，對糖友來說是弊多於利。

「不」要購買偏方或其他營養品來取代

Metformin 是經過臨床實證的控糖藥物，具有可靠的效果。相較之下，偏方或其他營養品缺乏臨床控糖實證，因此不建議用其取代二甲雙胍。

三要

「要」瞭解自己是否使用了 Metformin 作為糖尿病的治療藥物。

「要」詢問醫師關於使用的 Metformin 是否經過檢驗合格。在確認前，請繼續按照醫囑服用 Metformin 以控制血糖。

「要」與醫療團隊討論，若未使用 Metformin 且血糖未達到目標（糖化血色素＜ 7%），是否可以加入 Metformin 作為輔助控糖的選項。

在歐洲、美國和台灣等地的最新糖尿病藥物治療指引中，Metformin 通常是第一或第二線的推薦用藥。

因此，只要遵循上述的「二不三要」原則，糖友們可以安心使用二甲雙胍，不必過於擔心。

常用藥物 4：逆轉糖尿病前期的 AGIs

案例 1

朱先生是一位 60 多歲的糖友，已經患病 10 年。最近，他的餐後血糖偏高，於是醫生開始了他的 AGIs 藥物治療。結果，朱先生發現在飲食份量相同的情況下，只要加上 AGIs 藥物，他的餐後血糖可以保持在 180mg/dl 以下。然而，他也注意到服用藥物後會出現輕微的腸胃不適和脹氣。

儘管有一些藥物不適，朱先生仍然決定隨身攜帶 AGIs，這樣他可以同時照顧到生活品質和血糖控制的問題。如果他吃得多一些，他就可以使用藥物來控制血糖。他也分享了一個心得，當他服用兩顆藥物時，副作用更加明顯，而當他服用一顆藥物時，血糖可以保持在正常範圍內。

案例 2

唐女士是一位糖友，已經患病 2 年多，她在門診時提出了一個問題。「醫生，我在網上查到我正在使用的藥物會影響葡萄糖的分解。所以，如果我在低血糖的情況下飲用含糖漿的飲料，我的血糖會升不上去嗎？」其實，市售的手搖杯飲品是可以用來緩解低血糖的，即使是使用純糖漿製作的飲料，它還是含有一定量的葡萄糖。因此，在使用 AGIs 藥物的情況下，這些飲料仍然可以提升血糖水平。然而，果汁、糖包、牛奶等飲品將是更好的選擇來處理低血糖。

經過醫生的解答，唐女士對於低血糖的處理和應對方式有了更清楚的了解。同時，醫生還對 AGIs 類藥物進行了衛教，指出它是一種需要隨餐服用的藥物，建議在沒進食或進食量很少的情況下，可以暫時停止當次的 AGIs 使用。以上方式就解除了唐女士對於低血糖的疑慮。

降低餐後血糖

AGIs 藥物的作用機制是減少雙醣分解成單醣（葡萄糖），使得腸胃道無法吸收單醣，從而有效降低血糖。臨床上，這些藥物通常隨餐使用，用於降低餐後血糖。由於其作用機制的關係，AGIs 屬於難低血糖的用藥。因此，藥物使用上的順從性尤為重要。由於需要隨餐服用，實際上常常遇到一些糖友忘記服用藥物或忘記攜帶藥物出門的情況。

逆轉糖尿病前期

隨著劑量的增加，AGIs 藥物的副作用也會加強，因此建議從低劑量開始使用。在中國，AGIs 類藥物有著很高的市占率，因此也有一些重要的相關研究。根據中國的研究指出，AGIs 類藥物能夠有效延緩糖尿病前期進展為糖尿病。此外，根據美國糖尿病學會的治療指引，AGIs 類藥物確實也是治療糖尿病前期的一個選擇。

總而言之，AGIs 類藥物是一種能夠降低血糖的藥物，通常在餐後使用。儘管副作用可能增加，但透過適當的劑量和藥物使用的順從性，糖友可以有效地管理血糖並提高生活品質。

常用藥物 5：TZD 是被冤枉的好藥

案例 1 林先生是一位 50 多歲的糖友，已經患病 3 年。在門診中，他提出了關於糖尿病藥物的問題，詢問是否有某種藥物會增加心血管風險，以及是否有相關藥物曾經下架的情況。

經過確認，林先生指的是 TZD（胰嘧啶類）藥物。醫生解釋當林先生需要添加第三種藥物來穩定血糖時，詢問他願意使用自費還是給付的藥物。經過說明兩者之間的差異後，林先生選擇了給付的藥物，即 TZD。

醫療團隊向林先生進行健康教育，解釋以前提到增加心血管事件風險的論文已經得到推翻，目前的相關研究顯示 TZD 藥物不會增加心血管風險。然而，如果林先生對此類藥物仍然有疑慮，他可以選擇其他類型的藥物作為輔助，以降低血糖水平。

案例 2 陳女士是一位使用血糖藥物已經超過 10 年的 60 多歲糖友。最近她出現了腳部浮腫的情況。在門診評估和檢查後，醫生懷疑這可能是由 TZD 藥物引起的。醫生詢問陳女士是否可以將 TZD 藥物替換為其他藥物。然而，在陳女士沒有使用 TZD 後，她的血糖卻明顯升高，經常超過 200mg/dL。

隨後，醫生將 TZD 藥物重新納入治療計畫中，同時減少了藥物劑量，並建議她多做抬腳運動，以促進下肢血液循環，減少腳部水腫的發生。在 1 個月後的回診中，陳女士的血糖恢復到安全範圍內，腳部水腫也沒有之前那嚴重。

過去的誤解與平反

TZD 屬於難低血糖藥物，但是其中發生過一個誤解。在某年，美國一位心臟專科醫師投稿《新英格蘭醫學雜誌》的論文，指出某種 TZD 藥物因增加心血管風險，結果該論文導致該藥物被下架使用。然而，經過 10 年之後的研究，終於得到了平反，證實該藥物並不會提高心血管風險。

藥物特點與使用建議

TZD 是一種一天服用一次的藥物，主要禁忌症是心衰竭糖友（NYHA III、IV 級糖友）。常見的副作用是水腫，劑量越高副作用產生的機率越大。然而，它在穩定血糖方面效果不錯，尤其對某些族群的糖友反應相當好，甚至效果好到可以抵上兩種以上的血糖藥。

根據糖尿病指引的建議，TZD 被歸類為第二線用藥，適合在二甲雙胍之後使用。健保給付條件是，在使用足量的二甲雙胍或 SU 藥物後，可以開立使用 TZD。這種藥物幾乎都可以健保給付，並且藥價不高，副作用也能預測。加上有些人對 TZD 藥物反應很好，所以目前仍有一定比例的糖友使用。

此外，台灣也有加入 metformin 的複方藥物，可以一天服用 1 到 2 次，提供更方便的用藥方式。

總而言之，TZD 是一種曾被誤解並被下架的藥物，但經過長時間的研究後，證實它並不會增加心血管風險。雖然它屬於難低血糖藥物，但穩定血糖的效果不錯，目前台灣的 TZD 為 pioglitazone。

常用藥物 6：排糖藥，有多項穩糖好處

案例 1 何女士是一位 50 多歲的糖尿病患者，已經有六年多的病程。由於血糖逐漸升高，醫生建議她需要加藥以達到血糖標準範圍。在原本長期服用的 DPP-4 抑制劑基礎上，如果再加上排糖藥的使用，則需要自行支付額外的費用，大約增加了九百多元的藥費。

經過兩週的使用，她的血糖數值整體上有明顯改善，餐前血糖能夠保持在標準範圍內。然而，何女士反饋說，即使醫療團隊事先對排糖藥的副作用進行了衛教，她仍然偶爾感到私密部位有隱隱的搔癢感。

在與何女士討論了排糖藥的優缺點之後，她覺得雖然排糖藥對她的日常生活有些影響，但考慮到排糖藥穩定血糖、保護腎臟和心臟，以及減輕體重的好處，她決定繼續使用排糖藥，同時加強預防措施。

案例 2 李先生是一位 60 多歲的糖尿病患者，他同時有高血壓和高血脂的病史。在一次成人健康檢查中發現他的空腹血糖過高，糖化血色素測量結果為 8.2%，確定診斷為糖尿病，開始進行糖尿病治療。在原有的治療方案基礎上加入排糖藥後，他的血糖更加穩定，成功達到標準範圍。

然而，半年後，李先生經常夜間起床上廁所，這對他的睡眠造成了困擾。他尋求了泌尿科的幫助，並發現他有輕微的攝護腺肥大。但令人奇怪的是，即使使用了攝護腺藥物，情況並沒有改善。直到有一次回診時，醫生發現李先生將排糖藥也放在睡前服用。

146

原來，為了方便起見且避免漏藥，李先生自行將所有的血糖藥物都改成了睡前服用，包括排糖藥。隨後，醫療團隊建議李先生將排糖藥改為早上服用，而不再睡前使用。這樣的調整後，李先生的夜尿問題得到了改善，不再困擾他的睡眠。

排糖藥的發展

隨著近年來越多相關研究的發表，排糖藥作為一種新型糖尿病藥物逐漸受到關注。除了降低血糖的效果外，研究還發現排糖藥對於腎臟和心臟的保護作用。藥廠也相繼發展出加入二甲雙胍或 DPP-4 抑制劑的複方藥物。

給付規定

給付規定方面，使用足量的二甲雙胍或 SU 類藥物後，可以開始使用排糖藥作為第二線治療。目前仍不允許單獨給付 DPP-4 抑制劑，但如果糖化血色素超過半年且大於 7.5%，則可以給付含有 DPP-4 抑制劑的複方排糖藥。請注意「單方藥物不能同時獲得給付，但複方藥物可以」這一點很重要。

機制與作用

排糖藥的主要作用機制是在腎臟，通過增加尿液中的糖排泄來達到降低血糖的效果。如果血中糖濃度較高，則尿液中排出的糖也會較多（但有上限）；相反，如果血糖較低，則排出的糖量較少。因此，排糖藥被歸類為不易引起低血糖的藥物。由於其特殊的尿液排糖機制，建議患者攝取足夠的水分，以促進排糖藥的療效。

保險需知

在保險方面需要注意的是，對於沒有糖尿病的正常人來說，如果服用排糖藥後尿液中的糖呈現 +++ 或 ++++ 的異常情況，這常常被醫療檢查報告所發現。如果非糖尿病患者在進行保險體檢時服用排糖藥，有可能被保險公司視為糖尿病患者，進而加價、只能購買糖尿病患者專用保單，甚至可能被拒保。因此，非糖尿病患者在使用排糖藥時需要格外注意。可以參考《為減重吃排糖藥 當心保險拒保！》一文，有更多相關資料和細節說明。

療效與保護器官的效果

至於排糖藥的療效和保護器官效果，除了穩定血糖之外，研究顯示它能延緩腎病變的進展，減少心衰竭惡化和住院風險，具有顧腎護心的效果，如下示意圖。因此，目前的治療指引建議對於患有腎病變或心衰竭的糖尿病患者，優先考慮使用排糖藥來穩定血糖。

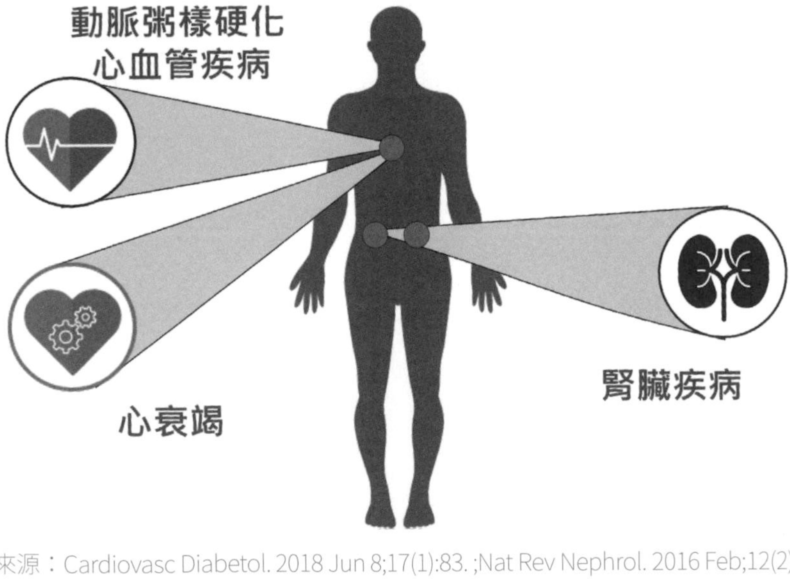

資料來源：Cardiovasc Diabetol. 2018 Jun 8;17(1):83. ;Nat Rev Nephrol. 2016 Feb;12(2):73-81

148

排糖藥副作用

關於排糖藥的副作用，根據日本的衛教資料顯示，主要副作用包括泌尿道和生殖器感染、脫水以及低血糖的酮酸血症（DKA）。此外，長期使用排糖藥還需特別留意其他副作用，例如增加白帶量、白帶顏色變化、殘尿感以及尿液混濁等。

以下排糖藥副作用列表，給大家參考。

脫水症狀	□喉嚨或口中乾渴感 □走路變慢、腳抖、眩暈、沒食慾 □尿量減少、色濃
泌尿感染症狀	□頻尿、排尿有痛感 □有殘尿感、尿濁
生殖感染症狀	□陰部癢或痛 □陰部潰瘍 **針對女性** □白帶量增加 □白帶的顏色有變、異味強烈

資料來源：《日本排糖藥衛教資料》

這些排糖藥副作用因應方式主有三點：

- **水要多喝。**（1500ml/ 天是基本盤，不要有口渴感也是另一個指標）
- **不要憋尿。**（有一定的尿意感，就去上廁所，或者可以每一個小時或一小時半去上廁所）
- **加強清潔。**（加強泌尿生殖道的清潔，男性的話，連包皮也要好好清潔）

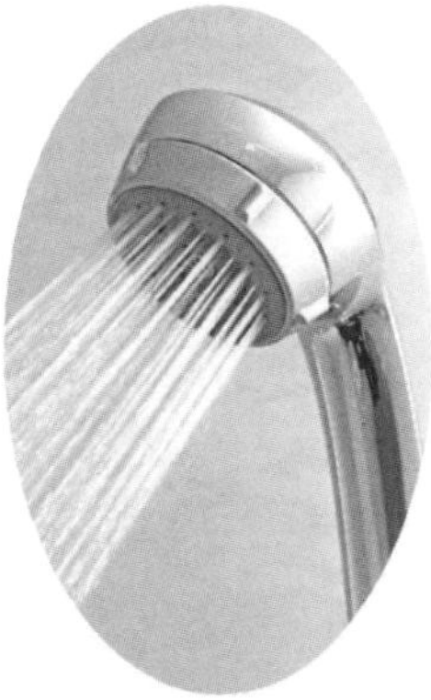

預防感染

保持泌尿生殖器清潔

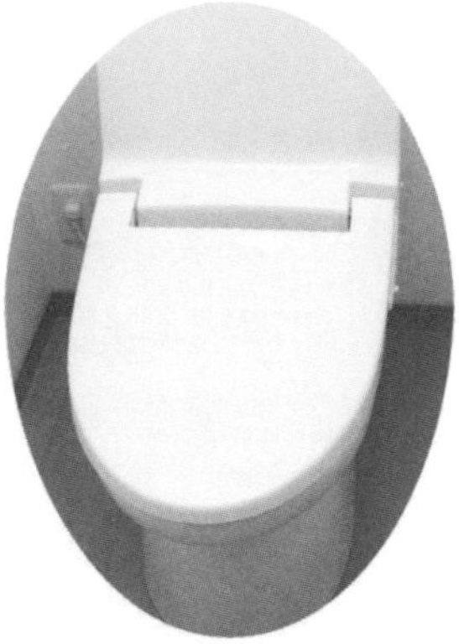

不要憋尿

有尿意時不要憋尿

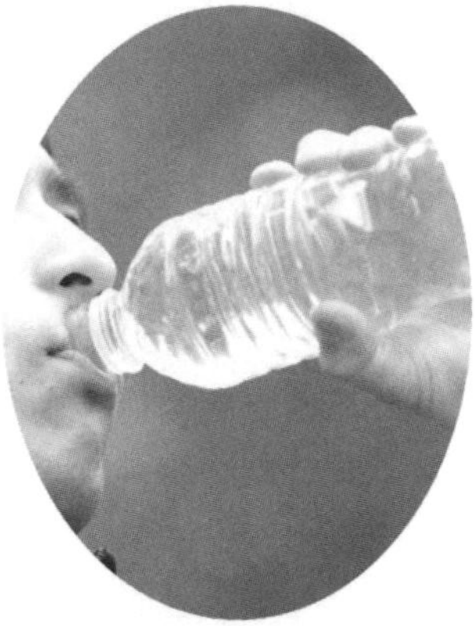

補充水分

分次補充不要口渴

資料來源：照片提供／余宜叡

臨床上常遇到患者治療一段時間後，就會忘記要做好上述三件事情之一，就會開始產生排糖藥的的副作用，身體不適。另外要注意的是，排糖藥因有利尿效果，不建議睡前或晚上使用，會造成夜尿，甚至男性患者會誤認為自己是攝護腺肥大造成。

150

常用藥物 7：
善用腸泌素，也能安心享受美食！

案例 1 錢女士是一位 50 多歲的糖尿病患者，已經有十年的病史。這次她因感冒不適前往門診就診，除了接受症狀治療的藥物外，也進行了血糖控制的評估。錢女士的 BMI 超過 38，她表示自從開始控制糖尿病以來，體重增加了近 20 公斤，但血糖一直無法達到標準。醫生檢視了她的用藥組合後發現問題所在，錢女士的基礎胰島素劑量超過了她體重的一半，使用的胰島素劑量過高。

醫生首先將高劑量的胰島素調整為低劑量，同時建議錢女士使用自費的腸泌素。在治療初期的兩週內，可能會出現噁心和嘔吐的症狀，但之後這些不適感會緩解，且不再那麼嚴重。經過兩個月的治療調整，減少了胰島素劑量，並搭配腸泌素和口服藥物，同時加強了飲食和運動，終於使錢女士的血糖達到了標準，同時體重也減少了近 16 公斤。

案例 2 黃先生是一位 60 多歲的糖尿病患者，患病已超過十年，血糖一直無法有效達到標準。家人介紹他前往門診求診。在醫生告知胰島素對於穩定血糖和維持生活品質的療效後，黃先生同意加入胰島素治療。很快，他的餐前血糖就能保持在 100-140mg/dl 範圍內，但餐後血糖仍經常超過 250mg/dl，有時甚至達到 300mg/dl。

原來，享受美食是黃先生持續工作和努力的動力，然而評估後發現他的飲食攝取過多。醫生建議黃先生使用腸泌素來限制享受美食的份量。醫生開始給黃先生使用兩週的低劑量腸泌素，這樣他的餐後血糖就能維持在 200mg/dl 以下。

接著，醫生讓他逐漸增加腸泌素的劑量，兩週後黃先生向醫生抱怨說，調高劑量後他感到更多的噁心和嘔吐，這讓他無法好好享受美食。醫生和黃先生討論後決定使用低劑量的腸泌素來穩定血糖。如果他在進食時攝取較多碳水化合物，黃先生願意在用餐後進行運動來降低血糖水平。

接下來，黃先生的血糖大部分時間能維持在標準範圍內，同時也能保持他的飲食品質。黃先生對目前的血糖治療方式非常滿意。

腸泌素的發現

早在 1986 年的研究中，人們發現葡萄糖液口服和點滴注射兩組的胰島素濃度有所不同。其中，口服組的胰島素濃度較高，血糖也更加穩定。研究人員推測，葡萄糖經過腸胃道時，身體可能產生某種物質，提高胰島素的濃度，進而穩定血糖。這種物質後來被稱為「腸泌素」。相關效果如圖所示。

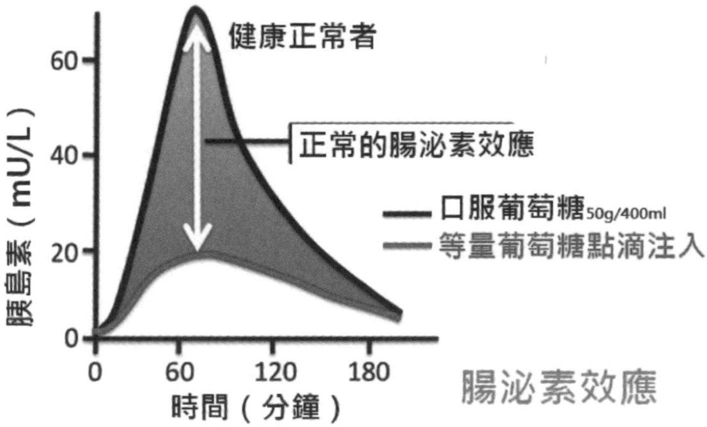

腸泌素效應

152

腸泌素的發展

藥廠從蜥蜴的口水中成功萃取出腸泌素，為後續腸泌素藥物的問世奠定基礎。目前，各大藥廠不斷發展和改良腸泌素藥物，分為兩大類：一類以人體腸泌素為基礎進行修正，另一類則以 Exendin 為基礎進行修正。至今，藥廠仍在研發更多類型的腸泌素，以作為穩定血糖和減重的利器。近期甚至出現了結合腸泌素系列 GIP 和 GLP-1 的複方藥物，具有更強效的穩糖和減重效果。

腸泌素的給付規定

根據腸泌素的給付規定，與排糖藥物併用時，需要選擇其中一種給付，另一種則需要自費。糖尿病患者必須使用口服血糖藥或胰島素，且血糖控制不佳半年後，糖化血色素濃度超過 8.5%才符合給付標準。

臨床困境與應用

然而，研究指出，只在糖化血色素超標時才加藥，血糖很快又會超過標準。此外，血糖超標（糖化血色素超過 1.5%，標準為小於 7%）時，血糖的穩定性更難以控制。如果能在早期介入，血糖更容易達到標準。這也引出了一個道德風險問題，即只要病患故意讓血糖不佳半年，就能獲得腸泌素藥物的給付，並且可能需要終身使用這種藥物。

這些問題反映了腸泌素的臨床困境和應用上的挑戰。雖然腸泌素在穩定血糖和減輕體重方面具有療效，但其高價格和供應短缺是目前的主要問題之一。此外，腸泌素的使用也需要謹慎考慮，因為它可能產生副作用，如噁心、嘔吐和頭暈。

在臨床上，腸泌素的應用通常需要與其他血糖藥物結合使用。它與 DPP-4 抑制劑有相似的作用機制，不建議同時使用這兩種藥物。然而，腸泌素與其他血糖藥物相容性較好，可以結合使用。

在選擇腸泌素劑量和使用頻率方面，臨床上也存在一些困境。例如，患者常常面臨選擇每天一次或每週一次的腸泌素使用。每週一次使用腸泌素可能會抑制整周的食慾，但如果在使用後出現身體不適或食慾降低，這種效果可能會持續一周左右。相比之下，每天一次使用腸泌素則只會持續一天。因此，在使用腸泌素的頻率上，建議與醫療團隊進行討論，根據個人情況做出適當的選擇。

口服腸泌素使用需知

近幾年台灣已有口服的腸泌素（瑞倍適），增加腸泌素藥物使用的方便性，不過目前口服腸泌素因使用了特別的藥物保護機制，使用時有特殊限制：

- **需早上空腹服用。**
- **用 120cc 以下的白開水吞服。**
- **半小時內不得飲食。**

如此，才能讓腸泌素被人體順利吸收，唯有足夠的腸泌素濃度，才能產生好的療效。也因其特殊的保護機制，此藥不可剝半。若是

154

剝半使用，會破壞保護機制，藥物失去療效，不可不慎。目前口服腸泌素仍屬自費藥物，健保尚未給付。

目前台灣已有的腸泌素相關藥物，整理如下表格，給大家參考。

商品名	Victoza	Trulicity	Ozempic	Rybelsus	Soliqua	Saxenda
中文名	**胰妥善**	**易週糖**	**胰妥讚**	**瑞倍適**	**爽胰達**	**善纖達**
使用	針劑	針劑	針劑	口服	針劑	針劑
頻率	一天 1 次	一週 1 次	一週 1 次	一天 1 次	一天 1 次	一天 1 次
穩定血糖	○	○	○	○	○	○
減輕體重	○	○	○	○	○	○ 已在台取得減重適應症
含胰島素	×	×	×	×	○	×
空腹用	不需	不需	不需	需要	不需	不需
給付	○	○	○	×	○	×
目前給付條件	6 個月以上的糖化血素＞8.5%			無	6 個月以上的糖化血色素＞8.0%	無

用藥提醒 1：血糖藥切半減量，先問醫師藥師

案例

「醫生，經過您的治療一段時間後，我的血糖非常穩定。我想試著減少藥物劑量，但又擔心停藥後血糖會上升。我可以自行用刀子將藥物切成一半來使用嗎？然而，我覺得長期這樣切藥會很麻煩，是否有其他不需要切割的藥物可以選擇？」

50 多歲的何女士最近被診斷出患有糖尿病，她非常積極地希望能夠穩定血糖。她目前使用的治療方式是口服一天一次的排糖複方藥物和腸泌素，但由於考慮到血糖的穩定性以及藥物費用等因素，她想詢問是否可以將口服的腸泌素藥物切成一半來使用。

有些藥物錠劑有特殊保護，若將藥物切半使用，藥物就會失去療效。特別是特定的排糖藥物有緩釋的特別作用，如果切半使用，可能藥物作用就會太快太強或是失效。

緩釋型藥物如果切半使用，易影響藥效緩釋作用，造成藥物濃度不穩定，甚至可能使藥效與副作用變得太強；而特殊劑型的藥物有外層的專利膜錠，保護藥中主要成分在體內合適的地方發揮作用，若切半破壞藥物結構，藥物將完全失去療效，因此需要謹慎處理。

在臨床上，糖友常擔心血糖藥物的藥效過強，因此自行減藥，將藥物切半，或覺得藥物太大顆，切半後服用。然而，自行切割藥物後的大小不一可能影響用藥效果。因此，建議糖友在確認藥物可

156

以剝半使用的情況下，採取以下三個步驟獲取一半劑量的藥物：

使用切藥器

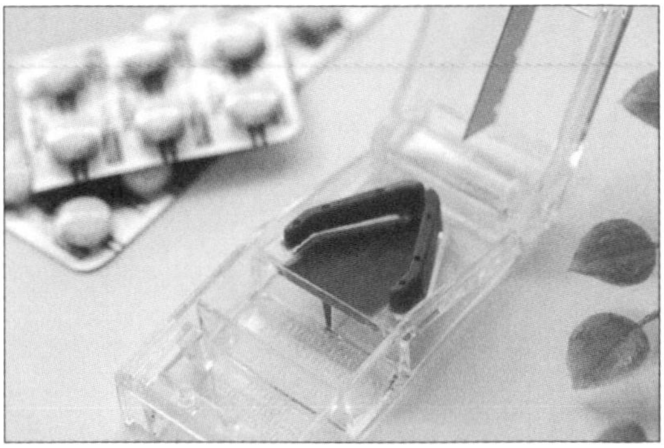
▲善用切藥器，利於藥物切一半。（照片提供／余宜叡）

將藥物放入切藥器中，將藥物放到適當的位置，輕輕按壓一下，藥物就會被切成一半。切藥器可以在藥局或醫療院所購買。

選擇有刻痕的藥物

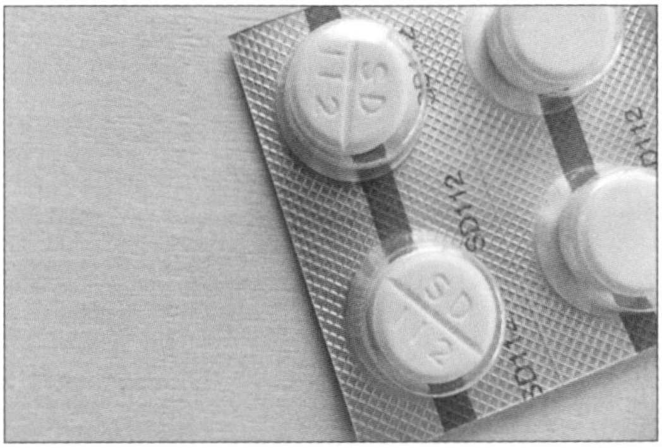
▲選用有刻痕的藥物，方便剝半使用。（照片提供／余宜叡）

一些藥物錠劑上有刻痕，通常只需輕輕剝去一部分，藥物就可以分成一半。這樣的設計表示該藥物可以剝半使用。

使用劑量一半的藥

例如，某些排糖藥物提供劑量一半的複方藥物選擇，您可以直接使用這種劑量一半的藥物，而無需自行切割藥物。

用藥提醒 2：特別注意複方藥使用

案例 1

45 歲的于先生患有糖尿病已經兩年多，最近在門診中提到他經常忘記服用醫生後來增加的血糖藥物的第二次劑量。此外，儘管他的糖化血色素仍未達標，但與醫生討論後，他的用藥方案被更改為一天一次的複方藥物。

雖然複方藥使藥物顆數減少，但它們的大小卻變大了。藥物的大小與一些保健品中的藥丸（如挺立或善存）相似。于先生服用複方藥物兩週後回診時表示可以接受藥物的大小，並且再也沒有漏服藥物的情況。

此外，他這兩週內量測的血糖值都在標準範圍內，身體也沒有出現任何不適。最終，他的糖化血色素值小於 7%。

案例 2

72 歲的嚴女士患有糖尿病已經十年多，她已經一段時間服用糖尿病、高血壓和高血脂的藥物。嚴女士的家屬在門診中抱怨她需要服用太多藥物。因此，醫生將她的血糖藥物轉換成了複方血糖藥。

回診時，嚴女士抱怨複方藥物太大顆，不方便吞服，希望改回原來較小的藥物。醫生向嚴女士確認後，複方藥物雖然顆數增加了，但藥物的大小變小了，但需要每天固定兩次服用。嚴女士表示她可以認真遵守這個藥物方案。

經過兩週的用藥，嚴女士表示可以接受藥物的大小，並且家中量測的血糖值保持穩定。

使用複方藥物時需要注意的事項：

頻率改變

轉換為複方藥物時，用藥頻率可能會有所改變。例如，原本一天一次的藥物可能變成一天兩次，或者原本一天兩次的藥物可能變成一天一次。對於複方胰島素，使用頻率的改變可能是一天兩次變成一天一次，或者一天四次變成一天三次。

藥物變大

轉換成口服複方藥物時，藥物的大小通常會變大。在臨床上，這可能會造成糖友對於吞服藥物的困難或心理障礙。建議可以將藥物分批服用。如果真的非常在意藥物的大小，可以考慮轉換為單一成分的小顆藥片，但要注意顆數會相對增加。

半量使用

部分複方藥物含有緩釋功能的錠劑。如果將其剝半使用，可能會導致藥效不穩定。可以與醫師或藥師討論是否適合進行半量使用。而有些複方藥物剛好是建議劑量的一半，因此不需要剝半使用，同時可以整合兩種血糖藥物，以達到一定的穩定降糖效果。

不易調整

複方藥物將兩種或以上的成分整合在一起，因此調整其中一種成分時會影響到其他成分。這使得藥物調整較為困難。因此，如果血糖仍未達到目標值，醫師可能會停止使用複方藥物，改用單一成分的藥物，以便更靈活地調整治療方案，特別是在血糖控制不佳的情況下。

先短期使用

在轉換為複方藥物時，由於緩釋劑型、用藥頻率的改變，以及不同藥廠的製程和添加物，可能會影響療效、引起過敏反應或產生副作用。建議在轉換複方藥物時，至少要監測血糖兩週以上。這樣可以掌握血糖的變化情況，同時注意身體是否有任何不適，以確定這個複方藥物是否適合長期使用。

二甲雙胍複方（＋ metformin）	
DPP-4 抑制劑	Sitagliptin, Linagliptin, Vidagliptin, Saxagliptin
排糖藥	Dapagliflozin, Empagliflozin, Canagliflozin, Ertugliflozin
TZD	Pioglitazone
排糖藥＋ DPP-4 抑制劑的複方	
Dapagliflozin ＋ Saxagliptin、Empagliflozin ＋ Linagliptin	
胰島素複方	
長效胰島素＋短效腸泌素、超長效胰島素＋速效胰島素、 長效胰島素＋短效胰島素、	

大魚醫師小叮嚀：台灣的注意事項

在使用複方藥物之前，請務必確認台灣目前的血壓藥物是否有三合一或二合一的選擇，以及血糖和血脂藥物是否有二合一的選項。在使用藥物之前，請與醫生進行詳細討論。

用藥提醒 3：排糖藥使用需知

案例 1

古先生是一位 50 歲多歲的糖友，已經患病 6 年。最近他因為泌尿道不適而就醫，檢驗尿液時發現除了細菌感染外，還有大量的尿糖。進一步檢查他的糖尿病用藥時發現他正在使用排糖藥。

排糖藥的作用是將血液中的糖分排出體外，以降低血糖濃度。然而，由於古先生的工作需要長時間在無塵室工作，常常憋尿，這已經是他第三次因為泌尿道感染不適而就醫。在向古先生提供關於使用排糖藥的衛教時，醫療團隊考慮到他的特殊職業，建議他將排糖藥換成其他種類的降糖藥。在接下來的三個月內，古先生沒有再因為泌尿道感染不適而就醫。

案例 2

林女士是一位 40 多歲的糖友，已經患病 3 年。醫師向她提供了有關使用排糖藥降低血糖並幫助減重的衛教。然而，在使用排糖藥兩週後，林女士抱怨她經常感到尿尿的地方不適。檢視使用排糖藥時需要注意的三件事情：多喝水、不憋尿、加強私密處清潔，林女士只有在加強清潔方面做到了，但在多喝水和不憋尿方面則存在困難。

由於她在櫃檯工作，通常需要工作1至2個小時才有機會去上廁所，有時忙碌時也會忘記。這導致了排糖藥的副作用。隨後，林女士請同事和主管幫助她定時上廁所，避免憋尿，結果不適感明顯改善。此時，她才體會到做好這三件事對於減少排糖藥副作用的重要性。

近年來，糖尿病用藥不斷更新，其中排糖藥根據目前的研究顯示除了有效降低血糖外，還具有護腎和顧心的額外效果。它們不僅適用於糖尿病治療，還適用於心衰竭和慢性腎病變的治療。然而，在使用排糖藥時，我們必須特別注意其副作用，尤其是與泌尿生殖道感染相關的副作用。

這些副作用包括尿尿部位的不適、小便不適甚至燒灼感。為了減少這些副作用，我們需要做好以下三件事：

多喝水

保持充足的水分攝取非常重要。適當的水分攝取可以稀釋尿液中的糖分，減少對泌尿道的刺激，降低感染風險。

不憋尿

避免長時間憋尿非常重要。憋尿會增加尿液在泌尿道中停留的時間，增加感染的風險。定期上廁所，避免憋尿，可以減少排糖藥引起的不適。

加強泌尿生殖道清潔

保持良好的個人衛生是預防感染的關鍵。加強泌尿生殖道的清潔可以減少病原菌的繁殖，降低感染風險。

對於一些需要長時間憋尿或不容易及時上廁所的特定職業，如長期在無塵室工作的人、櫃姐、櫃檯人員、長途駕駛等，我們需要仔細衡量是否將排糖藥納入他們的血糖治療計畫中。稍不留意，排糖藥的副作用就會產生，進而嚴重影響他們的工作和生活品質。

因此，在使用排糖藥時，要特別留意多喝水、不憋尿和加強泌尿生殖道清潔這三件事情。這些注意事項可以幫助減少排糖藥的副作用，提高病患的生活品質。對於那些需要長時間憋尿或不容易及時上廁所的人，可能需要考慮其他降糖藥物的選擇，以減少對泌尿道的負擔。

重要的是，醫療團隊在糖尿病治療中應該提供全面的衛教，特別是針對使用排糖藥的患者。患者應該了解這些副作用的可能性，並掌握如何有效地減少這些副作用的方法。此外，定期的追蹤檢查和與醫療團隊的溝通也是確保治療方案有效性和安全性的重要因素。

總之，對於使用排糖藥的糖友，多喝水、不憋尿和加強泌尿生殖道清潔是重要的注意事項，可以幫助減少排糖藥的副作用。同時，醫療團隊的指導和患者的積極配合也是確保治療效果和提高生活品質的關鍵。

用藥提醒 4：開車、送貨糖友的穩糖

案例 1 許先生是一名計程車司機，患有糖尿病已經五年多。儘管他在平時能夠控制血糖達到目標範圍，糖化血色素小於 7%，但後來才發現他常常因為載客關係而延後用餐，導致飢餓或無力感。他需要在車上服用牛奶或糖果才能緩解這些症狀。

在調整許先生的用藥組合後，減少易引起低血糖的藥物使用，他需要使用牛奶或糖果的次數減少了很多。建議許先生，如果他計畫延後用餐，應該在工作前先補充一些牛奶或小點心。

案例 2 嚴大哥是一名貨車司機，經常需要長途駕駛。他習慣性地在一趟駕駛結束後好好地大吃一頓，並且進食速度很快，不到 10 分鐘就能解決一餐。因此，他常常在進食後感到昏昏欲睡。

建議他在進食時可以添加一到兩份燙青菜，同時每口食物要咀嚼 20 到 30 下，以延長進食時間。起初，嚴大哥可能不太習慣，但隨著他執行這兩個建議的情況越來越好，他的昏昏欲睡感也得到了改善。

對於開計程車、送貨、快遞、外送員等糖友來說，常常誤餐、進食不定時、進食速度過快、攝取大量含糖食物，容易出現低血糖和高血糖，導致疲倦、嗜睡或頭腦昏昏沉的症狀。建議此族群糖友可以做以下幾件事情，以維持血糖的穩定：

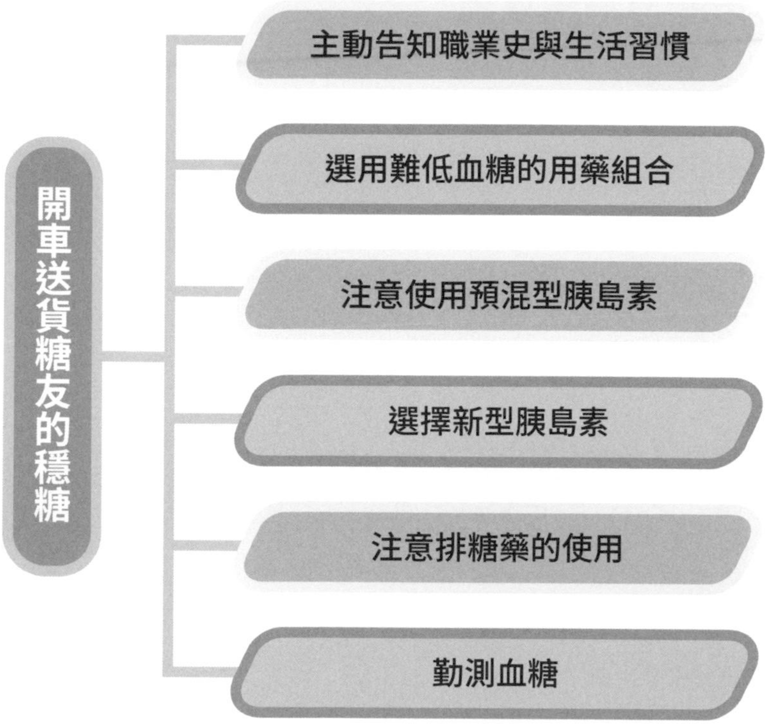
開車送貨糖友的穩糖
主動告知職業史與生活習慣
選用難低血糖的用藥組合
注意使用預混型胰島素
選擇新型胰島素
注意排糖藥的使用
勤測血糖

主動告知醫療團隊職業史與生活習慣

與醫療團隊保持密切聯繫，分享您的職業史和生活習慣。這樣他們可以根據您的情況提供相應的建議，並調整您的糖尿病治療計畫。

選用難低血糖的用藥組合

在藥物治療中，選擇難以引起低血糖的藥物組合，以減少低血糖的發生。諮詢您的醫生以了解可適合您的選擇。

注意使用預混型胰島素

如果您使用長效加短效的預混型胰島素，如 NovoMix 30、50 或 Humalog 25、50 等，請特別注意使用方法。這類藥物通常需要每天注射 2 至 3 次，且在使用前需要均勻搖晃 20 至 30 秒以上。遵循醫生的指示並確保正確使用。

選擇新型胰島素

新型的混合型超長效加速效胰島素 RYZODEG 和長效胰島素加速效腸泌素 SOLIQA，相對於其他藥物，其高低血糖的風險較低。請與醫生討論是否適合您使用這些藥物。

注意排糖藥的使用

對於開車送貨的族群，如果無法輕易停車上廁所，需注意排糖藥的使用。長時間憋尿或水分攝取不足，容易引起泌尿生殖道不適，例如會陰騷癢、小便灼熱感，這可能影響您的工作和生活品質。

勤測血糖

在血糖未穩定的情況下，建議頻繁測量血糖，以瞭解飲食和延後進食對血糖的影響。只有有效穩定血糖，才能減少意外事件和不適的發生。

CHAPTER 02 飲食對策

飲食原則：什麼都可以吃，但有技巧

「很多東西不能吃」是糖友常見的迷思，尤其是甜的東西不能吃；極端一點，甚至有糖友確診後就不吃飯、麵……等澱粉類，執行生酮飲食來穩定血糖。但其實糖友什麼都可以進食，不需禁糖，也不需禁醣，只要遵守以下相關原則。

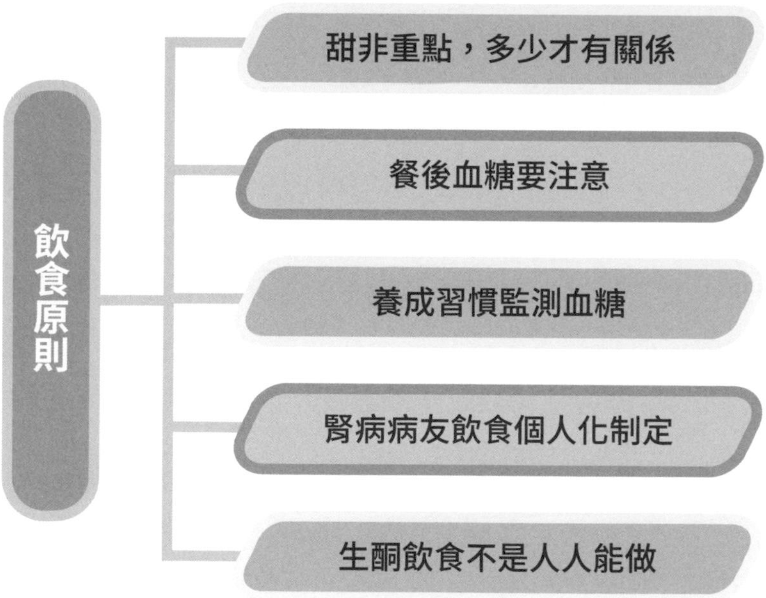
飲食原則
甜非重點，多少才有關係
餐後血糖要注意
養成習慣監測血糖
腎病病友飲食個人化制定
生酮飲食不是人人能做

甜非重點，多少才有關係

糖友其實什麼都可以進食，但要考慮份量。只要攝取適當的份量，即使是很甜的食物，仍可進食，並非什麼都不能吃，只不過很甜的食物，通常含醣許多，不要一次進食太多。糖友另一錯誤認知，飯與麵等不甜的主食，多吃無害，常常一餐可能不小心就攝取了一碗半或兩碗，血糖要不升高也難。不論吃進什麼食物，只要糖友量測的血糖在可接受的範圍內，表示是可以這樣吃。

餐後血糖要注意

臨床上常遇到糖友，一量測血糖高起來，超過標準，就非常緊張。其實只要一週不要超過三次的超標，都是可以接受的範圍，還是偶爾可以放鬆一下，若真的很在意超標，在進食較多的情況下，可以增加 10 ～ 20 分鐘的運動，或者加上穩定餐後血糖藥物。

養成習慣監測血糖

不論是使用自我監測血糖，或連續血糖儀，瞭解餐前餐後血糖，才能有效學習到，如何調整飲食份量，血糖能標準值內，一旦抓到對的份量，幾次之後，循序漸進地養成血糖合宜的飲食習慣，之後只要這樣吃，血糖都不太會超標，進而就可以減少如此飲食的血糖監測。此外，每週多了可以超標的額度，可以在別的飲食放鬆一下。

此外，定期監測血糖是非常重要的，它可以提供寶貴的資訊，讓糖友了解自己的飲食習慣對血糖的影響。通過持續監測血糖，糖友可以逐漸習慣適量的飲食，並找到自己身體所接受的食物範圍。

腎病病者飲食標準重新個人化制定

不過要特別注意，一旦發生糖尿病腎病變，腎功能惡化，需做出蛋白質攝取量的限制，若再進展到腎衰竭、洗腎程度，將會有更多飲食禁忌與限制，無法像上述放鬆飲食，會大幅影響到生活品質。因此，建議在糖尿病前期或早期糖尿病，好好穩定血糖至標準內，避免上述情況發生。

生酮飲食有前提，不是人人能做

生酮飲食早在一百年前就發明了，當下的時空背景，糖友身處在完全沒有糖尿病治療用藥的時代，沒有胰島素或口服藥，只能依靠生酮飲食來減少高血糖的危害與延命。此外根據最新的第二型糖尿病照護指引，需在醫療人員的監督下才執行生酮飲食，同時不要超過 2 個月，否則會造成腎功能的損害。

大魚醫師小叮嚀：正確飲食 隨心所欲

糖友飲食可以擁有越低的意志力考驗，越高的飲食自由度。

只要能夠循序漸近找出適合自己情況的飲食份量，就能擁有自由度越高的飲食習慣，越不用考驗意志力。越是做出許多限制，因應許多不適與不方便，越是考驗你的意志力，而越是嚴格考驗意志力的事情，就是越不易執行成功。

因此，只要可以找到隨心所欲，且血糖穩定的飲食方式，就能與糖共舞。

飲食重點1：控制血糖
食物「種類」和「份量」也要顧

案例　在周先生門診的那一天，他的飯後血糖值高達293mg/dL，而前幾天進行的糖化血色素檢查結果也顯示其值達到了8.9%，這些數值遠超過糖友血糖控制的目標範圍。

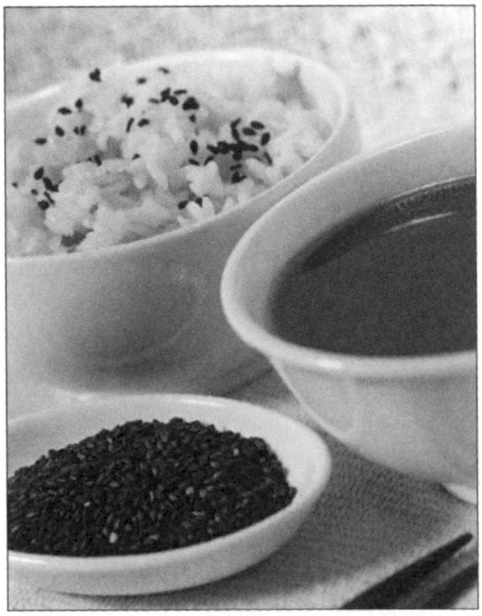

▲食物的重量和份量會決定血糖高低。

醫師問他是否按時服藥，周先生表示他確實按時服藥。

接著，醫師問了他早餐吃了什麼，周先生回答說：「只吃了一碗牛奶泡麥片，再加上4片白吐司，而且都不是甜的，為什麼血糖值會這麼高呢？」

然而，周先生所說的「一碗牛奶泡麥片」實際上是一大碗的份量，換算起來相當於兩碗飯的份量，再加上他還吃了4片白吐司。這樣的飲食份量過大，即使食物本身並不甜，血糖值也很難控制在正常範圍內。此外，從周先生的糖化血色素檢查結果來看，可以判斷出他在過去的3個月內並沒有穩定地控制血糖。

周先生的案例提醒我們，對於糖友來說，食物的種類和份量對於血糖控制至關重要。不僅需要注意食物是否甜味，還需要合理選擇食物種類並控制食物的份量。

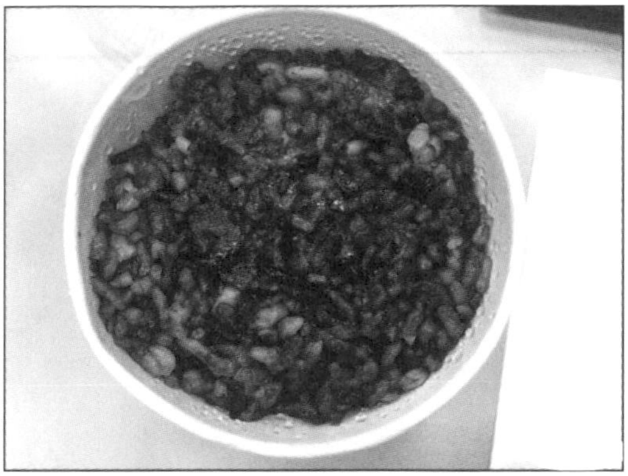

▲五穀飯雖可以輔助降血脂，但如果一次吃一大碗，也可能會影響血糖值。（記者羅碧攝）

因此，我們可以說食物的種類和份量會決定血糖高低，從以下三點來分別說明。

食物的份量和種類對血糖影響重大

許多糖友在追求控制血糖的過程中，往往只注重食物的甜度，忽略了食物的份量和種類對血糖的重要影響。一個典型的例子是周先生，他認為只要避免吃甜的東西，血糖就能夠得到很好的控制。然而，當他的血糖檢測結果出來時，卻發現血糖升高並且糖化血色素（HbA1c）也超過了標準範圍。這證明了食物的份量和種類對血糖控制的重要性。

周先生的例子告訴我們，食物的份量和種類會直接影響血糖的高低。即使食物不甜，如果份量過大，攝入的碳水化合物仍然會轉化為葡萄糖進入血液，導致血糖升高。因此，糖友在飲食選擇上不僅要注意甜度，還要控制食物的份量。

食物甜度不是衡量血糖的唯一因素

許多人誤以為只要避免吃甜的食物，血糖就可以得到有效控制。然而，事實並非如此。食物的甜度只是血糖影響的一個因素，還有其他因素需要考慮，例如食物的種類和份量。

以飯後血糖控制為例，不建議常吃的高糖食物，即使只吃一小塊，血糖的變動也不會很大。相反，建議的食物如果一次吃一大碗，未能適當控制份量，血糖反而會變動很大。這意味著食物的份量在血糖控制中起著關鍵作用。

此外，食物的種類也是影響血糖的重要因素。例如，五穀飯、糙米飯或含有輔助降血脂效果的麥片等食物可以作為建議的選擇，但如果一次吃一大碗，同樣會導致血糖升高。因此，糖友在選擇食物時，不僅要注意甜度，還要注意食物的種類和份量。

學習認識食物種類和計算份量是關鍵

為了達到良好的血糖控制，糖友需要學習認識食物的種類和計算份量。這意味著他們需要了解不同食物對血糖的影響程度，並能夠合理地控制自己的飲食份量。

透過了解食物的種類，糖友可以選擇對血糖影響較小的食物，並且避免過度攝入碳水化合物。此外，學習計算食物的份量可以幫助他們在進食時控制攝入的碳水化合物量，從而穩定血糖水平。

同時，監測飯後血糖也是非常重要的。僅僅監測飯前血糖是不足夠的，因為食物攝入後血糖會有一段延遲的反應。通過監測飯後血糖，糖友可以更好地了解自己的血糖變化情況，並在飲食中取得平衡點。

飲食重點 2：份量如何掌握？

案例 1 吃三顆芭樂的黃小姐，餐前血糖原本是 100，餐後血糖卻變成了 300，她大為驚訝，不明白為什麼餐後血糖會這麼高。因為一直以來，芭樂都被認為是較適合糖友食用的水果。

案例 2 另一位李先生，擔心吃不完浪費，早餐吃了兩顆肉粽後，測量餐前和餐後血糖，結果血糖直接飆升到 200 以上。「為什麼血糖會這麼高？」「在這麼高的情況下，為什麼我沒有任何不適或症狀？」

以上兩個案例中，份量對血糖的影響起著關鍵作用。只有透過自我血糖監測或連續血糖監測，才能更清楚地瞭解份量對血糖的影響。

對 GI 值的誤解

此外，關於低血糖指數（GI）的誤解，低 GI 飲食確實對血糖有較小的影響，但如果考慮到份量，情況就不一定了。例如，白飯的 GI 值較低，而糙米飯的 GI 值較高，但如果吃了一碗白飯和兩碗糙米飯，那麼餐後血糖可能比兩碗糙米飯更高。因此，在飲食中除了考慮 GI 值外，還需要考慮份量，但份量這一點往往容易被忽視。

在這個主題中，份量是最重要的因素。舉例來說，從年輕時就喜歡吃冰淇淋的邱先生，在罹患糖尿病十多年後，害怕吃冰淇淋後血糖過高，每次只敢吃一次冰淇淋。但在醫療團隊的教育下，他試著控制冰淇淋的份量，同時減少正餐中碳水化合物的攝取量，並測量血糖值，結果餐後血糖在 180 以內。

他終於了解只要控制適量的冰淇淋，並調整正餐中的碳水化合物攝取量，他的血糖值可以維持在標準範圍內。之後，他每個月都可以享受 3 ～ 4 次冰淇淋，他感到非常幸福。

類似的情況也發生在熱愛水果的戰女士身上。她每天都覺得身體不適，如果當天沒有吃到水果，她會感到怪怪的。營養師評估後建議她減少午餐的份量，並在午餐後食用水果，這樣對血糖的影響較小。

另外，唐先生也喜愛水果，他每次吃水果後都會再走路 20 分鐘，如果沒有走路，他的餐後血糖值就會超過 200，但只要有走路，血糖值可以維持在 180 以內。

GI 值和份量的搭配

對於對血糖影響較低的食物（如芭樂、糙米飯等），適量攝取仍然是可行的。同樣地，對於對血糖影響較高的食物（如冰淇淋、含糖飲料等），只要適量食用也是可以的。此外，減少碳水化合物攝取、在三餐中選擇攝取較少的一餐、攝取後進行輕微運動等，都是有助控制血糖的方式。

飲食重點 3：搭配藥物 & 運動，就可吃得輕鬆

案例

林先生是一位 40 多歲的糖友，已經患病三年。他以農務維生，主要是辛苦重型的工作。在罹患糖尿病時，他的血糖數值非常高，後來透過朋友介紹來門診求助。

在評估了他的血糖治療後，醫生決定只使用口服藥物治療。此外，林先生分享了因糖尿病的關係，妻子和孩子們在他的飲食上加以限制，這給他帶來很大的壓力。經過醫生和病人的討論後，他的治療方案加入了胰島素和腸泌素，減少了口服藥物的種類。

在不到六個月的時間內，他日常血糖監測的數值超過八成都在正常範圍內。這也讓關心他健康的家人們感到放心，不再對他施加說教或限制。林先生對目前的糖尿病治療非常滿意，他能夠達到血糖穩定和生活品質的平衡。

每個人對於吃得輕鬆的定義可能不同。有些人認為吃得輕鬆是指沒有太大的壓力，或者是能夠像其他人一樣吃自己喜歡的食物，或者是可以享受多一些食物的自由，或者是避免血糖劇烈波動等。但無論如何，共同的目標都是在不影響生活品質的前提下，自主輕鬆地進行飲食。

「吃得輕鬆」代表希望在飲食方面少一些節制，多一些彈性。要實現吃得輕鬆，需要加強運動和藥物的介入，這樣血糖才有機會保持在正常範圍內，減少糖尿病後續併發症的發生。

加強運動

除了每週至少 150 分鐘的運動量是基本要求外，還需要增加運動的時間或強度。例如，將每週的運動時間從 150 分鐘增加到 200 ～ 300 分鐘，或者從步行改為快走或慢跑等高強度運動。此外，也可以在餐後安排一段時間進行運動，例如餐後散步 10 ～ 30 分鐘，這有助於有效降低飯後血糖的升高。

至於餐後應該運動多久，可根據進食的量增減運動時間。

加強藥物

如果想要長期實現輕鬆進食，建議增加藥物的種類或劑量。例如，可以考慮配合穩定血糖的針劑藥物，如胰島素或腸泌素，以提高治療成功率。如果只是偶爾享受大餐或放鬆進食，可以使用一些餐後降血糖的藥物。

只要飲食增加一些或吃得盡興，可以在餐前使用 0.5 ～ 2 顆降血糖藥物。至於具體應該使用多少藥物，可以根據進食的量來增減藥物的劑量。

持續監測血糖

最後，請記得持續監測血糖，這樣才能知道加強運動和藥物導入是否真的使血糖保持在正常範圍內，並且能夠繼續享受輕鬆的飲食，同時維持目前的治療效果。

飲食重點 4：蔬菜可以多吃點

案例 1 王先生是一位糖友，常常在中餐之前感到飢餓並出現冒冷汗的症狀。經過檢視他的用藥、飲食和作息後，發現藥物使用沒有太大問題，但在飲食方面存在蔬菜攝取量過少的問題。因此，營養師建議他在早餐中改變原本的飯糰或鐵板麵，轉而選擇夾有青菜的漢堡或有青菜或小黃瓜的三明治。

這個建議使他的症狀顯著減少。隨後，王先生嘗試了另一種方法，即在前一晚保留一碗青菜，隔天早餐時加熱後食用。自從他每天早上都吃一碗青菜後，中午用餐前不再感到肚子飢餓的不舒服。

案例 2 白小姐是一位 50 多歲的糖友，患病已六年多。自從她增加了中餐和晚餐中一碗蔬菜的攝取後，她的體重減少了近 5%，同時血糖也達到了標準範圍。原來，增加蔬菜攝取不僅增加了飽足感，使她在中餐和晚餐中減少了飯麵的份量（從 1.5～2 碗減少到 1 碗）；同時，她在外食時也特別注意選擇不過油或經過去油處理的青菜，減少攝取的油脂量。白小姐很高興增加蔬菜攝取後，她的血糖達標，體重也減少了。

蔬菜的好處

蔬菜是六大類營養中最不會影響血糖的類別，因此建議每餐都攝取一碗蔬菜。蔬菜可以促進腸胃蠕動，幫助排便，同時增加飽足感，減少對碳水化合物的攝取，進而降低血糖的急升急降，同時也有助於減少攝取過多的熱量，使體重不再快速上升。此外，蔬菜還能維持血糖的穩定，降低餐前血糖過低或血糖急升急降所引起的不適症狀，例如飢餓、發抖等。

增加蔬菜攝取的方法

如果在家自己下廚，可以選擇川燙青菜作為菜餚。外出用餐時，可以在便當中增加 1 ～ 2 份的蔬菜。如果有機會選擇菜餚，可以要求不加滷汁或醬油。在自助餐店，可以主動選擇三種以上的青菜，並確保攝取一碗以上的份量。如果有機會，可以將菜餚過水，減少油脂的攝取。

不喜歡蔬菜的人，還是最少要吃三種

對於不喜歡吃蔬菜的人，醫師建議挑選三種最喜歡吃的青菜，輪流替換食用。當在餐廳只有炒青菜而沒有其他烹調方式時，仍然可以選擇點一份青菜，但記得要過水，以減少攝取過多的油脂。

大魚醫師的小叮嚀：偽裝的蔬菜

有些食物常被誤以為是蔬菜，但實際上不屬於蔬菜類。例如五穀根莖類或澱粉類食物如玉米、芋頭、地瓜、山藥，以及水果類中的小番茄（牛番茄才是蔬菜類）。建議可以拍照後向營養師諮詢，確保攝取足夠的蔬菜，以穩定血糖並控制體重。

飲食重點 5：營養品好好用，更穩糖

案例 1

胡小姐得知爸爸確診糖尿病後，每次回家都會帶一箱糖尿病專用營養品給爸爸，並叮嚀他要定時飲用，每天至少喝一罐，以輔助穩定血糖。然而，後續回診時，醫療團隊發現胡爸爸的血糖仍然居高不下。經過仔細詢問後，才發現多喝糖尿病專用營養品是造成血糖升高的主要原因。

醫生建議胡爸爸每週只需飲用 2～5 次糖尿病專用營養品，並將其作為早餐的部分飲食來替代，例如大杯奶茶或拿鐵等。這樣既能兼顧胡小姐的孝心，又能保持血糖在正常範圍內。

案例 2

60 多歲的沈女士已經患有糖尿病超過 10 年。孝順的兒女看到報紙上的廣告後，買了糖尿病專用飲品給媽媽，期望這些飲品能幫助媽媽穩定血糖，甚至減少對藥物的需求。然而，使用了三個月後，媽媽的糖化血色素值從原本的 6.7%上升到了 8.2%。

必須符合低 GI 值

糖尿病專用營養品主要符合低 GI（血糖上升緩慢）、營養均衡且份量計算過的特點。對於日常熱量攝取不足的糖尿病患者，建議使用這些營養品作為補充；對於攝取熱量足夠的患者，建議將其用來取代部分餐點；而對於攝取熱量過多的患者，則不建議使用。

然而，在臨床實踐中，許多糖尿病患者的家屬將糖尿病專用營養品視為保健營養品，誤以為多喝糖尿病專用營養品對血糖控制越好，甚至有些糖尿病患者血糖升高就歸咎於營養品攝取不足。然而，事實並非如此，除非糖尿病患者的熱量攝取不足，否則過量攝取糖尿病專用營養品只會導致血糖升高。

算入正常飲食 不應額外攝取

對於沈女士的情況，除了日常飲食外，她還每餐間飲用一罐糖尿病專用飲品，每天共兩罐。然而，在營養諮詢中，營養師向糖尿病患者和家屬解釋，根據沈女士的攝取情況，正確的使用方式是將糖尿病專用飲品作為替代某些餐點的選擇，而不是額外添加飲用。

糖尿病專用飲品與一般餐點相比，能夠使血糖波動更低，升高速度較緩慢，因此很適合取代那些血糖波動較大的飲料或水果等含有糖分的食物。修正使用方式後，沈女士的血糖又恢復到正常範圍內。

許多糖尿病患者希望能夠減少或停用血糖藥物，因此他們尋求糖尿病專用營養品的幫助。然而，僅僅依靠糖尿病專用營養品並不能改善或逆轉血糖情況。唯有正確地使用糖尿病專用營養品，才能夠獲得均衡的營養補充並保持血糖的穩定。

--CHAPTER--
03
運動、生活習慣及其他方面改善

做對運動 1：上班時間可做的運動

案例 1

林先生是一位糖尿病患者，他從事文書處理的行政工作，長時間處於靜態少活動的狀態。雖然他每週有規律的運動，但最近的體檢報告顯示血糖值有超出標準的情況。經過與醫療團隊的討論，他同意在工作的休息空檔進行運動，以幫助穩定血糖。

案例 2

何女士是一位長期患有糖尿病的患者，她在工作中的空檔時會進行原地踏步運動，但有時會因同事的關心或在場沒有執行而受到干擾。建議她在需要時告訴同事自己希望增加運動量，這樣或許能夠鼓勵同事們一起參與運動。

勞動不能取代運動

對於那些本來就需要走動的工作，例如巡視工廠或搬運貨物的工作，它們已經包含了一定的運動量。但是，我們建議不要將這些工作中的運動視為取代非上班或工作時間的運動。除非您的職業本身就是運動員，可以在下班後進行運動，否則仍然需要增加額外的運動時間來維持身體健康。

上班時間的運動主要是指在工作中進行的一些勞動，它們能夠增加熱量的消耗，並有助於穩定血糖。這些運動可以在工作的休息時間進行，不需要心情放鬆或愉悅的情況下進行，但仍然能夠為身體帶來益處。

長期靜態工作者可做的運動建議

對於長時間從事文書行政等靜態工作的人來說，建議每工作 1 小時就休息 5～10 分鐘，喝些水、進行一些簡單的運動，活動筋骨，讓身體得到放鬆，同時增加運動量。建議的運動如下：

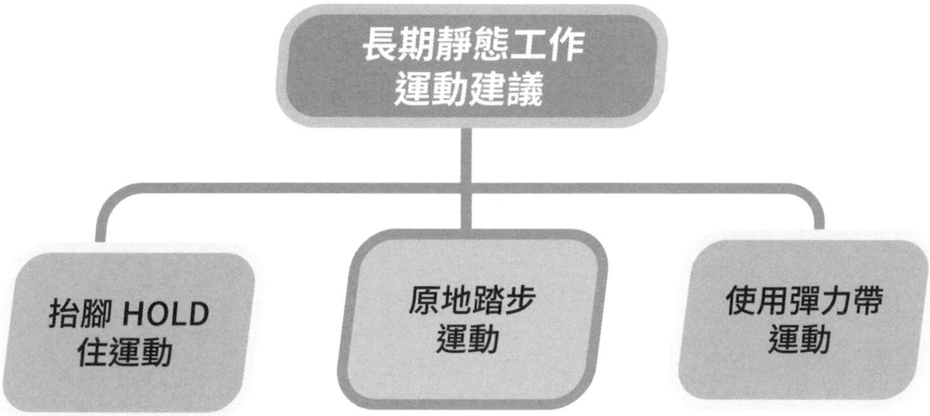

抬腳 HOLD 住運動

找一張固定且有椅背的椅子，一次抬一邊的腳至水平地面，同時 hold 住 5 秒以上。每次休息時間可以做 10 ～ 20 組，只需 1 分半至 3 分鐘。如果工作桌子下的空間很大，也可以在工作時三不五時做一下這個動作。

原地踏步運動

利用休息時間進行原地踏步。可以嘗試將膝蓋碰到胸部地抬腳，增加運動強度。每次休息空檔可以執行 10 ～ 20 組的原地踏步。

使用彈力帶運動

可以執行兩種運動：坐著動大腿和坐著動手臂。

- **坐著動大腿：**利用彈力帶固定在椅子上，以腿部肌肉為主進行運動。
- **坐著動手臂：**利用彈力帶固定在椅子上，以手臂肌肉為主進行運動。

不要擔心別人異樣的眼光

當在工作時間內進行運動時，不要擔心別人的眼光。可以在工作的休息時間內坦誠地告訴同事，運動是醫療團隊建議的，並且這樣做可以讓自己更健康。說不定您的積極態度會鼓勵同事們一起參與運動，共同維護健康。

做對運動 2：有氧運動 VS 阻力運動

案例

有氧運動與阻力運動，到底哪個對穩定血糖有幫助？！這是 30 多歲的糖友葉女士向醫師提出的問題。事實上，不論是有氧運動還是阻力運動，對於穩定血糖都有一定的幫助。

關鍵在於兩點：運動要足量，足夠以維持血糖在正常範圍內；培養運動的習慣，最好每週進行五次或更多次的運動。

因此，必須要確保運動時間足夠且持續，然後再逐漸增加運動強度。但要注意身體狀況，避免過度使用力量或逞強，同時在運動前做好暖身運動，在運動後進行適度的緩和活動。

有氧運動和阻力運動的好處

有氧運動

- 可增加血糖的消耗，降低血糖水平。
- 有助於減少體脂肪比例，減輕胰島素的阻抗性。
- 通常不需要任何器械，可以隨時隨地進行。

阻力運動

- 可增加血糖的消耗，降低血糖水平。
- 有助於維持身體一定的肌肉量，減輕胰島素的阻抗性。
- 通常需要一些器械的幫助進行。

足量的簡單運動

對於完全沒有運動習慣的人，建議從逐漸開始運動，逐步增加運動量，目標是每週進行五次或更多次的足量運動。所謂足量指的是運動的時間和強度。

以下是一些建議的簡單運動：

彈力繩運動

每天使用彈力繩進行 50 到 100 次的拉伸運動，可以使用手或腳拉動，並且每次持續 5 到 10 秒。

抬腳運動

每次抬起一隻腳，使大腿與地面平行，然後保持 5 到 10 秒（視個人身體狀況而定）。可以進行 50 到 100 組，每週進行 2 到 3 次。後續可以逐漸增加保持時間或組數。這項運動的好處是可以坐著執行，且不需要任何器材。

此外，個人還可以進行以下運動：

走路

每天走路 10 到 20 分鐘，每週三天開始，逐漸增加到每次走路 30 到 40 分鐘，每週五天進行。如果能從走路轉為快走或慢跑，那麼運動強度也會增加。

騎腳踏車

可以選擇騎腳踏車作為有氧運動的方式，這也是一種很有效的運動方式。

爬樓梯

利用日常生活中的樓梯進行爬樓運動，這對增加心肺功能和消耗能量都非常有益。

最重要的是，對於沒有運動習慣的人來說，重要的是開始行動。雖然起初可能感到困難，但逐漸培養運動的習慣，可以幫助穩定血糖並改善整體健康狀況。

生活習慣調整 1：症狀較重、有併發症糖友的穩糖

案例 1 蔡先生是一位 60 多歲的糖尿病患者，已經患病超過 10 年，並且還有高血壓和高血脂的問題。他中風兩次後需要長期臥床並接受照護。他的照護者每天給他管灌四餐，但是他的血糖值經常忽高忽低。

經過家訪醫師根據他的飲食和餐前餐後血糖記錄調整了預混型胰島素的劑量，低血糖情況得到了明顯改善，家屬也不用再過度擔心了。

案例 2 李女士是一位 70 多歲的糖尿病患者，已經患病超過 20 年。最近因肺炎住院，無法自行進食，需要使用鼻胃管進行營養灌食。每天她需要管灌 5 次，同時口服藥物和注射基礎胰島素來控制血糖，血

糖值通常在 150 到 220 之間。家屬詢問醫師這樣的血糖值是否過高？

經過檢視兩週的血糖記錄，醫師告知家屬這樣的血糖值是可以接受的，但是要特別監測早上空腹血糖是否過低，如果小於 100 就需要注意，甚至可以考慮減少基礎胰島素的劑量。

糖尿病是一種需要長期管理和控制的慢性疾病，特別對於症狀較重、有併發症的居家糖尿病患者來說，建立良好的穩糖的生活習慣尤為重要。以下將從各方面提供一些建議。

有鼻胃管者的穩糖

對於糖尿病患者來說，飲食和用藥通常是定時定量的，而且糖尿病患者的順從性往往比一般人更高，所以任何合適的藥物都可以用於穩定血糖。在管灌糖尿病患者中，需要特別注意餐後的反抽量，如果反抽量多，表示攝取吸收度較差，同樣劑量的藥物下低血糖的風險就會增加。

管灌糖尿病患者每天需要管灌 4 到 6 餐，使用液狀的營養品或自製食物來進行灌食。考慮到糖尿病患者的吸收程度有限，無法一次性大量灌食，為了滿足一天所需的熱量攝取，必須分多次進行管灌，這導致餐與餐之間的時間間隔較短。因此，餐前和餐後的血糖標準可以稍微寬鬆一些，例如血糖在 130 到 200 之間都是可以接受的。

然而，仍然建議監測血糖的三個月平均值，即糖化血色素（HbA1c），應該保持在小於 7%的範圍內。如果糖尿病患者有其他共病狀況，則可以放寬至 7.5%到 8.5%。同時，需要注意血糖是否經常過低或過高。如果血糖波動太大，可能需要調整飲食或藥物的劑量。

沒有鼻胃管者的穩糖

一般而言，糖尿病患者通常一天進食 3 到 4 餐，飲食內容與一般人相似，血糖控制可以按照正常人的方式進行，但仍需注意飲食的均衡和適量，避免過度攝取高糖、高脂、高鹽的食物。

加強血糖監測

居家糖尿病患者往往行動能力較差，缺乏運動，甚至長期臥床。因此，重點應該放在飲食和藥物的介入上，而運動對於穩定血糖的幫助有限。由於居家糖尿病患者運動量大幅減少，便秘是常見問題，這進一步影響了食慾。在飲食攝取量減少的情況下，血糖監測變得尤為重要，稍有不慎就可能發生低血糖。

預防便秘

建議居家糖尿病患者每天攝取 1500 毫升以上的水，如果體型較大或環境悶熱，則可增加至 2000 毫升以上。在飲食方面，可以增加纖維質的攝取量，無論是添加高纖營養品，還是增加蔬菜或水果（如蔬菜泥）都可以幫助增加排便順暢，減少攝取不穩定導致的血糖風險。

此外，儘管居家糖尿病患者的活動能力可能受限，但仍應根據自身情況進行適度的身體活動。這可以包括輕度的散步、伸展運動、家庭活動等。除了能夠增加排便的能力之外，還可以促進血糖代謝和減重，同時有助於提升心理和身體的健康狀態。

培養良好的心理狀態

糖尿病是一種長期的慢性疾病，患者需要面對長期的治療和管理。因此，培養良好的心理狀態對於維持穩定的血糖控制至關重要。患者可以尋求家人、朋友或專業輔導的支持，並積極參與興趣愛好和社交活動，以減輕壓力和焦慮。

大魚醫師小叮嚀：反抽量和胃造口

反抽量

先用灌食空針反抽，這是以鼻胃管灌食前必須做的動作。其目的有二：

一是確定鼻胃管是否在胃內。

二是觀察胃部內容物的多少與顏色，藉此評估胃部的消化狀況。如果少於 50 c.c 則可進行灌食；但如果是超過上一餐灌食量的一半以上，就先不要灌食，一個小時後再視狀況而定，同時要將反抽物灌回胃內，幫助消化。

胃造口

除了鼻胃管外，胃造口也是管灌外的一個選擇。

如果考慮使用胃造口，建議請腸胃科醫師進行專業的術前評估，確定居家糖尿病患者是否適合進行胃造口手術，這樣可以減少鼻胃管的頻繁置換，提高居家糖尿病患者的舒適度。

生活習慣調整 2：抽菸族群要戒菸

案例　近日，門診中遇到了一位主動要戒菸的 70 多歲的長者。醫師對他戒菸的動機感到好奇，他告訴醫師說：「這已經是我第 11 次嘗試戒菸了，我希望能夠減少抽菸的頻率，甚至完全戒掉菸，主要是為了減輕孩子們的負擔。他們幫我負擔了安養中心的費用，我不想再給他們帶來更多的負擔。」他補充道：「每年我都會使用兩次的戒菸療程，而且每次療程結束後，我確實有一段時間不再抽菸。」

醫師對他又抽菸的原因感到好奇，他解釋：「其實，有時朋友抽菸時，會順便請我抽一根菸，結果每次抽過之後，菸癮又回來了！」他有點不好意思地說：「希望這次是我最後一次的戒菸療程，這樣就不用一直來醫院了。」

醫師詢問了他之前的戒菸療程使用的藥物以及戒菸過程中是否有任何問題。他回答：「醫師，其實我試過嚼的、貼的和吃的三種戒菸方式，但我覺得吃的藥物對我來說更適合，能否開立一種口服的戒菸藥物給我？」

抽菸對健康的危害是眾所周知的。它不僅會引起咳嗽和痰液，還增加了罹患各種癌症（如肺癌、胃癌、大腸癌等）和心血管疾病（如心肌梗塞）的風險。對女性而言，抽菸更容易加速皮膚老化，看起來比實際年齡更老。

戒菸的多重好處

戒菸可以帶來多重好處。首先，戒菸有助於改善血液循環和降低血壓，減少心臟負荷，進而減少心血管疾病的發病風險。其次，戒菸能夠改善肺部功能，減少慢性肺阻塞等呼吸系統疾病的發展。此外，戒菸還可以改善血液中的氧合程度，有助於維持組織和器官的正常功能。

對於糖友而言，戒菸還有額外的好處。戒菸可以降低血糖波動，提高胰島素的敏感性，有助於更好地穩定血糖水平。考慮到糖尿病本身已經增加了心血管疾病的風險，戒菸是減少心血管疾病風險的另一個良好方法。對於糖友這樣的群體而言，戒菸更加關鍵，因為糖尿病本身已經增加了心血管疾病的風險。

抽菸會對心血管系統產生負面影響。菸草產生的煙中有害物質進入血液後，會導致血管收縮、血液凝結能力增強以及血壓上升，進而增加心臟負荷和心血管疾病的發病風險。糖友本身已經存在心血管疾病的風險因素，如高血糖、高血壓和高血脂，抽菸會進一步加重這些風險。

友善環境幫助戒菸成功

要成功戒菸，單靠意志力往往難以堅持。建議糖友與醫療團隊合作，制定一個個性化的戒菸計畫。在戒菸過程中，可以考慮使用戒菸藥物輔助，如口服的戒菸藥物或其他適合的方式。此外，親人和朋友的支持和鼓勵也對成功戒菸產生重大的動力。

60 歲前健康者，血糖標準嚴格點

案例 1

40 歲的關先生，糖尿病發病後積極地調整飲食運動，加上藥物規律地服用，三個月後，糖化血色素由原本的 11%降到 7.2%，後來幾次的糖化血色素一直在 6.9～7.5%之間。

下一次門診衛教和關先生說明，他需要與糖尿病最少和平共存 30 年以上，建議血糖標準是可以嚴格點，設定糖化血色素小於 6.5%以下，減少血糖超標的時間與機率。關先生想起家裡的妻小（五歲大的女兒及三歲大的兒子），同意在成功提升飲食運動的介入程度前，再多用一些糖尿病藥物。

後續他的糖化血色素，分別是 6.7%、6.8%，根據關先生的飲食記錄與監測的血糖數值，鼓勵他嘗試營養諮詢，以合適自己的日常與生活品質的前提下，做飲食調整，三個月後，第一次糖化血色素成功在 6.5%，之前也都維持在 6.0%～ 6.5%。

案例 2

同樣的情況也發生在 50 多歲的林女士身上，先前的糖化血色素都在 6.8 ～ 7.3%，而她想要身體不發生併發症，將來才可以照顧自己的孫子，因此將糖化血色素的標準設定在 6.5%。

原本不運動的她，開始了一週至少三天，每天萬步的運動計畫，最後養成一週五天運動習慣的她，體重減了快五公斤，而糖化血色素都在 6.5%。她對往後與糖尿病相處的時間，非常有信心！

糖化血色素的訂定標準，主要是根據糖尿病併發症產生的機率制定，大型研究顯示，一旦糖化血色素超標大於 7%，併發症機率會大幅提高，而且加上血糖藥的速度也會增加。

糖化血色素控制在 7% 以下是基本要求

該段文字置換如此：糖化血色素的訂定標準，主要是根據糖尿病併發症產生的機率制定的。大型研究顯示，一旦糖化血色素超標大於 7%併發症機率會大幅提高，而且加上血糖藥的速度也會增加。因此，對於 60 歲之前的患者群體，建議加強血糖的穩定控制，將糖化血色素控制在 7%以下是基本要求。對於年輕的患者來說，在不發生低血糖的情況下，血糖控制的標準可以更為嚴格，甚至可以達到 6%以下。

為了達到更嚴格的標準，飲食、運動和藥物的干預變得更加重要。在我個人看來，這三個因素的執行順序應該是飲食、藥物、運動。只要在飲食上做出一定程度的調整，血糖就會有所下降。但要培養這種習慣不是一蹴而就的，需要時間和意志力。在此之前，可以使用藥物來穩定血糖水準。如果只執行其中一項，達標會有一定的困難和考驗。建議根據實際情況與醫療團隊討論增強版穩糖計畫，選擇飲食、運動和藥物中的兩項或更多來執行。

減少藥物引起的低血糖風險

隨著新型血糖藥物的問世，如 TZD、DPP-4 抑制劑、排糖藥、腸泌素以及超長效基礎胰島素等，與 10 年前相比，藥物引起的低血糖風險已經大大降低。只要合理選擇血糖藥物，可以兼顧嚴格的血糖控制和降低低血糖風險的需求。

超過 70 歲者，血糖標準可較為彈性

案例 1

75 歲的胡先生，糖化尿已經超過 20 年。三年前中風臥床，需專人全天照護。這次回診的糖化色素為 7.4%，陪同就醫的孩子詢問：「這樣的血糖數值算可以的嗎？」「不是要小於 7% 才是血糖達標嗎？」

醫師則對他的孩子進行衛教，以胡先生的年齡與目前有的其他疾病來看，血糖算是穩定且標準可以寬鬆一點的，所以 7.4% 是可以的。孩子需幫忙的地方就是，留意爸爸是否有低血糖的不適症狀，如：肚子餓、脾氣變差……等，尤其在他進食量變少的時候。

案例 2

72 歲的王女士，糖尿病 5 年了，糖化血色素除了第一次確診的 8.3% 外，之後每次的糖化血色素都維持在 7% 以下，本身無其他共病。這次門診詢問她血糖的情況：「達標的情況下，會不會比較容易低血糖？」以年齡來說，她是可以寬鬆一點。不過王女士接著回應：「之前聽衛教師說過，糖化血色素大於 7% 會提高併發症的機率」

不過，由於她目前血糖達標，生活品質也不錯，醫病討論後，她決定繼續保持現行的治療目標。

與小於 60 歲罹患糖尿病的族群相反的情況是，確診糖尿病時，糖友年齡已經很大，與糖尿病共存的時間，沒有像小於 60 歲的族群那麼久，所以血糖標準可以設定寬鬆一點。

之前有新陳代謝科的老師分享，若年齡在 73 歲，糖化血色素就可以設定在 7.3%；78 歲，糖化血色素就可以設定在 7.8%。若身體還有其他共病，可以再放鬆一點，如：高血壓、洗腎、腦中風、癌症……等。

不過即使血糖標準放鬆一點，仍要注意低血糖的風險。很多人以為血糖標準或是糖化血色素提高，低血糖的風險就會降低，但實情卻不是如此。血糖標準或是糖化血色素提高，只能說是血糖的平均值拉高，但只要血糖的波動夠大，還是有可能發生低血糖。

低血糖的發生，與藥物種類與劑量、飲食進食時間與份量、運動的強度與時間……等，息息相關，糖友能做好的，就是留意低血糖不適、當下監測血糖，確認是否為低血糖、以及檢視發生低血糖的原因，做出相對處置，減少再次發生。

若年紀超過 70 歲，但無任何共病，身體硬朗得很，糖化血色素訂在 7%以下，其實也是可以的。但不論如何高齡或多重共病，根據糖尿病學會出版的《2019 年老人糖尿病臨床照護手冊》顯示，糖化血色素都不應大於 8.5%。建議醫病好好溝通討論，找到醫療團隊與糖友都可以接受的血糖標準。以下列表給大家參考：

健康	正常	中等	差
狀態	少共病症，認知及身體機能正常	多共病症，認知及身體機能輕微至中度異常	末期慢性病，認知及身體機能中等至嚴重異常
糖化血色素	<7.5%	<8.0%	<8.5%
空腹血糖目標	90 ～ 130 mg/dl	90 ～ 150 mg/dl	100 ～ 180 mg/dl

資料來源：《2019 年老人糖尿病臨床照護手冊》

糖友如何接種疫苗？

糖友血糖起伏較一般人高，且受飲食、情緒、運動、用藥順從性等眾多因素的影響，無法確保血糖一直維持在標準值內。若血糖持續偏高，糖友的免疫力可能會下降，使病毒和細菌有機可乘。因此，接種疫苗可以有效減少疾病的發生。

COVID-19 疫苗

建議按照指引的建議，完整接種 COVID-19 疫苗。接種疫苗的原因與肺炎疫苗相同。

流行性感冒疫苗

流行性感冒疫苗可以提高身體對流感病毒的保護力，減少引發肺炎或重症的機率，特別是對糖友而言，更建議接種。目前台灣公費接種流行性感冒疫苗的族群之一就是糖友（不論年齡）。

帶狀皰疹疫苗

當糖友的血糖不穩定且免疫力下降時，體內潛伏的水痘皰疹病毒可能會發作，初期會出現紅疹、不適感，伴隨著癢、痛，形成小水泡，後續可能出現難以處理的刺痛和神經痛。建議接種帶狀皰疹疫苗以增強保護力。

對於曾經患有帶狀皰疹的糖友，更強烈建議接種帶狀皰疹疫苗，原因有兩點：首先，身體內潛伏著皰疹病毒；其次，血糖升高不穩定會導致免疫力下降，復發的機會很高。

此外，糖友年齡越大，帶狀皰疹的症狀越嚴重。除了之前提到的不適感，還有更高的機會出現長期（6 至 12 個月）的神經痛症。此外，糖友年齡越大，帶狀皰疹的症狀越嚴重。除了之前提到的不適感，還有更高的機會出現長期（6 至 12 個月）的神經痛症狀。因此，對於糖友尤其是年齡較大的人，接種帶狀皰疹疫苗尤其重要。

目前帶狀皰疹疫苗分為活化和不活化兩種。若預算充足，或者年紀較大，尤其是超過 80 歲的糖友，建議優先考慮接種新型不活化的帶狀皰疹疫苗。

A 型肝炎疫苗

A 型肝炎可能引發肝炎，甚至造成猛暴性肝炎。與 B 型肝炎不同之處在於 A 型肝炎是透過食物傳染的。臨床上建議從事餐飲業的人或前往 A 型肝炎流行區的人應接種 A 型肝炎疫苗。對於合併患有 B 型或 C 型肝炎之一的糖友，建議接種 A 型肝炎疫苗，以減少肝炎發生並保護肝臟。

B 型肝炎疫苗

除非是 B 型肝炎帶原者，建議糖友接種 B 型肝炎疫苗以增強保護力，尤其是那些缺乏 B 型肝炎抗體或抗體不足的人。

大魚醫師小叮嚀：糖友疫苗接種順序和種類

糖友建議接種疫苗的順序和種類如下：

COVID-19 疫苗 = 流感疫苗 = 肺炎疫苗 > 帶狀皰疹疫苗 > B 肝疫苗 > A 肝疫苗

COVID-19 疫苗、流感疫苗和肺炎疫苗排名前三，建議優先接種。其次是帶狀皰疹疫苗，接著是 B 型肝炎疫苗和 A 型肝炎疫苗。如果還有餘力，請醫師評估糖友的身體狀況，並根據需要和醫師的建議，考慮接種其他疫苗，如百日咳三合一疫苗。

PART 3

拒絕糖胖的關鍵秘訣

CHAPTER 01 減重有助血糖穩定及減少用藥

體重管理對於血糖的穩定有著重要的好處，特別是當體重的BMI 超過 27 時，這部分資訊尤其重要。即使在 BMI 介於 23 至 27 之間的範圍內，仍然可從中學習如何有效管理體重，讓血糖更穩定。

此外，對於希望減少使用藥物的糖尿病患者而言，這也是一個重要的課題。體重管理的核心重點主要包括飲食調整、適度運動以及必要時的藥物輔助。

減重須知 1：3 妙招有助減重成功

案例 1 陳女士是一位不到 40 歲來求助門診體重管理的糖友。她分享了她以前的減重經歷，曾經花了近 20 萬元去健身房，成功減重了 16 公斤，但後來又復胖了 8 公斤。她嘗試以相同的方式再減掉這 8 公斤，但效果不佳，只減了 2 公斤。她非常擔心體重會回到原來的水平。

案例 2 30 多歲的張先生試過只吃蘋果的蘋果減重法，成功減掉了近 30 公斤，但後來因為對蘋果感到厭倦，恢復了原本的飲食習慣，體重又增加了 20 公斤。然而，當他再次嘗試使用蘋果減重法時，只能減掉不到 5 公斤的體重。最後，他放棄了痛苦的蘋果減重法，尋求減重門診的幫助，但體重比他減重前的 120 公斤又增加了 20 公斤。

減重後的反覆復胖是最令人擔心的問題，因為復胖所增加的體重往往是脂肪而非肌肉。過於激烈的減重方法，例如每週減重速度超過 0.5 至 1 公斤，會增加失去肌肉的風險。而不論是增加脂肪還是減少肌肉，都會降低身體的基礎代謝率，使減重變得更加困難。以下是 3 個避免反覆減重復胖的方法，可以維持基礎代謝率並降低復胖風險：

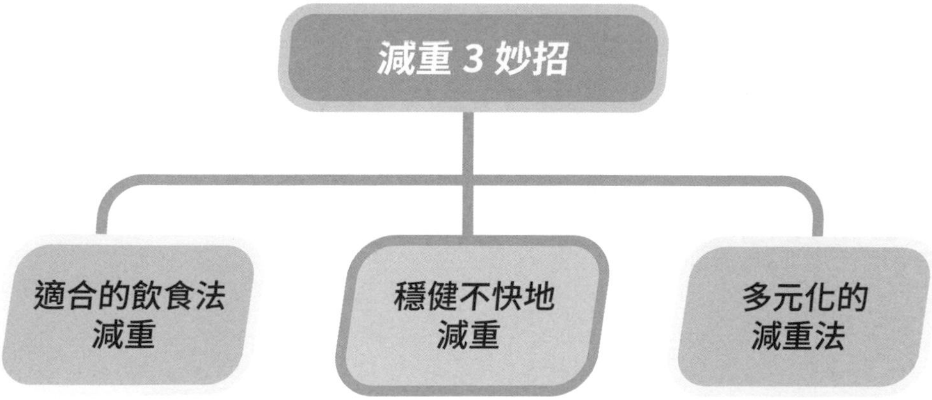

找到適合的飲食法

任何能夠產生熱量赤字（攝取熱量小於身體消耗）的飲食法都能夠有效減重。然而，只有營養均衡且不影響生活品質的飲食法才能夠持久地執行下去。建議尋求營養師的專業協助，共同找到最適合且營養足的減重飲食法。

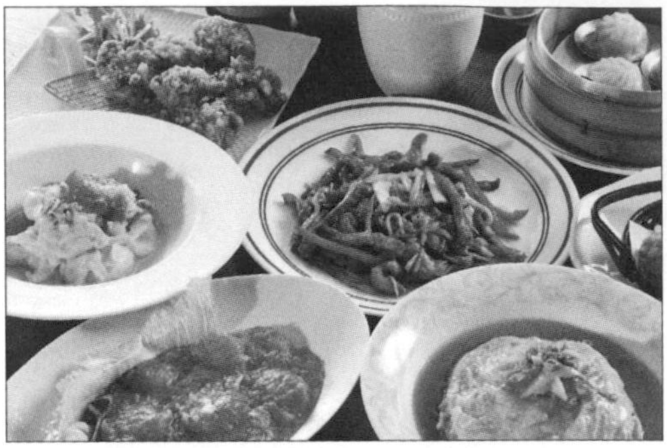

▲找到熱量赤字、營養且兼顧生活的飲食法。（照片提供／余宜叡）

穩健不快地減重

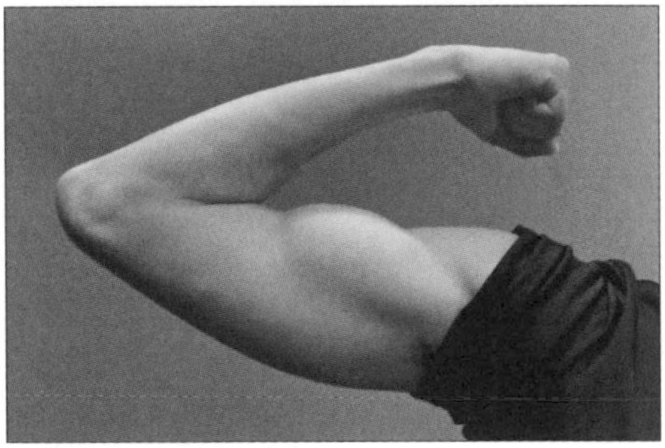

▲減重越快，越易減到肌肉。（照片提供／余宜叡）

減重速度越快，越容易損失肌肉，而且復胖速度也會更快。建議以逐步減少食量、選擇原始食物、增加運動量等健康方式來管理體重，不建議使用極端的飲食方法或減重藥物，以達到快速減重的目的。

多元化的減重法

除了飲食（產生熱量赤字）是減重中最重要的部分外，建議結合適量的運動（每週至少 3 次，每週運動總時長大於 150 分鐘）、減重藥物適應症、有效應對壓力等多種方式，以維持減重成果並避免復胖的發生。

減重須知2：別以為減重手術後不會復胖！

案例 1

黃女士是一位40多歲的糖尿病患者，她曾接受縮胃減重手術並成功減掉超過30公斤的體重。然而，最近她復胖了10公斤，感到非常焦急並尋求減重門診的幫助。進一步追蹤後發現，她已經超過一年沒有回診追蹤了。

案例 2

何先生是一位30多歲的糖尿病患者，他接受了減重手術後，期望體重不再超過100公斤。然而，他在回診後發現自己的食量已經回升。因此，建議他多吃原形食物，而非減重手術前的精緻加工食品。

案例 3

柯先生是一位50多歲的糖尿病患者，目前的身體質量指數BMI為30。雖然他接受了減重手術並成功緩解了糖尿病，但在五年的時間裡，他的體重逐漸回升，血糖也開始偏高。減重手術團隊三年前建議柯先生使用減重適應症用藥來維持減重成果，但他認為接受減重手術的目的就是不再依賴減重藥物，就沒有持續用藥，進而復胖了。

這些案例中都存在一些錯誤：

迷思 1：減重手術後，就不會再復胖？

事實上，減重手術僅能改變身體對食物的吸收程度以及內分泌狀態。雖然在手術後的一年內可以達到超過 30%的體重減輕效果，但糖尿病患者在手術後仍需要多方面的干預，包括飲食調整、適量運動、藥物治療和心理支持等，才能維持減重手術的成果。減重手術後並非一勞永逸的解決方法。

迷思 2：減重手術後，就不需要再定期回診？

接受減重手術的患者，在手術前會接受完整的評估和衛教，手術後的定期回診是非常重要的。

減重手術的醫療團隊會提供規律回診的服務，這不僅是為了檢視減重速度和身體狀況，還包括營養諮詢。回診時會評估食量的變化，確保營養攝取是否足夠。當食量回升時，也可以評估熱量攝取是否過多，並提供相應的調整建議。

迷思 3：減重手術後，就不需要使用減重藥物？

在飲食、運動和心理方面取得良好進展之前，適時搭配減重藥物可以獲得更多的時間進行調整和改變。此外，使用減重藥物還可以減少意志力消耗和增加自信心。對於接受減重手術的糖尿病患者來說，除了術前完整的評估外，術後的定期追蹤和遵循醫囑和飲食建議是保持減重手術成果、避免復胖的關鍵。

減重須知 3：壓力大、吃不停，須從「心」減重！

案例

40 多歲的王先生就是一個很好的案例。因為職場工作的不順利，他開始出現壓力性進食，體重比進入公司時增加了近 30 公斤。然而，透過減重團隊的幫助，從飲食、運動以及藥物協助下，並且以替代行為來因應壓力性進食，王先生的體重開始緩慢但穩定地下降，已成功減去了超過 10 公斤的體重。

最近，當他回診分享他轉換到新的職場後，雖然薪水減少了一些，但工作時感到很開心。以前當工作壓力大時，他總是會想要吃高熱量的食物來紓壓，但現在他不再像以前那樣有這樣的渴望。王先生深刻體會到壓力和情緒對體重的影響。

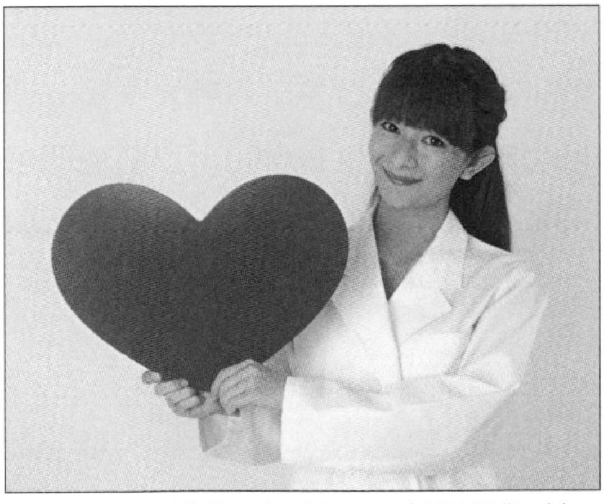
▲從心減重，減重，也要減壓。（照片提供／余宜叡）

除了大家熟悉的飲食、運動和藥物以外，抒發壓力和調整情緒對於減重和維持體重也是至關重要的。在減重的過程中，找出適合自己的減重方式至關重要，並且在減重過程中，不可忽略壓力和情緒的管理。

進食不能成為紓壓的方式之一

在減重過程中，許多肥胖糖友都有壓力性或情緒性進食的問題，導致攝取過多身體不需要的熱量。當壓力過大或情緒不穩時，他們經常會選擇某些特定的食物來緩解壓力或情緒，這些食物通常都是不健康且高熱量的食物，例如鹽酥雞、雞排、泡麵、洋芋片、花生等。這些食物提供了暫時的慰藉，但實際上我們的身體並不需要這些多餘的熱量，一旦形成這樣的進食習慣，體重就會不斷上升。

然而，在減重的實務中，人們常常忽略到心理介入的重要性。根據成人肥胖防治指引手冊，當身體質量指數（BMI）≧ 27 時，建議進行心理介入輔助減重。然而，一般民眾對於減重心理介入的認識相對較缺乏，這影響了減重成效和維持的效果。

從「心」減重

因此，從心減重成為一個重要的概念。對於肥胖糖友來說，建議他們首先自我察覺並意識到壓力和情緒的存在。這可以通過閱讀書籍、繪畫、運動、與他人聊天等非進食的正向方式來處理過大的壓力和情緒問題。這些替代行為能夠幫助他們轉移注意力，減少對食物的依賴。

心理師可以與糖友進行深入的訪談和評估，了解他們的壓力源和情緒狀態，並提供針對性的心理治療方法，例如認知行為療法、壓力管理技巧和情緒調節策略等。

減重須知 4：親友關心變壓力，小心越減越重！

案例 1

黃先生，年僅 23 歲，他的家人經常提醒他在看電視時應該多活動，這讓他感到很委屈。雖然他已經開始認真運動一段時間，但由於活動後感到氣喘嘘嘘，需要休息，他的家人的監督和壓力逐漸累積，加上他的體重停滯不前，這使他感到沮喪，覺得自己所做的努力還不夠好。

案例 2

黎小姐，年僅 19 歲，她的 BMI 為 30。她的媽媽經常說她在外面吃太多不健康的食物，應該多吃家裡健康的食物才容易瘦下來。媽媽的關心和愛心卻導致黎小姐外出就餐後還需要回家再吃一頓，結果攝取的熱量過高，她的體重一直超標。

然而，媽媽卻未考慮到黎小姐回家的時間較晚，導致她需要外食來避免餓得不舒服。媽媽的關心反而給黎小姐帶來了另一種減重壓力。

在體重管理的實踐中，人們常常忽略到親友的心理介入對減重的重要性。案例中的黃先生和黎小姐都面臨了親友關心所帶來的壓力，這對他們的減重過程產生了負面影響。

壓力是體重管理中常見且容易被忽視的障礙，也是導致復胖的重要因素。在臨床實踐中，我們經常遇到肥胖糖友受到家人善意關心所帶來的減重壓力。

要實現健康減重，需要從以下三個方面著手，讓親友的關心成為助力：

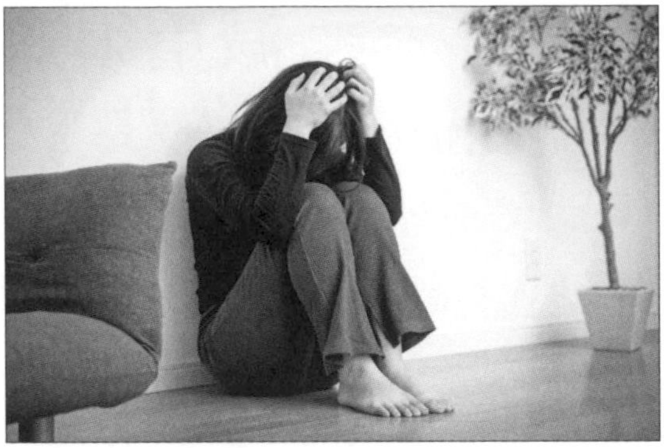

▲壓力是體重管理上常見且易忽略的障礙。（照片提供／余宜叡）

放下得失心

家人應該放下對減重結果的得失心，共同陪伴糖友建立健康有效的行為改變過程。

減重是一個長期的過程，並非一蹴而就，家人應該理解這一點並給予持續的支持和鼓勵。他們可以與糖友一同制定可行的目標，並關注糖友的努力和進步，而不僅僅關注減重的結果。這種正向的陪伴和支持將有助於減重者保持積極的心態和動力。

鼓勵與支持

減重涉及習慣的改變和建立，這是一個艱難的過程。

家人應該多給予糖友鼓勵的話語，以增強他們的自信心。他們可以讚揚糖友的努力、稱讚他們的改變和堅持，並表達對他們的支持和信任。透過正面的鼓勵，糖友將更有動力克服困難，堅持下去。

同理與配合

家人可以陪同糖友前往減重門診，瞭解糖友體重管理上的無助和壓力來源。醫療團隊可以提供專業的建議和指導，並讓家人了解減重的過程和策略。家人可以主動參與糖友的減重計畫，了解他們的需求和困難，提供適當的協助和支持。這種瞭解和參與將促進家人與糖友之間的溝通和合作，並建立更加支持和理解的關係。

透過有效的溝通和家人的助力，黃先生和黎小姐最終找到了解決減重壓力的方法。黃先生的家人放下對結果的期望，給予他肯定和鼓勵，並陪伴他建立健康的生活習慣。黎小姐在醫療團隊的協助下，學會了選擇合適的外食和增加中餐攝取量，同時她的媽媽也瞭解她的困難並不再強迫她吃多餐。

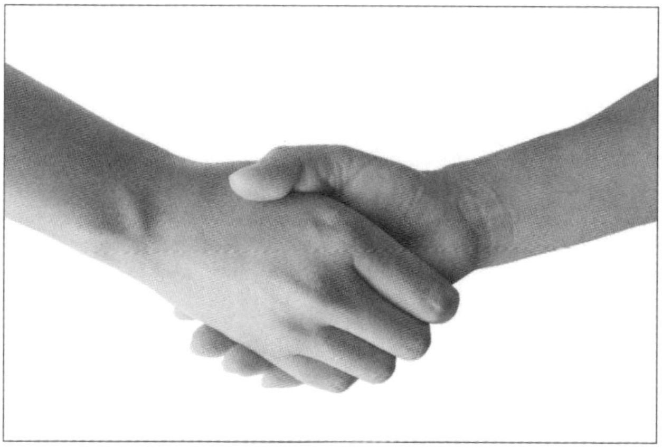

▲瞭解糖友無助與壓力源，給予適當協助。（照片提供／余宜叡）

減重須知5：
1不2要，防減重溜溜球效應

案例1

「為什麼每次只要一停減重藥物，體重就會回升？甚至增加更多？」43歲的蕭女士身高155公分，先前使用雞尾酒減重藥物，瘦了8公斤，但一停藥，體重便回升更多，如此反覆多次，體重已從68公斤增至75公斤，嚇得蕭女士趕緊到減重門診求助。

案例2

44歲的蔡女士以「少吃」與「間歇斷食」的方式減重，只要回復正常飲食，體重就會反彈，回升更多，形成體重越減越重的溜溜球效應。

經減重門診的幫助，她除了維持原本兩次的重訓外，另外增加3次的運動時段，此外，藉由營養師的指導建議，「吃對食物」的習慣漸漸上了軌道，輔以取得減重適應症的藥物，降低飲食的容錯率，終於順利讓蔡女士的體重從66.5公斤降至57.6公斤，後來停藥2個月後，還保持原來輕盈體重的戰果。

減重是許多人努力追求的目標，但很多人在減重後卻面臨一個問題，就是體重的反彈和復胖。這種反覆的體重波動被形容為溜溜球效應，讓人感到困擾和沮喪。為了避免這種情況的發生，我們應該注意以下「1不2要」三個要點即可：

不使用沒有取得減重適應症的藥物

有些減重方法使用未取得減重適應症的藥物，如利尿劑、瀉劑

和甲狀腺素等。這些藥物可能會在短期內產生減重效果，但一旦停止使用，體重往往會迅速回升。因此，我們應該選擇取得減重適應症的藥物，並在專業醫生的指導下使用。

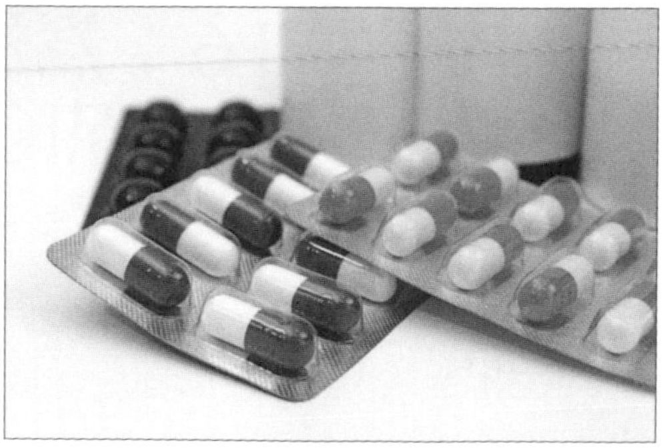

▲使用未取得減重適應症藥物減重，一停藥就易復胖（照片提供／余宜叡）

要規律運動

適量且規律的運動是保持體重的關鍵。建議每週運動5次以上，每次超過20分鐘。雖然運動本身的減重效果有限，但它可以保留肌肉並維持身體的基礎代謝率，降低復胖的機率。透過運動，我們可以燃燒卡路里、增加肌肉量，使得身體更有效地消耗能量，從而維持體重。

要吃對食物

不要盲目節食或完全放棄進食來減重。長期節食會使身體降低基礎代謝率，同時也容易導致肌肉流失。相反，我們應該尋求營養師的指導，制定適合自己的飲食計畫。這包括選擇營養豐富的食物、合理控制卡路里攝取量，並確保飲食均衡。通過吃對食物，我們可以提高基礎代謝率，促進脂肪燃燒，才能越吃越對，越吃越瘦。

減重須知 6：為減重吃排糖藥，當心保險拒保！

一位糖友在收到保險公司的拒保通知後，向醫師尋求幫助，希望了解報告中出現了什麼問題。檢視體檢報告後，發現尿液中的尿糖項目顯示 4 個正（＋）。醫師詢問糖友是否有使用任何特殊的藥物，糖友表示他聽朋友說吃排糖藥可以護腎顧心，並且朋友也在使用，因此他自行購買了這種藥物。結果，導致糖友體檢時出現尿糖的異常結果，其真正原因是服用排糖藥所導致的。

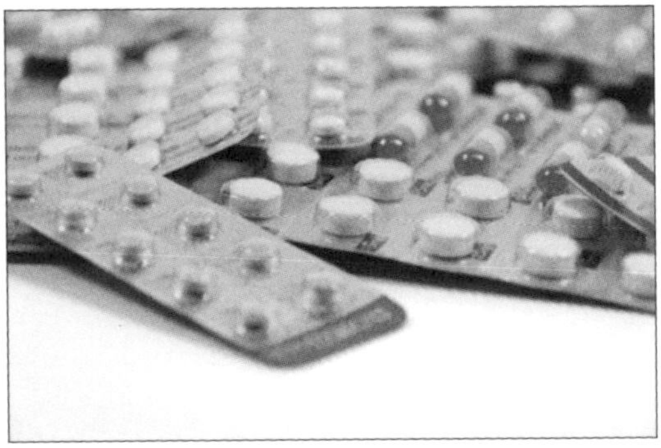

▲服用排糖藥，會產生尿糖，當心保險拒保。（照片提供／余宜叡）

排糖藥不是用於減重的適應症藥物。在第二個案例中，糖友看到尿糖報告異常後，擔心是否罹患糖尿病。檢視糖友的抽血報告並詢問平時使用的藥物後，發現他正在使用排糖藥物以減重。然而，排糖藥並不是用於減重的適應症藥物，而是針對糖友降低血糖和減輕體重效果的藥物。

無論出於何種原因使用排糖藥，都會導致尿糖的產生。然而，即使在臨床上並未確診為糖尿病的糖友，只要尿糖出現在保險公司的體檢報告中，保險公司目前的認定就是糖尿病。根據規定，保險公司對於投保的糖友可能會拒保，或者只能選擇糖友專屬的保單。

基於這些情況，以下是建議給糖友進行的三項措施：

考慮使用減重適應症藥物

糖友可以考慮使用減重適應症藥物，例如腸泌素的善纖達（Saxenda）、排油藥羅鮮子（Xencil）以及抑制食慾的康纖芙（Contrave）。這些藥物在減重過程中可能具有一定的效果，從0～5公斤不等，但仍需在醫師指導下使用，並注意可能的副作用和適應症。至於正常人使用目前則無減重相關研究與適應症的結果。

停止使用排糖藥物

如果糖友正在使用排糖藥物，特別是在進行保險體檢之前，建議至少提前一週停止使用該藥物。同時，增加水分攝取有助於在體檢時獲得正常的尿糖結果。但如果糖友已被確診為糖尿病，則不建議自行停藥，以免血糖升高並對健康造成影響。

與醫師或藥師討論

在使用任何減重藥物之前，建議糖友與醫師或藥師進行討論，了解該藥物的必要性、適應症和可能的副作用。專業的醫療指導和建議有助於確保糖友的減重計畫安全有效。

請注意，這些建議僅供參考，具體的治療和管理方案應根據糖友的具體情況和醫療專業人員的建議制定。建議您與醫生進一步討論這些選項，以制定最適合糖友個人情況的減重計畫。

減重須知 7：打胰島素變胖？——任意停藥更危險

案例

陳女士是一位 50 多歲的糖尿病患者，她的血糖控制一直不穩定。為了改善血糖控制，她嘗試使用胰島素，每天施打 4 次。雖然這一措施使她的糖化血色素從10.9%降至8.7%，血糖穩定了許多，但她的體重卻一直在增加。

陳女士開始擔心肥胖可能導致心血管疾病等相關問題，於是她決定停用胰島素，改為單純使用口服藥物控制血糖，這樣持續了 3 個月。在這期間，她沒有出現任何不適，因此她高興地回診向醫療團隊分享她停用胰島素後的情況，表示沒有任何症狀，血糖非常穩定。

然而，抽驗的結果顯示，她的糖化血色素從 8.7%急遽升高至 12.8%（平均血糖數值在 300mg/dl 以上）。在醫療團隊的衛教下，陳女士才意識到自行調藥會讓身體長期處於高血糖環境中，對各個器官造成極大損害，甚至可能導致腎功能衰竭或失明。因此，她遵從醫囑，重新使用胰島素來控制血糖。

同時，醫療團隊也運用口服血糖藥物來穩定陳女士在使用胰島素期間的體重。一週後的回診顯示，陳女士的空腹血糖在 100 ～ 150mg/dl 之間，飯後血糖在 130 ～ 200mg/dl 之間，而且體重沒有增加。陳女士對這樣的結果非常滿意，並承諾會定期回診、按時使用藥物和監測血糖。

在這個案例中，陳女士犯了幾個錯誤。

錯誤一：胰島素使用後體重一直增加，擔心肥胖不健康。

首先，她擔心使用胰島素會增加體重，誤以為肥胖對健康有害。雖然有些糖尿病患者在使用胰島素後可能會增加體重，但是若不使用胰島素，血糖控制將變得不穩定，對身體的傷害更為嚴重。

錯誤二：暗自擔心，自行調藥。

其次，陳女士私自停用胰島素並改用口服藥物，這是一個錯誤的做法。若擔心體重增加的問題，她應該及時向醫療團隊尋求幫助，而不是自行調藥。醫療團隊可以評估是否可以轉換使用其他口服血糖藥物，同時，糖尿病患者也可以通過調整生活方式、增加運動次數和飲食控制來維持體重的穩定。

錯誤三：沒有監測血糖的習慣。

最後，陳女士沒有培養監測血糖的習慣。她以為只要沒有出現明顯的症狀，血糖就一定穩定，這是不準確的觀念。實際上，血糖值必須達到 400mg/dl 以上才會出現症狀。建立定期監測血糖的習慣可以及早發現問題並回診追蹤，有助於糖尿病的管理和治療。

總結來說，戰勝糖尿病需要糖尿病患者與醫療團隊的積極合作。糖尿病患者應該遵從醫囑，定期回診，適時調整治療方案，並培養良好的生活習慣，如定時使用藥物、飲食控制和適量運動。這樣才能共同努力，找回健康。

減重須知 8：脖子黑黑髒髒，也和減重有關！？

案例

「脖子髒髒黑黑，我一直以為是沒洗乾淨造成的。」葛女士這次帶 40 歲體形肥胖的先生，至門診求助減重。經過兩個月的飲食、運動調整，同時搭配藥物的輔助，先生已經減了快 8 公斤。這次回診，剛好孩子陪同就醫。

葛女士也特別請教醫師，「孩子的脖子後面特別黝黑，是怎麼一回事？」檢視評估後，確認為臨床上所謂的「黑色棘皮症」，易發生在肥胖體型者身上。因此醫師建議孩子要像爸爸一樣力行減重，才能降低糖尿病或其他慢性病提早上門的風險。

體型肥胖的青少年，脖子上常可看到黑色棘皮。實務上，有許多家長以為是膚色黝黑或沒有認真清潔造成而不以為意，但已是黑色棘皮症上身。

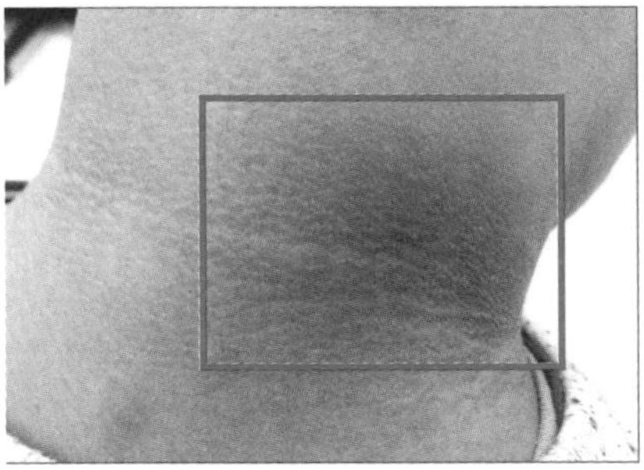
▲黑色棘皮症。（照片提供／余宜叡）

根據「兒童肥胖防治實證指引」資料顯示，青少年有肥胖症或黑色棘皮症等特徵者，應懷疑為第二型糖尿病。若放任肥胖與黑色棘皮症不管，除了可能成為糖尿病的高風險群外，也易引來同儕好奇、過度關心或嘲笑，進而影響孩子的社交與自信。

為維持健康，控制體重，改善症狀，建議做好以下三件事：

確認有無共病問題

就醫檢查，確認是否有其他共同疾病，如糖尿病、糖尿病前期、甲狀腺低下、多囊性卵巢等。這將有助於醫生針對個體狀況提供適當的治療和建議。

糖尿病和其他慢性疾病往往與肥胖有關，因此在減重過程中，確認是否存在共病是至關重要的一步。

就醫檢查可以幫助醫生評估身體狀況，並確定是否存在其他潛在健康問題。例如，糖尿病是一種常見的代謝疾病，而糖尿病前期是指身體的血糖控制已經出現異常，但尚未達到糖尿病的診斷標準。

甲狀腺低下和多囊性卵巢是其他可能與肥胖有關的潛在健康問題。通過確認共病，醫生可以針對個體的狀況制定相應的治療計畫和建議，從而更有效地管理體重和改善整體健康狀況。

進行飲食諮詢

對於黑色棘皮症的孩子來說，可能存在不良的飲食習慣，例如過度攝取飲料和零食，或者晚上吃消夜等。在減重過程中，尋求營養師的協助是非常重要的。

營養師可以幫助制定合理的飲食計畫，減少加工食品、飲料和零食的攝取量，並將飲食重點轉向全穀雜糧類、蔬菜類、豆魚蛋肉類、乳品類、水果類以及油脂與堅果種子類等六大類食物。

透過適當的飲食諮詢，孩子可以建立健康的飲食習慣，提供身體所需的營養，同時幫助控制體重並改善黑色棘皮症的症狀。

養成運動習慣

運動是減重和改善身體狀況的重要因素。對於青少年，建議以走路和快走作為起始運動，逐漸增加運動的強度和時間。一般而言，每週至少應達到 150 分鐘的運動量。

青少年可以從每天步行或快走開始，逐漸增加運動的時間和強度。一般而言，每週至少應該達到 150 分鐘的中等強度有氧運動，例如快走或慢跑。此外，青少年也可以參加其他有興趣的運動活動，例如籃球、足球、腳踏車等。選擇一種喜歡的運動有助於增加運動的動機和持續性。

適應運動頻率後，青少年可以進一步探索其他運動選項，例如參加健身班或團隊運動。這樣的運動活動不僅有助於消耗卡路里，增加身體活動量，還有助於塑造肌肉和提升心肺功能。通過運動，青少年可以改善身體組成，減少脂肪堆積，增加肌肉力量，並促進整體健康。

除了上述三個建議外，還有一些其他事項需要注意。首先，建立良好的睡眠習慣是重要的，因為睡眠不足可能與體重控制和代謝功能相關。確保每晚有足夠的睡眠時間有助於恢復和身體調節。其次，家庭和社會的支持也是成功減重的關鍵。親友的關心和支持可以提供動力和鼓勵，讓減重過程更加順利和愉快。

減重好處 1：
120Kg 胖叔減重 16Kg，高血壓好轉

案例 1

50 多歲的王先生身高 180 公分，體重 120 公斤，他的身體質量指數（BMI）為 37.0，屬於過度肥胖。王先生一直在使用四種降血壓藥物，但血壓仍然經常超過正常範圍。醫師建議他減輕體重，以便在不調整藥物的情況下達到穩定的血壓。

王先生選擇營養諮詢進行減重，在兩個月的時間裡調整了飲食並減少攝取高熱量的食物。在這期間，他成功減重了 6 公斤，且血壓已經回到正常範圍內。這大大提升了他的自信心。他繼續保持飲食調整的習慣，同時逐漸增加運動的強度和時間。一年後，他成功減重了 16 公斤，目前只需服用三種降血壓藥物。

案例 2

40 多歲的林小姐，身高 160 公分，體重 79 公斤，她的 BMI 為 30.9，屬於肥胖的範疇。林小姐已經服用兩種降血壓藥物三年了。這次門診中，她除了拿藥之外，還諮詢了醫師關於降血壓用藥的問題。

醫師建議她有效減重以維持健康。根據林小姐的情況，評估顯示若能減輕 10 公斤，有可能減少一種降血壓用藥的使用。

在經過醫療團隊一年多的飲食、運動和藥物調整後，當林小姐的體重下降到 5 字頭時，她已經不再需要使用降血壓藥物了。

在這兩個以減重為目標的案例中，我們可以清楚看到減重對健

康的好處。王先生和林小姐的個案都證明，減重不僅可以改善身體外觀和自信心，還能對高血壓病況產生正面的影響。

每減 10 公斤可減少一種降壓藥的使用

根據《成人肥胖防治實證指引》資料顯示，每減 1 公斤的體重，可以降低 1 毫米汞柱的血壓。而一種降血壓藥物，大約可以降低 10 毫米汞柱的血壓。因此，若能成功減輕 10 公斤的體重，就有可能減少一種降血壓用藥的使用。這是因為過重或肥胖狀態下的高血壓，一部分是由於體重過重導致的，減重可以減輕身體負擔，進而改善高血壓狀態。

在王先生的個案中，他成功減重了 16 公斤，從原本需要使用 4 種降血壓藥物，減少到現在只需使用 3 種藥物。這不僅減輕了他的體重負擔，也降低了對藥物的依賴程度。對於林小姐來說，她成功減重了 20 公斤，並且不再需要使用任何降血壓藥物了。這證明減重對於改善高血壓狀態具有重要的意義。

減重調整與減少降血壓用藥

「血壓藥吃了，不是要吃一輩子嗎？」臨床上常遇到高血壓糖友需要吃一輩子的藥，原因之一就是沒有減輕體重。這對於身形屬於過重或肥胖的高血壓糖友來說，是一個非常重要的好消息。

降血壓藥物的長期使用可能對身體產生一些副作用，例如頭暈、疲勞和消化不良等。因此，如果能透過減重達到降低血壓的效果，不僅可以改善血壓控制，還可以減少對藥物的依賴，同時減輕身體的負擔。

減重好處 2：小小減重 5%，大大有感變健康

根據成人肥胖防治證實指引指出，減重對肥胖糖友的好處不僅體現在減少共病的風險上，還能對特定的症狀進行改善。研究發現，只要減重達到體重的 5%以上，就能減少與肥胖相關的共病，例如膝關節炎、胃食道逆流等，同時還能提高受孕的機率。

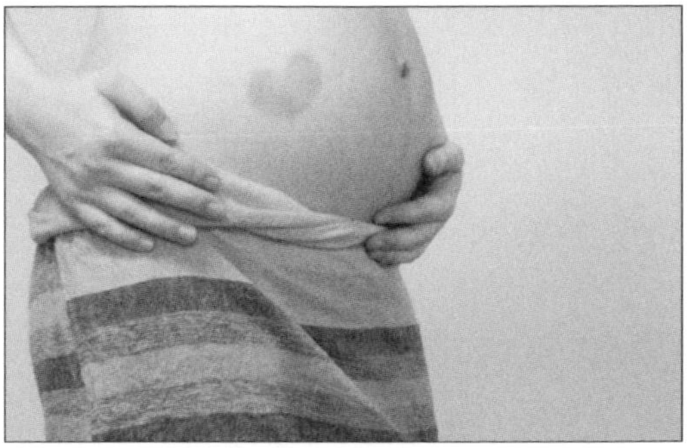
▲減重能增加受孕的機率。（照片提供／余宜叡）

膝關節走路不適減緩

減重對膝關節痛的緩解效果尤為明顯。

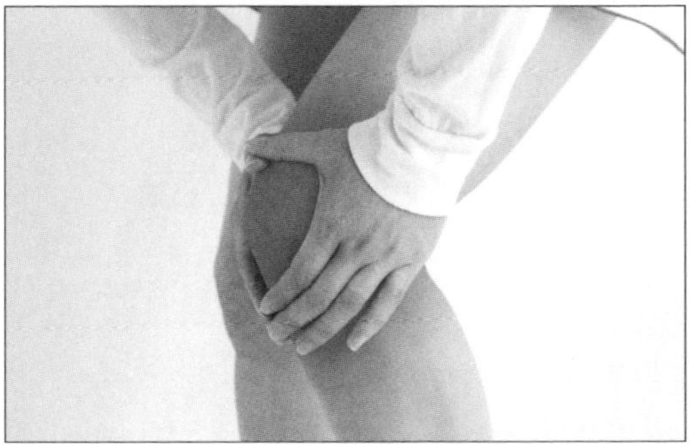
▲肥胖會造成走路一會後，膝部疼痛。（照片提供／余宜叡）

以 63 歲的趙女士為例，她原本體重為 89 公斤，屬於肥胖型的病例。在考慮置換膝關節手術之前，她試著減重，結果驚喜地發現，只要減重了 6 公斤，走路的不適症狀明顯減輕，可以走更長的時間而不感到疼痛。這樣的改善讓她對手術有了新的思考。

胃食道逆流頻率下降

另一位 40 多歲的黃先生也有類似的經歷。

他曾經感受到胸口燒灼感，特別是在躺下時更加明顯。儘管服用了胃食道逆流藥物，症狀只有部分改善。然而，當他努力減重，體重下降了 8%（9.6 公斤）後，他發現胸口燒灼感的頻率明顯減少，每週只有 3 到 5 次，且程度也不再那麼嚴重了。這樣的改善讓他更有動力繼續減重，以達到更好的健康狀態。

改善其他諸多病症

此外，減重對於改善其他共病也有顯著的幫助。例如，減重可以降低非酒精性脂肪肝的風險，改善肝功能異常。同時，減重還能夠減少睡眠呼吸中止症的發生，減輕打鼾等相關症狀。這些都是肥胖帶來的負面影響，而減重可以幫助我們減少這些風險並改善相關症狀。

這些症狀的改善並非僅僅基於單一的個案，而是經過廣泛的研究和臨床實踐得出的結論。當我們減少體重時，我們的身體結構和功能都會發生正向的變化，這些變化有助於改善各種肥胖相關的症狀。

因此，對於那些有肥胖相關症狀的人來說，減重是一個非常重要且有效的方法。不僅可以改善共病的風險，還可以緩解症狀，提高生活品質。當然，減重並非一蹴而就的過程，需要持之以恆的努力和適當的方法，例如飲食調整、適量運動以及醫療團隊的指導和監督。

總而言之，小小減重 5%可以帶來大大的好處，不僅能夠改善肥胖相關的共病風險，還能夠緩解膝關節痛、胃食道逆流等症狀。因此，對於那些有肥胖相關症狀的人來說，減重是一個重要且有效的策略。

減重好處 3：
4 步驟穩糖減重，不復胖

隨著糖尿病盛行率的增加，體重管理對於糖友來說變得越加重要。減重不僅可以改善血糖控制，還能降低心血管疾病風險和提高生活品質。

以下是糖友減重的 4 個步驟，讓我們一起與糖共舞，並保持穩定的體重。

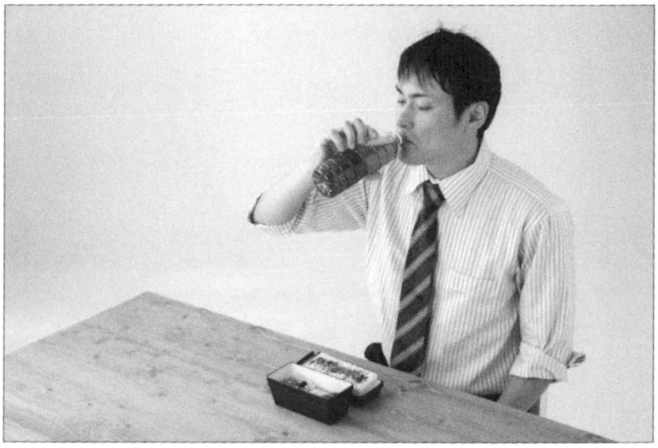

▲定時評估飲食的執行程度、後續力和生活品質。（照片提供／余宜叡）

每週至少量 4 次血糖

血糖監測是糖友體重管理的關鍵。建議每週至少測量 4 次血糖，特別是餐前和餐後的配對血糖。這有助於了解飲食對血糖的影響，並調整飲食計畫，以達到更好的血糖控制和減重效果。

量身個人飲食計畫

與營養師定期評估飲食計畫的執行程度，並討論後續力和生活品質。營養師的指導可以幫助您制定適合您的個人需求和目標的飲食計畫。如果執行程度不佳或對生活品質有不良影響，可以與醫療團隊一起討論替代治療方案。

依指示服藥

適當的藥物管理對於控制血糖和減重非常重要。按照醫生的指示，規律使用控糖藥物和減重輔助藥物。隨著體重減輕，可能需要調整藥物劑量或甚至停止某些藥物。這需要在醫生的指導下進行，並定期監測血糖和身體狀況。

每天固定時間量體重

定期量測體重是體重管理的關鍵。建議每天固定時間量測體重，以追蹤體重的變化並掌握減重進展。這將幫助您了解減重的效果，並提供動力和動力，以維持穩定的體重。

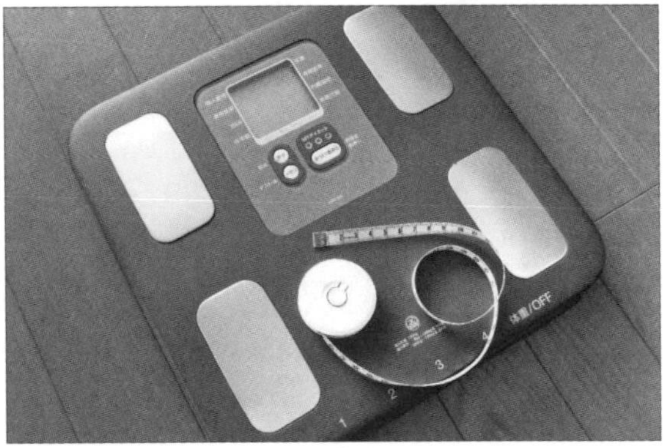

▲一天至少量一次，掌握體重的變化。（照片提供／余宜叡）

黃先生的案例也向我們展示了糖友減重的成功故事。

減重好處 4：「糖胖症」減重，降低罹癌隱憂

案例 1 60 多歲的何女士患有糖尿病超過 15 年。這次因持續腹痛就醫，安排超音波檢查，高度懷疑是胰臟癌，經進一步檢查後，確認是胰臟癌。

案例 2 50 多歲的林先生罹患糖尿病逾 10 年，BMI 超過 30。最近因糞便潛血檢查是陽性，進一步大腸鏡檢查，結果為大腸癌第二期。經手術切除大腸腫瘤後，持續門診追蹤大腸癌與使用降血糖藥，醫師也鼓勵他要減輕體重，以減少癌症的發生率。

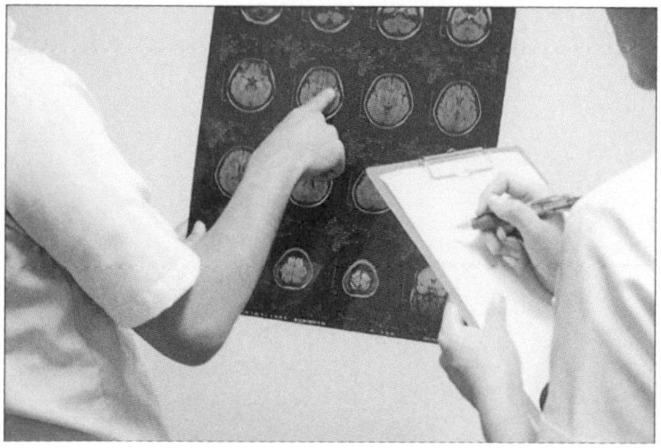

▲安排適切檢查，以期早期發現癌症。（照片提供／余宜叡）

糖友穩糖之外，需留意癌症的發生，其中糖胖症糖友罹癌機率增加。

根據《臺灣糖尿病年鑑 2019 第 2 型糖尿病》指出，癌症屬於糖尿病的共病之一，從 2000 至 2014 年第二型糖友癌症比例，由 3.4%穩定遞增至 5.3%，若要改善糖尿病人的癌症相關死亡率，可能需要各面向的努力，例如：癌症篩檢。

國健署「成人肥胖防治實證指引」提到，BMI 越高，罹癌風險性越大，例如：食道癌、胰臟癌、大腸直腸癌、腎臟癌、子宮內膜癌、乳癌及膽囊癌等，指引也建議過重及肥胖病人減重，可降低癌症發生率。

目前台灣執行的四癌篩檢，可以幫忙早期發現大腸癌、乳癌、口腔癌與子宮頸癌。建議糖友血糖穩定達標外，定期執行四癌篩檢，行有餘力，並且安排其他適切的癌症檢查，以期早期發現癌症，早期治療。

過重或肥胖族群的糖友是罹癌的高風險族群，除了做好檢查外，還要減輕體重，降低癌症發生率。

--CHAPTER-- 02 飲食與體重管理

飲食導入 1：營養諮商調飲食，健檢紅字變正常

案例 1 劉先生是一位 30 多歲的糖友，BMI 超過 35，同時也有高血脂和肥胖的問題。經過與醫師的討論後，他決定優先進行飲食調整以減重。劉先生尋求了營養諮詢，找出了需要改進的飲食習慣。令他高興的是，在完全遵照營養師的建議調整飲食的三個月後，他減重超過了 10 公斤。

此外，劉先生的膽固醇水平也有所改善。他的不好的膽固醇（LDL）從原本的 156mg/dl 下降了近 30mg/dl。此外，他在家量測的血壓平均值也下降了 5mmHg，相當於半顆血壓藥的效果。

案例 2 汪女士是一位 50 多歲的糖友，已經患有糖尿病 10 多年。儘管她使用了 3 種藥物，但她的血糖控制仍然不佳，沒有達到理想的標準。她感到困惑的是，明明她每餐的主食和菜都沒吃很多，為什麼血糖還是那麼高？

在被轉介給營養諮詢師後，營養師發現汪女士確實每餐的攝取量不

多，但她卻吃了不少「不甜的」零食或餅乾，導致攝取總量過高，這也解釋了為什麼她的血糖一直居高不下。

營養師找出這個問題，教導汪女士如何在三餐中吃得飽且有飽足感，從而不需要額外吃零食或餅乾來應對飢餓感。最近的回診中，汪女士的血糖終於達到了標準，而且不需要增加藥物的劑量。

這兩個案例向我們展示了飲食調整對於糖友的重要性。對於那些不想使用藥物或尋求營養諮詢幫助的糖友來說，飲食調整是一個非常重要的因素。在劉先生的案例中，他完全按照營養師的建議調整飲食，成功減重超過 10 公斤，並且改善了膽固醇和血壓指標。這顯示了飲食的影響力，即使沒有使用藥物，只通過飲食調整也可以達到良好的效果。

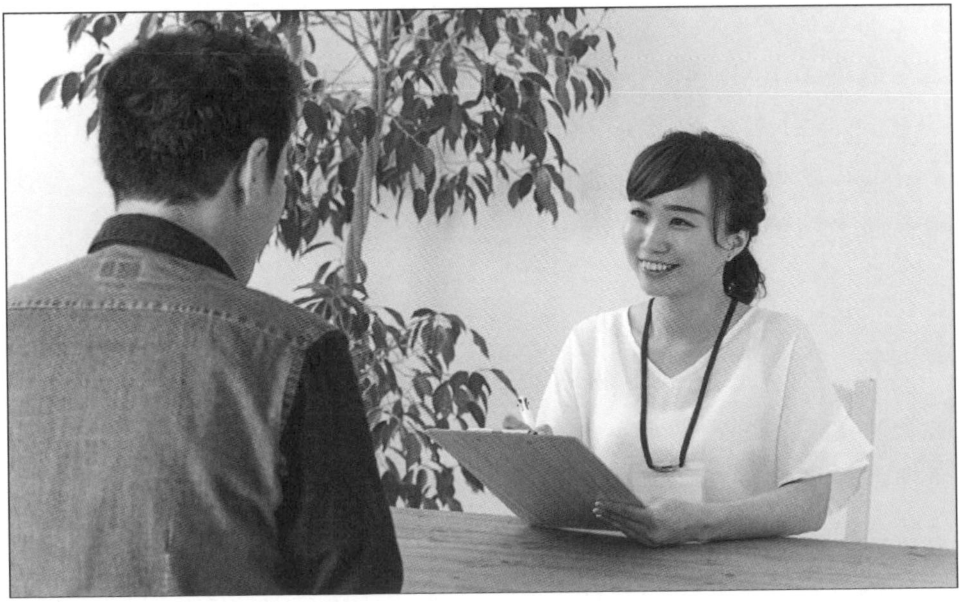

▲營養諮詢可找出飲食上許多問題。（照片提供／余宜叡）

在汪女士的案例中，她雖然每餐的攝取量不多，但卻常常吃一些「不甜的」零食或餅乾，這導致了攝取過量的問題，血糖無法控制。經過營養師的指導，她學會了如何在三餐中吃得飽且有飽足感，從而改善了血糖控制，達到了理想的效果。

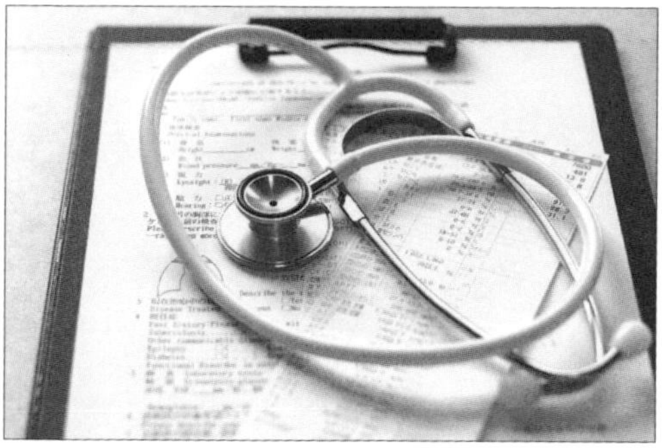

▲有效飲食調整，健檢紅字變正常。（照片提供／余宜叡）

這兩個案例告訴我們，飲食調整對於糖友來說是非常重要的。對於那些不想使用藥物或尋求營養諮詢幫助的糖友，他們可以開始關注自己的飲食習慣。這包括合理控制食物攝取量、選擇健康的食物，尤其是低 GI 指數的食物，避免過量攝取不健康的零食和加工食品。同時，定期監測血糖、血脂和血壓等指標，並根據情況進行調整。

然而，對於一些情況較為複雜的糖友，特別是那些已經使用藥物但血糖控制仍不理想的人，尋求營養諮詢的幫助是非常值得的。營養諮詢師能夠根據個人情況提供專業的建議，幫助制定適合的飲食計畫，改善血糖控制和其他相關指標。他們可以幫助糖友了解食物的影響，教授健康的飲食習慣，並提供實用的飲食建議和支持。

飲食導入 2：線上遠距營養諮詢，減重零距離

案例 1

「原本認為熱量不高的飲食，經營養師的線上提醒，才發現原來熱量這麼高！」使用遠距營養諮詢 1 個月的葉先生回診時分享。

在沒有使用藥物的情況下，第 1 個月他的體重減了約 2 公斤，接下來的 2 個月，分別減了 2 公斤與 0.8 公斤，3 個月以來，共減了 4.8 公斤，肚子真的小了一圈。

重點是他可以每餐都吃得飽，不用像以前那樣的節食餓肚子，同時體重持續地下降。

案例 2

「遠距諮詢加上藥物的輔助，真的不再易餓，也不會吃過多，1 個月以來減了快 3 公斤，而且幾乎沒有減到肌肉！」

40 多歲的鄧女士對自己的減重結果非常滿意。早餐常常只喝 1 杯咖啡的她，在中餐前會有嚴重的飢餓感，導致中餐食量不小，加上晚餐常與親友聚會，日積月累下，體重 1 年以來不自覺地增加了快 10 公斤，很多衣服與褲子都穿不下，經親友介紹至減重門診求助。

與鄧女士討論飲食導入的方式，她選擇上傳飲食照片與線上回饋的遠距營養諮詢，同時搭配減重藥物輔助。1 個月下來，她感覺食量變少，但沒有像以前那樣易餓。

線上諮詢的一個重要優勢是可以利用科技便利，例如上傳飲食照片，讓營養師能夠更準確地評估糖友的飲食習慣和營養攝取情況。透過照片的呈現，營養師能夠看到每餐的組成、食物份量、攝取的

熱量和營養素等重要資訊，並根據個人情況提供有針對性的建議。

在遠距營養諮詢中，糖友只需拍下每餐的照片，上傳至平台或透過通訊軟體分享給營養師。營養師會仔細分析這些照片，並針對其中的問題或不足之處給予回饋和建議。這樣的互動讓糖友能夠清楚地了解自己的飲食習慣，並且在日常生活中進行改善。與營養師的交流也能提供實時的指導，解答疑問，幫助糖友克服減重過程中的困難和挑戰。

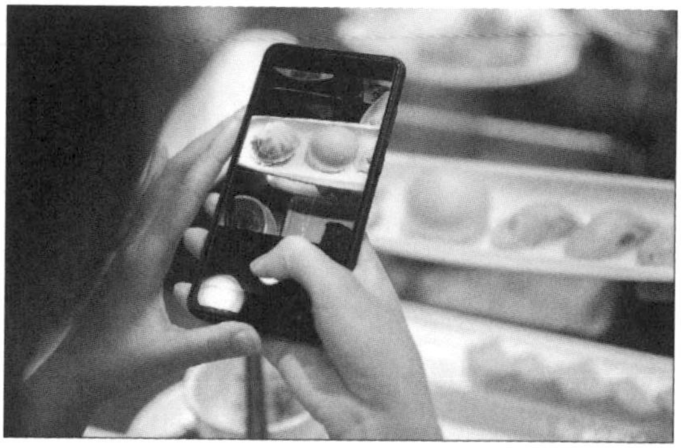

▲營養師根據上傳的飲食照片，給予飲食調整建議。（照片提供／余宜叡）

飲食習慣的改變需要時間和持續的努力。對於那些無法常去醫療院所找營養師進行面對面討論的減重糖友，選擇線上的遠距飲食諮詢是一個非常好的選擇。這不僅可以節省時間和交通成本，還能夠得到專業的營養指導，確保飲食調整的有效性和個人化。

在減重的過程中，飲食調整是最重要也是最根本的治療方法。無論是案例1的葉先生還是案例2的鄧女士，他們通過線上遠距營養諮詢，獲得了有效的減重成果，改善了飲食習慣，達到了體重控制的目標。

飲食導入3：節食總是復胖！醫師教戰「吃對飲食」無痛減重

案例

「每次節食減重，都能瘦10公斤，但最近幾次減重都只能瘦不到5公斤，而且復胖後，體重還增加得更多，是不是我的內分泌出了問題？」40多歲的邱女士到減重門診詢問時，做上述表示。

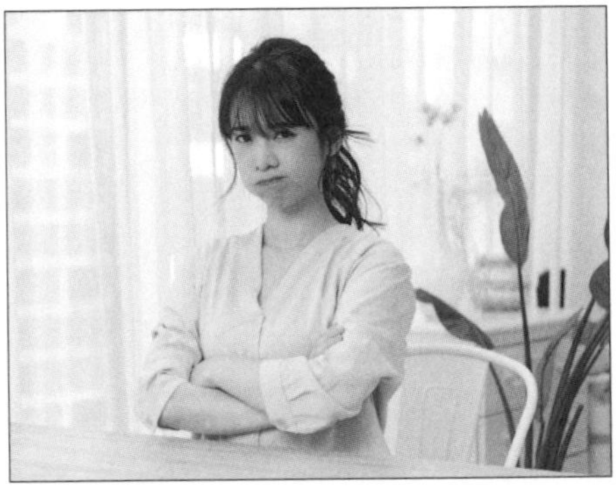

▲節食過程中易伴隨嚴重飢餓感、冒冷汗與易怒。（照片提供／余宜叡）

原來，邱女士主要靠少吃節食，產生飢餓感的方式減重。如此持續一段時間，體重數字確實會減少，但過程中伴隨嚴重飢餓感、冒冷汗與易怒，故而無法持續很久；一旦恢復原來飲食，不適感緩解，但也復胖更多的體重。如此反覆減了幾次，體重反而增加了快10公斤，致使邱女士趕快至減重門診求助。

運動+營養諮詢，2個月瘦6公斤

這次擬定的減重計畫，除了維持基本運動量、使用有減重適應症藥物輔助外，特別加入營養諮詢，學習「吃對飲食」減重。

剛開始時，因減重的速度沒有之前過度節食這麼快，每次回診，邱女士都會一直問：「這樣的減重方式真的有效嗎？」

隨著兩個月下來瘦了6公斤、卻不易有飢餓感、易怒生氣等情況發生，邱女士才體認到，吃對飲食原來可以這麼無痛地減重。

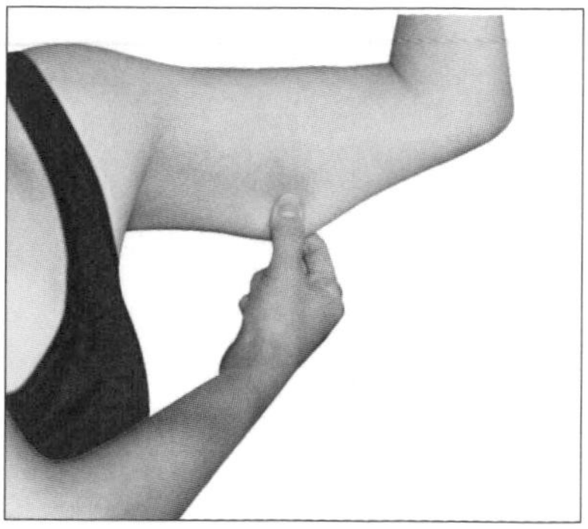

▲節食減重易減到肌肉而不是體脂肪。（照片提供／余宜叡）

追蹤的體組成分析，她的肌肉是少量增加。換言之，減下來的體重主要是體脂肪，不是肌肉。邱女士相當滿意這樣的減重方式與成果，並願意持續地執行。

節食減到肌肉，而非體脂肪

臨床上不少肥胖糖友像邱女士一樣，單純以節食來減重。初期可能成效不錯，但時間一久，有很高的機會復胖更多體重。其中最主要的原因在於，節食減重易減到肌肉而不是體脂肪，肌肉減少下，身體的基礎代謝率也下降。如此反覆發生，基礎代謝率越減越低，體重越減越難，減重就越減越易復胖更多，形成所謂的「溜溜球效應」。

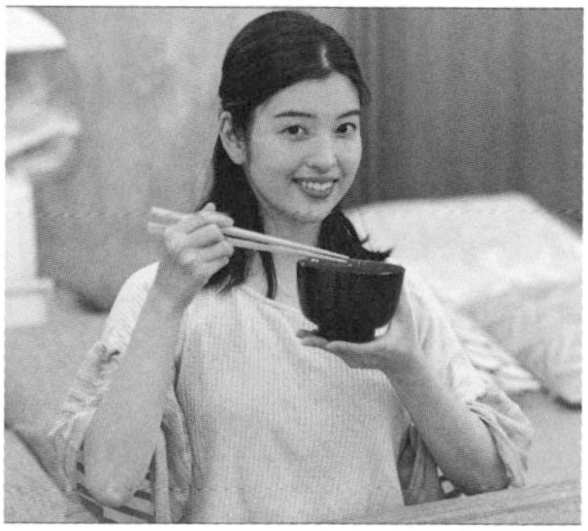

▲以吃對飲食取代過度節食，才能有效正確地減重且不復胖；圖為情境照，圖中人物與本文無關。（照片提供／余宜叡）

因此建議以吃對飲食取代過度節食，才能有效正確地減重且不復胖。

飲食導入 4：水果取代青菜，減重大不易

40 多歲的于先生，身高 172 公分，因減重回診，體重由原本的 92 公斤減至 86 公斤後，開始停滯不前。醫師詢問于先生的藥物、飲食與運動情況，瞭解于先生最近常吃夏季盛產的西瓜、芒果與鳳梨來增加水分與纖維質的攝取。

每餐水果份量，約一個拳頭

經營養師評估後，建議每餐水果份量要維持一個拳頭左右，而纖維質則以蔬菜為主要攝取，以減少熱量。後續一個月時間，追蹤于先生的體重變成 83 公斤。

另一方面，30 多歲的沈小姐，身高 158 公分，體重 77 公斤，身體質量指數（BMI）30.8，也尋求減重門診的幫助。她表示不太喜歡吃蔬菜，經常用水果來替代，以增加飽足感和促進排便。

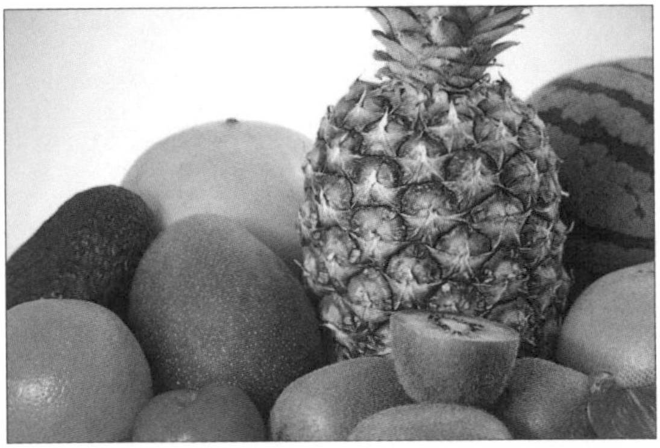
▲西瓜、芒果與鳳梨可增加纖維質攝取，但隱藏熱量。（照片提供／余宜叡）

為了兼顧健康和提升減重效果，沈小姐接受了營養師的建議，不再以水果取代蔬菜，而是增加她喜歡吃的 3 種蔬菜輪流替換。

在一開始的時候，沈小姐還會將玉米和小番茄誤認為蔬菜之一，放在她喜歡吃的菜單中。但在減重後的第一個月，只靠飲食調整，沈小姐的體重健康地減少了 4 公斤。

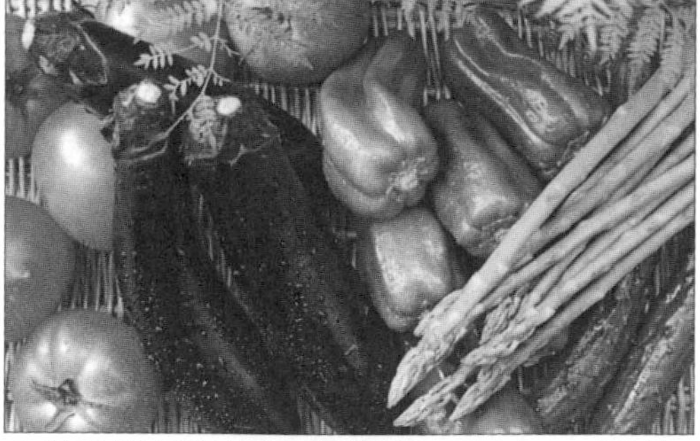

▲兼顧健康與減重，青菜攝取不可少。（照片提供／余宜叡）

注意水果熱量，減重不停滯

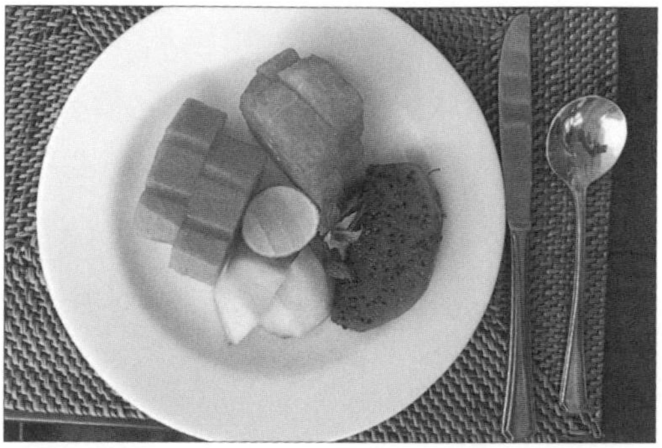

▲減重糖友經常會以水果餐取代三餐。（照片提供／余宜叡）

在減重門診中，經常遇到以水果餐取代三餐的糖友，許多個案在經營養師評估其水果攝取與熱量後，發現其熱量比原本的三餐還要高。

雖然水果含有許多纖維質和營養，但同時也隱藏著不少熱量。在臨床上常見一個迷思，即許多人認為水果屬於六大營養類別之一，建議每天攝取，認為多吃應有益健康，然而，建議每天攝取水果的概念容易讓人忽略水果中的糖分和熱量。如果攝取過多的水果，尤其是高糖水果，可能會導致熱量攝入過量，進而影響減重的進展。

因此，建議每日攝取水果時要注意控制份量，並將其納入整體飲食計畫中。若希望增加水果攝取量，可以諮詢營養師以替換其他高熱量食物，以確保飲食的整體熱量平衡。

飲食導入 5：168 飲食減重法夯，糖友執行前先問醫師

案例　「醫師，我可以使用 168 飲食減重嗎？」40 多歲的何女士在診間提出她的疑問；她身高 159 公分、體重 78 公斤、BMI 30.9，罹患糖尿病 1 年。

50 多歲的李先生則問說：「減重有機會讓我的血糖藥劑量減少，那我可不可使用同事介紹的 168 飲食來減輕體重？」他身高 172 公分，體重 83 公斤，BMI 28，糖尿病已經 5 年。

40 多歲的王女士則說：「醫師，我最近常常會有低血糖發生，是不是因為我用了 168 飲食減重的關係？」罹患糖尿病 8 年的王女士已瘦身超過 5 公斤，目前身高 162 公分，體重 59 公斤，BMI 22.5。

168 飲食的做法是：16 個小時不進食任何食物，只在 8 小時期間進食。糖尿病若使用 168 飲食，在 16 個小時禁食期，容易發生低血糖，尤其是治療藥物含易低血糖藥物的糖友們；在 8 小時的進食期，若是攝取大量醣類，會讓血糖升高太多，若是攝取太少醣類，亦會提高 16 小時禁食期的低血糖發生。

16 小時禁食期，恐怕低血糖

此外，減少體重，會降低身體的胰島素抗性，減少穩糖所需的藥量，考量糖尿糖友主要是 3 個月拿 1 次藥物，在藥量沒減的情況

下，減重更易讓糖友發生低血糖。

選對飲食，不僅減重，甚至還可穩糖，但若是用特殊飲食法減重，如 168 飲食，就要留意高低血糖的發生。建議想用 168 減重的糖友們，做好下列 2 件事：

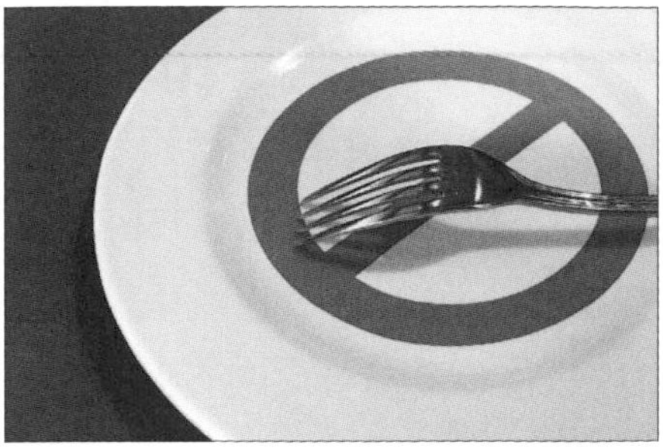
▲在禁食期，容易發生低血糖。（照片提供／余宜叡）

醫療團隊同意後才可以進行

事先評估

與醫療團隊討論，評估個人是否適合採用 168 飲食法，或是否需要尋找其他對糖友更安全的減重飲食方法，例如 211 飲食法（2 份青菜、1 份豆魚蛋肉和 1 份醣類）。這是為了確保選擇的飲食方式符合個人的身體狀況和需求。

做好飲食、血糖和體重的記錄

這樣可以檢視醣類攝取是否過多或過少，血糖是否過高或過低，以及體重的增減情況。這些記錄將成為調整血糖藥物劑量以及判斷是否繼續或中止 168 飲食的依據。

總之，透過事先評估，可以確保選擇合適的減重飲食方式，並且在執行過程中密切監控飲食、血糖和體重的變化。這樣的記錄和評估對於個人的血糖控制和減重效果至關重要，也有助於及時調整和調整飲食計畫，以確保安全和有效的減重過程。與醫療團隊合作並遵循他們的建議，將有助於糖友實現理想的減重目標。

飲食導入 6：
量身訂製飲食，健康減重不復胖

案例

「我第一次感受到有生活品質的飲食，同時體重還能一直減少！」50 多歲的柯女士回診時這樣說。

柯女士初到減重門診時，身高 155 公分、體重 98 公斤，身體質量指數（BMI）為 44，屬於重度肥胖。她表示，之前曾試過斷食法與蘋果減重法。其中斷食法讓她餓到手腳發抖，不到一週就放棄了；另一種只吃蘋果與喝水的蘋果減重法，則持續兩個月，雖然有變瘦，不過很容易覺得疲倦，而且只吃蘋果也吃到會怕，放棄後的結果，體重不知不覺就從原本的 68 公斤上升到現在的 98 公斤。

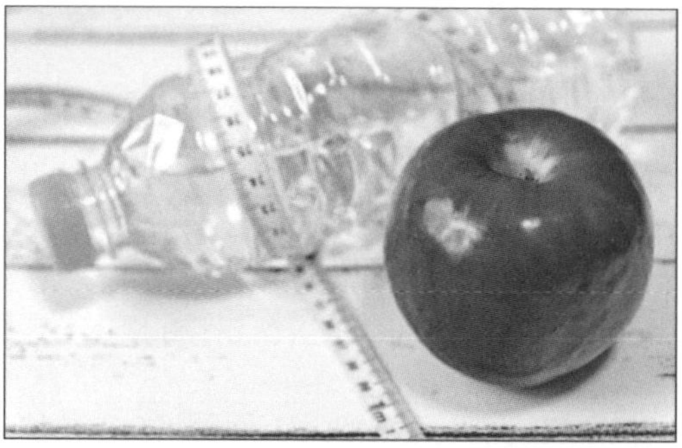

▲只吃蘋果與喝水的蘋果減重法，人很容易疲倦。（照片提供／余宜叡）

因考量她有不好的減重飲食經歷，多次減重又復胖，因此建議她此次減重需搭配營養師介入輔導飲食，同時輔以減重藥物輔助減重。

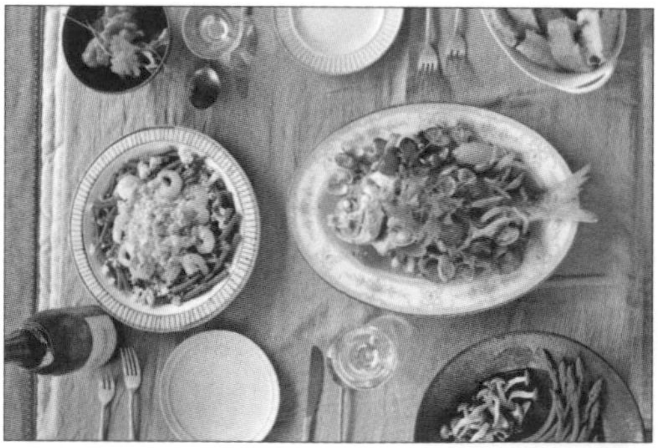

▲調整出可接受飲食，有時還是能吃些高熱量食物。（照片提供／余宜叡）

減重的過程中，她常常反應飲食調整的不習慣，以及有時會有飢餓感，不過在醫療團隊合作協助下，3 個月以來慢慢調整出她可以接受的飲食方式，有時還是能吃些炸物、喝點酒或含糖飲料等高熱量食物，體重目前已減至 83 公斤，重要的是，她沒有發生之前的身體疲倦，也不用特別害怕要一直吃某種食物。

現在她深深感受到飲食調整上軌道的魅力，也對繼續減輕與維持體重非常有信心。

考量個案個人與家庭飲食喜好、接受度、肥胖程度、健康與營養狀況，打造出個人化、可持久的飲食導入處方是健康減重能持續的關鍵。

坊間許多可減輕體重的飲食法，如果糖友嘗試後已發生不適或厭倦，則無法持久，也會再次造成減重又復胖，這時尋找專業減重團隊打造個人化的減重飲食，減重才能事半功倍，健康不復胖！

飲食導入 7：少吃一餐？多動甩肉？減重兩大迷思

迷思 1：只吃兩餐可減重？

一位約 30 多歲的女性糖友，BMI 為 30 的情況下，她每天只吃兩餐。當醫療團隊檢視她記錄的餐點內容後，才發現她一餐的份量是一個 80 公斤男性所攝取份量的 2 倍。換句話說，她一天攝取了相當於 4 份男性的食物份量。這讓她意識到過多的份量導致攝取過多的熱量，這才是影響她體重的關鍵因素，而不是減少一或兩餐。

減重的關鍵並不在於吃幾餐，而在於攝取的熱量是否過多。在減重門診中，求助的糖友常常會選擇減少餐數，例如只吃兩餐或一餐，但仔細瞭解每餐的內容後，我們會發現有時糖友減少餐數後，每餐的份量卻是一人份的好幾倍。

辦法：修正用餐習慣與內容，越吃越享瘦

此外，此類糖友，中間肚子容易餓，無意間就會吃些東西果腹，這也增加了熱量攝取。因此建議糖友使用軟體或手寫下來進行飲食記錄，找出飲食上的盲點，在營養師、衛教師與醫師的協助下，修正用餐習慣與內容，才能越吃越享瘦！

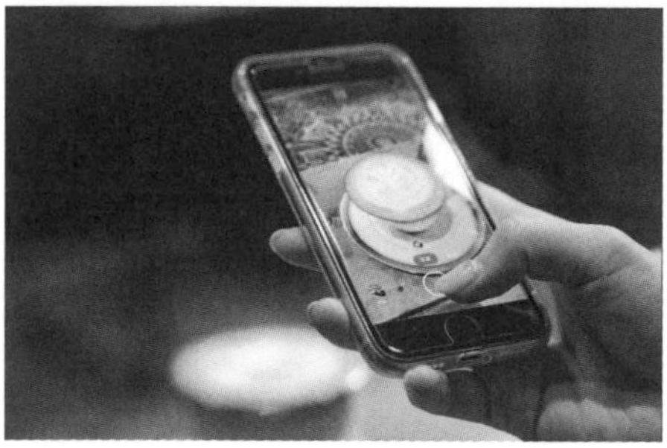

▲使用軟體做飲食記錄，找出飲食盲點。（照片提供／余宜叡）

迷思 2：好好運動就能減重？

在減重的過程中，糖友常常會詢問：「為什麼我這麼努力運動，體重卻沒有下降？」其中最常見的原因之一是，他們沒有在飲食上進行調整，仍然攝取了過多的熱量。

確實，運動可以增加熱量的消耗，但消耗的程度取決於運動的頻率、時間和強度。對於那些從沒有運動習慣逐漸增加到每週 1 到 3 次運動的人來說，他們的運動量確實有所增加。

然而，即使運動量增加了，如果他們的飲食習慣仍然沒有做出調整，攝取的熱量可能超過了他們消耗的熱量，導致體重無法下降。

辦法：熱量消耗，取決運動頻率時間強度

根據《成人肥胖防治實證指引》資料顯示，要實現運動不復胖的基本標準，成年人應該每週進行至少 5 次以上的運動，累積達到 150 分鐘的運動時間。對於年齡超過 40 歲的人來說，更應該每週累積至少 300 分鐘的運動時間，以確保減重的效果能夠持久。

單純依靠運動來減重並不容易實現目標。儘管運動可以增加熱量的消耗，但只有在適當的營養攝取和熱量控制的情況下，才能有效減重並預防復胖。

因此，建議糖友在減重的過程中，要遵循營養均衡且熱量不超標的飲食原則，並搭配適量的運動。這樣才能達到綜合調控體重的效果，同時減少脂肪的堆積，增加代謝率，促進健康的體重管理。

飲食導入 8：戒除 NG 飲食習慣，否則越減越肥

案例 1

60 多歲的蔡女士 BMI 超過 30，因長期膝關節痠痛就醫，醫師建議優先減重以減輕對膝關節的負擔。營養師發現，蔡女士的三餐熱量攝取不多，但問題在於她在追電視劇時經常吃過量的零食，導致熱量攝取過多。經過飲食調整，蔡女士一個月就瘦了超過 3 公斤。

案例 2

40 多歲的江先生身高 170 公分，體重接近 100 公斤。營養師發現江先生每餐食量不多，但一天吃 7 至 9 餐，每餐熱量則是正常人的 2 至 4 倍。營養師建議江先生固定三餐並控制熱量攝取。經過半年的努力，包括飲食習慣調整、適量運動和藥物輔助，江先生已成功減重近 20 公斤。

NG 習慣 1：三餐吃少，卻吃一堆零食

糖友常忽略三餐以外的飲食，例如大量進食零食、堅果或冰淇淋等高熱量食物。建議糖友應確保三餐飽足感，減少三餐以外的進食機會。

NG 習慣 2：養生食物過量，熱量驚人

某些所謂健康食物，如堅果和水果，雖然被《每日飲食指南手冊》

推薦，但攝取過量仍可能導致熱量攝取過多，阻礙體重減少的目標。

NG 習慣 3：少量多餐，攝取更多熱量！

糖友常誤解少量多餐的概念，導致每餐熱量攝取過多，無法達到控制熱量的效果，進而減重困難。

總結：與團隊合作，最能減重

這些案例和相關標題的整稿提醒了我們在減重過程中需要注意的一些重要因素。首先，減重並不僅僅是吃得少，而是要關注攝取的熱量是否過多，包括三餐以外的飲食。其次，飲食中養生食物的攝取也需要適量，過量攝取可能導致熱量攝入過多。此外，糖友需要正確理解少量多餐的概念，以避免每餐攝取過多熱量。

適當的飲食控制與熱量平衡是減重的重要基礎，並應該與適量的運動結合，以達到有效的減重效果並預防復胖。糖友可以尋求專業的減重團隊，獲得個人化的飲食建議，並可能需要進一步的運動調整或藥物輔助，以制定一個健康減重計畫。

最後，我們應該記住，減重過程需要耐心和持久的努力，與醫療團隊密切合作，並定期評估和調整計畫，以實現減重目標和維持健康體重。

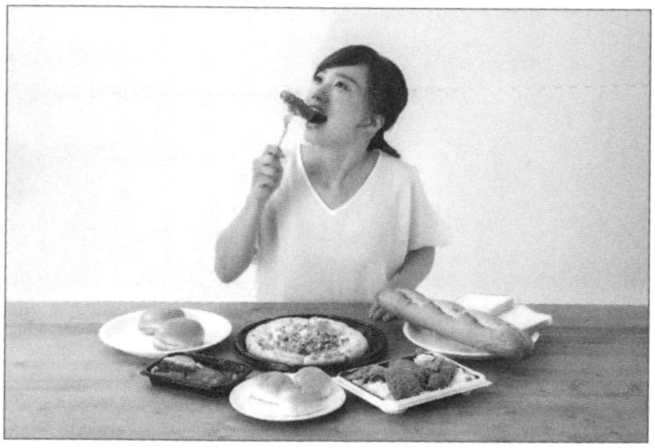
▲「不少量且多餐」易造成熱量攝取過多。（照片提供／余宜叡）

--CHAPTER-- 03 藥物與體重管理

藥物導入前須知：減重用藥常見的 4 大問題

即使大家在團隊指導下使用藥物減重，以下 4 大減重用藥常見的問題還是必須知曉，以便在有問題時可以隨時反應，讓團隊能夠隨時調整和改善。

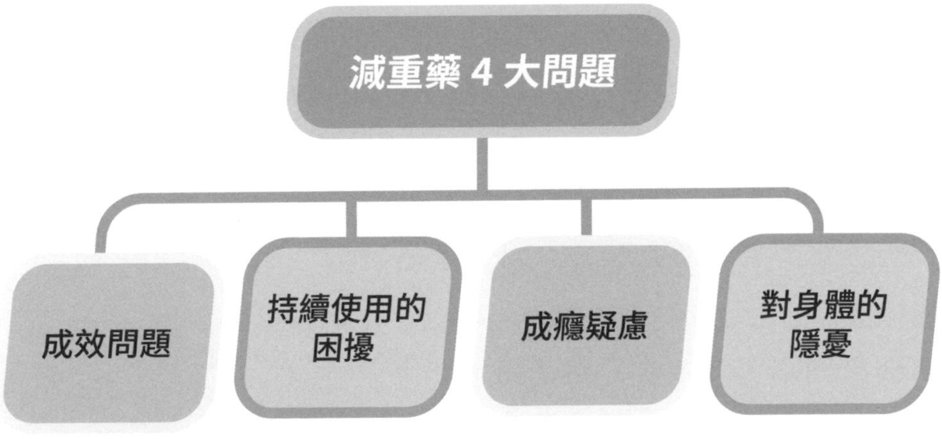

減重藥的成效問題

在減重過程中，人們常常會遇到這樣的問題：「為什麼家人吃了我的減重藥物，他卻沒有因此而抑制食慾呢？」或者「我和我的好朋友使用相同的藥物，我減了快 15 公斤的體重，但他只減重了 5 公斤。」

原因一：不同減重藥物，不同的減重機制

每個人增加體重的原因並不完全相同，而不同的減重藥物有著不同的減重機制。某些藥物可能針對特定原因引起的體重增加具有更好的效果。例如，某些藥物可能針對血糖問題進行調節，對於這種情況下的體重增加可能具有良好的減重效果。然而，當轉換成其他藥物時，效果可能不同。有經驗的醫師可以根據病人提供的資訊，建議適合的減重藥物。

原因二：藥物外，飲食、運動與心理影響減重成效

減重的成效不僅僅取決於藥物的使用，還受到飲食、運動和心理狀態的影響。那些在減重過程中綜合運用飲食控制、適度運動和心理抒壓等多種方法的人，往往能夠取得更好的減重效果。這並不意味著單純使用減重藥物的效果不佳，而是說綜合使用多種方法可以提高整體的減重成效。

持續使用減重藥的困擾

許多人會問：「減重藥物需要一直使用嗎？」這是一個臨床上

經常遇到的問題。實際上，減重藥物的使用是根據需要而定的。當需要減重時，才會使用藥物，而在不需要時可以停止使用。然而，當停止使用減重藥物時，飲食、運動和心理狀態也需要同步調整，否則可能面臨復胖的問題。

減重藥物通常用於幫助病人在餐飲和運動管理方面更容易控制自己，進而達到減重的目標。然而，這並不意味著減重藥物可以永遠解決減重的問題。在停止使用藥物後，病人仍然需要保持良好的飲食習慣、適度的運動和良好的心理狀態，以維持減重成果。

因此，減重藥物的使用應該與其他減重方法結合，形成綜合的減重計畫。這包括制定健康的飲食計畫，選擇均衡的食物，控制卡路里攝入量，適度增加身體活動，如散步、跑步、游泳等，並重視心理健康，適時釋放壓力，保持積極的心態。

減重藥的成癮疑慮

另一個常見的問題是關於減重藥物是否具有成癮性。所謂成癮性指的是使用藥物時會產生欣快感，而停止使用時會產生不適感，類似於吸菸的成癮狀態。然而，目前在台灣取得減重適應症的藥物並不會引起這樣的成癮問題，所以病人可以放心使用。

這些減重藥物通常是經過嚴格的臨床研究和安全性評估的，並且經過國內外藥物許可的。它們的作用機制通常是調節食慾、代謝或吸收，而非直接影響中樞神經系統或引起身體依賴。因此，使用這些減重藥物不會產生成癮的情況。

然而，即使這些藥物沒有成癮性，病人在使用減重藥物時仍應該遵循醫生的指示和劑量，避免濫用或長期依賴藥物。此外，減重藥物的使用應該與健康的生活方式相結合，包括均衡的飲食、適度的運動和良好的心理狀態。這樣的綜合方法才能取得長期的減重效果和維持健康的身體狀態。

減重藥影響身體的隱憂

有些人可能擔心使用減重藥物會對身體產生不良影響。特別是當使用非減重適應症的藥物時，例如甲狀腺藥物、血糖藥、瀉藥、利尿劑等，可能會導致身體不適或引發疾病，例如甲狀腺低下等問題。

另外，目前在台灣取得減重適應症的藥物已經經過大型且長期的臨床研究，證實了其減重效果、副作用、發生率以及安全性。這些藥物經過嚴格的監管和審批程序，取得了國內外的藥物許可，因此病人在醫師的指導下可以放心使用。

這些研究通常包括大量的受試者，持續觀察他們的減重效果和安全性。研究結果顯示，這些減重藥物能夠有效幫助病人減重，並在適當的劑量下並不會對身體產生明顯的不良反應。

然而，就像使用任何其他藥物一樣，減重藥物也可能引起一些副作用。這些副作用通常是輕微的，例如口乾、腹部不適、頭痛等，且大多數病人能夠忍受和適應。在開始使用減重藥物之前，醫師會評估病人的整體健康狀況，並根據個人情況選擇最適合的藥物和劑量。

藥物導入 1：選有藥證的減重藥，申請藥害救濟有保障

案例 1 在減重門診中，45 歲的張女士尋求幫助，她面臨著復胖的問題。張女士的身高為 158 公分，體重為 82 公斤，BMI（身體質量指數）為 32.8，顯示她屬於肥胖範疇。通過檢視她之前使用的減重藥物，發現這些藥物都沒有在台灣取得減重適應藥證。由於使用這些藥物期間，張女士經歷了心悸、利尿或持續腹瀉等不適症狀。當不適症狀嚴重時，她會自行減藥以緩解不適，然而，這反過來導致她的體重重新回升。因此，她尋求減重門診的醫療團隊幫助解決這個問題。

案例 2 另一位案例是王先生，他的身高為 172 公分，體重為 85 公斤，BMI 為 28.7。王先生使用針劑藥物作為減重的輔助，已經成功減重約 10 公斤。然而，在檢視他所使用的減重藥物時，發現這些針劑藥物仍未取得台灣的減重臨床適應藥證。儘管如此，王先生主張這些針劑藥物對減重有效。這引發了一個問題，即沒有藥證的藥物對減重的影響是什麼？

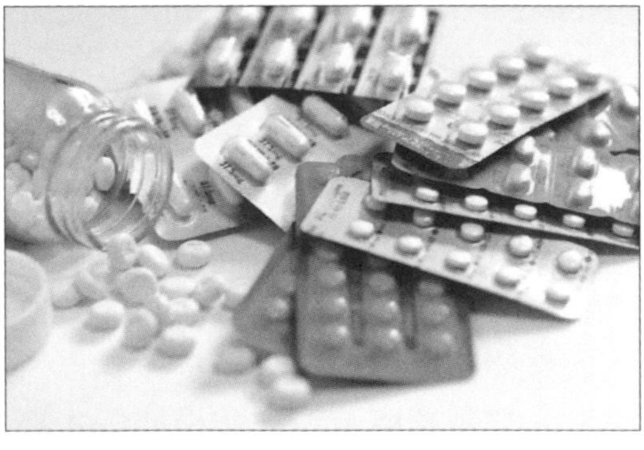
▲用非適應症使用（off label use）藥物減重，無法得到藥害救濟。（照片提供／余宜叡）

藥證藥 1：排油藥

目前在台灣，最常見的排油藥物是羅鮮子（Xencil）。這種藥物的作用機制是減少身體對油脂的吸收，進而減少熱量的攝取，達到減重的效果。副作用為油便、油屁和腸胃不適。

藥證藥 2：腸泌素

腸泌素最常見的是，一天一次針劑式的善纖達（Saxenda）。能夠抑制食慾，減少進食量，以達到減重的效果。

藥證藥 3：康纖芙

第三種臨床減重適應藥證的藥物是康纖芙（CONTRAVE）。這是一種一天使用 1 ～ 2 次的口服藥物，台灣最近才引進，能夠抑制食慾，減少對食物的渴望和攝取量，以達到減重的效果。

上述三種藥之外的其他藥品，若用來減重都屬於非適應症使用（off label use），若是發生藥物嚴重的副作用，是無法得到藥害救濟。

因此，經門診醫療團隊衛教建議後，張女士選擇有減重適應藥證的排油藥與腸泌素，而王先生則採用有減重適應藥證的腸泌素做為輔助的減重藥物。同時有效的營養諮詢，更讓兩人也改變飲食與增加運動量，不再單純只靠藥物來減輕體重。

藥物導入 2：飲食運動搭配處方藥，13 歲胖女孩瘦身有成

案例

林姓青少女，年僅13歲，因體重超過正常範圍，媽媽帶她到減重門診尋求幫助。儘管身高160公分，她的體重卻快要達到90公斤，而且走一小段路就會感到氣喘。她自行調整飲食和增加運動量，但減重效果仍然不佳。

糖友和她的媽媽進行了討論後，他們決定尋求專業醫療協助，包括使用藥物、營養師指導的飲食調整和增加基本運動量來幫助減重。考慮到糖友的飲食習慣，她選擇使用口服的排油藥物「羅氏鮮」（Xenical），這是一種適用於12歲以上減重適應症的藥物。

然而，在回診時，糖友反映使用這種口服藥物產生了副作用，包括油屁和油便。這些副作用對她的生活產生了嚴重影響，尤其在學校的課堂學習和與同儕的關係方面。她經常在不定時的時候需要上廁所，這使得老師甚至懷疑她的腸胃是否出現了問題。

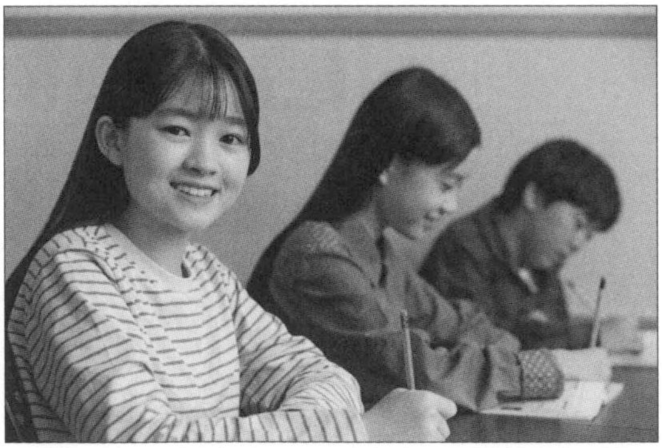

◀飲食運動搭配減重輔助藥，可助青少年找回自信。（照片提供／余宜叡）

使用針劑藥，克服口服藥導致油便的困擾

考慮到糖友對口服排油藥物的副作用無法忍受，醫生改用已取得 12 歲以上減重適應症的針劑藥物「善纖達」（Saxenda）。回診時，糖友告知使用針劑藥物時並沒有想像中那麼痛，也不再頻繁上廁所，而且她的食慾真的減少了。她的體重開始節節下降，終於得到了減重的成效。

此外，糖友還與營養師合作進行飲食上的改變，並保持基本運動量。每次回診時，她的減重進展持續取得進步。糖友開始充滿自信地分享她在學校的情況，與初診時的內向害羞相比有了很大的轉變。

根據台灣兒科醫學會的《兒童肥胖防治實證指引》資料顯示，青少年肥胖已被證實和成人疾病，如第 2 型糖尿病、高血壓等出現有關，也會影響青少年的社會心理健康。青少年常因體型而被同學嘲笑或排斥，甚至缺乏自信，影響社會關係，甚至產生退縮、內向或孤獨的個性。

台灣兩種取得減重適應症藥物　製表：余宜叡

羅氏鮮／羅鮮子 Xenical	商品名	善纖達 Saxenda
固定	調整劑量	可從低劑量調至高劑量
口服	使用方式	針劑
隨餐餐前	使用頻率	一天1次
減少油脂吸收	主要機制	抑制食慾
油屁、油便	主要副作用	噁心、嘔吐、腸胃不適
○	台灣取得減重適應症	○
○	12歲以上可使用	○

▲台灣兩種取得減重適應症藥物。（製表：余宜叡）

多元減重方式，事半功倍

為了解決青少年肥胖帶來的問題，減重門診結合了膳食、活動和行為的介入來幫助管理體重。同時，考慮到特定情況下的個人需求，可以考慮使用取得青少年減重適應症藥物，以加速減重進程。目前在台灣已有兩種獲得減重適應症藥物認證，同時適用於 12 歲以上的青少年。糖友可以主動與減重醫療團隊討論，考慮個人意願、使用方法、副作用和經濟能力等因素，制定出適合青少年的個人化減重治療計畫，以預防慢性病的發生。

青少年肥胖的問題不僅僅局限於身體健康，還會對社交和心理健康產生影響。因體型而受到同學嘲笑或排斥，常常使青少年缺乏自信，影響社會關係，甚至可能導致退縮、內向或孤獨的個性。因此，在減重治療中，除了身體健康的管理，也需要重視青少年的心理需求，提供心理支持和鼓勵，幫助他們建立積極的自我形象和心態，增強自信心，以促進整體的身心健康。

綜上所述，減重門診的綜合治療方法，包括針劑藥物、營養師指導的飲食調整和適度的運動，能夠幫助青少年克服肥胖困境。同時，重視青少年的心理需求和社會關係，提供全面的支持和指導，有助於預防慢性病發生，提升整體的身心健康。

藥物導入 3：
適量服用減重藥，無痛瘦身又健康

案例 15 歲的葉同學在學校因嚴重的噁心和嘔吐而尋求保健室的幫助。校護發現葉同學正在使用減重藥，因此建議他前往門診尋求醫生的協助，了解藥物的使用和相關的藥效副作用。

在門診中，醫生仔細詢問了葉同學的過去病史和用藥史，發現他最近因肥胖問題曾就診並開始使用減重藥物。

葉同學在使用藥物的第二個星期開始感到輕微的食慾抑制效果，而在第二個星期調整藥物劑量後，他已經感到非常飽足，許多食物已經吃不下去。這樣的情況持續了一個星期後，在第三個星期時，藥物劑量再次增加，然而只使用兩天後，葉同學在學校發生了嚴重的噁心和嘔吐，將胃中的所有食物都吐了出來。

門診後，醫生除了開立緩解症狀的藥物外，還建議葉同學停止使用減重藥物 1 至 2 天，讓身體恢復正常後再重新開始使用減重藥物。

並非藥物越強減重效果越好

很多人都有減重藥物越強，減重效果越好的迷思，但往往欲速則不達，或長久使用因藥物副作用而影響工作、求學與生活品質。其實每個人都有其最合適的減重藥物劑量，使用時，也可兼顧營養均衡與降低藥物副作用，適量使用減重藥作為藥物輔助，健康長久，更能無痛地減輕體重。

吃對飲食，提高健康減重勝率

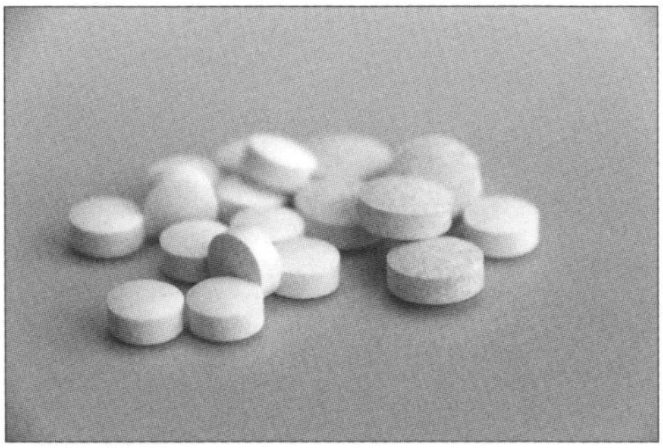

▲每位糖友都有其最合適的減重藥量。（照片提供／余宜叡）

減重藥的建議調整時程只是參考，實務仍需依照糖友反應來修正。目前取得台灣減重適應症的藥物只有3種，分別是Orlistat減少油脂吸收、Liraglutide抑制食慾與延緩胃排空，以及Bupropion/Naltrexone抑制食慾，在身體理想可接受下，3種都有建議的藥量調整時程與最大劑量。臨床實務上，仍需搭配糖友的生活作息、飲食內容，以及藥物反應情況，找出減重藥物的最合適劑量。

要提醒的是，減重藥物是輔助，而減重最重要也最有效仍是飲食導入，因此當下轉介葉同學做營養諮詢，唯有吃對飲食，不做食盲，才能食藥並行，提高健康減重的勝率。

藥物導入 4：瘦瘦筆缺貨！多元介入持續減重

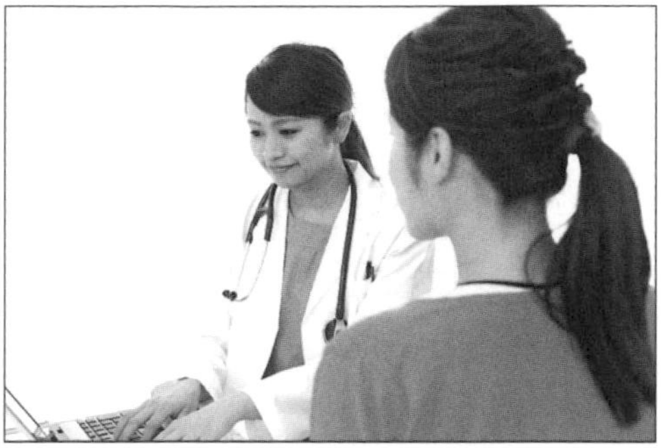

▲瘦瘦筆缺貨免驚！多元介入續減重。（照片提供／余宜叡）

自從腸泌素缺貨後，很多減重門診的病人開始詢問一些問題：「醫師，在別的醫院使用了一週一次的減重筆後，體重減輕了不少，但自從缺貨後，體重又漸漸上升，請問我該怎麼辦？還有哪些可以替代的減重藥物可供使用呢？」

面對這些疑問，我的建議是，在藥物部分可以考慮轉換，而在非藥物部分則建議多元介入，包括飲食、運動和心理方面的干預。

減重藥物轉換

一週一次的腸泌素在台灣，目前都是用在糖尿病的糖友，若用來減重都屬於非適應症使用（off label use），而目前在台灣取得減重適應藥物，有屬於腸泌素的善纖達 Saxenda、排油藥羅鮮子 Xencil，以及抑制食慾的康纖芙 Contrave。轉換輔助減重藥物時，建議由低劑量開始轉換，不要一次使用到最高劑量，避免噁心、嘔吐或排油等副作用產生。

非藥物導入

兼顧營養

糖友飲食調整中會遇到許多困難，營養師與醫療團隊能協助找出飲食的問題點，制訂可執行、熱量合適且兼顧生活品質的飲食方式，如：以蔬菜與原形食物、適量醣類攝取……等減少身體處於飢餓，控制熱量赤字（攝取的熱量小於消耗的熱量）、飲食方式，就能有效減重。

適度運動

運動頻率與時間要足夠，才能有效維持減重成果。建議運動提升至每週 3 至 5 次，一週達 150 分鐘以上。選擇走路或腳踏車通勤，提升達標機率，若實務執行困難，可調整為多動的生活型態，如多走一段路、多爬樓梯、使用手機時原地踏步等，達成運動目標。

舒緩壓力

臨床上許多體重過重或肥胖糖友，可能心理承受一定程度的壓力，這部分常被忽略。除了與減重團隊溝通討論出飲食之外合適的紓壓方法，與心理師或身心科醫師的會談，也是建議的方式之一。找到合適的情緒與壓力出口，有效減少壓力性進食，身體不再攝取過多熱量。

藥物導入 5：減重擅停胰島素，血糖不穩易疲倦

案例 1

李女士，50 多歲，罹患糖尿病 10 年，以胰島素加 3 種口服藥維持穩定血糖。最近她接受親友介紹前往某院所進行減重治療，結果在使用減重藥物的同時停止了會增加體重的胰島素。兩週後，李女士食慾減少，體重減輕了 10 公斤，但同時開始感到疲倦、多尿和口渴。她在早上回到原本的糖尿病主治醫師門診，空腹血糖量測結果高達 387mg/dl。

案例 2

湯先生，40 多歲，罹患糖尿病 5 年。在減重醫師的建議下，他使用了減重藥物並遵從去醣類的飲食。減重醫師告訴他可以先停用胰島素。然而，3 週過去了，湯先生雖然減重了 6 公斤，但自我量測的血糖數值從原本的 110 ～ 180mg/dl，直接跳躍到 200 ～ 300mg/dl，同時他也開始感到疲倦。

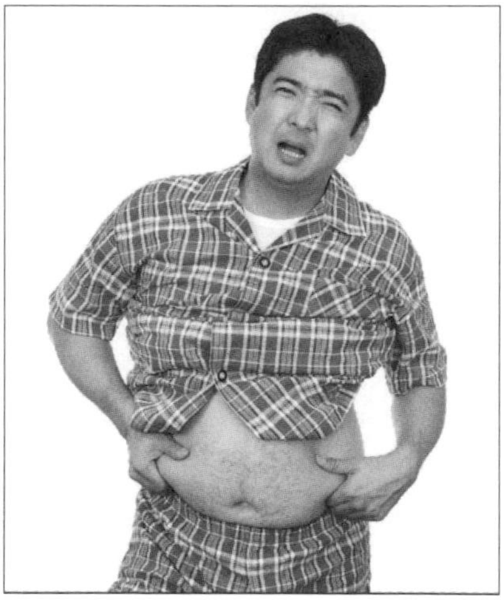
▲減重擅停胰島素，小心血糖不穩易疲倦。（照片提供／余宜叡）

體重雖減，但血糖數值飆高

根據《糖尿病臨床照護指引》一書顯示，胰島素雖然屬於會增加體重的藥物之一，但其具有良好的降低血糖效果。因此，對於希望減重又希

望維持血糖穩定的糖尿病患者，不建議直接停用胰島素。否則可能出現疲倦、多尿、食慾增加和口渴等症狀，嚴重的情況甚至可能導致昏迷甚至死亡。

做好 3 件事，瘦身穩糖可兼顧

為了在減重的同時保持血糖的穩定，建議糖尿病患者完成以下 3 個步驟：

1. 主動提出減重的需求，讓醫療團隊進行相關評估。
2. 與醫療團隊討論制定一個平衡穩糖、減重和提升生活品質的血糖治療計畫。
3. 在調整血糖治療計畫之後，務必自行監測血糖或安裝連續血糖監測器，同時定期量測體重，以掌握血糖和體重數值，以便判斷新治療方案的效果，確保血糖在正常範圍內且體重能夠持續下降。

胰島素作為已經問世百年的糖尿病治療藥物，具有穩定血糖的卓越效果。在李女士和湯先生重新開始使用胰島素之後，血糖迅速穩定達到目標範圍。在醫療團隊的協助下，他們成功地實現了減重目標。

PART 4

專業團隊讓減重&穩糖更有成效

--CHAPTER--
01 好團隊很重要

突破找團隊的 3 大迷思

案例 糖尿病超過 5 年的夫妻，年齡約 60 多歲，前來門診接種 COVID-19 疫苗。他們詢問醫生是否可以接種疫苗，考慮到他們都有糖尿病並使用藥物治療。經過評估，醫生確認他們可以接種疫苗。

同時，醫生還查閱了他們的雲端藥歷和檢驗結果，發現他們的糖化血色素水平，其中一位超過了 10%，另一位則超過了 8.5%。他們正在使用的藥物都是問世已有 10 年以上的糖尿病藥物，並沒有使用近 5 年問世的糖尿病藥物。

「可是之前幫我看的醫師已經開業超過二十年了……」

「可是之前幫我看的醫師每天門診都很忙碌，一次就診的糖友超過 80 人，看起來應該是很有經驗吧？！」

「自從我們告訴醫師我們不想使用胰島素之後，他非常配合地只讓我們使用口服藥物。」

以上是常見糖友對看診時醫療團隊的基本想法，其實當中存在著有 3 大迷思：

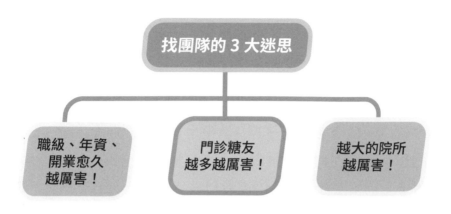

迷思一：醫師的職級越大，年資越高、開業許久就越厲害！

隨著糖尿病治療日新月異，若是沒有好好吸收新知，學習新型藥物使用，或跟上治療指引的更新，常常會治療就停留在之前的學習。一開始的糖尿病用藥，只有 MET、SU 與胰島素，持續了超過 10 年，後來才有 AGIs、TZD、DPP-4 抑制劑，最近則是排糖藥與腸泌素的問世，使用藥物的頻率也從一天 1 ～ 3 次，進展到一週 1 次，甚至已經在研發一個月 1 次的藥物。

因此，單純以醫師的職級、年資或開業時間來評斷其專業能力是不夠的。重要的是找一位不斷學習和跟上最新發展的醫師，確保病患可以受益於最新的治療方法和藥物。

迷思二：門診糖友越多的醫師越厲害！

糖友多常見的幾個原因：經營時間久累積了病患群體、有合適的口碑，讓人想來看診、能夠配合特定群體糖友的要求、除了看某疾病外，還能開立糖尿病用藥或其他藥物等。

然而，門診糖友多並不能直接代表醫師的專業能力和治療成果。血糖控制和生活品質是評估治療是否成功的關鍵指標。一位糖友多的醫師可能在病患數量的壓力下，無法充分關注每一位病患的個體需求，也無法提供充分的衛教和治療計畫。

因此，選擇一位能夠提供個體化關注和治療方案的醫師是非常重要的。這可能包括小型診所或專科醫師，他們通常能夠提供更貼近病患需求的治療方案。

此外，小型診所或專科醫師通常能夠提供更貼近病患需求的關注和治療。由於病患數量較少，醫師能夠花更多時間與病患交流，深入瞭解他們的生活習慣、飲食習慣和個人目標。這使得醫師能夠更好地制定個體化的治療計畫，並提供更多的衛教資訊和支持。

迷思三：越大的院所越厲害！

院所的規模大小對於糖尿病治療有其優勢和限制。大型院所通常擁有更多的人力和設備資源，可以提供全方位的照護和治療。然而，隨之而來的糖友數量增多可能導致討論和衛教時間的減少，這樣反而降低了照護和治療的效果。

在選擇醫療團隊時，我們應該根據自身的需求和情況來評估。治療的體驗、接受的衛教以及整體就醫感受是重要的參考指標。我們應該尋找對糖尿病治療給予重視、關心和實際行動的醫療團隊。這些團隊不僅僅關注血糖控制，還關注病患的整體健康和生活品質。

此外，對於接受衛教的效果，我們應該根據病患的當下聆聽和吸收能力來判斷。個別化的衛教計畫應該針對每位病患的需求，確保衛教重點的準確性和實用性。只有這樣，病患才能更好地理解和應用治療指導，從而提高與糖尿病共舞的勝率。

總之，糖尿病治療是一個長期的過程，達到良好的血糖控制和提高生活品質需要持續的努力和合作。只有醫療團隊對糖尿病治療的重視、關心和實務，才能提高與糖尿病的共舞勝率。案例當中的這對夫妻倆應該積極參與自己的治療，與醫療團隊緊密合作，共同制定適合他們的個體化治療方案，以達到良好的治療效果和生活品質的提升。

好的衛教團隊帶你與糖共舞

案例 1

王先生是一位 50 多歲的糖尿病患者，已經穩定控制血糖三年了。最近，他的血糖稍微超出了正常範圍。在營養諮詢時，王先生告訴營養師一個重要信息：他沒有按時用藥，經常減少每日的用藥劑量，導致一天只用一次藥物，並且減半了治療劑量。營養師在後續的 email 中向醫師、藥師和衛教師匯報了王先生的用藥情況。

下次回診時，醫師詢問王先生，他是否因為每天兩次用藥而容易忘記？是否一天一次用藥會更不容易忘記？王先生立即同意這樣的調整。這樣的調整對於工作繁忙的他來說，可以更容易記住用藥的時間。

當王先生去藥局拿藥時，藥師會詢問他的用藥情況，並強調規律用藥對於達到血糖目標的重要性。衛教師則稱讚王先生，他的血糖控制得很好，一直保持在正常範圍內。衛教師鼓勵他繼續保持規律用藥，這樣血糖可以長期穩定在正常值範圍內。

案例 2

鄭女士已經患有糖尿病八年了，她是一位 60 多歲的患者。除了口服藥物之外，她還使用每天一次的胰島素來控制血糖。這次，醫師與鄭女士討論添加腸泌素治療的可能性，最終鄭女士選擇了每天一次的腸泌素。

隨後，衛教師向她解釋了腸泌素的使用方法和需要注意的事項。藥師提醒醫師，要開立腸泌素所需的針頭數量，並提醒鄭女士腸泌素的保存方式。

衛教成效需要時間

在糖尿病衛教的臨床實務裡，糖友回饋醫療團隊的提醒與衛教，聽不懂或沒有用，如：講得太多、講得太快、講得都無法做到、沒機會或時間提問、聽不懂國語……等，其中有一個重要的原因是，給予醫療團隊的時間不夠。

老師教學需有一定的時間，與學生確認釐清、討論，甚至測試，才能瞭解學生吸收的吸收程度，同樣糖尿病衛教上，糖友帶著學習到的衛教重點回去執行，回診由醫療團隊追蹤成效，就很像老師一次教一個段落，定期舉行小考驗收教學成效；糖尿病的治療成績，就是平時的藥物使用與生活習慣衛教，最後以血糖監測或抽血報告當作衛教成效。

如果可以的話，請給予糖尿病團隊成員額外的費用與時間，討論糖尿病治療的各細項與注意事項。

好的衛教團隊 check list

以下列出優良衛教團隊的條件：

- 是否給予足夠的時間？
- 是否衛教清楚易懂、好執行？
- 是否使用合適言語？
- 是否有教具或模型示範？
- 是否讓糖友提問？

- 是否提供糖友可執行的建議？
- 是否越多醫療團隊成員執行？

糖尿病醫療團隊各司其職

一個標準的糖尿病衛教團隊必須由醫師、藥師、糖尿病衛教師和營養師等人組合而成。

醫師

與糖友討論糖尿病治療計畫、目前血糖數值的意義、可能的藥物副作用、開立檢驗檢查的結果、血糖目前情況，以及其他共病用藥，如：高血脂、高血壓、高尿酸…等。長期用藥，記得一年提醒醫師追蹤肝腎功能至少一次。行有餘力，詢問低血糖的發生與症狀……等。

藥師

審視醫師開立藥物間的交互作用、針劑藥物與附上的針頭是否足夠、用藥順從性：用藥方式、頻率與執行者、用藥上的不適與副作用、分享糖友提供的穩糖重要資訊給其他團隊成員。

糖尿病衛教師

筆劑藥的使用與衛教、教導量測血糖、建議的血糖機、安裝連續血糖儀、初步飲食資訊的收集、提供基礎的運動建議。

營養師

找出飲食上的問題點與滯礙難之處，提供可行好做的飲食調整、因應治療計畫與糖友的生活型態，給予個人化的飲食建議、以及提供基本的運動建議。

當然，醫療團隊若有成員缺少，可能會由其他成員補位。

如何尋找合適的院所做好穩糖？

案例 1 鍾小姐的媽媽 60 多歲，糖尿病快 20 年。最近她發現媽媽的血糖非常不穩定，加上她疫情時在旁聆聽醫師的電話問診時，發現醫師診療時間不到 5 分鐘，只是一直提醒媽媽要按時用藥與抽血，但對於偏高的血糖回應，只是大略式說要加強飲食與運動的調整，於是興起了她尋求其他院所就醫的念頭。

查到網路時，她發現有「台灣醫療院所糖尿病照護品質」的網站，發現目前的院所有在名單內，不過卻是黃紅燈居多；查詢此院所的醫療團隊，她發現只有醫師與衛教師，卻沒有營養師！因此，與媽媽討論後，她們決定至其他綠燈居多，且團隊陣容完整的院所，尋求控糖穩糖上的協助與建議。

案例 2 40 多歲的柯先生，最近做成人健檢，發現空腹血糖達到 156 mg/dl，複檢糖化血色素為 7.3%，確診為糖尿病。醫師鼓勵積極介入，有很高的機會與糖共舞。柯先生特別上網路搜尋了醫師名字，想要瞭解他的學經歷。

因此發現醫師有許多糖尿病衛教圖片與文章，醫師與其團隊都有加入糖尿病共照網，還有取得糖尿病衛教師，所屬的院所還在知名健康雜誌的推薦院所的名單內，另一個網站為台灣醫療院所糖尿病照護品質，發現許多都是取得綠燈的好成績，更確認自己要長期在此院所，好好學習與糖共舞。

你是否已經找到一個願意聆聽你對穩糖需求的醫療團隊？你是否找到願意努力調整治療方式以幫助你穩定血糖的醫療團隊？血糖控制和生活品質之間的平衡是糖友配合程度和與醫療團隊溝通能力的考驗。如果你的醫療團隊無法提供足夠的機會和時間來互相溝通和了解，那麼要實現血糖控制的好再更好就變得很困難。

在血糖控制的旅程中，不斷試驗和調整藥物治療、飲食替換和與醫療團隊密切合作是非常重要的。通過遵循這些原則，我們可以讓血糖與生活品質相輔相成，達到穩定達標的血糖並享受美好的生活。

如何尋找合適的院所做早期治療其實有一些相關指引可以參考。以下是一些方法和資源可以幫助您做出選擇：

查詢「台灣醫療院所糖尿病照護品質排行榜」

這是一個評估糖尿病照護品質的公開網站，使用紅黃綠燈來顯示院所照護糖尿病的成績。建議選擇綠燈越多的院所，或是對自己最在意的項目為綠燈的院所。

網路搜尋

除了醫療人員是否推薦外，還可以查詢院所或醫療團隊在糖尿病相關領域的專業程度。可以搜索醫師的學經歷、糖尿病衛教圖片與文章、糖尿病照護網相關的成績與是否得獎、糖尿病共照網的收案人數，以及是否有取得糖尿病衛教師資格的人數（包括醫師、衛教師與營養師）等。

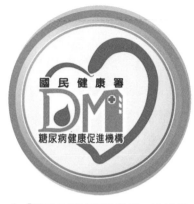

▲「糖尿病健康促進機構」是找尋合適的院所標準之一。

糖友就醫心得與口碑

可以尋找其他糖友的就醫心得與口碑，這些可以在糖尿病相關網站、討論區或社群平台上找到。

各大學會舉辦的血糖競賽

可以了解院所或醫療團隊是否參與各大學會舉辦的血糖競賽，以及是否有獲得獎項。

健康類雜誌評比或整理

可以參考健康類雜誌如康健雜誌、常春雜誌等對院所的評比或整理。

其他綜合考量

最後，還是要以看診的感受、血糖的成績以及交通的方便來做綜合考量，找到合適的醫療團隊和院所，讓您能夠進行早期治療並在控制糖尿病的路上不感到孤單。記得和醫師或專業團隊討論您的需求和期望，並確保您在選擇的院所中獲得全面的糖尿病照護，包括醫療指導、衛教資訊、營養諮詢等。

祝您找到合適的院所，並取得良好的糖尿病治療效果！

哪一種醫師最能幫助穩糖？

案例

「每次帶著血糖測量記錄去看醫生，他從來不正眼看一下；在聆聽衛教時，衛教師也從血糖記錄中沒有提出建議或說明，哪怕只是一句鼓勵或改進的話語。」

「每次我想和醫生多進行一些詢問或討論，醫生就會說：“到底你是醫師還是我是醫師？”但事實上，我只是想更深入地了解是否需要吃這麼多的血糖藥物。」

每次回診，醫生都會要求我測量血糖並記錄飲食。除了營養師和衛教師之外，醫生也會提供關於穩定血糖的基本而重要的建議。如果這些建議與營養師或衛教師的建議類似，那就表示這是經過多位醫護人員的確認和認可，現在應該優先進行調整和改善。

「等待兩個小時，只能見醫生兩分鐘。等待半小時，則只有 2 分鐘的時間。」我想這是許多糖尿病患者就醫時的共同經驗。那到底哪種情況比較好呢？沒有確定的答案，但對於受生活習慣（飲食和運動）影響較大的糖尿病患者來說，多一些門診時間進行衛教和討論可能是更好的選擇。

資深才好？

「醫師看起來太年輕，感覺糖尿病不會很厲害，我還是找資深點的醫師來治療我的糖尿病。」

資不資深只是參考。只要年紀夠或執業夠久就會資深，但重點是要端視醫療團隊在糖尿病上的學習與進修。隨著糖尿病治療的日新月異，差了一年的學習與更新，治療目標與方式，就能優先順序與選擇，就不一樣了。

屬性相投

「醫師你看起來就沒有一定的威嚴，而且也不會罵我血糖控制不好，我還是去找嚴格一點的醫師好了。」

每位醫師都有各自的看病風格與特色。相信喜歡被罵的糖友，一定可以找到開罵糖友的醫師；喜歡被鼓勵的糖友，一定可以找到鼓勵型醫師；喜歡與醫師討論交流的糖友，一定可以找到交流型的醫師。

類似情形

「我只是要拿一樣的血糖藥物，你問這麼多做什麼？我原來的醫師看了我很久！」同樣的，只是單純拿藥的糖友，也可以找到每次回診就是拿藥的醫師，沒有什麼不好。

但遇到筆者，若您的血糖有生活品質地達標，醫師不會再多問；當個照拿藥的醫師，其實不到 1 分鐘就可將處方開立完成，就可以拿到掛號費與診療費，但是若是達標或生活品質沒做好，醫師就會多問一些糖友的想法，而多問一些只是想要您能穩糖。

有效衛教

看診時間的長短並不是重點，重點在於在醫院就診時，糖尿病患者是否獲得了有效且具體的衛教和重要提醒。

例如，將運動時間從原本的 20 分鐘調整為 30 分鐘，將手臂舉重的負荷從0.6公斤調整為1.0公斤，每餐的白飯量從2碗減少到1.5碗，每餐的青菜量增加到半碗以上，將治療計畫中加入一天一次的半顆藥物，以及如果連續三天的空腹血糖超過 130mg/dl，則施打上週 2 單位的胰島素，同時繼續監測空腹血糖等等。即使在有限的門診時間內，仍然可以進行明確的衛教。

因材施教

不同的學生，需要不同的教導。不同的糖友，需要不同的衛教與討論方式，如：一切遵照醫師指示用藥、主要交給醫師與團隊處置，但會想問一些問題、想和醫療團隊討論治療計畫、醫療團隊好好督促或是寬鬆對待穩糖過程的調整與學習、有話直說，甚至可以念一下、委婉告知同時給予鼓勵……等。

找到合適

不同的糖友對糖尿病治療有不同的期許。試著找到合適您期許的醫師與醫療團隊，若是不合適的話，容易造成每次的回診或衛教，傷害到醫病雙方；當每次的看病或衛教感受不是很好，經反應也無法改善時，就是可轉換醫療團隊的時候，不論是請醫療團隊轉介，或是您或家屬尋找更合適的團隊。

大余醫師小叮嚀：與醫師互動良好很重要

現場的互動與討論、治療是否有達標，以及感受是否良好，對於需長期診療的糖尿病是相當重要的，尤其在這個看病快速的環境裡，益顯珍貴。

不復胖關鍵：多元減重 衝過停滯期不復胖

案例 柯先生是一位30多歲，身體質量指數（BMI）為32的患者。他一開始嘗試通過營養諮詢和調整飲食來減重。起初的成效還不錯，他在兩週內成功減重了2公斤。然而，一個月後，他的體重又回升了1公斤。

原來，柯先生在這個月的週末經常與親友一起光顧燒肉店或吃到飽餐廳，大快朵頤。此外，由於工作壓力增大，晚上他也不自覺地吃進了一些高熱量和重口味的食物，例如麻辣鍋、鹽酥雞等。

針對柯先生的個案，除了建議調整飲食方式和選擇更適合的食物之外，我們還建議他每週進行兩次肌力運動，同時考慮使用減重輔助藥物。

此外，柯先生已經開始學習在減重過程中尋找飲食以外的方式來紓壓，例如寫日記和閱讀等休閒娛樂。在過去的兩個月裡，柯先生已經成功減重了近5公斤，對目前的減重治療計畫感到滿意。

根據《成人肥胖防治實證指引》相關資料顯示，肥胖治療的主流概念在於多元介入，從飲食、運動、行為、藥物、外科手術等各個方面進行綜合考慮，制定個別化的治療計畫和建議。

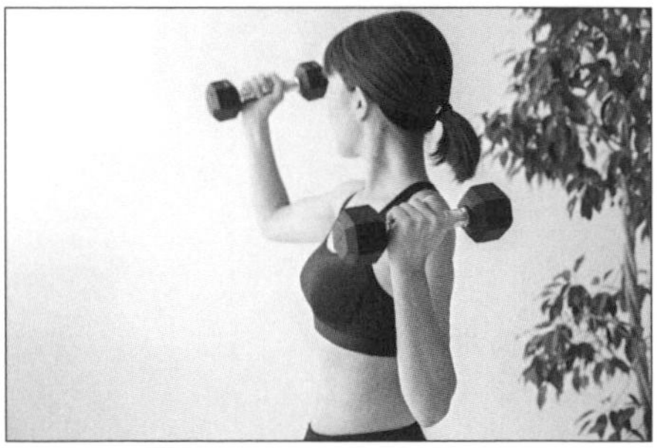

▲運動是多元減重方式之一。（照片提供／余宜叡）

在實踐中，採用多元化的減重方法可以增加減重的成功機率，同時降低復胖的風險。除了飲食方面的多元調整外，還可以考慮使用減重適應症藥物、進行有氧或無氧運動、接受心理諮詢以及尋找飲食以外的休閒活動等。這些方法都屬於多元介入的範疇。

專屬自己的多元減重專案

找出適合自己的減重方式至關重要，這樣才能有效地減重並避免停滯期或復胖的問題。建議尋找提供多元減重方法的醫療團隊，他們能夠根據個人的情況和需求，提供多種輔助減重方法和個別化的治療計畫。

這樣的醫療團隊可以結合專業的營養師、運動專家、心理諮詢師等，協助柯先生制定一個全面的減重計畫。營養師可以提供飲食指導，根據柯先生的喜好和需求，制定適合他的均衡飲食方案。運動專家可以設計適合柯先生的運動計畫，包括有氧運動和肌力運動，以增加卡路里消耗並提升新陳代謝率。心理諮詢師可以幫助柯先生處理壓力和情緒飲食的問題，提供情緒管理和壓力紓解的方法。

監測和定期回診

此外，減重過程中的監測和定期回診也是重要的一環。柯先生應該定期追蹤體重變化、血壓和其他相關指標，並與醫療團隊保持緊密的溝通和合作。根據柯先生的進展和需要，醫療團隊可以隨時調整治療計畫，確保減重效果的持續和長期成功。

--CHAPTER-- 02 案例分享

減重患者心得 1：
快樂 8 週，享瘦 10 公斤

門診患者基本資料

暱稱：蔡佳芸
年紀：44
性別：女
職業：教育單位主管

所有的人成功元素都相似，而深陷減重迴圈的人則敗因各不相同。

年輕時貌美如花，職場起步走後，工作與家庭雙重夾擊，體重跟體型齊步奔赴穩重中年的人多的是；而我也不例外。

跨過 40 歲之後，工作也進入任重道遠新階段，每天都以 8 小時油門踩到底的衝勁耕耘，回到家後難免也會犒賞自己。一回神來，體重從 56 公斤直升到 66 公斤，三、四年間已經胖了 10 公斤。

認知到骨感稱號有去無回的事實之後，我進入了第二個階段——挨餓耐力賽。畢竟運動是無比的讓人感到無趣。這段時間為期一年，我在無目標的挨餓和偶爾心理反彈間折返跑，體重也頑固地守在 64 公斤到 66.5 公斤間，不見其效。

一道曙光 門診學習

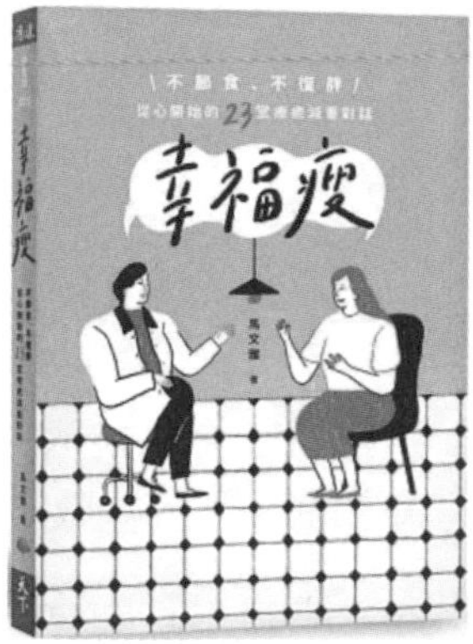

在第一次門診中，大魚醫師指定了必讀書目《幸福瘦：不節食、不復胖，從心開始的 23 堂療癒減重對話》一書。其中的一句公式：「你吃下去的熱量－你身體所需的熱量＝你心靈的匱乏程度」，絕對是一記黃金左鉤拳，徹底擊碎了我身陷減重迴圈的假面具。

門診過程，我學到以下幾點：

1. 無論遲或早，任何人都需要有控醣的覺醒，因為屆時都會需要用到。
2. 總熱量管控期間不一定要以一日為單位，以週為單位更具彈性，也更好操作。
3. 週總（熱）量控管，有助達成身體減醣目標與心理平衡需求，避免暴飲暴食。
4. 工作壓力下需要的大餐，吃完再來減容易失敗。反之，以預借熱量的方式，前幾餐就控制熱量，大餐就能放心吃（實際上會捨不得大吃）。
5. 只要能降低胰島素阻抗，對減重會有很關鍵的影響。

觀念先行 飲食管理

行為的改變需要觀念先行，減重的成功與失敗多涉及心理層面。每次與大魚醫師的門診就像輕鬆的聊天，他總能在不經意間揭示出我觀念上的錯誤，迫使我正視自己思維的盲點。改變觀念不是一蹴可幾的，尤其隨著年紀增長，越來越難。能夠讓糖友慢慢認清現況，並在適當時機給予引導，絕對是大魚醫師的超能力。

科技在營養監控中扮演了重要的角色。糖友可以使用「App 智抗糖」來控制飲食，並定期獲得營養師的回饋。對我來說，誠實且聰明地使用這些軟體，可以在一定程度上增加減重成功的機會。

誠實是關鍵

吃鹹酥雞或喝啤酒也照 Po，完全不隱瞞，因為減重的決定是我自己做的，自欺欺人說吃得很少是愚蠢的行為。

靈活運用谷歌（Google）大神

如果忘了拍照記錄飲食，我隨時可以透過谷歌搜尋來找到相同餐點的圖片補上。外出用餐如果不好意思拍照，也可以參考其他人的食記，找到同一間餐廳相似的餐點即可。

因此，記錄飲食變得零難度。

最後一哩 快樂享瘦

大魚醫師建議使用筆型注射器來穩定減重期間的血糖。減少熱量攝取不僅僅是毅力的問題，毅力再加上觀念的改變，在面對工作壓力時仍然可能無法承受。在醫學專業的監控下，正確使用藥物絕對是成功減重的關鍵。

腸泌素使我的血糖在專注攝取身體所需熱量時不會出問題，防止我吃下不必要的食物。而且，我一直保持腸泌素注射的最低劑量，因為我清楚知道腸泌素主要是被動地幫助我控制食慾，而不是主動地壓抑我的食慾。

進食是生活中的一大享受，減重的目標是獲得更多對自己的控制權，而不是放棄對快樂的追求。使用藥物的期間為 8 週，8 週後總熱量攝取明顯減少，停止使用藥物後，我個人深刻感覺到對於口腹之慾的控制不再像減重前那樣無法忍受。

在 44 歲的年齡下，透過大魚醫師的專業指導，在為期 8 週的時間內，草頭云成功地利用科技營養管理、藥劑、飲食觀念修正和最低強度的運動綜合應用的方法，將體重從 66.5 公斤降至 57.6 公斤。停藥後遭遇了三級疫情的影響，體重維持在 57 至 58 公斤之間約兩個月。在疫情降級後，重新啟動了最低強度的運動習慣，期待能夠緩慢而穩定地恢復到健康的 56 公斤。

減重患者心得 2：
從心開始，幸福瘦 10 公斤

門診患者基本資料

暱稱：蘋果魚
年紀：20 多歲
性別：女
職業：醫療人員

在開始減重之前，我做了一些功課，了解了各種減重方法（飲食、飲品、塗抹等），最終找到了適合自己且能負擔得起的方式。一路走來，我感到非常幸運和感激，因為我有一位非常用心且支持我的專業醫師、減重導師——余宜叡醫師。他不離不棄地陪伴我，給予我耐心的幫助，讓我享受到了優質的資源和醫療服務，而且我不需要跑遍各個城市，就能夠獲得這樣的待遇。我會繼續努力讓自己變得更健康。

起初，我沒有太大的感覺，直到漸漸發現自己真的瘦了近 10 公斤了，可以說以前我是大熊，現在則成了小熊。

給余醫師和自己身體與肥肉的一封信

因此，在有機會寫信給余醫師的時候，我毫不猶豫地寫了以下的內容。

余醫師您好，收信平安：

打開您推薦閱讀《幸福瘦：不節食、不復胖，從心開始的 23

堂療癒減重對話》一書的推薦序，我看到了作者馬文雅醫師所說的這樣一句話：「你吃下去的不只是熱量而已，還有那些無以名狀的空虛。」

的確如此耶！我覺得光是這段話就讓我很觸及內心。這要回溯到青少年時期，國中的階段，我想那一段日子真的很慘，家人忙於工作，在關係的陪伴上，有些疏忽，導致那一段日子我遇到了挫折及不知道該怎麼解決的事。我通通都用吃來去逃避問題。家人和朋友的鄙視讓我會想要報復性的吃更多。

直到進大學學習心理學後，才學會了為自己設置「天花板」心錨的方法，找到自己的「起胖點」，認真解決心因性的肥胖問題，並定期稱體重才能瘦下來。我覺得這個方法非常好，通過設定目標和適合的策略來解決心因性的肥胖問題是很有效的。關鍵在於將注意力放在內心的需求和情緒上，而不是僅僅關注外在的身體狀況。

同時，我利用老子的話作為開始改變的起點：「積思成言，積言成行，積行成習，積習成性，積性成命。」簡單講就是，只有真正想要改變的動機，行為改變才會發生。否則會原地打轉，耗掉彼此的能量。

最後，我還對那些曾經陪伴我度過難關的身體和肥肉，做了告別，顯示堅持瘦下去的決心。

敬祝　文安

蘋果魚

專業團隊的協助，幸福瘦的開始

這封信的內容主要是描述了我發胖的原因和過程，以及遇到余醫師團隊的高興和感動。同時，在接下來整個諮詢的過程中，余醫師分析了各種減重方法，讓我可以自行選擇。此外，他還希望我給他寫下閱讀書籍的心得，這讓我感覺像是參加了一個讀書會，我們討論了書籍的內容、心得和想法。他甚至送給我一個運動彈力帶，讓我可以隨時進行肌力訓練。他無所不用其極地幫助我變得更健康。

除了自身的專業知識，余醫師也明白「一個人走得快，一群人走得遠」的道理。他安排我與其他醫療專業人員，如營養師、物理治療師等專業人士交流，以尋求飲食和運動方面的建議，幫助我更深入了解自己的生活狀態，從身體和心理兩方面開始認識和了解自己。

雖然我還沒有達到完美的狀態，不過，由於余醫師的協助，能夠從心開始幸福瘦。重要的是，不要等到有了很厲害的狀態才開始，而是要從現在開始行動，才能取得卓越的成果。健康是一輩子的事情，我不會放棄讓自己變得更健康的目標，並願意與大家分享我的經驗和心得。

整體而言，我感到非常幸運能夠享受到如此出色的資源和醫療服務。感謝余醫師在這段時間的陪伴和支持，他的用心幫助讓我堅信自己能夠變得更加健康。我會持續努力，讓自己的健康狀態得到改善，加油！可以的！！

穩糖糖友心得：
連續血糖儀讓我與血糖共舞

糖友基本資料

暱稱：小美
年紀：50 多歲
性別：女
職業： 家庭主婦

以下是我歷經這段時間與糖共舞後體會到的精句，與大家共享：

「趁此時能隨時監測血糖的情況下，試著求找出合適的飲食及份量」

「從平日喜歡的食物開始」

「有生活品質地與血糖共舞」

原先抗拒

自醫生口中得知「CGMS 連續血糖儀」，對這新東西沒有特別感興趣，但因為自身的不忌口，血糖值忽高忽低，一直無法血糖有效穩定達標，讓我重新對此科技產品燃起興致。先前抗拒的原因是，預想裝機過程會如坐針氈，想著想著，就有種莫名悸動及恐懼感迎面而來。

裝機目的

醫生與衛教師囑咐，安裝 CGMS 連續血糖儀期間，要確實做好飲食、運動記錄及按時用口服與針劑藥。在如履薄冰的一週體驗過程中，很在意每次曲線的異常波動，對某些食物的食用量有所顧忌，但若不趁此時能隨時監測血糖的情況下，試著求找出合適的飲食及份量，就會失去了這次裝機的意義。

神奇體驗

從平日喜歡的食物開始。陸續吃進了平日喜愛的食物：包子、拿鐵咖啡、手搖果汁飲料、甜點，以及飯後水果：香蕉、鳳梨、芭樂、西瓜……等，透過血糖的即時監控，確實給了我不少震撼！但也從中學習到許多。

飯前血糖數據到飯後血糖波動，是如此起伏跳躍，同時伴隨著心跳加快與忐忑不安，到後續調整飲食與份量後，漸漸血糖數值平穩，情緒才得以心安神寧。

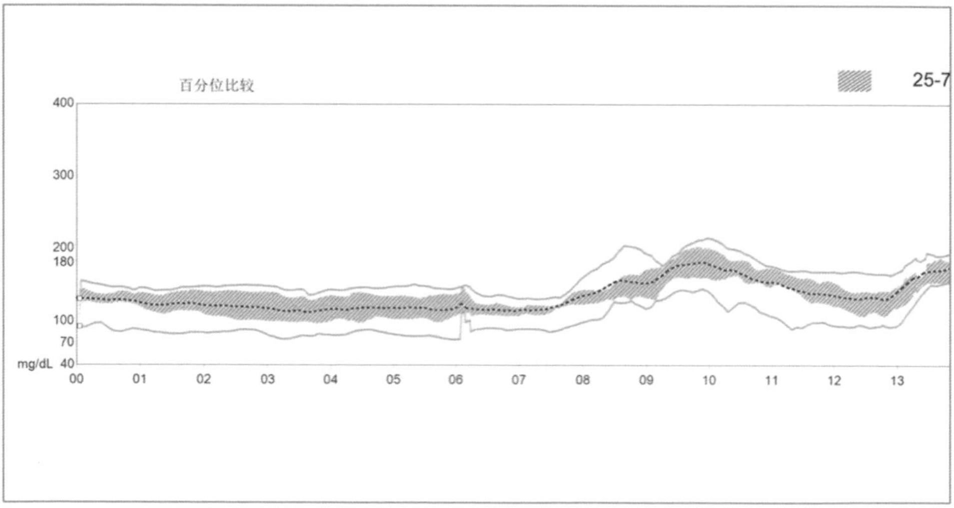

▲起伏跳躍的飯前血糖數據與飯後血糖波動，令自己理解到血糖與健康的神奇關係。

血糖高低

記得有一次晚餐前運動半小時，超過一個半小時未進食，竟然手機出現低血糖警報訊息，當下驚惶與不安。幸好衛教師及時教導低血糖處置。原來 CGMS 連續血糖儀不僅可以顯示，血糖的快速升高及驟降，並做出高低血糖的預知警示，讓使用者可以即時調整飲食及運動，適時穩定血糖值，減少長期高血糖及血糖過低的情況，不愧為實用的貼身小秘書。

與糖共舞

飲食的均衡營養、適度的運動，以及正常的作息，對血糖穩定真的很重要！藉由這次裝「CGMS 連續血糖儀」，透過即時的監測血糖變化，讓我對血糖與飲食、運動與藥物，有更深一層的認知。戰戰兢兢的體驗一週下來，瞭解懷著長期抗戰的堅毅精神，逐步調整飲食與運動，搭配合適的口服與針劑藥，是可以有生活品質地與血糖共舞。

工作坊學員分享 1：
用所學，助減重

學員基本資料

暱稱：小碩醫師
年紀：40 多歲
性別：男
醫護專業：基層院所醫師

以下是我學習到的四個最重要的穩糖的關鍵觀念：

學習減重、個別治療

一整天的課上下來，對於減重算是有較完整的了解。社會越進步，肥胖的人就越多，如何評估這些病人，有哪些武器可以來對付肥胖，都可在課程中學到。沒有單一方法適用於所有人。每一個減重的病人都需要仔細的評估，瞭解他的生活背景、飲食習慣、工作型態……等等，才能制定出一套可行的辦法，去幫助病人成功減重。

團隊協助、應用所學

減重最好還是有一個團隊，醫師、衛教師、營養師分工合作，一起跟病人配合，評估療效，即時調整，才更有機會達成目標。然後，體重減下來之後，更重要的是—如何不復胖，也是一個很重要的關卡。

上完這一整天的工作坊，深深覺得，減重真的是一門藝術，希望接下來，可以運用今天學到的知識，幫助更多病人達到心中理想的體重！！

工作坊學員分享 2：
誰說心理師不用懂糖尿病！

學員基本資料

暱稱：蘇琮祺心理師

年紀：40 多歲

性別：男

醫護專業：諮商心理師

這場具有實證精神、實用臨床經驗和邏輯架構清楚的分享，讓我這個有點像跑錯場子的心理師，卻可以有下列兩項統整吸收：

「從全然陌生，到上完課的略懂略懂」

「在跨界的學習體驗裡，我看見身為心理師的可能藍海」

調整飲食和運動要讓醫療團隊知道。在各單位帶領健康促進班的時候，總是會遇到幾位患有糖尿病的學員，這些學員經常是改善

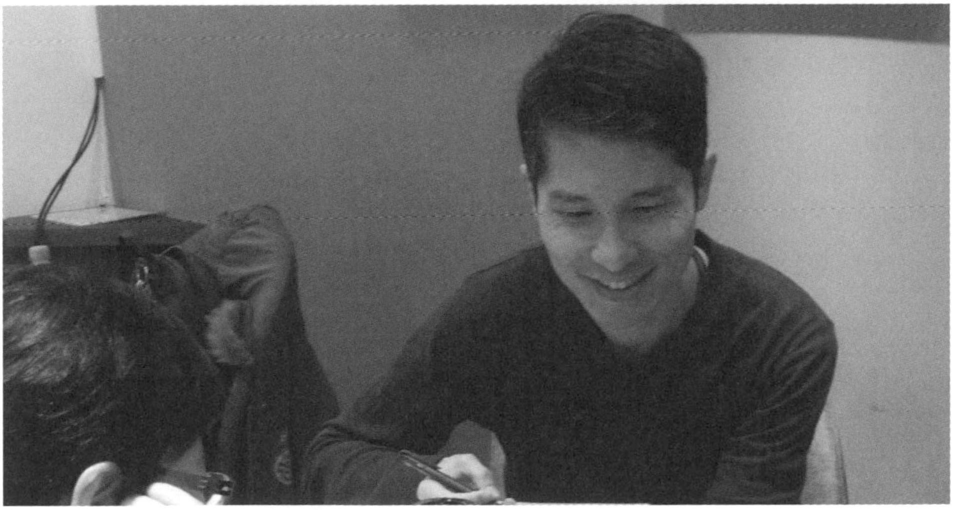

▲在跨界的學習體驗裡，我看見身為心理師的可能藍海，令人感動。

最明顯的一群，但每次面對學員的興奮回饋跟感謝時，我卻只想問：「你有跟醫師說你在調整飲食跟運動嗎？」因為我非常好奇「糖友與糖尿病共處的心態為何？」這區塊是有待補強的空白地帶。

因為心理師的專業，在於心理調適和行為改變，而糖尿病的治療卻需要更多的醫療專業。還好，每個學員都很配合，醫師護理師更是專業，讓大家的症狀可以有很好的改善。但我知道，這塊領域早晚還是要補起來。

為了臨床實務，我要的就是加強自己對於糖尿病的基本瞭解，因此如何系統性地學習關於糖尿病的知識、醫療處遇以及團隊運作，是我的最大需求。與余宜叡醫師的偶然接觸後，得知他在糖尿病治療上的專業及自我精進，所以報名了這次的講座，希望可以讓自己更有效率地進入這個陌生領域。

講座裡，認真專業的余醫師，透過具有實證精神、實用臨床經驗和邏輯架構清楚的分享，讓我這個有點像跑錯場子的心理師，可以有下列三項統整吸收：

學習糖尿病的概念

原來，我對糖尿病的誤解那麼多。三多一少，其實已經很嚴重了，更多時候，是沒有症狀的；飲料水果在有節制和監控的狀況下，是可以放心享用的；除了吃藥以外，更要調整飲食、增加運動和監控血糖。

這些糖尿病的基本概念，讓我釐清過去道聽途說的可怕迷思。

初探藥物治療邏輯

對於糖尿病藥物，我是陌生的。但透過課程內容及其他醫師學員的分享，我認識了糖尿病藥物的五大運作機制，可能的風險評估，也理解到健保制度之下許多醫師們的無奈。

從全然陌生，到上完課的略懂略懂，我知道我還有得學。

擴展心理介入可能

生理、心理、社會因素是相互連結的。很多同學們在課堂上所提出的實務困境，如果用心理社會角度來看，其實都有許多的可行切入，只是單從生理角度出發，很容易受困在知識詛咒之中。

在跨界的學習體驗裡，我看見身為心理師的可能藍海。如果您是需要瞭解糖尿病的心理師，鼓勵您參加余醫師的糖尿個案實戰初階班。

--APPENDIX--

附錄 成人肥胖治療流程與藥物重點重要圖表

以下相關圖表有三個重點，給大家參考：

1. 減重藥物各有其副作用，但不代表一定會發生。
2. 不同機制的減重藥物，各有其合適使用族群。
3. 台灣目前有其中三種藥物，而減重用的 semaglutide 也將引進。

AACE	分類	減重效果	機制	使用	費用
Semaglutide	腸泌素	15-18%	降食慾 延排空	注射 一週 1 次	$$$
Liraglutide	腸泌素	5-6%	降食慾 延排空	注射 一天 1 次	$$$
Phentermin/ Topiramate-ER	交感 Amine/GABA	9-10%	降食慾 增飽足	口服	$$
Naltrxone-ER/ Buproprion-ER	嗎啡拮抗 /DA-Norepi	4-6%	減嘴饞 降食慾	口服	$$
Orlistat	腸道脂肪 酶抑制	4%	減脂肪 吸收	口服	$$
Phentermine	交感	3%	降食慾	口服	$

製表：余宜叡 醫師

AACE	起始劑量	治療劑量	注意與禁忌症 × 懷孕＋泌乳
Semaglutide	0.25mg QW	2.4mg QW	甲狀腺髓質癌 / 第 2 型多發性內分泌腫瘤 MTC/MEN2、心跳加快、胰臟炎、膽囊疾病、糖尿病視網膜病變
Liraglutide	0.6mg QD	3mg QD	甲狀腺髓質癌 / 第 2 型多發性內分泌腫瘤 MTC/MEN2、心跳加快、胰臟炎、膽囊疾病
Phentermin/ Topiramate-ER	3.75/23 mg QD	7.5/46 QD max 15/92	青光眼、甲狀腺亢進、尿石症、代謝酸中毒
Naltrxone-ER/ Buproprion-ER	8/90 QD	16/ 180mg BID	癲癇風險、無法控制的高血壓、長期嗎啡使用
Orlistat	120mg TID	120mg TID	器官移植、尿石症草酸、膽汁鬱積
Phentermine	15mg QD	37.5mg QD	進行中冠心病、無法控制的高血壓、甲狀腺亢進、激動

製表：余宜叡 醫師

AACE	可能副作用
Semaglutide	噁心 / 嘔吐、腹瀉、便秘、頭痛、疲倦
Liraglutide	噁心 / 嘔吐、腹瀉、便秘、頭痛、疲倦
Phentermin/ Topiramate-ER	煩燥、失眠、頭痛、口乾、心跳快 / 血壓升、感覺異常、味覺障礙、腦霧、情緒改變
Naltrxone-ER/ Buproprion-ER	噁心 / 嘔吐、腹瀉、便秘、頭痛、疲倦、失眠、口乾、視力模糊、激動、情緒改變
Orlistat	脹氣、裡急後重、油便、脂溶性維他命或藥物吸收不良
Phentermine	煩燥、失眠、頭痛、口乾、心跳快 / 血壓升

製表：余宜叡 醫師

Contemporary Arabic Literature

For my beloved grandchildren
Tom, Maayan, Reut, Adam, and Carmel:
Be the masters of your fates,
Be the captains of your souls.

Contemporary Arabic Literature

Heritage and Innovation

Reuven Snir

EDINBURGH
University Press

Edinburgh University Press is one of the leading university presses in the UK. We publish academic books and journals in our selected subject areas across the humanities and social sciences, combining cutting-edge scholarship with high editorial and production values to produce academic works of lasting importance. For more information visit our website: edinburghuniversitypress.com

Edinburgh University Press Ltd
The Tun—Holyrood Road
12 (2f) Jackson's Entry
Edinburgh EH8 8PJ

Typeset in 10.5/13 pt Adobe Text
by Cheshire Typesetting Ltd, Cuddington, Cheshire, and
printed and bound in Great Britain

A CIP record for this book is available from the British Library

ISBN 978 1 3995 0325 9 (hardback)
ISBN 978 1 3995 0327 3 (webready PDF)
ISBN 978 1 3995 0328 0 (epub)

This book was published with the support of the Israel Science Foundation.

Contents

Preface

From the mid-1980s, my scholarship has concentrated on a series of topics serving a comprehensive research plan. My aim from the beginning has been to explore the internal dynamics of Arabic literature since the nineteenth century, the interrelations and interactions between its various sectors, and its connections with its cultural heritage and with other non-literary systems, as well as its interplay with foreign cultures. Based upon the general achievements of the field of historical literary poetics, in several studies I have outlined a theoretical framework that would make possible the analysis of the diverse texts that make up modern Arabic literature as a coherent system. For the purpose of a systematic investigation of the development of literary phenomena both synchronically and diachronically, this theoretical framework could not be closed, narrow, or static, but had of necessity to be open, broad, dynamic, flexible, and adaptable. And this much can be seen from the changes and updates to this framework that have I presented throughout my theoretical studies.[1] One of the advantages of such a framework is that it allows for a greater economy in analysis, in that it replaces large numbers of categories of a classificatory nature with a small number of parameters that can be viewed as governing rules. This feature can be considered a step toward accomplishing what has always been believed to be the goal of any scientific endeavor: the detection of those relatively few rules that govern the great diversity and complexity of phenomena both observable and non-observable. Such an endeavor is important for the study of any literature, but is certainly of the utmost importance for the study of a vast literature created and consumed among a population of as many as 467 million people.[2]

[1] Especially Snir 1994, pp. 61–85; Snir 1994c, pp. 49–80; Snir 1998, pp. 87–121; Snir 2001; Snir 2017.

[2] According to a study by Ulrich Ammon from the University of Düsseldorf, Chinese has more native speakers than any other language, followed by Hindi and Urdu, which have the same linguistic origins in northern India. English comes next with 527 million native

Using this theoretical framework, I have investigated and continue to investigate the relations between center and periphery in Arabic literature as a series of oppositions that actually make it possible to hypothesize more than one center, although in most historical cases the centers are stratified in such a way that only one center succeeds in any specific time in dominating the whole. Each text is placed, at each given period of time, at a particular point in the system, which is its synchronic value. Diachronic value, on the other hand, is assigned to it by its paradigmatic position in the succession of synchronic systems, which acquire retrospective significance. Consequently, the diachronic correlativity of a given text is to be considered alongside its synchronic orientation toward other texts.

During the last four decades, I have participated in numerous conferences and scholarly seminars and taught dozens of courses on the topics discussed in the following pages, focusing on different periods and on varying fields but always being aware of the main parameters, criteria, and guidelines of the previously mentioned comprehensive research plan. My published studies, books, and articles in several languages reflect this scholarly investigation. At the beginning of my academic career, my fluctuating movements, shifts, and leaps between different areas of interest—sometimes in the same time period—were generally perceived by scholars in my field as a "lack of focus." They thought that my wide-ranging scholarly interests reflected arrogance and that it was not appropriate for a beginner to cover so much territory. However, that "lack of focus" in my studies was necessary at the time, for it afforded me the opportunity to explore the common denominators of various literary phenomena and to probe the depths of the ambiguous relationships between the various sectors of Arabic literature and to examine its connections with other cultural systems.

During my BA studies, I was an ardent student of medieval Arabic literature; my MA thesis focused on an ascetic Muslim manuscript from the eighth century;[3] and my PhD dissertation studied the common links between the medieval and the modern literature related to various mystical conceptions and themes.[4] Not once in my undergraduate and graduate studies did I possess divided loyalties. I always thought that the study of contemporary Arabic literature must rely on its medieval heritage, if only because we cannot find even one Arab author whose education does not include the medieval literary heritage. In fact, we cannot find even one literary text in Arabic that

speakers. Arabic is used by nearly 100 million more native speakers than Spanish (Noack and Gamio 2015. Cf. http://istizada.com/complete-list-of-arabic-speaking-countries-2014 [last accessed December 28, 2020]).

3 Snir 1982.

4 Snir 1986.

does not conduct any dialogue with the medieval literary tradition, if only because the latter is written in the same Arabic language. Focusing in the later stage of my academic career on the study of Arabic literature of the last two centuries, I have a deep awareness of the importance of the medieval literary works for the study of contemporary literary Arabic texts. Against this background, the relationship of the Arabs' literary creativity since the nineteenth century with that of other cultures, Western culture included, and the extent of the impact that the latter has made on the former over the years have become a conundrum that I have tried to explore and resolve. I have come to perceive the various dimensions of Arabic literature and the relationships between Arabic literature and other cultures as one dynamic system, whose components retain their correlation on all levels of analysis. Reviewing the studies that I published during the last four decades, I recently decided to embark on a new project: I updated several studies, wrote new ones, united their method of presentation, and incorporated them all into one overarching framework in the belief that such a framework would make it easier for readers to understand the aforementioned relationships. In addition, this new framework is more than merely a sum total of my previous work. The present book is complementary to my *Modern Arabic Literature: A Theoretical Framework* (2017), but, unlike the latter's macro-conception, which at times could be subject to the charge of ignoring the nuances and details of the topic, the emphasis here is on the texts themselves and specific literary activities—in other words, on the micro-systems that make up the entire system of Arabic literature.

Acknowledgments

I wish to thank the editors and publishers of the following journals for permission to reuse material published in them (in alphabetical order): *Acta Orientalia, Arabic Language & Literature, Der Islam, Edebiyāt, HaMizrah HeHadash, Hebrew Studies, Hispanic Issues, Jamaʿa: Interdisciplinary Journal of Middle East Studies, Jusūr, al-Karmil: Studies in Arabic Language and Literature, Mamlūk Studies Review, Middle Eastern Studies, Orientalia Suecana, Quaderni di Studi Arabi, Virginia Woolf Miscellany*, and *Yearbook of Comparative and General Literature*. My thanks go out as well to the following publishers of the books from which material has been reused in the present study (also in alphabetical order): Ben-Zvi Institute for the Study of Jewish Communities in the East, Brill, Dār al-Sāqī, Edinburgh University Press, Harrassowitz Verlag, Harvard University Press, Reichert Verlag, Routledge, and York Press.

This book is the result of research projects that I have been conducting for the last three decades. The projects have been supported by grants and fellowships that I obtained from the Israel Science Foundation (ISF) (1992–1995 and 2021), Memorial Foundation for Jewish Culture (1993 and 1998), Oxford Centre for Hebrew and Jewish Studies (2000 and 2008), Seminar für Sprachen und Kulturen des Vorderen Orients and Hochschule für Jüdische Studien at Heidelberg University (2002 and 2017–2018), Wissenschaftskolleg zu Berlin—Institute for Advanced Study (2004–2005), Seminar für Semitistik und Arabistik at the Free University of Berlin (2004–2005), Radcliffe Institute for Advanced Study at Harvard University (2009–2010), Simon Dubnow Institute for Jewish History and Culture at Leipzig University (2015), Department of Languages and Literatures at the University of Gothenburg (2017–2018), Herbert D. Katz Center for Advanced Judaic Studies at the University of Pennsylvania (2019), and IMéRA—Institut d'études avancées—at Aix-Marseille University (2020).

Finally, as in several of my previous volumes, a special word of thanks and appreciation is due to the editor Michael Helfield for his excellent work on the manuscript and for his significant contribution to the final shaping of this book.

Technical Notes

1. Translations are mine unless otherwise indicated.
2. Quotations (generally, but not solely, in poetry) in the original appear wherever the Arabic text is important for the understanding of the arguments presented. The aim is by no means to provide a poetically parallel text in English, especially with regard to verses in the *qaṣīda* form—an elaborately structured ode maintaining the same meter and a single end rhyme that runs through the entire piece, in which each verse is divided into two paired hemistichs, the first being the *ṣadr* and the second being the *ʿajuz*. The generally independent nature of the meaning of each verse usually allows them all to stand alone, and thus these verses have been translated as separate verses, with each hemistich being translated on a separate line.
3. The epigraph appearing at the opening of the book and the epigraphs appearing at the start of its two parts appear in the original and in translation. The epigraphs appearing at the start of its chapters appear in English only; if they are translations, the original Arabic text will appear within the main text of the chapter.
4. Titles of Arabic books and articles are transliterated into English. Titles of Hebrew books and articles are translated into English and identified as such at the end of the translated title. The transliterated Arabic titles are accompanied by their translation immediately afterward in the body of the text but not in the References. For the system of transliteration from Arabic, see Notes on Transliteration below.
5. In the titles of one chapter and several subchapters, I have incorporated parts of verses that I believe are relevant to the chapter content. For example, in Chapter 4's title, I have incorporated the words "I Saw My God," which is part of a mystical poem, and the title of Section 3 in Chapter 2 is "The Guitar Is Aflame" from a poem by Samīḥ al-Qāsim. I have generally done this when I am discussing literary texts and

offer my own close reading of them. Of course, I am well aware that other scholars or laypersons may offer different readings of the texts in question.

6. The definite article ال appears as *al-* throughout the entire book before solar and lunar letters. In the beginning of a surname in the References, it is not taken into consideration with regard to alphabetical order.
7. Works with one author/editor or two authors/editors will appear with the name or names fully cited. For works with more than two authors/editors, "et al." will be used.
8. In case of a subsequent edition of a book, the year of the first edition is mentioned only when it is significant for the arguments made in previous research—for example, when referring to studies related to the emergence of new modes of literary genres: al-Malā'ika, Nāzik. 1983 [1962]. *Qaḍāyā al-Shi'r al-Mu'āṣir*. Beirut: Dār al-'Ilm li-l-Malāyīn.
9. When referring to sources on the Internet that are being continuously updated, I mention the last time I accessed the relevant website. Readers are encouraged to access the relevant websites themselves in order to familiarize themselves with the most recent information.

Notes on Transliteration

أ؛ ؤ؛ ئ	’i; ’u; ’a	ط	ṭ
ب	b	ظ	ẓ
ت	t	ع	‘
ث	th	غ	gh
ج	j	ف	f
ح	ḥ	ق	q
خ	kh	ك	k
د	d	ل	l
ذ	dh	م	m
ر	r	هـ	h
ز	z	و	w
س	s	و (long)	ū
ش	sh	ي	y
ص	ṣ	ي (long)	ī
ض	ḍ	ِ; َ; ُ (short)	i; a; u

1. The definite article *al-* is used before solar and lunar letters. The *waṣla* over silent *alif* is systematically ignored.
2. ’ (أ) is not indicated when it is at the beginning of a word. ا or آ or ى are transcribed as *ā*.
3. ة at the end of words and names is not transliterated (i.e., *ḥikāya* for حكاية). When it occurs in the first word of an *iḍāfa* (construction), it is transcribed as *t*.
4. A *shadda* (ّ) is represented by doubling the relevant letter.
5. Final *nisba* is transcribed as *ī* (masculine, i.e., *‘Arabī* for عربيّ) and *iyya* (feminine, i.e., *‘Arabiyya* for عربيّة).
6. Arabic words or letters transcribed into Latin characters are generally given in *italics*, except for personal names and names of places and publishers.

7. Anglicized spellings of commonly used names and locations have been retained, and foreign names in transliterated passages generally appear in their English form. In English quotations, transliterated Arabic words appear as is, even if they differ from our preferred system.

كانت القبيلة من العرب إذا نبغ فيها شاعر أتت القبائل فهنّأتها بذلك وصنعت الأطعمة واجتمع النّساء يلعبن بالمزاهر كما يصنعن في الأعراس وتتباشر الرجال والولدان لأنّه حماية لأعراضهم وذبّ عن أحسابهم وتخليد لمآثرهم وإشادة لذكرهم وكانوا لا يهنّئون إلّا بغلام يولد أو شاعر ينبغ فيهم أو فرس تنتج.

– ابن رشيق القيروانيّ

When a poet appeared in a family of the Arabs, the adjacent tribes would gather together and wish that family the joy of their good luck. Feasts would be got ready, the women of the tribe would join together in bands, playing upon lutes, as they were wont to do at bridals, and the men and boys would congratulate one another; for a poet was a defense of the honor of them all, a weapon to ward off insult from their good name, and a means of perpetuating their glorious deeds and of establishing their fame forever. And they used not to wish one another joy but for three things: the birth of a boy, the coming to light of a poet, and the foaling of a noble mare.

– Ibn Rashīq al-Qayrawānī

Introduction

Without fear of exaggeration, one could say that the changes that Arabic literature has seen since the mid-nineteenth century are as momentous or even radical as the ways in which Arabic literature had been transformed following the rise of Islam in the seventh century. These changes have been accompanied by a dramatic increase in readership, first, throughout the Arab world and, second, since the mid-twentieth century, throughout the entire globe. With regard to the latter case, the writing and publishing of contemporary Arabic literature, in the original as well as in translation, have taken flight, as has the concomitant increase in literary consumption by Arab and foreign reading publics. Arabic literature has become such a huge field; the number of literary texts produced in recent decades is so enormous that they cannot be covered in any meaningful way by any traditional scholarly tool. This is why it is our duty as scholars of this literature to constantly revise the way we approach our material, which has not only grown quantitatively but qualitatively as well, as can be seen by its readers. Referring to the need to rewrite the literary history of the Arabic novel, Roger Allen (b. 1942), the most experienced contemporary scholar of modern Arabic literature, proclaims—in the words of the Irish poet and playwright Oscar Wilde (1854–1900)—that "the one duty that we owe to history is to rewrite it." Allen then adds the following:

> I wish to challenge many of the premises and organizing principles that have governed research and publication that I have done previously, not so much in order to suggest that they were not relevant or even useful for their time, but rather that the changing nature of Arabic fiction—a primary facet of its very essence, of course—requires a continuingly [sic] changing perspective in order to reflect both the creativity of Arab littérateurs and the kind of studies now being devoted to it.[1]

[1] Allen 2007, p. 248. On the need to challenge the premises and organizing principles of Arabic literary history, see also Sacks 2015 and the review of the book by Terri DeYoung (DeYoung 2016).

Given the recent expansion of Arabic literary texts and the need to change our perspective on their study, I have proposed a shift in approach, that is, a new theoretical framework or model that would make possible the comprehensive study of the diverse and multifarious texts that make up Arabic literature.[2] In the present book, I would like to offer an approach that will be in line with the proposed theoretical framework, but that will also deal more closely and in much more detail with various texts selected for their wider literary and cultural implications. This approach will enhance our understanding of all the elements that together make up Arabic literature, and it may throw light on traditionally neglected aspects of literary production. In this sense, I hope this book will succeed in stimulating others to take up the fascinating challenge of mapping out all those areas of contemporary Arabic literature that are as yet unexplored.

Within the aforementioned proposed theoretical framework, there are three principal components: the first looks at the literary dynamics in the synchronic cross-section. Inventories of canonized and non-canonized literary texts are presented separately in three sections or subsystems: texts for adults, texts for children, and translated texts for adults and children. The resulting six subsystems—three canonized and three non-canonized—are seen as autonomous networks of relationships and as interacting literary networks on various levels. The internal and external interrelationships and interactions between the various subsystems need to be studied if we want to arrive at a comprehensive understanding of the Arabic literary system.[3]

The second component, which is most relevant to the present book, refers to the outlines of the diachronic intersystemic development of the Arabic literary system. Semiotically, a literary text is an utterance made by someone to someone else in a pre-existing language at a certain time and within a certain social and cultural context.[4] The space between the text, its author, and the reader is understood as constituting both an economic environment

[2] Snir 2017.

[3] In her review of Snir 2017, Anna Ziajka Stanton argues that its portrait of the contemporary Arabic literary field is in some respects out of date as it "overlooks a rich body of recent work on blogs, comics, graffiti, pop music, protest poetry, and Twitter feeds," and "a number of significant recent developments in the Arabic literary field receive only passing mention or are omitted entirely from Snir's discussion" (Stanton 2019, p. 682). However, being aware when writing the book of such possible critical comments, I indicated in the book's conclusion that my proposed model "is not in any way a closed, narrow, static, and finished framework, but an open, flexible, adaptable, and dynamic one. The tools for the study of modern Arabic literature, like those for the study of any other literature, which include the intersection between the investigation of text and theory, will never be complete and will always involve a constant rewriting of literary history as part of the study of Arab culture" (Snir 2017, pp. 273–4).

[4] Based on Sebeok 1986, I, pp. 453–9.

(e.g., literary markets, publishing) and a sociocommunicative system that passes the meaning potential of the text through various filters (e.g., criticism, literary circles, groups, salons, public opinion) in order to concretize and realize it. All the other spaces related to literary production and consumption, including the linguistic, spiritual, social, national, and economic spaces, are also considered. Therefore, even if Arabic literature is regarded as an autonomous system for the purpose of its study as *literature,* we must also consider the various ways in which it interacts with other external literary and non-literary systems. Literary works are never fully intelligible in and of themselves. According to Terry Eagleton, "you have to see them as belonging to a global literary space, which has a basis in the world's political landscape, but which also cuts across its regions and borders to form a distinctive republic of its own."[5] For example, in order to determine the general characteristics of the historical development of Arabic literature from the start of the nineteenth century, we should look at the interaction of literature with, for example, religion, territory, state nationalism, language, politics, the economy, gender, electronic media, and philosophy, as well as with foreign literatures and cultures.

The third component, which is relevant as well to the present book, concentrates on the historical, diachronic development that each genre underwent and the relationships that exist between them. As with any scholarly treatment of genre, it refers to the developing innovations and discussions of genre theory and the question "What is genre?" Crucial in this regard is the concept of periodization, that is, how one is to delimit and define "literary periods." Since literary genres do not emerge in a vacuum, the issue of generic development cannot be confined to certain time spans, and emphasis will be placed on the relationship between modern literature, on the one hand, and classical and medieval[6] literature, on the other. The complete study of the historical, diachronic development of literary dynamics requires an analysis of every genre and subgenre, of the interrelationships and interactions between the genres, and of the interactions and interrelationships between the genres and the subgenres.

With the metaphor of the system serving as our primary frame of reference,[7] all of the chapters in the present book are based, in one way or another, on the

[5] *New Statesman,* April 11, 2005. For more on the concept of the "republic of letters," see the Epilogue.

[6] The terms "classical" and "medieval" are used here and throughout the present book to refer to periods of literary creation prior to the nineteenth century. As for the demarcation between classical, medieval, postclassical, and premodern periods, see al-Musawi (= al-Mūsawī) 2015b, p. 323, n. 1. See also Bauer 2007, pp. 137–8.

[7] Steiner 1984, p. 99.

dialogue between the literary texts and the dialogue between the literary texts and other texts, mainly those in Arabic, but also in other languages. These multilayered dialogues have been perhaps most compellingly described by the American-English poet and literary critic T. S. Eliot (1888–1965) in his well-known essay "Tradition and the Individual Talent" (1919):

> No poet, no artist of any art, has his complete meaning alone. His significance, his appreciation is the appreciation of his relation to the dead poets and artists. You cannot value him alone; you must set him, for contrast and comparison, among the dead. I mean this as a principle of aesthetic, not merely historical, criticism. The necessity that he shall conform, that he shall cohere, is not one-sided; what happens when a new work of art is created is something that happens simultaneously to all the works of art which preceded it. The existing monuments form an ideal order among themselves, which is modified by the introduction of the new (the really new) work of art among them. The existing order is complete before the new work arrives; for order to persist after the supervention of novelty, the whole existing order must be, if ever so slightly, altered; and so the relations, proportions, values of each work of art toward the whole art readjusted; and this is conformity between the old and the new. Whoever has approved this idea of order, of the form of European, of English literature will not find it preposterous that the past should be altered by the present as much as the present is directed by the past. And the poet who is aware of this will be aware of great difficulties and responsibilities.[8]

The French literary theorist Roland Barthes (1915–1980) mentions such multilayered dialogues, in which we "will not find it preposterous that the past should be altered by the present as much as the present is directed by the past," by referring to texts as "a tissue of quotations drawn from the innumerable centres of culture," when the author's "only power is to mix writings, to counter the ones with the others, in such a way as never to rest on any one of them."[9]

Speaking of "innumerable centres of culture," one cannot ignore the new virtual centers of culture that have been causing, since the late twentieth century, seismic changes in society and culture throughout the world. The rapid growth and proliferation of sophisticated forms of media, particularly social media, and Internet-related technologies, such as blogging, techno-writing, and interactive literature, have changed culture and literature in the forms known to previous generations. Fresh possibilities for literary voices have been opened for Arab writers to imagine new realities, and these possibilities have provided additional forums and stages for literary and

[8] Eliot 1950, pp. 4–5.
[9] Barthes 1977 [1967], pp. 146–7.

critical texts to be presented and discussed side by side with the traditional ones.[10] Revolutionizing virtually every aspect of how our lives function now, including our literary lives, the Internet has catapulted us into an immediate, collaborative, and interconnected existence that is characterized, as Cathy Davidson suggests, by the sudden breakdown of barriers, such as those between private and public, work and play, domestic and foreign, and office and home: "With the Internet, we have seen dramatic rearrangements in the most basic aspects of how we communicate, interact, gather knowledge of the world, develop and recognize our social networks and our communities, do business and exchange goods, understand what is true, and know what counts and is worthy of attention."[11] Referring to the technological developments and the new modes of communication in Islamic countries, Amy Ayalon writes that the impact "might well prove to be as revolutionary as that prompted by printing ... the internet rewrote the rules of access, application and consumption of information. In Islamic countries, where the public sphere [is] monitored by governments and free expression [is] determined by political oscillations, the significance of such new devices [is] perhaps greater than in other places."[12] Also, the technological revolution in mass media of communication has been one of the most powerful engines of globalization in the Arab and Islamic world as illustrated, for example, by the worldwide reaction to the publication of *The Satanic Verses* by Salman Rushdie in 1988:

> The protests and burning of his book by indignant Muslims began in Bradford, England. These were broadcast throughout the world and stimulated violent

[10] Among the numerous studies dealing with the impact of Internet-related technologies on Arab culture, see Kirchner 2001, pp. 137–58; Eickelman and J. Anderson 2003; J. Anderson 2005, pp. 252–63; Sakr 2007; al-Buraykī 2008; Abdel-Messih 2009, pp. 515–23; El-Ariss 2010, pp. 533–48; El Sadda 2010, pp. 312–32; Raven 2010, pp. 201–17; Sabra 2010, pp. 32–5; Daoudi 2011, pp. 146–63; Armbrust 2012, pp. 155–74; El-Ariss 2012, pp. 510–31; El Sadda 2012; Pepe 2012, pp. 547–62; Dūs and Davies 2013, pp. 365–9; El-Ariss 2013, pp. 145–71; Pepe 2015, pp. 73–91; Cook 2017; Ramsay 2017; Wheeler 2017; El-Ariss 2019; Lenze 2019; Pepe 2019; Jacquemond and Lagrange 2020; Abu-Remaileh 2021, pp. 68–96; De Blasio 2021, pp. 91–117; Junge 2021; Otterbeck 2021. On the role of Internet technologies in the development of Arab liberal discourse, see Hatina 2011, pp. 8–9 . On interactive Arabic literature, see al-Buraykī 2008, pp. 123–56. One of the literary expressions of the new horizons opened up by Internet technologies is the cultural magazine *Bi-Dūn/Bidoun* (*Without*) (http://bidoun.org). Lisa Farjam, the magazine's founding editor, had this to say about its creation: "When I came up with the name, I was struggling. I felt like I was without a place. I belong to many places and none. That was when I found that word. It meant a lot to me" (*New York Times*, December 26, 2015). For analogies and differences between the advent of the periodical press during the *nahḍa* period and the computer and Internet-related technologies in our time and their impact on the Arabic literary field, see Winckler 2018, pp. 27–64.

[11] Davidson 2011, p. 11.

[12] Ayalon 2011, p. 595.

> protests in Pakistan and India. In a particularly low point of the Iranian post-revolutionary politics in February 1989, after the book had been banned in India, South Africa, Bangladesh, Sudan, Sri Lanka and Pakistan, Iran's supreme leader Khomeini broadcast his famous *fatwā* condemning Rushdie, a non-Iranian writer who lived in England, to death for apostasy, and clerically controlled Iranian foundations immediately put a bounty on his head.[13]

Around the turn of the twenty-first century, the Internet became a virtual library for billions of Arabic literary texts housed on millions of websites. In addition, we have seen a sharp rise in the amount of research on Arabic literature being published online by both Arab and non-Arab academic and cultural institutions. Browsing on the Internet, one could input Arabic script into a variety of search engines and get results rather easily. Also, the notion of a cultural and literary center has disappeared from the Arab world. Instead, there are many local centers, but none of them could claim that it is a center whose influence could be compared with the influence that Cairo, Baghdad, Damascus, or Beirut once held in the past.

In the introduction to a report within the project "Multilingualism and Diversity as a Resource in the Cultural Field—Employment and Integration through Literature in the Nordic Countries," Ahmed Al-Nawas writes:

> "Cairo writes, Beirut publishes, and Baghdad reads" is an old Arab saying, which has been widely used in the past to illustrate the transnational circle of knowledge production in the Arabic-speaking world. After decades of ongoing disasters, i.e. civil wars, dictatorships, economic and political inequalities and mass migration, the triangular Cairo-Beirut-Baghdad network has become outdated. Today, an Arabic book of poetry could be written in Tampere, published in Milano [sic] and translated into several languages, awarded with the PEN Prize in London, and censored in Jordan and most of the Gulf States. In their search for social and economic justice and prosperity, many Arabic speakers have found refuge in Nordic countries. It is from such circumstances that Arabic literature has been written and published in the Nordic region and crossed multiple genres for the last three decades.[14]

However, it seems that the changing definition of a literary and cultural center has much to do with the decreasing status of literature as such, as well as with the marginalization of printed literary texts in the Arabic cultural system: one can easily discern the emerging influence of satellite mass media and Internet communication outlets, whose notion of culture is much broader. The speedy development of Internet technologies has fostered politically and aesthetically subversive transformations in Arabic literature

[13] Arjomand 2011, p. 194. On the Rushdie affair, see Snir 2019, pp. 138–47.
[14] al-Nawas 2018, pp. 160–83.

and the emergence of new generations of writers. The Internet, as one of the factors and manifestations of globalization, has been embraced so far by 69 percent of the world's population and 78.9 percent of the Middle East's population.[15] As with any other technological invention, the Internet makes our lives easier—human beings, even those of us who speak out against technology and science in favor of spirituality and a natural life—tend to adopt and adapt to new inventions immediately after they become available.

The speedy development of Internet technologies has done much to change the way culture is perceived, and they have changed dramatically the way literature in general—and Arabic literature in particular—is created and consumed. Other developments have accelerated this process, such as the wide migration, globalization, deconstruction, and fragmentization of the concept of identity, the cosmopolitan turn, and the classlessness of the bourgeoisie: all have freed human beings from many limitations and chains, real or imagined. They have exerted as well their impact, in various ways, on Arab culture, even if that impact is still not parallel to that on Western culture and even if scholarship has not been able so far to properly assess the results of the current processes that Arabic literature has been undergoing. Also, the Internet has changed the relationship between Arab culture and the West:

> With the accessibility of the Internet via inexpensive, handheld devices that operate as bodily extensions, and that make conversation and confrontation in colloquial Arabic accessible to all, the idea that the Internet is a product of the West that makes its "users" complicit in Western identities, if not political projects (as traitors or foreign agents), no longer holds. A new relation to technology and language ushers in epistemological frameworks that allow us to gauge the kinds of consciousness, subjectivity, and political contestation emerging from street and online performances of leaking and scene-making in the Arab digital age.[16]

For lack of space, we will not be able to refer here in detail to these changes, but one of the most important conclusions of the preliminary studies that I have conducted shows that the impact of the Internet on Arabic literary writing has been gradually intensifying and that there are signs that Arabic literature is changing in many respects. First, it is the quantity of the literary texts, including translations—particularly of poetry—that is increasing, and I have no doubt that quantity will make quality in the long run. Where the

15 Internet usage statistics available at: http://www.internetworldstats.com/stats.htm (last accessed August 11, 2022). The statistics in 2016 stated that the Internet had been embraced by 49.2 percent of the world's population (in the Middle East, 57.4 percent of the population) (last accessed September 4, 2016).

16 El-Ariss 2019, p. 11.

Internet is available (without strict governmental interventions), there is no censorship, no publishing limitations, no need for literary editors, and no need for financial resources to publish whatever you want. The temporal distance between writing and publishing has now become shorter, if it really exists now at all. Poets use the Internet not only to publish new works but also to show works that they wrote yet never published and/or to republish what they consider to be their best works. Complaints against publishing limitations and/or restrictions are now essentially mute.

Internet technologies are also behind what seem to be essential poetic changes in literary writing, such as the preference for short texts and the blurring of the boundaries between prose and poetry. These gradual changes deserve to be researched, and such research has yet to be conducted. One can easily see in the field of poetry, for example, the sheer superiority of the prose poem known as *qaṣīdat al-nathr* over *al-shiʿr al-ḥurr* (free verse) and certainly over the traditional *qaṣīda*. Also, because the prose poem has become the leading contemporary poetic genre, poets tend to publish prose poems that they had already published many years ago in order to prove their pioneering role in the field.[17] And, also, thanks to the Internet, there are daily literary discussions on various topics, such as the literary activities that followed, since January 2011, the advent of what the international media dubbed the "Arab Spring."[18] Also, the Internet has accelerated the controversies over whether we are still living in "the time of the novel" or returning to "the time of poetry." For example, the Palestinian author Saḥar Khalīfa (b. 1942) wrote in a Facebook post what has been already well known for several decades,[19] which is that the novel is "the new public register of the Arab people,"[20] and, in one of the comments to Khalīfa's post, the Syrian poet Ḥamza Rastanāwī (b. 1974) immediately gave the following response:

[17] On the prose poem and relevant references, see Fakhreddine 2021.

[18] On the "Arab Spring" as an invention against the background of imperial policies, see Massad 2014, pp. 129–54; Massad 2015, p. 100. The English reader may have a glimpse at the contribution of the Internet to the distribution of the literary expressions of the Arab Spring in the various issues of *Arablit & Arablit Quarterly: A Magazine of Arabic Literature in Translation*—one recent example is the summaries of thirteen books (six novels, three works of literary non-fiction, a graphic novel, a poetry collection, a short-story collection, and a collection of playtexts), which provide a not insubstantial literary landscape of contrasting visions and emotions of Egyptians after 2011, available at: https://arablit.org/2021/11/24/13-books-in-translation-a-literary-history-of-egypt-after-2011, last accessed November 24, 2021).

[19] See Snir 2017, pp. 223–4.

[20] See سحر خليفة 8 August 2016, available at: https://www.facebook.com/permalink.php?story_fbid=120591025051960&id=100013031880075 (last accessed December 27, 2020).

لم تعد الفنون الكتابيّة بكلّ أشكالها ديوانا للعرب! كم نسبة القراءة؟ الصّورة والفضائيّات ومواقع التّواصل الاجتماعيّ هي ديوان العرب! ربّما تكون الرواية ديوانا للنّخبة العربيّة المثقّفة القارئة وهي شريحة ضيّقة، نعم هذا صحيح، ولكن ليس العرب بإطلاق!

Writing arts are no longer the public register of the Arabs! What is the percentage of [literary] reading now? The picture and satellite and social media are the true public register of the Arabs! Perhaps the novel is the public register of the reading intellectual elite; yes, indeed, that is correct, but this elite is a small group. [The novel is not the public register] of all the Arabs.[21]

More importantly, poetic creativity has never been so rich and spontaneous as it has been in recent years online; in some sense, it is reminiscent of the poetic activities of the pre-Islamic period, the Jāhiliyya, and the medieval period, when poets used to recite verses on every occasion they deemed suitable according to the famous saying, *li-kull maqām maqāl* ("every session has a different discussion"). Arab writers and poets are aware of the dramatic change in Arabic literary writing. The Iraqi poet Ṣalāḥ Fā'iq (b. 1945), who between 1994 and 2019 had been living in the Philippines before he moved to Britain, recently started to be active on Facebook and made it, in his words, "a daily occupation." And he has testified to this change:

بفضل الفيسبوك، لي الآن أصدقاء وقرّاء
أتقدّم بجزيل الشّكر إلى نفسي
لأنّي أنجزت هذا!

Thanks to Facebook, I now have friends and readers.
Many thanks to myself,
Because I have made it![22]

Without the Internet, Fā'iq would have been totally excluded from the Arabic literary scene, but for several years I have been reading his poetic texts on a (more or less) daily basis.[23] His compatriot Hātif al-Janābī (b. 1952) has

[21] Cf. also what the Saudi scholar 'Abd Allāh al-Ghadhdhāmī (b. 1946) argues:

"في هذا العصر لم يعد الشعر هو الأهم، بل أصبح الخطاب الاتصال العام، خطاب التفاعل وشرائط الأخبار والتلفزيون والتواصل والفضائيات"

It is ironic that al-Ghadhdhāmī expressed his view in a discussion broadcast on Twitter, available at: https://twitter.com/search?q=%D8%AC%D9%86%D8%A7%D9%8A%D8%A9%20%D8%A3%D8%AF%D9%88%D9%86%D9%8A%D8%B3%20%D8%A3%D9%88%20%D8%A7%D9%84%D8%BA%D8%B0%D8%A7%D9%85%D9%8A&src=typed_query&f=top March 1, 2022 (last accessed March 20, 2022).

[22] See Salah Faik, August 12, 2016, available at: https://www.facebook.com/salah.faik/posts/859439700855905 (last accessed December 27, 2020).

[23] He justifies his daily poetry publication as a kind of compulsion (أنشر كلّ يوم لأنّي مرغم على ذلك); see Salah Faik, August 22, 2021, available at: https://www.facebook.com/salah.faik/posts/2333698093430051 (last accessed August 23, 2021). On Ṣalāḥ Fā'iq's poetry published on Facebook, see comments by the 'Umānī poet Fāṭima al-Shīdī (b. 1973) (al-Shīdī 2021).

stated that the "Internet brought about a great leap, facilitating our writing and its checking and revising; it enables us to be familiar over the net with the experiences of others; it makes easy our connection with intellectuals and writers so we can see them on the palm of our hand. The advantages of the Internet are innumerable despite its disadvantages."[24] On the occasion of publishing a new anthology of Arabic poetry, the Iraqi poet Naṣīf al-Nāṣirī (b. 1960) wrote the following:[25]

في سنوات الثَّمانينيّات من القرن الماضي، كان أكثر الَّذين يُهيمنون على الإعلام طبعًا أصدقاء
وأساتذة أجلاَّء، رئاسة تحرير المجلاّت الأدبيَّة، الصّحف، دوائر الإبداع، الخ، يتَّهمون الشُّعراء
الشُّباب آنذاك بقلَّة الثَّقافة وقلَّة الوعي، وعدم الموهبة، والسَّعي إلى تدمير التُّراث. طبعًا من غير
المعقول أن يسعى الشّاعر الشّاب الَّذي يحاول ويُجرِّب أن يسعى إلى هدم تراث عمره أكثر من
1700 سنة. الآن وأنا أغطسُ في أعماق هذا التُّراث الكبير منذ أكثر مِن 36 سَنَة، أشعرُ أنَّ آبائي
الشّعراء الكُثار آلهة عُظماء، تجارب كبيرة ومختلفة، وأجملُ ما في الشّعر العربيّ، هي الدَّيمومة.
ماكو شاعر أحْسَن مِن شاعر. لكلّ شاعر تجاربه وأساليبه وموضوعاته وأحلامه.

In the 1980s, most those who controlled the media were, of course, friends and great scholars, such as editors of literary magazines, of departments of literary creation; they accused the young poets at the time of lack of culture and lack of awareness and talent and an attempt to destroy the heritage. Of course, it is unreasonable for a young poet who is trying and experimenting to be able to destroy a heritage of 1,700 years. Now, when I have been diving for the last 36 years into the depths of this great heritage, I feel that my many ancestors, the great poets, they were great gods and they had great and various experiences. Each poet has his own experiences, styles, themes, and dreams. (Facebook, September 10, 2016)

Internet technologies were also behind the Arab Spring revolution: on January 15, 2011, the Tunisian poet Muḥammad al-Ṣaghīr Awlād Aḥmad (Mohamed Sghaïer Ouled Ahmed) (1955–2016) posted the following graffiti-like text on his Facebook wall:

كنتُ أنوي كتابة قصيدة جديدة،
وجدتُ جنازة محمّد البوعزيزي.
مشيتُ وراءها
فاذا بي أشارك في انجاز ثورة بأسرها

I was planning to write a new poem,
I found Muḥammad al-Būʿazīzī's funeral.

---

[24] See his essay "The Exile Has Lost Its Glory," available at: https://www.alaraby.co.uk (last accessed August 16), 2016. See also Hatif Janabi, August 16, 2016, available at: https://www.facebook.com/hatif.janabi/posts/1043869042358323 (last accessed December 28, 2020).

[25] I have made only minor modifications to the punctuation.

I walked behind [the coffin]
All of a sudden, I was participating in the creation of a whole revolution.[26]

Muḥammad al-Bū'azīzī (Mohamed Bouazizi) (1984–2011) was the Tunisian street vendor who on December 17, 2010 set himself on fire in front of the municipal headquarters in Sidi Bouzid. It was a desperate act of protest against the confiscation of his merchandise by a municipal official. Soon, the incident set the social networks ablaze, and Bouazizi became the symbol of social and economic injustice in Tunisia, a catalyst for the Tunisian Revolution and the wider Arab Spring against autocratic regimes. The Tunisian uprising has enacted a spatial revolution that accommodates hitherto incongruent geographies, namely, the virtual space of social media and the real space of the street. Poetry, revolution, and technology lace together and negotiate a new aesthetics wherein poetics and politics engage in a dialogue in a porous virtual space. The new and innovative turn in Muḥammad al-Ṣaghīr Awlād Aḥmad's literary work, continuing until his death, was his unremitting use of Facebook as a channel of writing and protest. In a study of his poetry by Hager Ben Driss, she refers to his blurring of the lines between the private and the public, and the personal narratives about his oppression by the regime became a testimony to collective trauma:

> Facebook was his headquarters, a location of poetical and political activism ... Facebook was not a site to indulge in private socialization; it was an official place for militant activities. As a place maker, Ouled Ahmed transformed the virtual space of social network into a place of poetry and revolution. As he complicated the lines between poeticizing the revolution and revolutionizing poetry, he created a poetics of the virtual, a new geo-poetics combining virtual geography with poetry. The result is a type of writing that trespasses across the traditional borders between prose and verse, online texts and printed ones.[27]

The Egyptian Ṣabrī Ḥāfiẓ (Sabry Hafez) (b. 1942), one of the few scholars of his generation who has deeply understood the major impact the explosion of the Internet has had on Arab culture, alluded to his personal experience in editing one of the most widely read online cultural journals, *al-Kalima*,[28] which was launched in January 2007:

> When I embarked on this project, I was aware of a number of factors that contributed to the launching of this online journal. These include: the rapid growth of reading on the internet in the Arab world, particularly among

[26] See at: https://www.facebook.com/hamadi.elleuch.7/posts/171764252866590 (last accessed June 13, 2021). For another translation, see Ben Driss 2021, p. 83.
[27] Ben Driss 2021, p. 99.
[28] See at: http://www.alkalimah.net (last accessed June 30, 2021).

> the younger generation; the dwindling market of print literary journals, on account of the delays in their appearance which wrecked their regularity, the *raison d'être* of journalism; the growing cost of print journals, which priced their reader, particularly the young, out of the market; the tightening of various boundaries—geographical, political and censorship-related—which deterred their movement and decreased their dissemination; the urgent need for a truly independent literary forum that was regular and free from censorship and co-option; the need for a critical forum capable of "speaking truth to power," following Edward Said; and, finally, the fact that the young writers and the marginalized were already flocking to the internet and creating their own blogs.[29]

According to Hafez, cyberspace has become the space for literary and cultural publication in the twenty-first century, and any investigation of literary journalism in the present century needs to look closely at it as it requires, for example, "a different theoretical approach based on the Deleuzean concept of the *rhizome* besides Bourdieu's concept of the cultural field. The internet itself seems to embody the six principles of the Deleuzean *rhizome* with its connection, heterogeneity, multiplicity, signifying rupture against the over-signifying breaks separating structures or cutting across a single structure, and the principle of cartography and decalcomania."[30]

In short, Arabic literature is now in another place, but its scholarship needs time to adapt to the dramatic changes it has been undergoing. And I write this without ignoring the negative aspects of the Internet, which Arab writers are aware of.[31] For example, the Moroccan writer Fāṭima al-Zahrā' al-Rayūwī (Fatima al-Zohra al-Rghioui) (b. 1974) says:

> تلك النّصوص الفايسبوكيّة شبه اليوميّة، فأنا لا أسمّيها كتابة حقّا. لا أعرف كيف أسمّيها. إنّها كتابة قلقة أيضا، وملحّة، ولكنّها لا تشبع رغبتي في الكتابة، وإنّما تزيد الظّمأ.

> Those Facebook texts, I cannot refer to them as real [literary] writing. I do not know how to call them. This is a restless writing, pressing, but it cannot satisfy my desire for writing, only intensify the thirst.[32]

[29] Hafez 2017, pp. 38–9.

[30] Hafez 2017, p. 32. For a delineation of the Deleuzean concept of the *rhizome*, see Deleuze and Guattari 1987, pp. 3–25.

[31] On the negative approach to the Internet and the fear of the tremendous damage it could inflict on visitors to the virtual world side by side with its importance in allowing people to cross barriers of time and place and overcome obstacles of religion, race, and ethnicity, see Younis 2021, pp. 224–43.

[32] See at: http://elmawja.com/blog (September 2, 2016). Cf. critical remarks by the poet Ḥusām Ma'rūf (b. 1981) regarding prose poem texts published on social media websites (see at: https://www.eremnews.com/culture [November 2 , 2022] [last accessed November 7, 2022]).

And the Iraqi poet Zaʿīm Naṣṣār (b. 1960) considered the "Facebook's poets" terrorists because they "destroyed the life of my Arabic words."[33] Furthermore, a deep nostalgia for the simple and unsophisticated past has given birth to such poems as "My Mother Does Not Have a Facebook" by the Syrian poet Ibrāhīm Qaʿdūnī:

ليسَ لدى أمّي فيسبوك
ولا واتساب،
إنّما لديها قلبٌ سُرعانَ ما يهبِطُ كلّما رنَّ جرسٌ بعد التّاسعة
ويدان مفتوحتان على السّماء، تبعثان برسائل محروقة الأطراف
تسألُ فتجاب،
هي الّتي لازمت حياتنا بمنبّه صوتها الصّباحيّ،
قبلَ ديكة الحيّ تداهم نومنا

My mother does not have Facebook
And not WhatsApp,
But she has a heart that immediately falls down when the bell rings after 0900,
And she keeps her hands open to the sky, sending letters the edges of which are burned.
She asks and is being answered,
She accompanied our life with her morning awakening voice,
Before the neighborhood's roosters invaded our sleep.[34]

But it seems that a post by the Iraqi poet ʿAlī Nwayyir (b. 1950) on Facebook, whose title is "I Salute You, I Am the Facebook Poet," is representative of most Arab writers who have started to be active on the Internet. Among what Nwayyir has written is the following:

قالوا: شاعرٌ فيسبوكيّ.
وقالوا: شاعرةٌ فيسبوكيّة.
وأقول: ليس ثمّة أجمل من فضائهما الأزرق هذا، من قبلُ وربّما من بعدُ. هذا الكائن الخرافيّ بأجنحته السّحريّة ومداه اللامنتهي هو أكثر واقعيّةً ممّا نعتقد ويعتقدون، حيث يضعنا في قلب العالم الحيّ، ويُدخِل العالم كلّه بلا استئذان الى القلب والرّوح والوجدان.

They say: A Facebook poet.
And they say: A Facebook poetess.
And I say: There is nothing more beautiful than their blue space, there was not before and will perhaps be not even after. This mythological creature with its magic wings and its infinite space is much more realistic than we and

[33] See زعيم نصّار, August 27, 2021, available at: https://www.facebook.com/zaeemalnassar/posts/10159905517514407 (last accessed August 27, 2021).

[34] *Jarīdat Zaytūn*, June 5, 2017. See also at: https://baytalnas.blogspot.com/2020/06/AnthologyofSyrianpoetry.html?hl=en (last accessed December 28, 2020).

> they think; it puts us in the heart of the living world and inserts, without any permission, the whole world into [our] heart and spirit and emotional life.[35]

As its subtitle indicates, the present book has two main axes relevant to contemporary Arabic literary production: the first axis is *heritage*. Modern Arab authors have been drawing inspiration from their rich ancient heritage whether it has been embodied in texts or concrete experiences, real or imaginary. This is why the way we view the relationship between modern and medieval Arabic literature is highly essential for our understanding of the nature of the contemporary Arabic literary system. Moreover, the *literariness* of any text cannot be isolated from the history of the literature in the language in which the text is written, and, at the same time, it cannot be isolated from the history of literatures in other languages. No literary text can be read in isolation from other texts, certainly when it comes to Arabic literary texts.

The second axis is *world literature*. The relationships and connections between Arabic literature and other literatures are essential for our understanding of the nature of the contemporary Arabic literary system, whereby Arabic literature may become a source of direct or indirect loans for another literature and vice versa. What may move, be borrowed, and/or taken over from one culture to another is not just an item of repertoire, but also a host of other literary features used in that repertoire. The role and function of literature, the nature of literary criticism and scholarship, the relations between religious, political, and other activities within culture and literary production—all may be modeled in a given culture in relation to some other culture or cultures.

The book is structured in line with these two axes: it consists of two parts, each of which has four chapters. Each chapter includes an introduction, three additional sections, and a conclusion. The following is a short description of the parts and chapters of the book.

Part I, "Heritage, Myth, and Continuity," discusses four cases representing the strong connections between the various periods of Arabic literature and the significance of medieval cultural heritage for Arabic literary authors. *Chapter 1*, "Topos: *Mundus Inversus*," discusses the tendency found in various modern Arabic literary texts to represent reality as topsy-turvy, which in Western criticism is known as the topos of *mundus inversus* (world upside down). This topos' widespread literary use in all genres of contemporary Arabic literature—fiction, poetry, and theater alike—necessarily raises the possibility of commonly known and shared models or sources of inspiration.

35 See علي نوير, Septemebr 1, 2016, available at: https://www.facebook.com/ali.nwayyir/posts/1068901856559144 (last accessed December 27, 2020).

Chapter 2, “Challenge: The al-Andalus Experience,” deals with the way in which the experience of al-Andalus, Muslim Spain, is used in modern Arabic poetry as a vehicle to challenge Western cultural hegemony. Since the nineteenth century, Arab poets have been invoking the image of al-Andalus in a conscious effort to highlight the benefits that Western civilization has gained through its interaction with Arab civilization—the al-Andalus experience is seen as an epitome of that interaction, the Arabs’ greatest and most enduring success on European soil. *Chapter 3*, “Glory: Baghdad in Verse,” refers to the role of Baghdad in Arabic poetry since its foundation in 762 AD and throughout the history of Arabic literature. Baghdad was founded at a time when Arabic poetry was at its peak, and its development thus coincided with and was inspired by the creative imagination of the poets who were associated with what was a cultural urban center during the Golden Age of medieval Arabic culture. The discussion in this chapter refers as well to the period from the city’s downfall until modern times. *Chapter 4*, “Religion: ‘I Saw My God,’” refers to the role that Islam, especially Muslim mysticism (i.e., Sufism), plays in Arabic poetry. Even from the time of early Islam, we can find mystical dimensions in non-religious poetry, for this was a time when poets started to express spiritual feelings and the desire to be absorbed by nature together with pantheistic revelations. And following the Second World War, which undermined the belief that technology and science would be able to bring about human salvation, one could sense a strong tendency in Arabic poetry to return to the early and pure values of Muslim mysticism.

Part II, “East, West, and World Literature,” deals with the impact of Western culture on Arabic literature since the nineteenth century against the backdrop of its deflated self-image. *Chapter 5*, “Self-Image: Between ‘Decadence’ and Renaissance,” concentrates on the decline of the self-image of Arabic literature against the backdrop of its relationships with the West. Examining the repeated lamentations by Arab intellectuals and writers about the status of Arab culture throughout the last two centuries, the nuances and wording of each of their plaints enable us to understand their complicated attitude toward the West in light of the huge gap between the august status enjoyed by Arab culture in the Middle Ages and its feeble modern counterpart. *Chapter 6*, “Existentialism: The Frightened Mouse,” discusses the significant existentialist impact of Franz Kafka on Arabic literary writing, which was at least partially due to the fact that his work was torn between the tragic conviction that the destiny of human existence is determined and the frustrated desire to change it. Such impact can be found, for example, in the fiction writing of Najīb Maḥfūẓ, who resembles Kafka especially in his intensive use of the absurd. Here, I will explore the interactions between Kafka’s works and Arabic poetry, discussing the inspiration that the

Egyptian poet Ṣalāḥ ʻAbd al-Ṣabūr drew from him. *Chapter 7*, "Reception: Stream of Consciousness," deals with the process of reception of Western authors in Arabic literature not as an example of direct interference, but of indirect interference through intermediaries, especially via translation. The case study here is the reception of English literature in Arabic literature as illustrated by the writings of Virginia Woolf, whose inspiration later opened the way for Arab authors, female writers included, to write original fiction in Arabic in her spirit. It goes without saying that many other foreign authors exerted their impact on Arab authors directly or indirectly through translations. *Chapter 8*, "Import: Science Fiction," deals with the genre of science fiction (SF) as a new and emerging imported genre in Arabic literature. Initially, this growth came as a result of translations and adaptations, but later it came as a result of an increase in original Arabic SF texts, which eventually entered the process of canonization. The emergence of SF in Arabic literature is the most evident illustration of imported genre—at least from the point of view of the beginnings of the genre: it grew by borrowing the relevant Western patterns. At a later stage, the genre would pass through a process of Arabization and even Islamization.

The *Epilogue*, "Arabic Literature and World Literature," deals with the place of Arabic literature within world literature, referring to the issue of the continuity of Arabic literary writing and the relationship between modern, premodern, and classical Arabic literature, which is essential to our understanding of the nature of the contemporary Arabic literary system. Summarizing my studies published during the last fifty years, I discuss the conceptions and insights provided by one of the major contributions to the study of Arabic literature in recent years in order to provide students, scholars, and readers with the necessary theoretical tools to critically examine various issues in the field.

PART I

Heritage, Myth, and Continuity

ريشتُك المسمومة الخضراءْ
ريشتُك المنفوخةُ الأوداج باللّهيبْ
بالكوكب الطّالع من بغدادْ
تأريخنا وبعثنا القريبْ
في أرضنا — في موتِنا المُعادْ.
– **أدونيس**

Your green poisonous quill
Your quill whose veins swelled with flame
With the star rising from Baghdad
Is our history and our immediate resurrection
In our land—in our recurring death.
– Adūnīs

What is the relationship between cultural heritage, on the one hand, and contemporary literature, on the other? And what do we mean when we speak about myth and continuity in literature in our current age of globalization? While the historical circumstances of a contemporary literary text seem sometimes to be "essential" for its understanding, at least by the estimation of some schools of literary studies, the remote history and heritage of a society or a culture, or even a literature written in a specific language, are generally not considered "important." Why should we be familiar with a text's cultural heritage and its myths, or even the poetry written some centuries ago, in order to read and understand the text? First, there is no need to be familiar with anything if you want to read a poem or a novel in a language you know: you can read and even unconditionally enjoy them with your own understanding, even if it is limited, using "objective" criteria. Critics and literary historians, however, refer to these questions and offer several models as answers. Among the various models dealing with the relationship between literary texts and history, scholars mention a model that considers literature as aesthetically autonomous and universal, as transcending the contingencies of any particular historical time or place, and as having its own laws. Another model sees literary texts as being produced within specific historical contexts that are necessary for their proper understanding but, at the same time, remain separate from these texts. A third model refers to literature, especially realist works, as providing imaginative representation of specific historical events and periods. A fourth model, associated with the new historicist criticism, refers to literary texts as being bound up with other discourses and as being a part of a history that is still in the process of being written.[1] These four models, which characterize various schools of literary studies, are not contradictory, and critics belonging to each school can easily present examples of literary works that represent their specific approach.

But there is another aspect relevant to the aforementioned issues concerning cultural heritage, associated myths, and continuity with regard to literature. The *literariness* of any given text cannot be isolated from the history of the literature in the language in which the text was written, and it cannot be isolated from the history of literatures in other languages. No literary text can be fully understood in isolation from other literary texts, and this is certainly the case when speaking about contemporary Arabic literary texts. This is why the way in which we view the relationship between modern and medieval Arabic literature is essential to our understanding of the nature of the Arabic literary system. In this regard, the Egyptian author and scholar

[1] This section is inspired by Bennett and Royle 2004, pp. 18–26, 113–23. Cf. Snir 2019, pp. 191–202.

Ṭāhā Ḥusayn (1889–1973) expressed in the mid-1940s a very clear position: in his article "al-Adab al-ʿArabī Bayna Amsihi wa-Ghadihi" ("Arabic Literature between Its Past and Future"),[2] which in October 1945 opened the first issue of his journal *al-Kātib al-Miṣrī*,[3] he asserts the continuity of Arabic literature. Unlike Greek and Latin literatures, which have no direct contemporary extensions, modern Arabic literature, according to Ḥusayn, is a direct linear extension of classical Arabic literature:

> The historical existence of Arabic literature has never been cut off, and it seems that it will never be cut off. The connection between this literature and contemporary generations in the lands of the Arab East, from the Persian Gulf to the Atlantic Ocean, and in various Arab lands here and there, is still strong and fertile, like the connection between Arabic literature and the Arab nation during the period of al-Mutanabbī and Abū al-ʿAlāʾ ... Arabic literature is very traditional and at the same time very modern. *Its ancient past has been directly mingled with its modern present without any break or bend* ... Our Arabic literature is a living being and resembles, more than anything else, a huge tree, the roots of which have been consolidated and extended into the depths of the earth, while its branches have risen and spread out in space. The water of life is still ample and running in its steady roots and its high branches ... Our Arabic literature is definitely a traditional one, possessing an old Arab-Bedouin character that it never relinquished, nor will it ever do so ... The way in which we see things might change as ages, regions, and circumstances change. But our way of portraying things, even if it takes different shapes, will always go back to a set of traditional principles which cannot possibly be avoided, because such avoidance means killing this literature and breaking the connection between it and the new time as well as deterring it from the road of the continuous life of the living literatures [and moving it] onto the road of cut-off life that the Greek and Latin literatures took.[4]

This direct extension of classical into modern literature has been guaranteed, according to Ḥusayn, by the continuous equilibrium that Arabic literature maintained until modern times between aspects of continuity and aspects of change:

> The revival of ancient Arabic literature[5] was, and still is, turning modern Arab minds toward the past, highlighting elements of stability and steadfastness. On the other hand, the contact with modern European literature has been pushing

[2] Ḥusayn 1945, pp. 4–27. The article was also incorporated into Ḥusayn n.d. [1958], pp. 5–32.
[3] The publisher was the Jewish Harari Brothers—the journal was closed down following the 1948 War. On the journal and its conceptions, see Micklethwait 2011, pp. 155–92.
[4] Ḥusayn 1945, pp. 10–11; Ḥusayn n.d. [1958], pp. 11–13 (my emphasis).
[5] That is, through the editing and disseminating of classical texts since the mid-nineteenth century.

> Arabic literature in a different direction, stressing elements of mobility and change. It is surprising that the Arab mind has maintained its equilibrium in spite of this fierce conflict. Indeed, it has benefited from it immensely.[6]

By preserving some traditional principles to ensure its distinctive identity and, at the same time, incorporating a variety of innovations both in form and content, Arabic literature has proven its vitality down through the ages.[7] In the following chapters of *Part I* of the book, I will discuss four cases in which the cultural heritage and the contemporary form of Arabic literature are intermingled—in other words, in these cases the direct linear extension between modern and medieval Arabic literature is vital if we want to fully understand contemporary literary texts.

Chapter 1, "Topos: *Mundus Inversus*," discusses the tendency found in various modern Arabic literary texts to represent reality as topsy-turvy, which in Western criticism is known as the topos of *mundus inversus* (world upside down). This topos' widespread literary use in all genres of contemporary Arabic literature—fiction, poetry, and theater alike—necessarily raises the possibility of commonly known and shared models or sources of inspiration. There exist some similarities between the various renditions of the topos of *mundus inversus* and certain thematic elements in Western literary schools, such as Surrealism, the Absurd, and Nonsense literature; however, these similarities are predominantly external compared with the specific literary use of that topos and its contexts. In this chapter, I will present the employment of this topos and its literary Arabic renditions in some genres and among various writers with clear allusions to the figure of the *Dajjāl* (the Deceiver), namely, the False Christ—the Antichrist and Armillus from the Christian and Jewish traditions, respectively—that evil personage endowed with supernatural powers who, according to Muslim tradition, will come forth before the end of time and rule in heresy and tyranny for a limited period of either forty days or forty years, and who will be followed by the universal conversion of humanity to Islam. The *Dajjāl*'s appearance is one of the proofs of the end of time, and he will die at the hands of the *Mahdī* (the Rightly Guided) or Jesus. In ancient Muslim traditions, the appearance of the Antichrist is preceded by *Ashrāṭ al-Sāʿa* (The Signs of the Day of Judgment) mentioned in the Qur'ān. Some of these signs are frequently presented in the form of what is described as the topos of *mundus inversus*.

Chapter 2, "Challenge: The al-Andalus Experience," deals with the way the experience of al-Andalus, Muslim Spain, is used in modern Arabic poetry as a vehicle to face the decline of the Arabs' self-image and to challenge Western

[6] Ḥusayn 1945, p. 17; Ḥusayn n.d. [1958], p. 20.

[7] Cf. Semah 1974, p. 122. For a discussion of this topic, see Snir 2017, pp. 175–93.

cultural hegemony (which will be discussed in a separate chapter). Since the nineteenth century, Arab poets have been invoking the image of al-Andalus in a conscious effort to highlight the benefits that Western civilization has gained through its interaction with Arab civilization—the al-Andalus experience is seen as an epitome of that interaction, the Arabs' greatest and most enduring success on European soil. But even more so, when poets recall the cultural achievements of the Andalusian Arab heritage during nearly 800 years of Muslim rule, they do so to remind their audience that their present bitter state is only a transitory period, a temporary clouding of the skies between a glorious past and a splendid future. Also, modern Arab writers and artists have been reviving the Andalusian past, especially for its achievement in the fields of literature and music, in order to counter those who claim that Arab culture has become excessively Westernized. Inspired by nostalgia, the picture that most frequently appears in modern Arabic literary writings is that of al-Andalus as the "lost paradise" (*al-firdaws al-mafqūd*) or "God's paradise on earth" (*jannat Allāh 'alā al-arḍ*). As Muslim Spain is generally associated in contemporary Arabic literature with images intended to play off Arab culture against Western culture, it is not surprising that most literary expressions of al-Andalus have appeared in poetry. Unlike other modern genres of Arabic literature, the genre of poetry was not introduced into the Arabic literary system only as a result of the impact of Western culture. Poetry recorded the very appearance of the Arabs and has been the principal channel through which Arabic literary creativity has been flowing from the pre-Islamic period, through the Middle Ages when it reached a peak both in the East and in al-Andalus, to the present day.

Chapter 3, "Glory: Baghdad in Verse," is about the role that Baghdad has played in Arabic poetry since its foundation in 762 AD and throughout the history of Arabic literature. Baghdad was founded at a time when Arabic poetry was at its peak, and its development thus coincided and was inspired by the creative imagination of the poets who were associated with what was a cultural urban center during the Golden Age of medieval Arabic culture. The glorious image of the city perched on both banks of the Tigris ignited the imagination of subsequent generations of poets to carve it in verse and enshrine it in the mantle of universal myth. "Poetry and Baghdad are indivisible, flowing together. One reflects, then feeds the other and so on," as one contemporary Baghdadi poet writes: "The very nature of Baghdad strikes the match that ignites the poetic imagination of the Iraqis, and, in a sense, of poets in the Arab world." During several periods, Baghdad became known for its remarkable religious tolerance, multicultural cosmopolitan atmosphere, and peaceful cohabitation between all components of the local society. There were also periods when Baghdad claimed attention because of its dramatic decline and disintegration (such as following the destruction of the city in 1258 by Hulagu—see below), as well as for being a theater for bloody wars (such as during the American-led occupation in 2003), but even in such tragic times the image of an alternative, utopian Baghdad, as a metaphor, remained immune to the vicissitudes of time and the dreary reality of the earthly city. The sway of Baghdad, the fabled city of Hārūn al-Rashīd and the enchanted land of *A Thousand and One Nights*, continues to capture the imagination of successive generations of poets, writers, and artists the world over. Neither East nor West seems immune to its irresistible charm.

Chapter 4, "Religion: 'I Saw My God,'" explores the role that Muslim mysticism, Sufism, plays in modern Arabic poetry. Early mystic Arabic poetry arose along with the development of Ṣūfī theory at the beginning of the ninth century AD and flourished during the next several centuries. Its origins were rooted in the spontaneous utterances of early Ṣūfī mystics, who poetically expressed their love of God and, at the same time, rejected worldly pleasures. The birth of modern Arabic secular poetry in the second half of the nineteenth century paved the way for the appearance of mystic dimensions in non-religious poetry, especially after the First World War, when poets started to emphasize personal experiences and feelings, the desire to be absorbed by nature, and pantheistic revelations and mythological elements. Following the Second World War, which undermined belief that technology and science would be able to bring about human salvation, one senses a strong tendency to return to the early pure values of Muslim mysticism. Contemporary secular Arab poets have closed a circle originally opened by the first Ṣūfī poets more than twelve centuries ago. The simplicity and spontaneity that characterized the early Muslim works of mysticism are revived in contemporary poetic expressions of mystical love, especially with the emergence of new poetic models. As secular poets, contemporary Arab poets, who make frequent use of early Ṣūfī terms and figures, rarely concern themselves with the precise original meanings of the ancient terms, concentrating rather on the expression of their experiences and feelings as well as their social views. Unlike the early Ṣūfī poets, they are not solely committed to Ṣūfī themes, and Sufism is not a practical way of life for them. All poets of this trend are united in their sensitivity to the dialectical tension between language and silence, and all of them occupy themselves with the alchemical metamorphoses and transformation of the despised body into the pure divine essence. That is why most of them adopt the metaphor of the poet as a mystic constantly advancing on the path toward the divine essence. Poetry for them is a *safar* (journey) that only winds up leading you to a new *safar*.

[illegible]

[illegible] Chapter 3, "Religion, [illegible]," explores the [illegible] Arabic [illegible] Arabic poetry. [illegible] along with the development of Sufi [illegible] the beginning of the ninth century AD [illegible] during the next several centuries. [illegible]

[illegible]

Chapter 1

Topos: *Mundus Inversus*[1]

The sheep forgets the face of its aged shepherd
The son turns against his father, and the tear-soaked loaf of bread
Tastes of ashes, and a glass eye
In a dwarf's head, denies the free light.
– 'Abd al-Wahhāb al-Bayyātī

1. INTRODUCTION

It is not rare to find a peculiar literary phenomenon or pattern in modern Arabic literature that has a rough equivalent in Western literature. Though frequently the tendency is to see the Arabic phenomenon as being inspired by its Western equivalent, one has to be careful enough not to make a hasty conclusion. Such is the case concerning the frequent representation of reality in Arabic literary texts as topsy-turvy. In Western criticism, this is known as the topos of *mundus inversus* (world upside down). The topos, generally, is "a commonplace appropriate for literary treatment, an intellectual theme suitable for development and modification according to the imagination of the individual author."[2] Originally, *topoi* were rhetorical concepts used in composing orations, but when rhetoric loses its original meaning and purpose, they acquire a new function and "become clichés, which can be used in any form of literature."[3] Ernst Robert Curtius (1886–1956), who discussed the adaptation of *topoi* to literary use, has illustrated this particular topos of the world upside down with one of the pieces

[1] This chapter uses material that first appeared in Snir 1991b, pp. 88–107; Snir 1994b, pp. 51–75; Snir 2007, pp. 181–208.
[2] Preminger 1974, p. 282.
[3] Curtius 1952, p. 70. On *topoi* in general, see Curtius 1952, pp. 79–105.

among the *Carmina Burana*, a collection of Goliardic poems whose underlying theme is the Horatian *carpe diem*.[4] The poem begins as follows:

> Once Learning flourished, but alas!
> 'Tis now become a weariness.
> Once it was good to understand,
> But play has now the upper hand.
> Now boyish brains become of age
> Long before time can make them sage,
> In malice too of age become,
> Shut wisdom out of house and home.
> In days long gone and passed away
> A scholar hardly dared to say
> When he had reached his ninetieth year,
> "My hour of rest from toil is here."
> But now see little boys of ten
> Lay down the yoke, strut out as men,
> And boast themselves full masters too.[5]

Starting out as a complaint about the times, the whole world represented in the next lines of the poem is topsy-turvy: birds fly before they are fledged; the ass plays the lute ("the ass is deaf to the lute," according to the Greek proverb); the Fathers Gregory, Jerome, Augustine, and Benedict are to be found in the alehouse, in court, or in the meat market;[6] Mary no longer delights in the contemplative life nor Martha in the active; Leah is barren and Rachel is bleary-eyed; Cato haunts the stews; and Lucretia has turned into a whore. The basic formal principle of the poem is a stringing together of impossibilities—that is, *adynata*[7]—whose first appearance seem to be, according to Curtius, in the work of the Greek poet Archilochus. The eclipse of the sun on April 6, 648 BC would seem to have given him the idea that nothing was any longer impossible now that Zeus had darkened the sun. This frequent and common topos in the Latin Middle Ages has worked its way into Western literature, and figures in the descriptions of the times, denunciations of and complaints about them, satire, and criticism leveled against different targets.[8]

This topos' widespread use in modern Arabic literature necessarily raises the possibility of commonly known and shared models or sources of

4 Preminger 1974, pp. 103–4, 324–5; Shipley 1972, pp. 49, 200; Cuddon 1986, pp. 103–4, 288.
5 Curtius 1952, pp. 94–5.
6 Cf. Nietzsche 1941, pp. 50–1.
7 Canter 1930, pp. 32–41; Shipley 1972, p. 3; Preminger 1974, p. 5; Cuddon 1986, p. 16.
8 Curtius 1952, p. 96.

inspiration. There exist, for example, some similarities between the various renditions of the topos of *mundus inversus* and certain thematic elements in Surrealism,[9] the Absurd,[10] and Nonsense literature;[11] however, these similarities are predominantly external compared with the specific literary use of that topos and its usual context. In the following sections, I will present the employment of the topos in various genres and its origins, starting with two of the most famous writers in modern Arabic literature, the first in poetry and the second in fiction.

2. "SON TURNS AGAINST HIS FATHER"

In his poem "Abārīq Muhashshama" ("Broken Pitchers"),[12] the Iraqi poet ʿAbd al-Wahhāb al-Bayyātī (1926–1999)[13] provides a clue to the roots of the topos of *mundus inversus* in Arabic literature. As in the entire collection by the same title (1954), al-Bayyātī abandons in that poem the romantic conception to which he had adhered in his first collection, *Malā'ika wa-Shayāṭīn* (*Angels and Devils*) (1950), and joins the pathbreakers to modernism in Arabic poetry.[14] Expressing his "boundless hope for the emancipation of the proletariat,"[15] he points to the awareness of servitude among the unliberated and their hope for change:

اللّه، والأفق المنوّر، والعبيد
يتحسّسون قيودهم:
"شيّد مدائنك الغداة
بالقرب من بركان فيزوف، ولا تقنع
بما دون النّجوم
وليضرم الحبّ العنيف
في قلبك النّيران، والفرح العميق."

God and the blazing horizon, and the slaves
Are feeling their chains:
"Tomorrow you must build your cities
Close to erupting Vesuvius, and not be satisfied

9 Shipley 1972, p. 403; Preminger 1974, pp. 821–3; Abrams 1981, p. 194; Cuddon 1986, pp. 668–9.
10 Abrams 1981, pp. 1–2; Taylor 1984, p. 7.
11 Preminger 1974, pp. 571–4; Shipley 1972, pp. 282–3; Cuddon 1986, pp. 425–8.
12 Al-Bayyātī 1954, pp. 82–3; al-Bayyātī 1979, I, pp. 157–9. On the poem, see also Thompson 2017, pp. 218–22.
13 In many scholarly publications (including in his English Wikipedia entry!), his name is transliterated as *al-Bayātī*. However, in all the collections of his poetry I have checked, the name on the cover is البيّاتي with a clear *shadda* on the letter *yā'* (ي).
14 Jayyusi 1977, p. 560.
15 Badawi 1975, pp. 210–11.

With anything beneath the stars
Let violent love and deep joy
Set your hearts aflame."[16]

Across from the slaves, who are aware of their slavery and have decided to break their chains, stand others:

والبائعون نسورهم يتضوّرون
جوعا، وأشباه الرّجال
عور العيون
في مفرق الطّرق الجديدة حائرون:
"لا بدّ للخفّاش
من ليل، وإن طلع الصّباح
والشّاة تنسى وجه راعيها العجوز
وعلى أبيه الابن، والخبز المبلّل بالدّموع
طعم الرّماد له، وعين من زجاج
في رأس قزم، تنكر الضّوء الطّليق."
وأرامل يتبعن أشباه الرّجال
تحت السّماء، بلا غد، وبلا قبور.

Whoever sells his eagles dies of
Starvation, and the impotent men
The one-eyed
Stand at the new crossroads confused:
"The bat must have
Night though it is daybreak now
The sheep forgets the face of its aged shepherd
The son turns against his father, and the tear-soaked loaf of bread
Tastes of ashes, and a glass eye
In a dwarf's head, denies the free light."
Widows follow the impotent men
Beneath the sky, without a future, and without graves.[17]

The above lines are steeped with descriptions that could be perceived as a reversal of the desired reality: the sheep does not remember the face of its good aged shepherd, the son rises up against his father,[18] the tear-soaked loaf of bread, whose dough the mother had kneaded with her tears, a motif

[16] The translation of the poem is based on Badawi 1975a, p. 133. See also Asfour 1988, pp. 84–5. For a study of the poem, see Snir 1995a, pp. 7–53.

[17] *Bilā qubūr* according to the first edition (al-Bayyātī 1954, p. 83). In several editions (e.g., al-Bayyātī 1969 [1954], p. 7; al-Bayyātī 1979, p. 159), it was printed wrongly as *bilā quyūd*, and Asfour (1988, p. 85) translates it as "without chains."

[18] Cf. "And brother will deliver up brother to death, and the father his child, and children will rise against parents and have them put to death" (Mark 13:12). See also Matthew 10:21; Bousset 1896, pp. 8, 122; Chekhov 1929, p. 492; Ibn Kathīr 1966, p. 203.

familiar from other nations' poetry as well,[19] tastes of ashes, and the widows follow no one but the impotent men. But there is also a mention of the one-eyed men and "a glass eye in a dwarf's head," which are clear allusions to the *Dajjāl* (the Deceiver) from the Muslim medieval tradition. This is the False Christ—Antichrist or Armillus from the Christian and Jewish religions, respectively—that evil personage endowed with miraculous powers who will come forth before the end of time and rule in heresy and tyranny for a limited period of either forty days or forty years and who will be followed by the universal conversion of humanity to Islam. His appearance is one of the proofs of the end of time, and he will die at the hands of the *Mahdī* or Jesus. According to early Muslim traditions, he is blind in his left eye[20] or right eye[21] and one of them is "like green glass."[22] The reversal of reality in the poem alludes to the *Ashrāṭ al-Sāʿa* ("The Signs of the Day of Judgment") mentioned in *sūrat Muḥammad* (47:18):

فَهَلْ يَنْظُرُونَ إِلاَّ السَّاعَةَ أَنْ تَأْتِيَهُمْ بَغْتَةً فَقَدْ جَاءَ أَشْرَاطُهَا فَأَنَّى لَهُمْ إِذَا جَاءَتْهُمْ ذِكْرَاهَا

> Are they looking for nothing but the Hour, that it shall come upon them suddenly? Already its tokens have come; so, when it has come to them, how shall they have their reminder?

Some of these signs are presented in the medieval Muslim tradition in the pattern of the aforementioned topos:

النبيّ، صلّى الله عليه وسلّم، قال: إنّ من أشراط السّاعة أن يرى رعاة الشّاء رؤوس النّاس، وأن يرى الحفاة العراة الجوع يتبارون في البناء، وأن تلد الأمة ربّها وربّتها.

> The Prophet, may God bless and save him, said: Among the Signs of the Day of Judgment, shepherds will become leaders; the naked, barefoot and hungry, will compete among themselves in building houses; and the slave girl will give birth to the master.[23]

19 Cf. a poem by the Hebrew poet Hayyim Nahman Bialik (1873–1934) (Bialik 1966, p. 113).

20 For example, Ibn Ḥanbal n.d., V, p. 38. Cf. Bukhārī 1927, IV, p. 143.

21 For example, Bukhārī 1927, IV, p. 142.

22 Ibn Ḥanbal n.d., V, pp. 123–4. About the *Dajjāl*, see also Wensinck and Mensing 1936–1969, II, p. 111; Abel 1965, pp. 76–7; Cook 2002, pp. 93–120; Livne-Kafri 2006, pp. 49–53, and the references mentioned there. Cf. the Antichrist in Jewish and Christian sources (Bousset 1895; Bousset 1896; Roth 1934; Hill 1971; Emmerson 1981).

23 Ibn Ḥanbal, n.d., II, p. 394. See also I, p. 27; III, pp. 151, 176, 202, 213, 273, 289; Bukhārī 1927, III, pp. 108, 164, 198; IV, pp. 137, 142; Shulman 1984, pp. 186–7; Cook 2017. For a selection of Muslim apocalypses translated into English, which include some aspects of this topos, see Cook 2002, pp. 333–85. One of the earliest Islamic sources in which the topos is found is *Kitāb al-Zuhd* by al-Muʿāfā ibn ʿImrān (Ibn ʿImrān n.d., 236b–237b. Cf. Snir 1982: traditions 13–19). Cf. the signs and events preceding the Antichrist's rule (Emmerson 1981, pp. 83–9).

In order to challenge a state of affairs demanding immediate reform, this Prophetic tradition combines realistic unaccepted conditions from the time it came into being and presents them hyperbolically as topsy-turvy.[24] The similarity between that reversal of the created order and the rhetorical hyperbole common in Arabic literature, with its various kinds (*mubālagha, ighrāq, ghuluww*), is only external.[25] The hyperbole is a figure or trope in which serious or comic effect is achieved by deliberate and extravagant bold exaggeration "with a tendency toward proverbial or quasi-proverbial form."[26] Conversely, the reversal of reality as represented by the *mundus inversus* topos is a hyperbolic display of unaccepted and rejected actual conditions. It differs as well from the aforementioned *adynaton* (sg. of *adynata*)—a form of hyperbole involving the magnification of an event by reference to the impossible, of which the two most common varieties in Greek and Latin literature are the "sooner than" type and the "impossible count."[27] While the *adynaton* strings together impossibilities as a limited rhetorical device with a local aim in the literary work, the topos generally proves to be pivotal for the presentation of the author's comprehensive worldview. It is presumably born when the committed author witnesses an actual and dangerous deviation from the desired reality, as he sees it. Out of his passion to restore that reality and in order to illustrate the dangers entailed by that deviation, unless it is corrected at once, he creates a fictional reversed rejected reality, which is in fact non-existent in the over-exaggerated presentation of the deviation. Not aware of the Islamic allusions, critics have failed to reach a full understanding of the comprehensive vision presented by al-Bayyātī's poem.[28] Though such interpretations are legitimate, they may be seen as based on the fallacy of considering modern Arabic poetry as lending itself to Western modes of composition. By means of the allusions to the ancient Arabic heritage, the committed al-Bayyātī apocalyptically illustrated the imminence of the revolution in accordance with his social realist views, which he was adhering to in the early 1950s and for which he has served

[24] Cf. also in Jewish and Christian sources, for example Micha 7:6; *Talmud Bavli*, Sotah, pp. 49a–49b (English translation: *The Talmud of Babylonia*, XVII, Tractate Sotah, pp. 284–5); Mark 13:12; Matthew 10:21. See also literary works with religious motifs, for example, Auden 1970, pp. 409–18; Eco 1984, pp. 75, 77–83, 401–5.

[25] Cf. Dana 1982, pp. 159–61, and also 97–105, in which the hyperbole is interwoven with the pseudo-Aristotelian aphorism "the best poem is the falsest" (Brann 1987, pp. 39–54); Ḥusayn 1983, pp. 82–9.

[26] Canter 1930, p. 41. Cf. Shipley 1972, p. 216; Preminger 1974, p. 359; Abrams 1981, pp. 77–8; Cuddon 1986, p. 316; Beckson and Ganz 1990, pp. 115–16.

[27] Preminger 1974, p. 5.

[28] Badawi 1975, p. 211; Jubrān 1989, pp. 72–4.

ever since as one of the most important Arab representatives.[29] The reversed order is the omen that presages the coming revolution in the aftermath of which a new era shall arrive:

والله والأفق المنوّر، والعبيد
يتحسّسون قيودهم:
"نبع جديد!
نبع تفجّر في موات حياتنا
نبع جديد
فليدفن الموتى موتاهم
وتكتسح السّيول
هذي الأباريق القبيحة، والطّبول
ولتفتح الأبواب، للشّمس الوضيئة والرّبيع."

God and the blazing horizon, and the slaves
Are feeling their chains:
"A new spring!
A spring has gushed forth in our dead life
A new spring
Leave the dead to bury their own dead[30]
And let the deluge sweep
Those ugly pitchers, and the drums
And let the gates be opened for the spring and the bright sun."

The poem was written in a period during which the poet believed that Communism would cure all ills, a belief he subsequently relinquished, as did other intellectuals in the Arab world following the exposure of Stalinist crimes in the Soviet Union. Ironically, in his poem "Madīnat al-Sindbād" ("The City of Sindbād"), al-Bayyātī's compatriot Badr Shākir al-Sayyāb (1926–1964) describes the chaos brought about in Iraq by the Communists during ʻAbd al-Karīm Qāsim's (1914–1963) regime in terms of a *mundus inversus*, in which Adonis is impotent and spring comes without flowers:

وفي القرى تموت
عشتار عطشى، ليس في جبينها زهر،
وفي يديها سلّة ثمارها حجر
ترجم كلّ زوجة به.

And in the villages
Astarte has died of thirst; there are no flowers on her forehead,

29 Cf. Moreh 1976, pp. 267–72; Jayyusi 1977, pp. 574–83.
30 Based on Matthew 8:21–22; cf. the use of this verse from the New Testament by the poet Yūsuf al-Khāl (1917–1987) (al-Khāl 1979, p. 201).

And in her hands she holds a basket, its fruit are stones
Stoning every wife with them.[31]

As in the case of al-Bayyātī's poem, unawareness of the Islamic roots of the topos has caused difficulties in the interpretation of the poem and in perceiving its overall vision.[32]

About twenty years after al-Bayyātī published his "Abārīq Muhashshama," the world of the persona in his poems was still in chaos, and the revolution whose omens had been envisioned still lingered in coming, as evidenced in his mystical poem "Qirā'a fī *Kitāb al-Ṭawāsīn* li-l-Ḥallāj" ("A Reading in *Kitāb al-Ṭawāsīn* by al-Ḥallāj") from the collection *Qamar Shīrāz* (*The Moon of Shīrāz*) (1975).[33] The world according to al-Bayyātī, who since the late 1950s has stood at the forefront of the neo-Ṣūfī trend in modern Arabic poetry, has yet to be freed from the tyrant's yoke. Wondering whether all that actually remains are only words, he presents a reality in which

تصير الكلمات
طوق نجاة
للغرقى في هذا اليمّ المسكون بفوضى الأشياء

The words become
A lifesaver
To those who drown in this ocean of chaos.

This poem has none of the assertiveness and optimism of his earlier poems, when the committed al-Bayyātī believed that the "upside-down world" was on the brink of reform and that the new world stood at the threshold.[34]

3. "TAIL ABOVE THE HEAD"

Awareness of the Islamic allusions of the *mundus inversus* pattern might be a powerful tool not only in interpreting a single literary work, but it may also shed new light on the comprehensive worldviews of some poets and writers. Such is the case of the Egyptian writer Najīb Maḥfūẓ (1911–2006). The most striking work in which images of an inverted order of creation frequently figure is the short story "Taḥt al-Miẓalla" ("Under the Bus Shelter") from the

[31] Al-Sayyāb 1971, I, pp. 463–73. On al-Sayyāb's attitude to Qāsim's regime, see also a series of articles he published during 1959 in *al-Ḥurriyya* titled "Kuntu Shuyū'iyyan" ("I Was a Communist"); the articles were later incorporated into al-Sayyāb 2007.

[32] For example, see Moreh 1976, pp. 250, 254–5; Moreh 1984, pp. 182–3; Moreh 1988, pp. 157–8.

[33] Al-Bayyātī 1984 [1975], pp. 21–34; al-Bayyātī 1979, III, pp. 423–36.

[34] For a full interpretation of both of al-Bayyātī's poems, see Snir 1992a, pp. 7–54; Snir 1993b, pp. 49–93.

eponymous collection.[35] Although it seems on the surface of the story that Maḥfūẓ is taking it in the direction of the Absurd,[36] or in the words of Rashīd al-ʻAnanī (Rasheed El-Enany) (b. 1949) "it is a world depicted in the best traditions of the literature of the absurd,"[37] under no circumstances should we treat Maḥfūẓ as a writer of that literary school. Such writers have a vision of life "without apparent purpose, out of harmony with its surroundings, sad to the point of anguish."[38] But Maḥfūẓ has always been a realist, his work featuring a concrete actuality with temporal dimensions and a very specific geographic framework.[39] Furthermore, if his works do have glimpses of the Absurd, then it serves for him as one of the contrasting poles from which it is necessary to stay away.[40] Maḥfūẓ himself unequivocally rejects any attempt to categorize him as belonging to this school:

> The meaning of the Absurd, briefly, is that there is no meaning to life, while to me life has meaning and purpose. All of my literary experience has been a battle against the Absurd. It could be that I sense the diffusion of absurdity, but I fight against it, try to make it rational, to explain it, to defeat it. Some of the heroes of [the novel] *al-Ḥarāfish*[41] look as though their lives were in vain, but in the context of the greater family they were not.[42]

Elsewhere, Maḥfūẓ further elaborates his views on the subject:

> I am definitely not a writer of the Absurd, but rather a writer committed to certain questions, which have always been a great concern to me. I began with them and I will end with them ... a writer of the Absurd does not believe in any values or any truth. This literature has no meaning of any kind.[43]

"Under the Bus Shelter" features a Cairene street in which people under a bus shelter witness a succession of events that contradict the order of a regulated world. A man, chased by men and boys yelling "thief," has been caught and beaten, but then dances naked while his pursuers clap their hands and dance around him; a couple indulge in sex in the open, while the woman's

35 Maḥfūẓ 1978 [1969], pp. 5–14 (for English translations, see Mahfouz 1969, pp. 50–5; Mahfouz 1973, pp. 141–9).
36 In 1997, even the author himself referred to the story as written "in the absurd mode" (Mahfouz 2001, p. 84).
37 El-Enany 1993, p. 201.
38 Cuddon 1986, p. 693. Cf. Hinchliffe 1981, pp. 35–44.
39 Cf. Badīr 1982, p. 87.
40 Anders 1965, p. 9; Myers 1986, p. 95.
41 Maḥfūẓ n.d. [1977].
42 Al-Ghīṭānī 1980, p. 54.
43 ʻAṭiyya 1970, pp. 27–8; ʻAṭiyya 1977, p. 19. About Maḥfūẓ's attitude to the Absurd, see also his story "al-Ḥubb wa-l-Qināʻ" ("Love and Mask") (Maḥfūẓ n.d. [1979], pp. 145–90 and esp. pp. 182–6). Cf. Snir 1989, pp. 135–6. On the "Absurd" in Maḥfūẓ's plays, see Riad 2000.

head lies on the corpse of one of the victims of a fatal traffic accident; from the south, a caravan of camels advances with a group of Bedouin men and women; from the north come foreign tourist buses; the two love-makers are buried, while still alive, in a tomb dug in the middle of the street, while the accident victims are laid upon a bridal bed erected nearby; the appearance of a judge reading what seems to be a verdict leads to fights, killing, dancing, and a sexual orgy on the tomb and around it; the policeman, who should be upholding the law, calmly watches all these reversed events. The onlookers under the bus shelter wonder whether they are witnessing a nightmare or a segment in the shooting of a movie with the policeman awaiting his turn to appear in the coming scene. When a man seems to be issuing orders, they are confident they have found the director, but he is chased off by the others. Viewing all these deviant events, including a severed human head rolling in the street toward them, the people under the bus shelter refrain from intervening, making every effort to justify their unwillingness to be involved. When they are finally driven to yell for the policeman, he asks for their identification cards, and although they deny any conspiracy he accuses them of lying and of subversive motives, and he shoots all of them to death.

The story, written presumably with the concrete aim of criticizing the regime of Egypt's then President Jamāl 'Abd al-Nāṣir (Gamal Abdel Nasser) (1918–1970), reflects, as the critics have pointed out, "condemnation of despotism,"[44] the sense of dismay among Arab intellectuals after the 1967 War, and the "dreadful anarchy and bloody climate in which our contemporary world lives."[45] It is also "an expression of the destructive forces in society. The violence of political authority is commensurate with the violence of anarchy."[46] But the interpretation of the story might acquire deeper significance by considering its Islamic allusions of the chaotic, bizarre events. The fictional point of view of the people under the bus shelter may be taken as corresponding to the realistic point of view of the intellectuals, even of Maḥfūẓ himself, in Egypt of the 1960s. Furthermore, the significance of the story cannot be confined to criticism of the regime, especially in light of the observation in the opening of the collection, in which this story is the first, that "these stories were written between October and December 1967."[47] Undoubtedly, the conflict in the Middle East is hovering over the stories even if the author himself indicates that "Under the Bus Shelter" is related

[44] Somekh 1987–1988, p. 10.
[45] Shukrī 1982, pp. 446–7.
[46] Myers 1986, p. 92.
[47] On Maḥfūẓ's political awareness as it relates to the conflict, see Snir 1989, pp. 120–5.

to the conflict on an abstract level "for a realistic portrayal of the problem is difficult, since we do not have a full understanding of reality."[48]

The story should be considered in view of the limitations placed on freedom of expression in Egypt in the 1960s, which required Maḥfūẓ, among others, to develop allusive literary modes.[49] These indirect modes, according to the author himself, were necessary even prior to the 1960s,[50] but the 1967 War made them urgent, as the fear among the intellectuals became greater. Keeping in mind the previously mentioned limitations on freedom of expression and being aware of the religious allusions of the topos, the significance of the story before us becomes strikingly clear. There is no better testimony to that significance than the climax of the reversal of order represented in the story:

> في أثناء الحديث تربّع فوق القبر رجل يرتدي روب القضاء. لم يرَ أحد من أين أتى. من عند الخواجات أو من عند البدو أو من حلقة الرّقص، لم يعرف أحد. بسط صحيفة بين يديه وراح يتلو نصًّا كأنّما ينطق بحكم. لم يميّز كلامه أحد إذ غطّى عليه التّصفيق وضوضاء الأصوات بشتّى اللّغات والمطر. ولكنّ كلماته غير المسموعة لم تضع فانتشرت في الطّريق حركات كالأمواج الصّاخبة في عنف وتضارب. نشبت معارك في محيط البدو وأخرى في مواقع الخواجات. واشتعلت معارك بين بدو وخواجات. وجعل آخرون يرقصون ويغنّون. وأقبل كثيرون حول القبر وراحوا يمارسون الحبّ عرايا. وأخذت النّشوة اللّصّ فتفنّن في رقصه وأبدع. واشتدّ كل شيء وبلغ غايته، القتل والرّقص والحبّ والموت والرّعد والمطر.

> A man wearing a judge's robe sat down cross-legged on the grave. No one had noticed where he had come from; the foreign tourists, the Bedouins, or the dancing circle, no one had any idea. He spread a sheet of paper in front of him and began reciting a text as though he were pronouncing judgment. No one could understand his words, since his voice was drowned by the clapping, the noises of people speaking in a variety of languages, and the rain. Yet his inaudible words were not lost, for the street suddenly seethed with movement and actions as violent and fraught with conflict as roaring waves. Battles broke out

48 ʿAṭiyya 1977, p. 158.

49 Cf. ʿAṭiyya 1977, p. 180; Milson 1977, pp. 437–8; Shukrī 1982, pp. d–h (introduction); *al-Jumhūriyya*, March 4, 1989, p. 8. On the indirect writing in Egypt in this period, see, for example, the novel *Shayʾ min al-Khawf* (*A Shred of Fear*) (Abāẓa 1983 [1967]) about whose meaning the author Tharwat Abāẓa (1927–2002) said that Fuʾāda symbolizes Egypt and ʿItrīs symbolizes ʿAbd al-Nāṣir, and the shout "The marriage of Fuʾāda and ʿItrīs is void" refers to the invalidity of the regime of ʿAbd al-Nāṣir (*al-Aḥrār*, January 8, 1990, p. 9). Among the classical meanings of the word ʿItrīs are "despotic," "tyrant," "demon," and even "the Devil" (Ibn Manẓūr n.d., VI, p. 130). On proper names as means of characterization, see Gordon 1917; Rudnyckyj 1959, pp. 378–82; Auden 1970, p. 267 (see also below). Still, it is an exaggeration to attribute the development of symbolic language in modern Arabic literature to the lack of political freedom (Ṭarābīshī 1972, p. 91. Cf. Idrīs 1973, p. 7; ʿAṭiyya 1977, p. 171).

50 For example, see Maḥfūẓ n.d. [1957], p. 209. Cf. ʿĀmir 1970, p. 26; ʿAṭiyya 1977, pp. 174–5. See also Milson 1989, p. 4; Snir 1989, pp. 125–8.

in the ranks of the Bedouins, and fights flared up among the tourists. Battles also raged between the Bedouins and the tourists. Others started dancing and singing and many turned to the grave and began making love, completely naked. The thief was overwhelmed by ecstasy and began to dance with consummate perfection. Everything grew in intensity and reached its climax: killing, dancing, love-making, death, thunder and rain.[51]

The similarity between this passage and the disorder described in the early Muslim traditions of *Ashrāṭ al-Sāʿa* is striking, as, for example:

لا تقوم السّاعة حتّى يقتتل فئتان عظيمتان يكون بينهما مقتلة عظيمة [...] وحتّى يبعث دجّالون قريب من ثلاثين كلّهم يزعم أنّه رسول الله [...] وحتّى يقبض العلم، وتكثر الزّلازل [...] وتظهر الفتن، ويكثر الهَرْج [...] وحتّى تشرق الشّمس من مغربها.

The Day of Judgment will not come until two large groups fight with one another, with great massacres between them ... and until about thirty false Antichrists make their appearance, each claiming to be the Prophet ... and until knowledge disappears and the earthquakes increase ... and the temptations appear and the sexual activity (*harj*)[52] increases ... and until the sun rises from the West.[53]

Like the identification of the Antichrist with a specific pope or political figure in the Middle Ages,[54] the Islamic allusions in the story may indicate that the Egyptian regime was perceived by the author as directed by the spirit of the *Dajjāl*. The same social and political message was delivered by writers not only after the war but also before it as, for example, in the verse drama *Maʾsāt al-Ḥallāj* (*The Tragedy of al-Ḥallāj*) (1964) of Maḥfūẓ's compatriot, the poet Ṣalāḥ ʿAbd al-Ṣabūr (1931–1981). In Scene III, Act I, the Ṣūfī al-Ḥusayn ibn Manṣūr al-Ḥallāj (858–922) says:

وخلف القحط، جيش الشّرّ والنّقمة
خلائقهم مشوّهة، كأنّ الذّيل فوق الرأس
يقود خطاهمو إبليس، وهو وزير ملك القحط
وليس القتل والتّدجيل والسّرق
وليس خيانة الأصحاب والملق
وليس البطش والعدوان والخرق
سوى بعض رعايا القحط، جند وزيره إبليس.

And behind poverty, under its unfurled banner,
March poverty's soldiers, the legions of evil vengeance;
Those malformed creatures, as though the tail above the head
Led by the devil, Vizier of the kingdom of poverty

51 Maḥfūẓ 1978 [1969], p. 11.
52 Ibn Manẓūr n.d., II, p. 389. The traditional meaning of this word is *qatl* (killing) (cf. Wensinck and Mensing 1936–1969, VII, pp. 82–3).
53 Bukhārī 1927, IV, p. 142.
54 Emmerson 1981, p. 7.

Murder, concealing the truth with falsehood and theft
Betrayal and flattery
Violence, aggression and violation:
These are nothing but the citizens of poverty's realm, the battalions of its Vizier the Satan.[55]

The appearance of the *Dajjāl* is the omen boding the coming revolution, which will remove oppression and tyranny, and launch a new era.[56] But the finger is also put on the people under the bus shelter, that is, the intellectuals who were aware of the disorder but chose to overlook it. Passing through a process of bestialization, they lost the ability to distinguish between good and evil. Maḥfūẓ's *Amāma al-'Arsh* (*Before the Throne*) (1983), whose subtitle defines it as "a conversation with Egyptian personalities from Mīnā to Anwar al-Sādāt," helps to elucidate the significance of "Under the Bus Shelter." Putting Egypt's rulers on trial before history, when Anwar al-Sādāt (1918–1981) comes before the bench, we find the following dialogue between him and his predecessor:

سأله جمال عبد النّاصر:
— كيف هان عليك أن تقف من ذكراي ذاك الموقف الغادر؟
فقال أنور السّادات:
اتّخذت ذاك الموقف مضطرّا إذ قامت سياستي في جوهرها على تصحيح الأخطاء الّتي ورثتها عن عهدك.
— ولكنّي عهدتك راضيا ومشجّعا وصديقا؟
— من الظّلم أن يحاسَب إنسان على موقف اتّخذه في زمن رعب أسود خاف الأب ابنه والأخ أخاه!
— وما النّصر الّذي أحرزته إلا ثمرة استعدادي الطّويل له!
فقال أنور السّادات:
— ما كان لمنهزم مثلك أن يحقّق انتصارا، ولكنّي أرجعت للشّعب حرّيّته وكرامته ثمّ قدته إلى نصر أكيد.

Jamāl 'Abd al-Nāṣir asked him:
—How could you be so treacherous toward my memory?
And al-Sādāt replied:
—I was forced to take this stand against my will, as my policies were based largely on reforming the mistakes I inherited from your period:
—But I knew you as satisfied, supportive and a friend?

55 'Abd al-Ṣabūr 1965 [1964], pp. 76–7. The translation is based on 'Abd al-Ṣabūr 1972a, p. 28, with some modifications. About the strategy of the *Qinā'*, see also Snir 1994d, pp. 245–56. On the power struggle reflected in the verse drama "between tyranny and aspirations for fear-free life, freedom and justice," see Ouyang 2012, p. 122.
56 Cf. Ṭāqa 1969, pp. 91–5.

—It is unjust to blame a person for a position taken in a dark period of terror, during which a father fears his own son, and a brother fears his own brother.[57]

Unlike "Under the Bus Shelter," in which Maḥfūẓ used an indirect mode of writing, in *Before the Throne* he alludes to the horrible rule of the secret police, and he directly describes that "dark period of terror." But that description in terms of *mundus inversus,* in which "a father fears his own son, and a brother fears his own brother," is more than "the most direct, systematic and concentrated attempt by Maḥfūẓ to challenge the myth of Jamāl 'Abd al-Nāṣir."[58] It also sheds light, in both intratextual and intertextual ways,[59] on the early story as well as providing "justification" for the behavior of the intellectuals in that "world upside down," as reflected in the behavior of the people under the bus shelter. It may even "justify" Maḥfūẓ's own behavior and his own poetics in the writing of "Under the Bus Shelter."

Maḥfūẓ's criticism of 'Abd al-Nāṣir did not begin after the 1967 War but long before, although he always emphasized that he had not rejected the July Revolution but had only been trying to draw attention to its faults.[60] This criticism, however covert, appears one way or another in almost all of his works written after the Revolution. The long allegorical novel *Awlād Ḥāratinā* (*Children of Our Alley*) (1959),[61] his first to be composed after the Revolution, was published after a period of silence on the part of the author following his Cairene trilogy (it was first published in 1956–1957, although it was concluded before the Revolution). The writer and his critics give several explanations for this silence,[62] but it is not improbable that it was due mainly to his feeling that he was not free to say what he wanted to. Ghālī Shukrī (1935–1998) asserts that when Maḥfūẓ resumed writing he was still under the impact of "the crisis of freedom and cultural backwardness," and that he "turned to symbolic form in *Awlād Ḥāratinā* only because he had not yet freed himself from the stress of that crisis."[63] A close reading of this novel, with the indispensable assistance of the author's public

[57] Maḥfūẓ n.d. [1983], p. 202. Cf. Maḥfūẓ n.d. [1982a], p. 63.
[58] Milson 1989, p. 21.
[59] Cf. Fitch 1982, pp. 89–108.
[60] For example, see al-Ghīṭānī 1980, p. 78; *al-Mustaqbal,* July 14, 1989, p. 58.
[61] Serialized in *al-Ahrām* from September 21 to December 25, 1959. It was first published as a book in 1967 (Maḥfūẓ 1967). According to Ghālī Shukrī (*al-Waṭan al-'Arabī,* March 17, 1989, p. 22), the English translation (Mahfouz 1981) is the only complete version of the book.
[62] See Duwāra 1963, p. 17; Duwāra 1965, pp. 283–4; Milson 1970, p. 177; Somekh 1970, p. 25; Somekh 1973a, pp. 51–2; al-Ghīṭānī 1980, pp. 100–1; Shukrī 1982, p. 235; Peled 1983, pp. 97, 171; Brugman 1984, p. 303.
[63] Shukrī 1982, p. 239. Cf. Peled 1983, p. 171.

declarations in the mid-1970s, reveals not only "a parable of authority and power ... the strong-arm men, the *futuwwāt* ... as the absolute monsters,"[64] but also a sharp criticism of the new regime in the 1950s.[65] Furthermore, according to Shukrī, Maḥfūẓ himself censored the Arabic version of the novel,[66] and in a way helped in directing the attention of the readers and critics to its conventional religious dimensions.[67] We might assume that

64 Abu-Haidar 1985, p. 119. Wen-chin Ouyang considers the novel "as a national allegory premised on parody ... and at the same time a history of the nation-state focalised around the question of power, or more appropriately, tyranny. This national allegory reads to me more like a biography of tyranny" (Ouyang 2013, p. 170).

65 Maḥfūẓ admitted this in an interview with *al-Qabas*, December 31, 1975, in which some of his sharp remarks were omitted. The interview was published again in its entirety in *al-Usbūʿ*, January 24, 1976 (cited in Peled and Shamir 1978, pp. 104–15). As to Milson's remark that this work's "political significance has been generally unnoticed" (Milson 1989, p. 5), it should be noted that the books and articles that he mentions were published before Maḥfūẓ admitted the existence of this criticism in his fictional writings. Milson himself did not notice it in his relevant studies published after Maḥfūẓ's admission (Milson 1976, pp. 158, 162–4, 179; Milson 1977, p. 459). Ghālī Shukrī appears to be the first critic, to my knowledge, who correctly noted, albeit only in vague terms, the immediate political relevance of *Awlād Ḥāratinā* (Shukrī 1982, pp. 239–40). Other critics who noticed it are mentioned in Ronnow 1984, pp. 89–90.

66 *Al-Waṭan al-ʿArabī*, March 17, 1989, p. 22. Gretchen Ronnow, who used only Stewart's translation of the novel, points out that "the descriptions of the social conditions could lead the reader to surmise that Maḥfūẓ is criticizing the political or sociological atmosphere of Egypt" (Ronnow 1984, pp. 88–9).

67 The novel, whose publication in Egypt was forbidden for many years, was published in Cairo only after its author's death (Maḥfūẓ 2006), owing to the outcry in the religious circles that claimed it did not treat the sanctities of Islam with the appropriate reverence (cf. Maḥfūẓ 1968, pp. 85–6. On the novel, see also Schuman 1965; Somekh 1971, pp. 49–61; Vatikiotis 1971, pp. 169–84; Somekh 1973a, pp. 137–55; Shalaq 1979, pp. 119–40; Shukrī 1982, pp. 238–66; Peled 1983, pp. 170–96; Ronnow 1984, pp. 87–118; Snir 1989, p. 127; Snir 2017, pp. 138–43; Shuʿayr 2018; Shoair 2022). The international furore engendered by *The Satanic Verses* by Salman Rushdie (b. 1947) and the death sentence passed down on the author again agitated the radical religious circles against *Awlād Ḥāratinā* (e.g., *al-Iʿtiṣām*, April 1989, pp. 5–7), perhaps because of Maḥfūẓ's determination in denouncing the death sentence against Rushdie, although he rejected any similarity between it and his book (*al-Ahrām*, March 2, 1989, p. 7). The Mufti of the radical Egyptian group *al-Jihād*, ʿUmar ʿAbd al-Raḥmān (1938–2017), delivered in April 1989 a *fatwā* of a death sentence against Maḥfūẓ himself (*al-Ahālī*, April 12, 1989, p. 13), which aroused many protests in the Arab world (e.g., *al-Hadaf*, April 9, 1989, pp. 40–3; *al-Shirāʿ*, May 15, 1989, p. 52; *al-Akhbār*, May 17, 1989, p. 9; *al-Wafd*, May 30, 1989, p. 9; *al-Ahālī*, June 7, 1989, p. 11). The Grand Mufti of Egypt, Muḥammad Sayyid Ṭanṭāwī (1928–2010), absolutely rejected this *fatwā* (*al-Ahālī*, May 3, 1989, p. 3). However, *Awlād Ḥāratinā* was published in Egypt in book form only in 2006 (Maḥfūẓ 2006) and has even in general been omitted from the list of Maḥfūẓ's works appended to his books. Censorship of books in the Arab world has been very frequent (e.g., fifty-five books were banned in Egypt in the first five months of 1989, according to *al-Ahālī*, June 7, 1989, p. 11) and included even classical works, such as those of the Ṣūfis (e.g., Schimmel 1982, p. 39). For the issue of censorship in the Arab world for religious reasons, see Snir 2006, pp. 41–57; Snir 2017, pp. 118–21.

Maḥfūẓ in that period of silence was in the process of searching for another mode of literary expression that would provide him with the necessary tools to criticize the regime without having to expect any retribution from the state. Turning to the genre of allegory, in which the author "may disguise his criticism or satire for fear of reprisal,"[68] he made abundant recourse to this mode of writing,[69] though its value has declined in the world of literature. Consequently, his "quest for meaning" novels of the 1960s might be interpreted on three levels: the surface story and references to the unsavory realities brought about by the new regime;[70] the allegorical and symbolic meaning;[71] and the poetic and even meta-fictional or meta-structural meaning produced by the very act of turning to that genre as an escape from the surrounding rejected political and social realities "in quest of fullness of experience."[72]

Against that background, we can understand why, unlike ʿAbd al-Nāṣir, Maḥfūẓ sees al-Sādāt as one of the greatest Egyptian heroes of all time. Representing in *Amām al-ʿArsh* (*Before the Throne*) (1983) the striving for peace, Akhenaton, the ancient Egyptian pharaoh of the 18th Dynasty, says to him: "I bless you as a seeker of peace, and I am not surprised that your enemies accuse you of treason. They made similar accusations against me for the same reason."[73] On the last page of the book, Maḥfūẓ lets al-Sādāt declare that the path of Egypt "must be civilization and peace."[74] Still, confronted with the popularity of ʿAbd al-Nāṣir, who had become a trope that connotes specific images constantly invoked whenever he is mentioned,[75] Maḥfūẓ tries in his public declarations to play down his great appreciation of al-Sādāt.[76]

Maḥfūẓ's use of the *mundus inversus* topos comes in a multilayered ethical social and political context befitting a writer who is engaged in the social and political problems of his people and land. His starting point is the idea of the political and social order—he "is committed to an ordered world, where order reflects the inherent good of the universe." Furthermore, "the idea of order is inevitably fixed on the point of authority. Someone or something must establish and perpetuate a system of order."[77] Reflecting the extreme

68 Beckson and Ganz 1990, p. 9.
69 Snir 1989, p. 126, n. 25.
70 Somekh 1987–1988, p. 10.
71 Milson 1989, pp. 6–7.
72 Shipley 1972, pp. 144–5.
73 Maḥfūẓ n.d. [1983], p. 201.
74 Maḥfūẓ n.d. [1983], p. 207. Cf. Snir 1989, pp. 150–3.
75 See Khalifah 2018.
76 For example, see *al-Mustaqbal*, July 14, 1989, p. 58.
77 Myers 1986, p. 82.

deviation from the desired order, the use of the topos implies the necessity of a quick action for the restoration of the proper order.

This topos has been frequent in the work of Maḥfūẓ ever since his first collection of short stories, *Hams al-Junūn* (*The Whisper of Madness*) (1938),[78] as in the story "al-Sharr al-Maʿbūd" ("The Worshipped Evil").[79] In the novel *al-Ḥubb Taḥt al-Maṭar* (*Love under the Rain*) (1973), one of the characters, ʿAshmāwī,[80] whose proper name is used as a kind of characterization,[81] is stereotypical of the type the writer deplores and scorns. After the 1967 War, when he hears that a released prisoner has just received an appointment in the civil service, he marvels at the change:

ماذا جرى للدّنيا؟ نسوان عرايا في الشّوارع، مساجين موظّفون، ويهود غزاة!

> What has happened to the world? Naked women in the streets, prisoners become officials and Jews have become invaders![82]

Women in Arab society should go about in the streets covered from head to toe, according to Islamic law,[83] but here they are walking about naked in the streets, a probable allusion to the "mini" fashion in Egypt in the early 1970s; prisoners become officials in the government service, and the Jews who had been known, according to ʿAshmāwī, as cowards, have become invaders—that is, the created order has been reversed. Although this use seems to be for the aim of amusement,[84] one cannot overlook the inner significance

78 On its publication date, see Brugman 1984, p. 297.

79 Maḥfūẓ 1973 [1938], pp. 135–41.

80 "Antonomasia"—the use of a proper name to refer to somebody with associated characteristics (cf. Shipley 1972, p. 26; Preminger 1974, p. 41; Cuddon 1986, p. 50): Ashmāwī is the name of a famous hangman in Egypt, whose name became synonymous with "hangman." It should be noted that in recent literary fiction the use of proper names is much more sophisticated and ironical; for lack of space suffice it to refer to the saying (in fiction!) that "[a] charming name never stopped anyone from being a bastard" (Perrin 2018, p. 13; Perrin 2020, ch. 2).

81 Cf. Gordon 1917; Rudnyckyj 1959, pp. 378–82; Auden 1970, p. 267. See also above.

82 Maḥfūẓ 1977 [1973], p. 136. Cf. the sense of shame touching Arab males after the trauma of the 1967 War as illustrated by Naṣr Ḥāmid Abū Zayd (1943–2010): "Following defeat (*hazīma*) in 1967, Arabs increasingly felt a sense of shame. To compensate for his impotence (*injirāḥ*), the Arab male self (*al-dhāt al-ʿarabiyya al-rajuliyya*) resorted to escaping to the past, to his original identity, to the illusion of manhood ... I heard story after story from my friends about how they were unable to engage in regular sexual intercourse with their wives—it was as though they were castrated (Moch 2017, pp. 90, 103).

83 Qur'ān 24:31.

84 Cf. a similar use with a meta-fictional significance in *El Ingenioso Hidalgo Don Quijote de la Mancha* by Míguel de Cervantes (1547–1616) (Cervantes 1972, pp. 262–3; Cervantes 2003, p. 195).

it bears for the ethical, social, and political contexts found elsewhere in Maḥfūẓ's work.[85]

4. "REFUSAL WILL BE A VIRTUE"

A very short and selective journey in typical works of twentieth-century Arabic literature may demonstrate the widespread circulation of the *mundus inversus* topos, the diversity of its literary renditions, and its reinvestment with new life in prose and poetry. For example, it is already found in *Zaynab* (*Zaynab* [name of the heroine]) (1913) by the Egyptian Muḥammad Ḥusayn Haykal (1888–1956), which is regarded as the first Arabic novel.[86] First published under the pseudonym *Miṣrī Fallāḥ* (*Egyptian of Peasant Origin*),[87] the novel concentrates on the male–female relationship in Egyptian society. Discussing the subject of marriage with four of his friends,[88] Ḥāmid, whose character contains autobiographical elements of the author himself, claims that, after the first few days of illusions, married people regret their hasty decision to wed. In contrast, a Prophetic tradition is cited:

85 For example, see Maḥfūẓ 1973 [1938], p. 78; Maḥfūẓ n.d. [1977], p. 330; Maḥfūẓ n.d. [1979], pp. 70, 344; Maḥfūẓ n.d. [1982], p. 107.

86 Haykal 1968 [1913], p. 7 (English translation: Haikal 1989. On the pioneer role of *Zaynab* in the history of the Arabic novel, see Barrāda 1996, pp. 32–3). On Haykal and his novel, see Badr 1983, pp. 322–37; Brugman 1984, pp. 234–43; Elkhadem 1985, pp. 26–8; Allen 1987, pp. 31–5; Badawi 1992, pp. 190–2, 223–6; Allen 1998, pp. 303–4; Selim 2004, pp. 58, 62, 92. A film based on the novel was directed by Muḥammad Karīm (1896–1972) and presented in Cairo in 1930 (Shafik 1998, p. 133; Qāsim 2002, p. 16). *Zaynab* has been generally regarded as the first Arabic artistic novel, albeit, as Roger Allen indicates, "the ascription of 'firstness' to such a work and the total confusion in placing its antecedents into some sort of narrative categories or developmental sequence provide an excellent illustration of the consequences of the unbalanced picture presented by the failure of the scholarly community to come to terms with the nature of generic change as it was affected by attitudes to modernity and pre-modernity during the 19th century" (Allen 2007, pp. 253–4. See also Allen 2018, p. 20). For more on "how *Zaynab* became the first Arabic novel," see Colla 2009, pp. 214–25. The Egyptian critic Ṣabrī Ḥāfiẓ (Sabry Hafez) (b. 1942) indicated that when Haykal wrote Zaynab "it was under the hypnotic lure of the occident ... He was not aware that by mediating his culture through the Western genre, and subjecting it to its rubrics, he was adopting from the West a form of writing, a way of seeing, and a mode of thinking, much more than he would like to admit. The Arabic novel, which he inaugurated, continued to interact with its European counterpart for the first seventy years of its history. It did not discover the enriching process of conducting a dialogue with its rich heritage of Arabic narrative until the arrival of the innovative strategies of the 1960s generation" (Hafez 2014, p. 18).

87 Out of the author's fear that his career as a lawyer may be in jeopardy if he were to use his real name (Haykal 1968 [1913], p. 7).

88 Haykal 1968 [1913], pp. 131–7.

تناكحوا تناسلوا، فإنّي مباهٍ بكم الأمم يوم القيامة

> Marry, be fruitful and multiply, for thus will I be proud of you among the peoples of the world on the Day of Final Judgment.[89]

Arguing that all his married acquaintances are tormented and miserable, one of Ḥāmid's friends emphasizes the importance of marriage by demonstrating the unbearable condition into which the anti-marriage perspective would lead:

تصوّر تلك الحال الّتي تريد أن ترى النّاس فيها! تصوّر أبناء ضعافا لا يعرفون آباءهم، ونساء لا يجدن من يعولهنّ أيّام ضعفهنّ المطلق وسط مدينتنا الحاضرة الكثيرة الحاجات والمطالب!

> Just picture the condition into which you want to cast people! Imagine weak little children who do not know their fathers, and women who can find no one to support them in their absolute weakness in the midst of our civilization, which has so many needs and demands.

Alluding to the chaos into which society would enter without marriage, the reversal of the desired order stresses the importance of that social institution as one of the fundamental elements of human society.[90]

Mīkhā'īl Nu'ayma's (1889–1988) essay "al-Maqāyīs al-Adabiyya" ("Literary Criteria")[91] indicates the need for strategies "to reconcile between our limited senses and the limitlessness of life ... in this upside-down world." Thus, man has measured time, distance, and weight within the framework of inventing unchanging criteria by which to measure and appraise various aspects of life, among them literature. Calling for the rise of a literary criticism capable of judging works by standards that will not change with the changing of the times, Nu'ayma concludes his essay as follows:

حاجتنا إلى شعراء وكتّاب يقيسون ما ينظمون ويكتبون بهذه المقاييس، فيسيرون وتسير معهم آدابنا في الصّراط القويم، وإلى ناقدين ممحّصين يميّزون بين غثّ الأدب وسمينه، فلا يحسبون الأصداف دررا ولا الحباحب كواكب.

> We are in need of poets and writers who measure what they compose [with certain criteria] and write according to such criteria, and this way they progress and our literature turns toward the straight path, and [we are in need] of critics who can examine closely and distinguish between what is bad in literature and what is good, and who will not consider the seashells as pearls nor the fireflies as stars.

89 On the origin of this tradition, see Hujwīrī 1999 [1926], p. 470. Cf. Wensinck and Mensing 1936–1969, I, pp. 142–3. On the Prophet's injunctions against celibacy, provoked in part by the influence of Christian monasticism, see Goldziher 1910, pp. 145, 150–1, 187, n. 11; von Grunebaum 1953, p. 125.

90 On similar use of the topos with Christian allusions, see Heym 1981, p. 158.

91 Nu'ayma 1951 [1923], pp. 54–61.

Criticism of Arabic literature in the 1920s, according to Nu'ayma, is an "upside-down world" that requires a fundamental change.

In the opening of *al-Raghīf* (*The Loaf of Bread*) (1939), the Lebanese writer Tawfīq Yūsuf 'Awwād (1911–1989) dedicates the novel, in which he describes his childhood during the First World War, to his father:

إليك، يا أبي، أقدّم هذا "الرّغيف".
وإذا كنت سكبت له الحبر وراء مكتبي الوثير فقد قدّمت أنت إليّ في أيّام الحرب الكبرى، وإلى إخواني وأخواتي، أرغفة سكبت لها عرق جبينك ودم قلبك، عهد تخلّى الآباء عن أبنائهم وأنكر الأخ أخاه.

> To you, my father, I present this "loaf of bread." And while I poured out ink for it behind my comfortable desk, you provided me and my brothers and sisters, during the First World War, with loaves for which you poured the sweat of your brow and the blood of your heart, when fathers abandoned their sons and a brother pretended not to know his brother.[92]

Against the background of the collapse of ethical standards during the war, the topos of the world upside down is used as a tool for emphasizing the author's appreciation for his father.

At the close of his poem "al-Ẓill wa-l-Ṣalīb" ("The Shadow and the Cross"),[93] published in his second collection *Aqūlu Lakum* (*I Say to You*) (1961), the aforementioned poet Ṣalāḥ 'Abd al-Ṣabūr says:

هذا زمن الحقّ الضّائع
لا يعرف فيه مقتول من قاتله ومتى قتله
ورؤوس النّاس على جثث الحيوانات
ورؤوس الحيوانات على جثث النّاس
فتحسّس رأسك!
فتحسّس رأسك!

> This is the time of the lost right
> In which the slain knows neither who slew him nor when
> People's heads lie on corpses of animals
> And heads of animals lie on corpses of people
> Touch your head!
> Touch your head!

Inspired by the Absurd dramatist Eugene Ionesco (1912–1994), the reversal of reality in the poem emphasizes the disgust with modern civilization; the spiritual emptiness that it has generated has brought human beings to the brink of despair. Fearing the loss of his soul and of his human individuality

92 'Awwād 1984 [1939] (the dedication).

93 'Abd al-Ṣabūr 1965 [1964], pp. 60–71; Abdel Sabour 1970, pp. 28–41; 'Abd al-Ṣabūr 1972, pp. 148–54.

in the world of the machine, the computer, and the atom bomb, the poet indicates in another place: "In this poem, I spoke about the emptiness of human society and I wanted to point to the reason."[94] Exposing a world of chaos in need of quick reform, mainly on a personal-existential level, ʿAbd al-Ṣabūr combines in other works that level with the social one. In the poem "Mudhakkirāt al-Ṣūfī Bishr al-Ḥāfī" ("Memoirs of the Mystic Bishr al-Ḥāfī"), published in his third collection, *Aḥlām al-Fāris al-Qadīm* (*Dreams of the Ancient Knight*) (1964),[95] he adopts the strategy of the *qaṣīdat qināʿ* (mask poem)—the presentation of ideas and feelings through a well-known figure generally from Arab heritage using the image of the Muslim mystic Bishr al-Ḥāfī ("the barefooted") (d. 841).[96] Characterizing a repugnant reality in need of fundamental reform, the poem describes the period as follows:

هذا اليوم الموبوء هو اليوم الثّامن
من أيّام الأسبوع الخامس
في الشّهر الثّالث عشر.

This miserable day is the eighth day
Of the fifth week
Of the thirteenth month.

Interestingly, though the poem refers to a social condition in urgent need of reform, on the personal level the escape from the gloomy reality presented by the poem lies in the desire for God and the mystical experience.[97]

An interesting use of the topos of *mundus inversus* is found in the work of the Sudanese poet Muḥammad al-Faytūrī (1929–2015), whose Blackness—and his life as a Black man in a world of Whites—has been a source of inspiration for a large part of his work. His work *Suqūt Dabshalīm* (*The Fall of Dabshalīm*) (1968) includes a segment called "al-Ghathayān" ("Nausea"):

تبّا لعصر تمطر السّماء فيه
— قال بيدبا لدبشليم —
جرذانا وأغربة
وتلد الرّجال فيه
ويعانون من المحيض
ويلتقي النّقيض بالنّقيض
وتستمدّ القبب المذهّبة

[94] ʿAbd al-Ṣabūr 1969, pp. 88–9; ʿAbd al-Ṣabūr 1981 [1969], pp. 123–4. Cf. Ismāʿīl 1978, pp. 269–76; Mīkhāʾīl 1968, pp. 206–7.

[95] ʿAbd al-Ṣabūr 1964, pp. 113–25; Abdel Sabour 1970, pp. 54–67; ʿAbd al-Ṣabūr 1972, pp. 261–9.

[96] See al-Sulamī 1953, p. 39; Arberry 1979 [1950], pp. 40–1. On the biography of Bishr, see Cooperson 2004, pp. 154–87.

[97] Cf. Snir 1984, pp. 12–13; Snir 1985, pp. 129–46; Snir 1989a, pp. 31–43; Snir 1992a, pp. 24–6. See also below, Chapter 4.

طلاءها اللّمّاع
من أعين الجياع.

May the time perish, in which the heavens rain
—So says Baydabā to Dabshalīm[98]—
Rats and ravens
And the men give birth
And suffer in menstruation,
And two opposites meet
And the golden domes draw
Their glittering gilt
From the eyes of the hungry people.[99]

Emphasizing in the last line the social injustice of our reality, the poet describes our epoch as reversed reality in need of urgent reform.

In his poem "al-'Aṣāfīr Taltāḥu fī al-Dhākira" ("The Birds Are Thirsty in the Memory"),[100] from the collection *Alif Lām Mīm* (the title refers to the letters of the word *alm* [pain]) (1979), the Palestinian poet Muḥammad Ḥamza Ghanāyim (1953–2004) is longing for a better future ("Oh dawn come"), but his tongue is manacled:

إنشقّت كلّ شواطئ هذا لبحر وحيفا تأتيني
بالرّعد ولا تطلقني من سجن لساني!

All the shores of this sea have been breached and Haifa brings to me
The thunder and does not free me from the jail of my tongue!

Dreaming of Palestine's children as "birds passing the bridge of return," the poem concludes as follows:

يأتيكم زمن تتقلّب فيه نساء السّلطان على جمر الشّهوة
يتسوّر فيه العطش الشّفّاف على أقنعة الجدران
ويصير الرّفض فضيلة.

The time will come when the sultan's women will toss and turn on the ember of lust
The translucent thirst will scale the masks of walls
And refusal will be a virtue.

As appeared in the Prophetic traditions combining the signs of the Day of Judgment, these days of reversed reality that the poet-prophet speaks of as

98 An allusion to the moralizing animal fables of *Kalīla wa-Dimna* translated into Arabic from the Middle Persian version of the Indian *Panchatranta* by Ibn al-Muqaffa' (d. 759[?]).
99 Al-Faytūrī 1979, pp. 560–1.
100 Ghanāyim 1979, pp. 47–50.

coming in the future are in fact in the here and now. The world in which the vices are turned into virtues[101] needs quick reform.[102]

As mentioned above, the rapid growth and proliferation of sophisticated forms of media, particularly Internet-related technologies, such as blogging, techno-writing, and interactive literature, has opened new possibilities for literary expression for Arab writers to imagine new realities, and these possibilities have provided additional forums and stages for literary and critical texts to be presented and discussed side by side with the traditional ones. The topos of *mundus inversus* has been imbued with new life. Here is just one example from the poet Bashīr Shalash:

من علامات السّاعة أنّه:
الشّراميط أوّل من يتنطّح للتّنظير للأخلاق،
العملاء ينظّرون للوطنيّة ويمنحون صكوكا،
التّافهون ينظّرون للمعنى،
والمرتشون لنظافة اليد،
الخانعون ينظّرون للحرّيّة،
البخلاء ينظّرون للبذل والعطاء،
وإذا تجرّأت وسألت: ولكن كيف؟
تجد جيوشا من التّافهين في جوق واحد يقولون:
حرّيّة تعبير!

Among the Signs of the? Day of Judgment:
The whores are the first thrusting to theorize for ethics,
The collaborators theorize for patriotism and grant checks,
The worthless people theorize for meaning,
The bribed people theorize for incorruptibility,
The submissive people theorize for freedom,
The misers theorize for sacrifice and generosity,
And if you dare and ask: but how?
You will find armies of worthless people in one orchestra saying:
Freedom of expression![103]

101 Cf. Emmerson 1981, p. 53.

102 Cf. works by other Palestinian writers: Ḥabībī 1985a, pp. 87–8; Abū Ḥannā 1988, pp. 95–6; Qaʿwār 1988, pp. 75–9. See also the film *Maqlūba* (*Maklouba*) (*Upside Down*) (2000) by the Palestinian filmmaker Rashīd Mashaharāwī (b. 1962). It is interesting to find also the same topos in the writing of the Iraqi-Jewish writer Samīr Naqqāsh (1938–2004); for example, in the story "Dunyā al-Makhālīf" ("The World of the Opposites") from the collection *Nubū'āt Rajul Majnūn fī Madīna Malʿūna* (*Prophesies of a Madman in a Cursed City*) (1995), the narrator plays the role of a prophet in a topsy-turvy world (Naqqāsh 1995, pp. 85–105). See also his novel *Shlūmū al-Kurdī wa-Anā wa-Zaman* (*Shlomo al-Kurdī, Myself, and Time*), when the narrator had to escape with his family from his hometown of Ṣablākh, in Iranian Kurdistan, during the First World War, because of the world upside down created in the town (Naqqāsh 2004, p. 36).

103 Facebook, April 18, 2018.

5. CONCLUSION

Until the mid-twentieth century, the topos of *mundus inversus* was generally not of interest to Arab poets and men of letters, and appeared only in religious traditions, in historical texts,[104] and popular sermons of preachers.[105] The traditional nature of Arabic poetry and the late development of the Arabic novel had confined the literary use of this topos, even in the first half of the twentieth century, to the constraints of the historical texts and popular sermons. An example of this is the use of the Prophetic tradition in *Zaynab* as well as the allusion to the signs of the Day of Judgment in *al-Ayyām* (*The Days*) (1926–1927) by Ṭāhā Ḥusayn (1889–1973).[106] However, since the 1950s this topos, like apocalypticism in general,[107] has become extremely popular in Arabic *belles lettres*, generally acquiring new functions in the field of committed literature. Indicating the diversity of its literary renditions, the present chapter has shown the ways in which the topos is imbued with new life by alluding to the Islamic signs of the Day of Judgment accompanied by a hyperbolic presentation of a concrete ejected reality—be it personal, political, social, ethical, national, rhetorical, or even aesthetico-critical. The basic concept of *Ashrāṭ al-Sāʿa* is closely associated with the concept of *Fasād al-Zamān* (The Deterioration of the Times), which has been used by muftis as a basis for legal decisions.[108] Also, the topos of *mundus inversus* frequently appears in postcolonial Arabic literature, such as with the intertextual reference to the Qur'ānic earthquake that will convulse the Earth at the end of time (*surat al-Zalzala*).[109] That the same pattern appears abundantly in Western literature by no means implies that the Arab authors were inspired by imported models. In fact, without denying the great impact of Western culture on Arab culture, the case of this specific topos, among others, firmly supports the view that, in general, the present literary Arab creation is a direct extension of the ancient Arabic literary heritage.

As the *mundus inversus* pattern is inherent in the literary imagination of Arab poets and writers, it comes to mind when they witness a deviation from the desired reality, as they see it. Out of their desire to restore this reality, they create a non-existent reversed rejected reality in order to illustrate the

104 For example, see Ibn Kathīr 1966, p. 203; Ibn Ṭabāṭabā 1966, p. 141.

105 For example, see Shoshan 1991, p. 84.

106 Ḥusayn n.d. [1929], pp. 107–9.

107 Cf. Emmerson 1981, p. 3.

108 Cf. Gerber 1999, pp. 124–8.

109 For example, see Waṭṭār 1977 (English translation: Waṭṭār 2000). Cf. Toorawa 2006, pp. 241–2.

dangers entailed by that deviation if it is not corrected at once. One of the advantages of the topos is that it conceals the writer's own confusions and shifted opinions as he slowly faces reality.[110] Another advantage is its vagueness: it can conceal attacks on more than one target. The poets and writers who use its symbolism might have presumably no consciously evasive purpose in mind. Like those who used the symbolism of the Antichrist in seventeenth-century England,[111] they draw on allegorical habits of mind inherited from the past. Nevertheless, its imprecision allows differing interpretations to be put upon it, either by different people or by the same person in appealing to different groups. This vagueness has security advantages: in Egypt in the 1960s, critics of the "world upside down" were in fact attacking the regime. But even the supporters of the regime could hardly object to the denunciation of this reversed reality as long as it was not too clearly defined: "Like sin, everyone was against him."[112]

The religious allusions of this topos cannot be ignored, even when poets and writers adapt it to literary use without cognitive awareness of these allusions. Like an archetype, the religious significance is the product of some "collective unconscious" of the Arab authors—Muslim, Christian, and Jewish—inherited from the ancient Arab heritage. The signs of Judgment Day alluded to through the topos are no longer in the distant future, but are here and now. Thus, the hyperbolic presentation of the reversed reality in a way that is reminiscent of these signs powerfully challenges a state that demands immediate reform, as manifested in Cassius' words in Shakespeare's *Julius Caesar* (I, 3: 62–71):

> But if you would consider the true cause,
> Why all these fires, why all these gliding ghosts,
> Why birds and beasts, from quality and kind,
> Why old men, fools, and children calculate,
> Why all these things change, from their ordinance,
> Their nature, and pre-formed faculties,
> To monstrous quality; why, you shall find,
> That heaven hath infused them with these spirits,
> To make them instruments of fear and warning,
> Unto some monstrous state.[113]

110 Cf. Hill 1971, p. 66.
111 Hill 1971, pp. 44–5.
112 Hill 1971, p. 45. See, for example, 'Abd al-Ṣabūr 1965 [1964], pp. 158–9; 'Abd al-Ṣabūr 1972a, p. 58.
113 Shakespeare 1971, p. 723. Cf. Ibn Ṭabāṭabā 1966, p. 141.

But this topos in modern Arabic literature is not only a complaint about the times or a warning "unto some monstrous state." Alluding to the religious urgency of destroying the existing reversed order as a necessary transition to the kingdom of heaven, it is also the gates of hell through which the road to a better future passes, the gutters from which salvation shall spring,[114] sometimes even the "redemption through sin," to use the words of the sinister Jewish prophet, or Antichrist, Jacob Frank (1726–1791):

> No man can climb a mountain until he has first descended to its foot. Therefore, we must descend and be cast down to the bottom rung, for only then can we climb to the infinite. This is the mystic principle of Jacob's Ladder, which I have seen and which is shaped like a V.[115]

[114] Cf. Shoham 1980.
[115] Scholem 1974, p. 130.

Chapter 2

Challenge: The al-Andalus Experience[1]

Who silenced the poet's voice
With treacherous nightly bullets?
O Lorca, the adored features
O soul, the clearest of mirrors
Vanished from the lands of al-Andalus.
– Fu'ād al-Khashin

1. INTRODUCTION

Al-Andalus, the medieval Arab state in the Iberian Peninsula, acquired a legendary status in Arab culture—its literary trajectory in time and place contains a utopian vision, similar to the dream of the homeland in modern exile literature. It is viewed as a golden age, or a paradise lost, or the hunt for the hidden treasure. When contemporary Arab authors, artists, and intellectuals recall the cultural achievements of the Arab heritage in al-Andalus during nearly 800 years of Muslim rule, they do so to remind their audience that their present bitter state is only a transitory period, a temporary clouding of the skies between a glorious past and a splendid future. And they do so and revive the Andalusian past and its achievements in order to counter those who claim that Arab culture has become excessively Westernized. Such "Arab patriotism" has infiltrated the literary texts as well. For example, in the mid-1980s, the Palestinian poet Maḥmūd Darwīsh (1941–2008), who was born in the village of Birwa, near Acre (Akka), which was destroyed by Israeli forces in June 1948 after they had expelled all its inhabitants, asks himself what he would do if he were given the chance to start his life all over again. He has no doubts:

[1] This chapter uses material that first appeared in Snir 2000, pp. 263–93.

إِذَا كَانَ لِي أَنْ أُعِيدَ البِدايَة أَختارُ ما اخْتَرْتُ: وَرْدَ السّياج
أُسَافِرُ ثَانيةً فِي الدَّرُوبِ الّتِي قدْ تُؤدِّي وقَدْ لا تُؤدِّي إِلَى قُرْطَبهْ.

If I were to start all over again I'd choose what I have chosen now: the roses on the fence
I'd set out again on the road that may or may not lead to Cordova.

But reaching this homeland may always remain an illusion:

أَعُودُ، إِذَا كَانَ لِي أَنْ أَعُودَ، إِلَى وَرْدَتِي نَفْسِهَا وإِلَى خطْوَتِي نَفْسِهَا
وَلَكِنَّنِي لاَ أَعُودُ إِلَى قُرْطُبَه.

I will return, if I can, to my roses, to my steps
But I will not go back to Cordova.[2]

Andalusian Cordova here is the paradise the poet was driven from, the mythological homeland to which he is longing to return.[3] Darwīsh is among numerous Arab authors, mainly poets, who, since the nineteenth century, have been invoking the image of al-Andalus, Muslim Spain, in their writings in a conscious effort to highlight the benefits that Western civilization has gained through its interaction with Arab civilization.[4] The al-Andalus experience—the Arabs' greatest and most enduring success on European soil—is seen as the epitome of that interaction. But even more so, when authors recall the cultural achievements of the Arab heritage in al-Andalus during nearly 800 years of Muslim rule, they do so to counter those who claim that Arab culture has become excessively Westernized and to remind their audience that their present bitter state is only, as I mentioned above, a transitory period, a temporary clouding of the skies between a glorious past and a splendid future.[5] As such, they are a part of a wider phenomenon: a conscious effort on the part of contemporary Arab authors to highlight the benefits that Western civilization has gained through its interaction with Arab civilization—the al-Andalus experience is seen as the epitome of that interaction, the Arabs' greatest and most enduring success on European soil.[6] Surprisingly,

[2] Darwīsh 1987a, p. 9.

[3] Darwīsh 1987a, p. 9.

[4] On al-Andalus in Arabic and Muslim culture, see 'Uthmān 1988, pp. 5–72; Montávez 1992; Noorani 1999, pp. 237–54; Snir 2000, pp. 263–93; Anidjar 2002; Shannon 2007, pp. 308–44; Elinson 2009; Eksell 2011, pp. 103–26; Jarrar 2011, pp. 361–93; Brann 2013, pp. 119–34; Calderwood 2014, pp. 27–55; Arslan 2016, pp. 278–97; Hermes 2016, pp. 433–52; Wien 2017, pp. 48–79; Calderwood 2018; Cruz 2018, pp. 103–23; Fernández-Parrilla 2018, pp. 229–42; López-Calvo 2019, pp. 274–8; Civantos 2020, pp. 598–619; Corrao 2020, pp. 121–30; Brann 2021, pp. 172–94; Ziter 2021, pp. 394–424.

[5] Noorani 1999, pp. 237–54; Snir 2000, pp. 263–93.

[6] On the role of al-Andalus in the movement of ideas between Islam and the West, and the arguments that trace the beginnings of the Renaissance in Europe to al-Andalus, see Chejne 1980, pp. 110–33; Recapito 1998, pp. 55–74.

we find something similar in Miguel de Cervantes' (1547–1616) *Don Quixote* (published in two volumes in 1605 and 1615), which is considered a founding work of modern world literature and one of the earliest canonical Western novels. According to Cervantes, he acquired a book and then looked around for a Moor, a Muslim, to translate it: this was the Arabic manuscript written by an Arab historian named Cide Hamete Benengeli, who is the fictional Moorish author created by Cervantes and listed as the chronicler of the adventures of Don Quixote.[7] Paradoxically, the novel chronicles the demise of Arabic Andalusian literature, shedding light on an era when al-Andalus' Islamic culture forcibly came to an end.[8]

Looking closely at the way al-Andalus appears in modern Arabic literary works, we find that they reflect a number of aspects of Muslim Spain's historical developments from the time the Arabs along with Berber troops crossed the Straits of Gibraltar into the Iberian Peninsula in 711 AD and overthrew the Visigoths there. Though the period that followed was one of political fragmentation that saw the creation of local dynasts—known as *Mulūk al-Ṭawā'if* (Party Kings)—it was also a period of great cultural efflorescence that lasted uninterrupted until the fall of Granada to the Christians in 1492 AD. Undoubtedly, the Arabs left their mark on Spain: "In the skills of the Spanish peasant and craftsman and the words with which he describes them, in the art, architecture, music and literature of the Peninsula, and in

7 See Soons 1959, pp. 351–7; El Saffar 1968, pp. 164–77; Forcione 1970, pp. 155–6; Stewart 1997, pp. 111–27; Rothstein 2005. Based on the phonetic rule that Cervantes frequently uses in his invention of names, it was suggested that the name Benengeli is derived from Ben-Engelis ("Angel's Son") with intertextual allusions, among others, to the symbolic meaning of the Islamic primordial pen and Qur'ānic *Sūrat al-Qalam* (*The Pen*) (López-Baralt 2006, pp. 579–93).

8 Cf. a similar reading by the British-Pakistani novelist and historian Tariq Ali (b. 1943) in his Globalization Lecture given on December 1, 2010 at SOAS, University of London, available at: https://www.youtube.com/watch?v=NaP0KEwdGro&t=1222s (last accessed August 3, 2020). In her keynote address "The Secret Literature of the Last Muslims of Spain," given at the International Conference at the American University of Beirut titled "Latin America, al-Andalus, and the Arab World" (April 17, 2018), Luce López-Baralt referred to the "underground authors' manuscripts," written in Spanish but transliterated with Arabic script, as a last sign of loyalty to the Arabic language, providing "a first-hand testimony of what it was like to experience the decline of Islamic culture." Those manuscripts were written by the sixteenth-century Moriscos, or Moors, in the midst of their collective misfortune as a strangled minority. The term "Moor" was first used by Christian Europeans to designate the Muslim inhabitants of the Maghreb, the Iberian Peninsula, Sicily, and Malta during the Middle Ages. The Moors initially were the indigenous Maghrebine Berbers. The name was later also applied to Arabs and Arabized Iberians. The "Moriscos" were former Muslims and their descendants whom the Roman Catholic Church and the Spanish Crown commanded to convert to Christianity or compulsory exile after Spain outlawed the open practice of Islam by its sizeable Muslim population in the early sixteenth century. See: https://www.youtube.com/watch?v=WhizgnMTtyg (last accessed April 25, 2021).

the science and philosophy of the legacy of antiquity faithfully guarded and increased."[9]

Inspired by nostalgia, the picture that most frequently appears in modern Arabic literary writings is that of al-Andalus as the lost paradise (*al-firdaws al-mafqūd*) or God's paradise on Earth (*jannat Allāh 'alā al-arḍ*). As Muslim Spain is generally associated in modern Arabic literature with images intended to play off Arab culture against Western culture, it is not surprising that most literary expressions of al-Andalus appear in poetry. Unlike other modern genres of Arabic literature, no one can claim that poetry was introduced to the Arabic literary system in the nineteenth century as a result of its interaction with Western culture. Poetry recorded the very appearance of the Arab nation and has been the principal channel through which Arabic literary creativity has been flowing from the pre-Islamic period, through the Middle Ages, when it reached a peak both in the East and in al-Andalus, to the present day. Poetry has been the true "public register" of Arab cultural and political history (*al-Shi'r Dīwān al-'Arab*).[10] That we see a change in the second half of the twentieth century is partially explained by the universal decline of the status of poetry in modern society together with the increasing impact of mass media. Still, in the Arab world, even in this period when social media over the Internet control human interactions, it is overwhelmingly poetry to which people turn when they seek a vehicle for expressing their national sentiments, their trials and frustrations, their hopes and aspirations. It is in such contexts that we find the image of al-Andalus appearing in Arabic poetry, much more frequently than in modern Arab prose and theater, although the Andalusian theme has featured also in the Arabic novel from its earliest stages.[11]

[9] Lewis 1970, p. 130.

[10] This saying is found in different forms in various medieval works (e.g., Ibn Qutayba 1928, II, p. 185; al-Suyūṭī n.d., II, p. 470). Cf. Lyall 1930, p. xv. For an examination of the above saying with regard to the change in perception of poetry and its function during the emergence of Arabic-Islamic society, see Ouyang 1997, pp. 56–60.

[11] See, for example, the historical novel *Budūr* that Salīm al-Bustānī (1848–1884) published serially in his periodical *al-Jinān* (vol. 3, 1872) as well as the novels *Fatḥ al-Andalus aw Ṭāriq ibn Ziyād* (*The Occupation of al-Andalus* or *Ṭāriq ibn Ziyād*) and *'Abd al-Raḥmān al-Nāṣir* by Jurjī Zaydān (1861–1914) (Zaydān 1905; Zaydān 1910–1911). Much more modernist employment of the Andalusian history and myth is found in *Thulāthiyyat Ghranāṭa* by Raḍwā 'Āshūr (1946–2013) ('Āshūr 1998). For the connections between the temporal and spatial significations of al-Andalus and how they function within Arabic novels, see Granara 2005, pp. 57–73. In the dramatic field, see the plays *Fatḥ al-Andalus* by Muṣṭafā Kāmil (1874–1908) (on the play, see Najm 1956, pp. 310–14) and *Amīrat al-Andalus* (*al-Andalus' Princess*) by Aḥmad Shawqī (Shawqī 1932; on the play, see Boudot-Lamotte 1977, pp. 296–302). An interesting use of the figure of 'Abd al-Raḥmān al-Dākhil is found in the play *al-Muharrij* (*The Jester*) by the Syrian poet and dramatist Muḥammad al-Māghūṭ (1934–2006) (al-Māghūṭ 1981, pp. 495–614. On the play, see Ziter 2015, pp. 21–4, 205–9).

2. "AL-ANDALUS ARISING FROM DAMASCUS"

Neoclassical poetry set out to cleanse impurities that had come to cling to it during previous centuries and to revert to the grand poetic style that had characterized the Abbasid Golden Age of Arabic poetry during the Middle Ages.[12] Adhering to the rigid structure of meter (*baḥr*, *wazn*) and rhyme (*qāfiya*) of the ancient Arabic poetic form, the *qaṣīda*, traditional poets included many direct and indirect allusions to al-Andalus. Among these poets we find Maḥmūd Sāmī al-Bārūdī (1839–1904), Aḥmad Shawqī (1868–1932), Ḥāfiẓ Ibrāhīm (1871–1932), Aḥmad Muḥarram (1878–1945), ʻAlī al-Jārim (1881–1949), Ismāʻīl Ṣabrī (1885–1923), Maʻrūf al-Ruṣāfī (1875–1945), Jamīl Ṣidqī al-Zahāwī (1863–1936), and Muḥammad Mahdī al-Jawāhirī (1900–1997).[13] Al-Andalus' contribution, the neoclassical poets claimed, was not confined to the Arab civilization, but, in the words of Ḥāfiẓ Ibrāhīm, "through it the world acquired the dress of civilization."[14] Significant is the tendency among neoclassical poets to frequently use the practice of *muʻāraḍa* (a contestatory emulation), that is, writing a poem for which rhyme, meter, and sometimes even topic are borrowed from a particularly well-known classical, or in our case Andalusian, poem.[15]

One of the prominent poets who frequently called up the image of al-Andalus in his poetry was Aḥmad Shawqī (1868–1932), "The Prince of Poets" (*Amīr al-Shuʻarā'*), in the first quarter of the twentieth century. As a court poet closely associated with the Khedive ʻAbbās II (1874–1944), he was given the title of Bey. When, at the start of the First World War, the British ousted ʻAbbās II and prevented him from returning to Egypt from Istanbul, Shawqī remained loyal to the Khedive. Following a poem he wrote in honor of the deposed ruler, he was exiled from Egypt in 1915. Shawqī preferred to go to

We also find the image of al-Andalus in Arab comic strips (e.g., Douglas and Malti-Douglas 1994, pp. 143–9). On the limited presence of al-Andalus in Palestinian prose, see al-Juʻaydī 1997, p. 2; al-Juʻaydī 2000, p. 9.

12 According to Michael Cooperson, the prominence of this era in later memory as a golden age is traced to the adoption of paper, which supported, on the one hand, the simplification and vulgarization of Arab language, lore, and religion, and, on the other, the appearance of the first reliably contemporary eyewitness accounts in Arabic literature. These productions made the period the first Islamic space to be imaginable in almost granular detail, as well as the source of much of what we know about antecedent "Arab" and "Islamic" history (Cooperson 2017, pp. 41–65).

13 On the neoclassical trend in Arabic poetry, see Moreh 1973, pp. 155–79; Badawi 1975, pp. 14–67; Moreh 1976, pp. 1–2; Boudot-Lamotte 1977; Jayyusi 1977, pp. 46–54; Brugman 1984, pp. 26–56; Somekh 1992, pp. 36–81, 491–4.

14 Ibrāhīm n.d. [1937], I, p. 99.

15 On the *muʻāraḍa*, see Nawfal 1983; Montgomery 2013, pp. 155, 252–4; Fakhreddine 2015, pp. 164–6, 179–81, 190–1.

Spain, where he stayed until 1920. During his Andalusian exile, Shawqī spent much of his time visiting the great ancient Arab monuments and reading the works of famous Andalusian writers. Especially remarkable was the inspiration he drew from *Nafḥ al-Ṭīb fī Ghuṣn al-Andalus al-Raṭīb* (*The Breath of Perfume on the Fresh Branch of al-Andalus*) by the Moroccan man of letters Aḥmad ibn Muḥammad al-Maqqarī (1578?–1632), which many regard as the main source for all subsequent works on Andalusian music.[16] While in Spain, Shawqī wrote a series of poems in which he commemorated the glories of the Andalusian Arab civilization and described its enduring heritage.[17] Among these poems, titled *Andalusiyyāt*, is a *mu'āraḍa* of a poem that the Andalusian poet Ibn Zaydūn (1004–1070) wrote to his beloved Wallāda after he had escaped from prison in Cordova and was heading toward Seville. Ibn Zaydūn's poem opens with one of the better-known verses in medieval Arabic poetry:

أَضْحَى التَّنَائِي بَدِيلًا مِنْ تَدانِينا وَنَابَ عَنْ طِيْبِ لُقْيانَا تَجَافِيْنَا

The great distance between us replaced our intimate relationship
Distancing from one another has replaced our sweet encounter.[18]

Shawqī's poem opens with the following verse:

يا نائح الطّلح أشباه عوادينا نشجى لواديك أم نأسى لوادينا؟

O mourner of the valley, our tragedies are so similar,
Would I mourn your valley or mine?[19]

Shawqī's inspiration from Ibn Zaydūn's poetry is evident not only in form but also in content. When the *Dīwān* of this medieval Andalusian poet first appeared in print, Shawqī published a poem praising his eloquent lines.[20] In "al-Riḥla ilā al-Andalus" ("The Journey to al-Andalus"),[21] Shawqī describes the great Andalusian sites through a *mu'āraḍa* of a poem by the classical poet al-Walīd ibn 'Ubayd Allāh al-Buḥturī (821–897) about the ruins of Khosrau's palace. Shawqī's Andalusian poems became so well known that, in a poem written on the eve of Shawqī's return to Egypt from Spain, his compatriot Ḥāfiẓ Ibrāhīm coined the term *Andalusiyya Shawqiyya*, that

16 Al-Maqqarī 1968; al-Makkari 1967.
17 On Shawqī's Andalusian exile, see Mandūr 1970, pp. 60–5; Badawi 1975, p. 29; Boudot-Lamotte 1977, pp. 53–64. On the attitude of the poet to al-Andalus before and after his exile, as well as on the circumstances that led to the writing of these poems, see al-Miṣrī 1994, pp. 85–193; al-Miṣrī 1999, pp. 57–126.
18 Ibn Zaydūn 1958, pp. 141–8.
19 Shawqī 1964, II, pp. 104–8. Cf. Adūnīs and Sa'īd 1982, pp. 174–80.
20 Shawqī 1964, IV, pp. 78–9; Boudot-Lamotte 1977, p. 376.
21 Shawqī 1964, II, pp. 44–52.

is, a poem containing an image of al-Andalus written by Aḥmad Shawqī.[22] Subsequently, the term *Andalusiyya* was applied to poems by other poets as well and now stands for the general use of Andalusian themes in Arabic poetry.[23]

While most of Shawqī's *Andalusiyyāt* describe the poet's longing for his homeland, it was the rich heritage of al-Andalus that inspired him: when he describes the great Andalusian remains, he finds in them proof that the ancient glory will be revived in the near future, so much so that the adjective *Andalusī* becomes a synonym for glorious: "Time would become Andalusian"[24] is an expression that connotes the splendor that al-Andalus' culture and society evokes in the minds of modern Arabs. The figure of the first Umayyad king in al-Andalus, 'Abd al-Raḥmān I (731–788), who was later called *al-Dākhil* ("The Incomer"), was used by Shawqī in his poem "Ṣaqr Quraysh" ("The Hawk of Quraysh," the epithet of the Andalusian king).[25] Shawqī praises 'Abd al-Raḥmān al-Dākhil with the following words:

فـي كتـاب الفخـر للدّاخـل بـــاب لـم يلجـه من بَنِي الملك أمير

In the book of praises, al-Dākhil has a chapter
No prince of the men of authority can enter into.

Significantly, Shawqī chose to write the poem in the form of *muwashshaḥ*, a postclassical poetic form arranged in stanzas that flourished in al-Andalus but never succeeded in acquiring canonization.[26] This was presumably Shawqī's way of highlighting the unique literary heritage of al-Andalus.

22 Ibrāhīm n.d. [1937], I, pp. 98–103.

23 For example, see al-Bur'ī 1978, pp. 67–8. The Lebanese singer Fayrūz (Nuhād Ḥaddād) (b. 1934) released an audio-cassette titled *Andalusiyyāt*, whose songs used the broader sense of the term—the longing for a lost paradise. For example, the first song is "Irja'ī Yā Alf Laylā" ("Come Back, One Thousand [and One Nights]").

24 Shawqī 1964, I, p. 242.

25 Shawqī 1964, II, pp. 171–8.

26 The non-canonical status of the *muwashshaḥ* is illustrated by the fact that by the mid-twelfth century knowledge of early *muwashshaḥāt* had already disappeared (Ibn Bassām 1979, I, p. 469. Cf. Jones 1988, pp. 11–13; Abu-Haidar 1991, pp. 115–16). Moreover, it was not customary to include *muwashshaḥāt* in highly regarded literary or historical works (al-Marrākushī 1963, p. 146. Cf. 'Abbās 1985, pp. 217–18). The non-canonical status of the *muwashshaḥ* should be viewed in the framework of the canonical status of Arabic literature in the East, which Andalusians themselves saw as the example of excellence. Ibn Ḥazm (994–1064) illustrates this attitude when he writes: "I am the sun shining in the spheres of sciences, / but my shortcoming is that I rise in the West" ('Abbās 1969, p. 321. Cf. Nykl 1946, p. 102). About the non-canonical status of the *muwashshaḥāt*, we can also learn from the popular models (whether Eastern, according to M. Hartmann, or Spanish, according to García Gómez) that inspired the Andalusian poets who composed them (Monroe 1974, pp. 30–3; and Kennedy 1991, pp. 68–69). James Monroe considers the *muwashshaḥ* as the daughter of the non-canonical genre of the *zajal* (Monroe 1993, p. 413). On the close

Shawqī's Andalusian poems may be seen as typical for the way the image of al-Andalus appears in neoclassical poetry, abounding as they do in sensuous descriptions of the heritage and using referential patterns consciously taken from medieval Andalusian poetry. Most of the modes in neoclassical poetry that refer to al-Andalus derive particularly from memories associated with medieval contexts, be it Andalusian Arabic poetry, Arabic historical medieval chronicles, or, as was actually the case for modern poets, the famous Andalusian sites that inspired them. Some neoclassical poets even used the remnants of the Andalusian past as rhetorical figures. For example, in a poem by the Egyptian author Ismāʿīl Sarā al-Dahshān (1882–1950) from his collection *Bayna al-Jidd wa-l-Jayyid* (*Between Seriousness and Excellence*),[27] *al-Ḥamrā'* (Alhambra), the Citadel of Granada, rather than alluding to an Andalusian theme, stands for the opposite of poverty, which is illustrated by the word *kūkh* (hut). Neoclassical poetry, as may be expected, is on the whole backward-looking, and thus we will not find here any attempts to use the sensuous impressions inspired by al-Andalus as a vehicle for new and complex human experiences. This was to happen in the late 1940s, when poets began deviating from classical metrics and adopting *al-shiʿr al-ḥurr* (free verse), thus breaking the patterns of the ancient sacrosanct form of Arabic poetry.[28]

Inspired by English poetry, the central concept of Arabic free verse is a reliance on the free repetition of the basic unit of conventional prosody—that is, the use of an irregular number of a single foot (*tafʿīla*)—instead of a fixed number of feet. This was not simply an innovation in metrics: writers and literary critics from the center of the literary system claimed that the new poetry was not a superficial reflection of modern life but a profound expression of the spirit of the age; that the new aesthetic concept sprang from the heart of the literary work itself, which sought to explore the essence of life and to reflect the culture of the age on a universal basis; and that, given that changing perceptions had inspired new forms and techniques, poetic experiences were no longer limited to personal emotions. The new forms were seen as the only ways in which Arabic poetry could be revived; their acceptance was vital if poetry was to remain for the modern Arab world the

relationship between these two genres, see Einbinder 1995, pp. 252–70. On the intimate association of the *muwashshaḥāt* with folk music, see Shiloah 1995, p. 77. On *muwashshaḥāt* as a simple development from the Arabic literary tradition of the East without any outside influence, see Abu-Haidar 1992, pp. 63–81; Abu-Haidar 1993, pp. 439–58 (both studies were incorporated in Abu-Haidar 2001, pp. 126–38, 147–67, and see also other chapters of the book on that issue). On the *muwashshaḥat* in general, see Stern 1974.

27 Al-Dahshān 1983, p. 107.

28 On the issue of terminology regarding the "free verse," see al-Tami 1993, pp. 185–98.

vehicle of artistic and intellectual expression that it had been in the past. Hence, the image of al-Andalus together with the metric innovations that poets had incorporated proved to be crucial in shaping the development of the new poetry, in that they enabled it to rediscover various dimensions of the Arabic poetic heritage.

Al-Andalus, as the lost paradise, has been used in Arabic poetry since the 1950s as a twofold metaphor: while its glory and splendor is used to allude to the huge potential of the Arab nation, the period of local dynasties (*Mulūk al-Ṭawā'if*) epitomizes the fragmentation of the Arab world in the twentieth century. These direct allusions to al-Andalus in Arabic poetry can be found in the poetry of the Syrian Nizār Qabbānī (1923–1998).[29] However, there are also indirect techniques. One such technique, which has been much favored since the late 1950s, is the employment of Andalusian figures as literary masks and the creation of the so-called *qaṣīdat qinā'* (mask poem). That is, through an artistic mask the poet seeks to reconcile "the mortal and the eternal, the finite and the infinite."[30] Thus, the Syrian 'Alī Aḥmad Sa'īd, better known as Adūnīs (b. 1930), in his *Kitāb al-Taḥawwulāt wa-l-Hijra fī Aqālīm al-Nahār wa-l-Layl* (*The Book of Changes and Migration in the Regions of Day and Night*)[31] invokes the figure of 'Abd al-Raḥmān al-Dākhil to express the contemporary human condition but makes no attempt to imitate the use of neoclassical poetry often made by the same figure:

والصّقر في متاهه، في يأسه الخلاّقْ
يبني على الذّروة في نهاية الأعماقْ
أندلس الأعماقْ
أندلس الطّالع من دمشقْ
يحمل للغرب حصاد الشّرقْ

The Hawk in his labyrinth, in his creative despair
Builds on the peak at the end of depths
Andalus of the depths
Andalus arising from Damascus
Bearing to the West the harvest of the East.[32]

For Adūnīs, "Ṣaqr Quraysh" ("The Hawk of Quraysh," 'Abd al-Raḥmān al-Dākhil) is one of the links in the chain of transmission through which the achievements of medieval Arab civilization reached the West.[33] He was not

29 Cf. al-Waṣīfī 2002, pp. 229–49.
30 Al-Bayyātī 1968, p. 134. Cf. Badawi 1975, p. 214.
31 Adūnīs 1965; Adūnīs 1988 [1983], I, pp. 431–597; Adūnīs 2012–2015, II, pp. 7–166.
32 Adūnīs 1988 [1983], p. 458; Adūnīs 2012–2015, II, p. 32.
33 See also the aforementioned play *al-Muharrij* (*The Jester*) by Muḥammad al-Māghūṭ in which the figure of *Ṣaqr Quraysh* was used in order to criticize the contemporary Arab condition (al-Māghūṭ 1981, pp. 495–614). Cf. also the poem "Thawrat al-Manāqīr Amāma

the first to use it in this sense: Muḥammad ʻIzzat Darwaza (1888–1984), one of the major figures encouraging dramatic performances in Palestine before 1948, wrote the play *Ṣaqr Quraysh* (*The Hawk of Quraysh*), in which he used this figure in order to prompt his Arab audience to challenge the contemporary Western hegemony.

In his collection *Tanabba' Ayyuhā al-Aʻmā* (*Prophesy, O, You Blind!*), Adūnīs included twelve poems he wrote while visiting Granada in 1996, titling the series *Ithnā ʻAshar Qindīlan li- Ghranāṭa* (*Twelve Lamps for Granada*).[34] The series, whose poems are without titles but have only numbers, concludes with the following text:

أصغِ، أيّها الشّاعر، إلى غرناطة
أنتَ لم تَعْشَقْ مساءَ ما مَضَى
إلاّ لأنّكَ مأخوذٌ بصباحِ ما يأتي.
المساءُ يُهيّئُ الفجر —
جذْرًا يفتح لك الأفقُ
وعمقًا يُغذّيك بالعلوّ.
ولكَ مثل الشّمس، ومثل غرناطة،
خَدّان:
خَدّ على الشّرق،
وخَدّ على الغرب.

Listen, O poet, to Granada
You did not love the evening of what had passed
But because you are possessed by the morning of what will come.
Evening prepares the dawn—
A root that opens for you the horizon
And depth that feeds you with heights.
And you have, like the sun, and like Granada,
Two checks:
One on the East,
And another on the West.

In 2007, Adūnīs visited Cordova and concluded a poem he wrote following the visit of the city as follows:

يكفي، أيّها الحاضر العربيّ، أن "تنسى" قرطبة:
الجسد والفنّ. يكفي أن "تكتب" تأريخك بالقتل!
وانظر إلى الخريطة العربيّة-الإسلاميّة: جسمها كوكب
ضخم، لكنّ صوتها صوت عصفور يكاد أن يختنق.

Ṣaqr Quraysh al-Mujawwaf" ("The Revolution of the Beaks in front of the Hollow Hawk of Quraysh") by the Lebanese Ilyās Laḥḥūd (b. 1942) (*al-Ādāb*, February 1972, p. 69). See also al-Qāsim 1987, pp. 481–2. On the use of the figure ʻAbd al-Raḥmān al-Dākhil in Palestinian poetry, see al-Juʻaydī 1997, pp. 6–12; al-Juʻaydī 2000, pp. 14–21.

34 Adūnīs 2012–2015, VI, pp. 47–61.

It is about time for you, the Arab present, to stop "forgetting" Cordova:
The body and the art. It is about time to stop "writing" your history with murder!
Look at the Arab-Islamic map: its body is a huge
Star, but its voice is of a bird being almost suffocated.[35]

The poem, titled "A Cloud above Cordova," hardly refers to the link between past and present, with the exception of the aforementioned concluding lines as if to show that, even if you try, the Arab tragic present cannot be ignored.

Apart from "Ṣaqr Quraysh," another figure mentioned in Arabic poetry is that of the conqueror of al-Andalus, Ṭāriq ibn Ziyād (670–720), which has become popular in Palestinian poetry. For example, Mu'īn Bsīsū (1927–1984) uses it in both his poetry and poetic drama: in his "Qaṣīda min Faṣl Wāhid" ("A Poem with One Chapter"), Ṭāriq ibn Ziyād is in prison,[36] while in his verse drama *Thawrat al-Zanj* (*The Revolution of the Negroes*) Ṭāriq is called to participate in the *jihād*, the holy war.[37]

The Iraqi poet 'Abd al-Wahhāb al-Bayyātī (1926–1999) in his poem "Ziryāb"[38] speaks through the mask of the gifted Baghdadian musician 'Alī ibn Nāfi', also known as Ziryāb (d. 857), whose jealous teacher had him driven from the court of Caliph Hārūn al-Rashīd (763–809). Ziryāb made it to the Cordovan court of 'Abd al-Raḥmān II in 822, where he introduced innovations they had not heard before and became chief court musician.[39] Through the device of the artistic mask reconciling "the present and that which transcends the present,"[40] al-Bayyātī considers Ziryāb as representing the continuous progression that leads from past through present to future in unifying "all man's experience throughout history ... proving the endless capacity of human experience for reproducing itself."[41] Ziryāb, in the figure of the new Arab, cries in the "desert of nothingness":

أندلس المجهول
ماذا يختفي وراء هذا الصّوت؟
هل عاد المحبّون من السّفر؟
أم نذر أدلت بها عرّافة القدر؟

[35] Adūnīs 2012–2015, VIII, pp. 82–5. In another poem Adūnīs wrote after he visited Granada in 2009 (Adūnīs 2012–2015, VIII, pp. 309–16), he does not mention the Arabs' past or present at all, conducting instead a personal dialogue with Granada and the poet Federico García Lorca (1898–1936), whose presence in Arabic poetry is frequently related to al-Andalus.

[36] Bsīsū 1988, pp. 331–2.

[37] Bsīsū 1988a, p. 285.

[38] First published in *al-Dustūr*, July 31, 1989, p. 52; republished in al-Bayyātī 1995, pp. 123–5.

[39] Shiloah 1995, pp. 74–5. On Ziryāb and his contribution to the musical heritage of al-Andalus, see Reynolds 2020, pp. 822–52; Reynolds 2021, pp. 115–51.

[40] Al-Bayyātī 1968, p. 134.

[41] Jayyusi 1977, p. 745.

زرياب كان صوتها
ووجهها الآخر والشّبح؟

O Andalus of the unknown
What is hidden behind that voice?
Did the lovers return from the journey?
Or is it warnings uttered by the fortune teller of fate?
Was Ziryāb her voice,
Her other voice and nightmare?[42]

That al-Bayyātī chose Ziryāb as an artistic mask with which to express his own emotional and intellectual aspirations is again testimony to the great cultural impact that the Andalusian past has had on Arab culture. This does not mean that, alongside this new technique, neoclassical techniques are no longer used by contemporary poets. For example, ʻAlī al-Ḥusaynī's poem "Sifr ʻAbd al-Raḥmān al-Dākhil" ("The Book of ʻAbd al-Raḥmān al-Dākhil") from the collection with the same title[43] reflects in clear neoclassical style the longing of contemporary Arabs to see the ancient glory of the past revived through the figure of ʻAbd al-Raḥmān al-Dākhil:

أنت العربيّ القادم من الشّرقِ أو الغربِ
وأنت اللّهب الكامن في أهليها.

You are the Arab man coming from the East or the West
And you are the fire hidden among the people.[44]

Likewise, for the Israeli Palestinian poet Fārūq Mawāsī (1941–2020), the impression Spain left on him led to a long poem called "Andalusiyyāt" from his collection *al-Khurūj min al-Nahr* (*The Exodus from the River*).[45] Written in August 1987, the poem consists of seven parts: (1) "A Smell of Perfume"; (2) "Cordova"; (3) "Seville"; (4) "Malaga"; (5) "Far from Gibraltar"; (6) "Alhambra"; and (7) "All Over Again." Mawāsī's poem, like most poems that concentrate on this kind of sensuous employment of Andalusian sites and places, was written following a visit to Spain, and its parts generally correspond to the stages of his visit.[46]

Another technique that modernist poets have employed is to use names of Andalusian sites not for sensuous external descriptions, but to give voice to deeper, more inner experiences. For example, al-Bayyātī, who spent many years in exile in Spain, in the last collection he published, *Kitāb al-Marāthī*

[42] Al-Bayyātī 1995, pp. 124–5.
[43] Al-Ḥusaynī 1980, pp. 107–14.
[44] Al-Ḥusaynī 1980, p. 114.
[45] Mawāsī 1989, pp. 51–79.
[46] Cf. Mawāsī 2002, p. 52.

(*The Book of Elegies*) (1995), includes a poem titled "al-Dukhūl ilā Ghranāṭa" ("Entering Granada")[47] in which the emotional attachment to the streets of that Andalusian city moves beyond the sensual into the realm of myth:

لم أدخل غرناطة، لكنّي كنت بها شبحا
أتجوّل في قصر الحمراء
أصغي لنحيب الماء
وأنين جذور الأشجار
أتسلّق أبراج السّور المهدومة
— — — — — — —
وماذا قال العرّاف؟
لن تدخل غرناطة إلا بعد الموت
— — — — — — —
ها أنذا أسقط من أعلى البرج
أطير قليلا
أدخل غرناطة من كلّ الأبواب.

I did not enter Granada, but I was a ghost there
Wandering in Alhambra
Listening to the weeping water
And the wailing roots of the trees
Climbing the towers of the destroyed walls
— — — — — — — — — — —
And what did the fortune teller say?
You will never enter Granada
— — — — — — — — — — —
Here I am falling from high above the tower
I am flying for some time
I am entering Granada through all its gates.

Granada here is no longer the actual Andalusian city but has become a symbol of the longed-for utopian city that the poet realizes he will never enter during his earthly life.[48] In this sense, Granada is mentioned by many other modern poets for whom the distant past serves as a backdrop to their own current emotional experiences.[49] Thus, it could happen that for many of them one of the major connecting links between Granada's past and the present has become the legendary image of the Spanish poet and dramatist Federico García Lorca (1898–1936), whose murder by the Nationalists at the start of the Spanish Civil War brought him posthumous world fame.

[47] Al-Bayyātī 1995, pp. 99–104.
[48] Cf. the poem "al-Ḍaw' Ya'tī min Ghranāṭa" ("The Light Comes from Granada") (al-Bayyātī 1979, II, pp. 395–7), in which the poet uses the mask of the Prophet Muḥammad (on this poem, see Athamneh 2017, pp. 78–85).
[49] Shalḥat 1989, p. 51.

3. "THE GUITAR IS AFLAME"

Lorca is frequently described by Arab authors as the son of Granada:

> Lorca, before anything else, is the son of the ancient Arab city of Granada, which once upon a time was one of the radiant cultural oases, that is, he is the son of al-Andalus. This is al-Andalus, the myth whose civilization and culture were created by the Arabs, especially as his poetry is so highly influenced by the Arabic writings of al-Andalus.[50]

The image of Lorca captivated Arab poets not only because of his reputation as a revolutionary poet, or because he was a son of Granada, but especially because of the "Andalusian" nature of so many of his poems. Aware of the close relationships (for example, in his arabesque *Casidas* and *Gacelas of Diván de Tamarit* [1940]) between his poetry and Arabic poetry, some Arab poets even detect links between Lorca and Andalusian Arab culture.[51] In fact, the hold Lorca has had during the past few decades on the minds of poets in the Arab world has turned him into a symbol of their struggle for freedom and justice, as the Egyptian poet Ṣalāḥ 'Abd al-Ṣabūr (1931–1981) does in his poem *Lorca*:[52]

لوركا
نافورة ميدان
ظلّ ومقيل للأطفال الفقراء.
لوركا أغنية غجريّة،
لوركا شمس ذهبيّة،
لوركا ليل صيفيّ منعم،
لوركا سوسنة بيضاء
مسحت خدّيها في الماء.
لوركا أجراس قِبابْ،
سكنتْ في جوف ضبابٍ،
قرب النّجم المفرد،
آنا تشدو، آنا تتنهّد.
لوركا سعف العيد الاخضر
لوركا حلوى سكّر
لوركا قلب مملوء بالنّور الرّائق

[50] Al-Akhḍar 1986, p. 4.

[51] For example, see the argument of the Iraqi poet Buland al-Ḥaydarī (1926–1996) in his essay in *al-Majalla* (London), September 19, 1989, p. 75. On Lorca and Arab Andalusia, see Puccetti 1956, pp. 22–5.

[52] See 'Abd al-Ṣabūr 1972, pp. 228–30. For other poems using the image of Lorca, see al-Bayyātī 1979, I, pp. 605–9; II, pp. 225–7, 249–51, 258–61, 332–7, 344–54; III, pp. 221–42, 321–7, 331–40, 407–19; al-Sayyāb 1971, I, pp. 333–4, 355–8. Cf. Moreh 1976, p. 268; Badawi 1975, pp. 210, 224, 250, 262; Jayyusi 1977, pp. 565, 577, 691–2, 749; Shukrī 1978, pp. 49, 149; Badīr 1982, pp. 129, 177; 'Abd al-'Azīz 1983, pp. 271–99; 'Abd al-Ṣabūr n.d., pp. 167–75.

Lorca
Is a fountain in the square
A shelter and resting place for the poor children
Lorca is gypsies' songs
Lorca is a golden sun
Lorca is a tender summer's night
Lorca is a woman bearing twins
Lorca is a white lily
Rinsing her cheeks in water
Lorca is bells of domes
Dwelling in the midst of the fog
Near the lone star
Sometimes singing, sometimes sighing
Lorca is the green palm of the feast day
Lorca is sweet candy
Lorca is a heart filled with pure light.

The Lebanese-Druze Fu'ād al-Khashin (1925–2009) concludes his "Qamar Ghranāṭa wa-l-Ḥaras al-Aswad" ("Granada's Moon and the Black Patrol")[53] with the following lines:

من أسكت حنجرة الشّاعر
برصاص ليليّ غادر
يا لوركا، يا وجها يُعبد
يا نفسا، أصفى مرآة
غابت عن أرض الاندلس!

Who silenced the poet's voice
With treacherous nightly bullets?
O Lorca, the adored features
O soul, the clearest of mirrors
Vanished from the lands of al-Andalus.

In a poem titled "Layālī Ghranāṭa" ("Granada's Nights"), the Egyptian poet Fatḥī Sa'īd (1931–1989) says:

نافورة لوركا في الميدان
تبكي الشّعراء وتهزأ بالأوزان
تتناثر حرفا عربيّ الدّيوان
وزنا أندلسيّ العنوان
لوركا في دمنا العربيّ وإن جنح
إلى الأسبان

Lorca's fountain in the square
Is weeping over the poets and laughs at the [poetry] meters

[53] Al-Khashin 1972, pp. 155–7. Cf. also pp. 213–16.

Its [water] scattering about letters whose poetry is Arabic
A meter whose title is Andalusian
Lorca exists in our Arab blood even if he inclines
to the Spanish people.[54]

In his collection *Andalusiyyāt Miṣriyya* (Egyptian *Andalusiyyāt*), Saʿīd published the same poem under a new title, "Ḥānat Lorca" ("Lorca's Tavern") together with several textual changes.[55] The collection includes other poems recalling the memory of al-Andalus and connecting it with the Arab present and the poet's own experiences. For example, in "Layl Ghranāṭa" ("Granada's Night") he describes the night of Granada as:

يجهش بالبكاء
ينساب كالرّقطاء
يصبّ في دمي
— — — — —
ونهر غرناطة
سطر على لسان صاحب الإحاطة
جداول على مروجها الخضراء
جدائل على قبابها الخرساء
تستر بعض عورة الرّداء!

Breaking into tears
Flowing like speckled snake
Into my blood
— — — — — — — —
Granada's river
A line uttered by the writer of *al-Iḥāṭa*[56]
Water streams on its green pastures
Braids on its silent domes
Covering part of its nakedness![57]

For Palestinian writers, and especially poets, Lorca has become a catalyst triggering a widespread use of al-Andalus as a metaphor for the lost paradise. As a mythical figure, Lorca has inspired them to search the rich Andalusian Arab heritage for connections between past and present that could serve them as links in the chain of their own collective and cultural memory. That the glory of the Andalusian past and the fame of the modern Spanish poet are the products of the same spatial context made the act of mythologizing

[54] *Al-Ahrām* January 21, 1983, p. 11.
[55] Saʿīd 1994, pp. 47–50.
[56] The allusion is to *al-Iḥāṭa fī Akhbār Ghranāṭa* (*The Comprehension of the News of Granada*) by Lisān al-Dīn ibn al-Khaṭīb (1313–1374), a historical lexicon including biographies of famous men of Granada (Ibn al-Khaṭīb 1901).
[57] Saʿīd 1994, pp. 39–40.

Lorca seem almost self-evident. For example, Samīḥ al-Qāsim (1939–2014), after he visited Spain, wrote a poem titled "Laylan, 'alā Bāb Federico" ("At Night, At Federico's Door").[58] Unlike other poems he wrote,[59] this poem nowhere alludes directly to al-Andalus, but a sense of the splendor that was Arab Andalusia and the atmosphere that pervades Andalusian Arabic poetry hover unmistakably above the lines:

فدريكو ...
الحارس أطفأ مصباحَه
انزل
أنا منتظر في السّاحة

فد - - ري - - كو
قنديل الحزن قمر
الخوف شجر
فانزل
أنا أعلم أنك مختبئ في البيت
مسكونًا بالحمّى
مشتعلًا بالموت
فانزل
أنذا منتظر في السّاحة
مشتعلًا بلهيب الوردة
قلبي تفّاحة.
الدّيك يصيح على قرميد السّطح
فدريكو
النّجمة جرح
والدّم يصيح على الأوتار
يشتعل الجيتار
فد - - ر - - يكو
الحرس الأسود ألقى في البئر سلاحه
فانزل للسّاحة
أعلم أنّك مختبئ في ظلّ ملاك
ألمحك هناك
زنبقة خلف ستارة شبّاك
ترتجف على فمك فراشة
وتمسّد شعر اللّيل يداك
انزل فدريكو
وافتح لي الباب
أسرع

[58] Al-Qāsim 1986, pp. 49–53. On the poem, see also the interpretation of Fārūq Mawāsī in *al-Ittiḥād*, January 5, 1996, pp. 20–1. Cf. the poem "Lorca" by Maḥmūd Darwīsh (Darwīsh 1988, pp. 68–70).

[59] For example, his poem "Andalus" (al-Qāsim 1992, IV, pp. 567–75). On the poem, see Fatḥ al-Bāb 1992, pp. 505–16.

أنذا أنتظر على العتبة
أسرع
في منعطف الشّارع
جلبة ميليشيا مقتربة
قرقعة بنادق
وصليل حراب
افتح لي الباب
أسرع خبّئني
فدريكو
فد - - ري - - كو

Federico ...
The guard turned off his flashlight
Come down
I am waiting in the square

Fede - - ri - - co
The lamp of sadness is a moon
The fear is trees
Come down
I know, you are hiding in the house
Gripped with fever
Burning with death
Come down
I am waiting in the square
Burning with the flame of the rose
My heart is an apple

A rooster calls on a tiled roof
Federico
The star is a wound
And the blood is screaming on the strings
And the guitar is aflame

Fede - - ri - - co
The black patrol threw its weapons in the well
Come down to the square
I know, you are hiding between the wings of an angel
I see you
A lily behind a curtain
And between your lips trembles a butterfly
And your hands caress the hair of the night
Come down, Federico
And open the door for me
Quickly
I am waiting in the doorstep

Quickly
At the street corner
The din of an approaching militia
The clatter of rifles
And the clangor of lances
Open the door for me
Quickly
Hide me
Federico
Fede - - ri - - co

"Moon," "trees," "rose," "apple," "strings of a guitar," "lily," and "butterfly," all allude to Andalusian nature poetry, while "black patrol," "weapons," "militia," "rifles," and "lances" allude to the powers of darkness responsible for what Antonio Machado (1875–1939) described in his elegy for Lorca as "the crime in Granada."[60] Death reigns in the poem's image of Lorca: he is hiding "between the wings of an angel," and a butterfly trembles between his lips, his soul about to leave his body.[61] Al-Qāsim's poem alludes to Lorca's poem "La guitarra" ("The Guitar"):

Empieza el llanto
de la guitarra.
Se rompen las copas
de la madrugada.
Empieza el llanto
de la guitarra

Es inútil callarla.
Es imposible callarla.

Llora monótona
como llora el agua
como llora el viento
sobre la nevada.

Es imposible callarla.
Llora por cosas lejanas.
Arena del Sur caliente
que pide camelias blancas.

Llora flecha sin blanco,
la tarde sin mañana,

[60] Machado 1973, pp. 252–3. For an Arabic translation of the poem, see *al-Ṭalīʿa*, August 1976, pp. 163–4.

[61] Cf. al-Bayyātī 1979, II, pp. 258–61.

y el primer pájaro muerto
sobre la rama.

¡Oh, guitarra!
Corazón malherido
por cinco espadas.

The weeping of the guitar
Begins.
The glasses of the early morning
Break
The weeping of the guitar
Begins.
Useless to silence it
Impossible to silence it.

It weeps monotonously
As water weeps
As the wind weeps
Over snowfall.

Impossible to silence it.
It weeps for distant things,
Yearning for white camellias
Of southern sands

Weeps like an arrow without target,
Evening without morning,
And the first dead bird
On the branch.

Oh guitar!
Heart mortally wounded
By five swords.[62]

Lorca appears as well in the works of Arab poets writing in other languages, such as in English. For example, the French-American Palestinian poet Nathalie Handal (b. 1969) published *Poet in Andalucía*,[63] in which she recreated Lorca's *Poeta en Nueva York* (written in 1930; published posthumously in 1940).[64]

As the annals of the Palestinian people's history, especially after 1948, Palestinian poetry, apart from the image of Lorca, contains such a wide range of neoclassical and modernist techniques using the image of al-Andalus

[62] Lorca 2014, pp. 22–3.
[63] Handal 2012 (Arabic translation: Handal 2019).
[64] Lorca 1940 (English translation: Lorca 2008).

that one of the first scholars who studied comprehensively the presence of al-Andalus in modern Arabic poetry concentrates solely on Palestinian literature.[65] For Maḥmūd Darwīsh, the main Andalusian sites (Cordova, Granada, Toledo, and Seville) are icons that stand for experiences that go on beyond the historical, external meanings or sensuous dimensions of these places. In a poem titled "Idhā Kāna Lī an Uʿīda al-Bidāya" ("If I Were to Start All Over Again"), he says:

إذَا كَانَ لِي أَنْ أُعِيدَ البِدايَة أَختارُ ما اخْتَرْتُ: وَرْدَ السّياج
أسَافِرُ ثَانيةً فِي الدَّرُوبِ الّتِي قدْ تُؤدِّي وقَدْ لا تُؤدِّي إِلَى قُرْطَبهْ.
أُعلِّقُ ظِلِّي عَلَى صَخرَتَيْنِ لِتَبْنِي الطُّيُورُ الشَّرِيدَةُ عُشًّا على غُصْنِ ظِلِّي
وأُكسرُ ظِلِّي لأَتْبَعَ رَائِحَةَ اللَّوْزِ وَهِيَ تَطِيرُ عَلَى غيْمةٍ مُتْربَهْ
وَأتعبُ عنْدَ السُّفوحِ: تَعَالَوا إِليَّ اسْمَعُونِي. كُلُوا مِنْ رَغِيفِي
اشْربُوا مِنْ نَبِيذي، ولا تَتْرُكُونِي عَلَى شَارِعِ العُمْرِ وَحْدِي كَصَفْصَافَةٍ مُتْعبَهْ.
أُحِبُّ البِلاَدَ الِتي لَمْ يَطَأهَا نَشِيدُ الرَّحِيلِ ولمْ تمْتَثِلْ لدمٍ وامْرَأَهْ
أُحِبُّ النِّسَاءَ اللَّواتِي يُخَبِّئْنَ فِي الشَّهَوَاتِ انْتِحَارَ الخُيُولِ عَلَى عتبَهْ.
أَعُودُ، إِذَا كَانَ لِي أَنْ أَعُودَ، إِلَى وَرْدَتِي نَفْسِهَا وإِلَى خطْوَتِي نَفْسِهَا
وَلَكِنَّنِي لاَ أَعُودُ إِلَى قُرْطُبَهْ.

If I could to start all over again I'd choose what I have chosen now: the roses on the fence
I'd travel again on the road that may or may not lead to Cordova.
I'd hang my shadow on two rocks for fugitive birds to build a nest on my shadow's branch
I'd break my shadow to follow the scent of almonds as it wafts on a cloud of dust
And feel tired at the foot of the mountain; come and listen to me. Have some of my bread
Drink from my wine and do not leave me on the road of years on my own like a tired willow tree
I love the country that's never felt the tread of departure's song, nor bowed to blood or woman
I love women who in their desire conceal the suicide of horses dying on the threshold.
I will return, if I can, to my roses, to my steps
But I will not go back to Cordova.[66]

The allusion in the aforementioned lines to Lorca's poem "Canción del jinete" ("The Rider's Song") can hardly be overlooked:

Córdoba.
Lejana y sola.

65 See al-Juʿaydī 1997; al-Juʿaydī 2000, pp. 7–52.
66 Darwīsh 1987a, p. 9 (English translation is based on Al-Udhari 1984, p. 23).

Jaca negra, luna grande,
y aceitunas en mi alforja.
Aunque sepa los caminos,
yo nunca llegar é a Córdoba.

Por el llano, por el viento,
jaca negra, luna roja.
La muerte me está mirando
desde las torres de Córdoba.

¡Ay qué camino tan largo!
¡Ay mi jaca valerosa!
¡Ay, que la muerte me espera,
antes de llegar a Córdoba!

Córdoba.
Lejana y sola.

Cordova.
Lonely in the distance.

Little black horse, giant moon—
And olives in my saddlebag.
Even if I know the way,
I never will reach Cordova.

Over the plain, into the wind,
Little black horse, red moon—

Death is watching for me
From up in the towers of Cordova.

Oh, such a long road!
Oh, my valiant little horse!
Oh, but death awaits me
Before I ever reach Cordova.

Cordova.
Lonely in the distance.[67]

Cordova, as the famous center of Andalusian learning and culture, is not just the historical Andalusian city but a vehicle for the "Palestinian" experience of the 1980s, signifying the lost Palestinian paradise, or even Jerusalem, as the Palestinian critic Muḥammad 'Abd Allāh al-Ju'aydī (b. 1948) says: "If the circumstances prevented the poet from reaching Jerusalem, and he was

[67] Lorca 1994–1996, I, pp. 368–9.

forced to go to Cordova, the idea is that his journey stopped on the boundaries of his creative work and remains a dream with no chance to ever be fulfilled."[68]

4. "I AM ONE OF THE KINGS OF THE END"

Cordova, like other Andalusian sites, appears in Darwīsh's poetry on the same level as "tears, dance and the long embrace of a woman. Al-Andalus is a universal esthetic and artistic property, but Jerusalem is an esthetic, spiritual and juristic property."[69] In Psalm 16 from his *Mazāmīr* (*Psalms*) from the collection *Uḥibbuki aw lā Uḥibbuki* (*I Love or I Do Not Love You*),[70] Darwīsh says:

أداعب الزّمن
كأمير يلاطف حصانًا.
وألعبُ بالأيّام
كما يلعب الأطفال بالخرز الملوّن.

إنّي أحتفل اليوم
بمرور يوم على اليوم السّابق
وأحتفل غدًا
بمرور يومين على الأمس
وأشرب نخب الأمس
ذكرى اليوم القادم
وهكذا أواصل حياتي!

عندما سقطتُ عن ظهر حصاني الجامح
وانكسرت ذراعي
أوجعتني إصبعي الّتي جرحت
قبل ألف سنة!

وعندما أحييت ذكرى الأربعين لمدينة عكّا
أجهشت في البكاء على غرناطة
وعندما التفّ حبل المشنقة حول عنقي
كرهت أعدائي كثيرًا
لأنّهم سرقوا ربطة عنقي!

I flirt with time
As a prince caresses a horse
And I play with the days
As children play with colored beads.

68 Al-Juʻaydī 1997, p. 9; al-Juʻaydī 2000, p. 17.
69 Al-Juʻaydī 1997, p. 25; al-Juʻaydī 2000, p. 36.
70 Darwīsh 1988, pp. 396–7.

Today I celebrate
The passing of a day on the previous one
And tomorrow I shall celebrate
The passing of two days on yesterday
I drink the toast of yesterday
In remembrance of the day to come
And thus I carry on my life!

When I fell from my indomitable horse
And broke an arm
My finger, wounded a thousand years ago,
Caused me pain!

When I commemorated the passing of forty days on the city of Acre,
I burst out weeping for Granada
And when the rope of the gallows tightened around my neck
I felt a deep hatred for my enemies
Because they stole my tie.[71]

The poem is about the attention that modern Arabs pay to marginal matters while neglecting the essence, as illustrated by Acre of the East and Granada of the West. The most prominent motive in Darwīsh's poetry, as in the entire corpus of modern Palestinian poetry in general, specifically between the 1982 Lebanon War and the outbreak of the *Intifāḍa* in the West Bank and the Gaza Strip in December 1987, is the use of al-Andalus as a mirror for Palestine.[72] The despair and frustration that formed the psychological background for the outbreak of the *Intifāḍa* have been deeply etched into the poetry and writings of Darwīsh, whose own fate may equally be seen as a metaphor for the Palestinian tragedy. Darwīsh's series of poems titled "Aḥada 'Ashara Kawkaban 'alā Ākhir al-Mashhad al-Andalusī" ("Eleven Stars on the End of the Andalusian Scene") from the collection *Aḥada 'Ashara Kawkaban* (*Eleven Stars*) is one long repetition of the equation al-Andalus = Palestine = paradise lost.[73] The general title illustrates the tragedy that the end of the Andalusian scene represents in the overall history of the

71 Translation following Darwīsh 1980, p. 50.

72 It seems that one of the first uses of al-Andalus as a mirror for Palestine appears in 1910, when the Damascene *al-Muqtabas*, edited by Muḥammad Kurd 'Alī (1876–1953), wrote: "We fear that the new settler will expel the indigenous and we will have to leave our country en masse. We shall then be looking back over our shoulder and mourn our land as did the Muslims of Andalusia" (*al-Muqtabas*, March 15, 1910 [according to Yazbak 1998, p. 221]). In 1948, the Iraqi poet Muḥammad Mahdī al-Jawāhirī (1899–1997) published "Filasṭīn wa-l-Andalus" ("Palestine and Andalus"), in which he implores God not to "let Palestine be like Andalus" (*al-Ḥaḍāra*, July 31, 1948. Reprinted in al-Jawāhirī 1982, II, p. 313).

73 Cf. Ismael 1981, pp. 43–5.

Arabs. Significantly, Darwīsh published the collection in 1992, that is, 500 years after the end of Arab rule in al-Andalus. It was on January 2, 1492 that the combined armies of Castile and Aragon captured the city of Granada. This was followed by a royal edict that decreed the expulsion of all non-Catholics from the Peninsula. Darwīsh sees himself as one of the last kings of the Andalusian era; the fourth star-poem is called "Anā Wāḥid min Mulūk al-Nihāya" ("I Am One of the Kings of the End"):

...وأَنا واحِدٌ مِنْ مُلوكِ النِّهايةِ. أَقْفِزُ عَنْ
فَرَسي في الشِّتاء الأخير، أنا زَفْرَةُ الْعَرَبيِّ الأخيرَةْ
لا أُطِلُّ على الآسِ فَوْقَ سُطوحِ الْبُيوتِ، ولا
أتطلَّعُ حَوْلي لِئَلاَّ يراني هُنا أحَدٌ كانَ يَعْرِفُني
كانَ يَعْرِفُ أنّي صَقَلْتُ رُخامَ الْكلام لتَعْبُرَ امْرأَتي
بُقَعَ الضَّوءِ حافَيةً، لا أُطِلُّ على اللَّيْل كَيْ
لا أرى قَمَرًا كان يُشْعِلُ أَسْرارَ غَرْناطةٍ كُلَّها
جَسَدًا. لا أُطِلُّ على الظِّلّ كَيْ لا أَرى
أَحَدًا يَحْمِلُ اسْمي وَيَرْكُضُ خَلْفي: خُذِ اسْمَكَ عَنيّ
وَأعْطِني فِضَّةَ الْحَوْرِ. لا أتلَفَّتُ خَلْفي لِئَلاّ
أَتَذَكَّرَ أَنّي مَرَرْتُ على الأرْضِ، لا أَرْضَ في
هذهِ الأرْضِ مُنْذ تَكَسَّرَ حَوْلي الزَّمانُ شَظَايَا
لَمْ أكُنْ عاشِقًا كَيْ أُصَدِّقَ أَنَّ الْمياه مَرايا
مِثْلمَا قُلْتَ لِلأصْدِقاءِ الْقُدامى. ولا حُبَّ يَشْفَعُ لي
مُذْ قَبِلْتُ «مُعاهَدَةَ التِّيهِ» لَمْ يَبْقَ لي حاضِرٌ
كَيْ أَمُرَّ غدًا قُرب أَمْسي. سَتَرفَعُ قَشْتالَةُ
تاجَها فَوْقَ مِئْذَنَة الله. أَسْمَعُ خَشْخَشَةً لِلْمَفاتيحِ في
بابِ تاريخنا الذَّهَبيَّ، وداعًا لِتاريخنا، هَلْ أَنا
مَنْ سَيُغْلِقُ باب السَّماءِ الأَخيرَ؟ أَنا زَفْرةُ الْعربَيِّ الأخيرَةْ.

... And I am one of the Kings of the end, jumping off
My horse in the last winter, I am the last gasp of an Arab.
I do not look for myrtle over the roofs of houses, nor do I
Look around, so that no one who knew me should recognize me,
No one who knew that I polished marble words to let my woman step
Barefoot over dappled light. I do not look into the night, so that
I will not see a moon that once lit up all the secrets of Granada
Body by body. I do not look into the shadow, so as not to see
Somebody carrying my name and running after me: take your name away from me
And give me the silver of the white poplar. I do not look behind me, so I won't
Remember I've passed over this land, there is no land
In this land since time broke around me shard by shard.
I was not a lover believing that water is mirrors,
As I told my old friends, and no love can redeem me,
For since I've accepted the "peace accord," there is no longer a present left
To let me pass, tomorrow, close to my yesterday. Castile will raise
Its crown above God's minaret. I hear the rattling of keys in the

Door of our golden history, good-bye our history, will it be me
Who will close the last gate of heaven? I am the last Arabs' sigh.[74]

As against the glory of the past, which elicits the image of al-Andalus in the present, the only remaining hope is survival ("the most important thing is to survive. Our survival is a victory"),[75] but, as the poet describes in an earlier collection, there will be harder days ahead:

هُنَالِكَ لَيْلٌ أَشَدُّ سَوَادًا هنالك وَرْدُ أَقَلُّ
سَيَنْقَسِمُ الدَّرْبُ أَكْثَرَ مِمَّا رَأَيْنَا، سَيَنْشَقُّ سَهْلُ
وَيَنْهَدُّ سَفْحٌ عَلَيْنَا، وَيَنْقَضُّ جُرْحٌ عَلَيْنَا، وَيَنْفَضُّ أَهْلُ
سَيَقْتُلُ فِينَا القَتِيلُ لِيَنْسَى عُيُونَ القَتِيلِ وَيَسْلُو
سَنَعْرِفُ أَكْثَرَ مِمَّا عَرَفْنَا، وَنَبْلُغُ هَاوِيَةً بَعْدَ هَاوِيَةٍ حِينَ نَعْلُو
عَلَى فِكْرَةٍ عَبَدَتْهَا القَبَائِلُ ثُمَّ شَوَتْهَا عَلَى لَحْمِ أَصْحَابِهَا حِينَ قَلُّوا
سَنَشْهَدُ فِينَا أَبَاطِرَةً يَحفِرُونَ عَلَى القَمْحِ أَسْمَاءَهُم كَيْ يَدُلُّوا
عَلَيْنَا. أَلَمْ نَتَغَيَّرْ؟ رِجَالٌ عَلَى دِينِ خِنْجَرِهم يَذْبَحُونَ، وَرَمْلٌ لِيَكْثُر رَمْلُ
نِسَاءٌ عَلَى دِينِ مَا بَيْنَ أَفْخَاذِهِنَّ وَظِلَّ لِيَصْغرَ ظِلُّ ...
وَلَكِنَّنِي سَأُتَابِعُ مَجْرَى النَّشِيدِ، وَلَوْ أَنَّ وَرْدِي أَقَلُّ.

There will be blacker night. There will be fewer roses
The trail will split even more than we have seen till now, the plains will be sundered
The foot of the mountain will heave upon us, a wound will break down over us, families will be scattered
The slaughtered among us will slaughter the slaughtered, to forget the slaughtered's eyes, and forget
We will know more than we knew; we will reach an abyss beyond the abysses, when we rise above
A thought which the tribes worshipped, then roasted on its originators' flesh, when they had grown fewer
We will see among us emperors etching their names in wheat in order to refer to ourselves.
Haven't we changed? Men who slaughter with faith in their daggers, and increasing sand
Women with faith in what they have between their legs, and a shadow to lessen shadows
Still, I will follow the poems, even if I have fewer roses.[76]

In the poem "al-Kamanjāt" ("Violins"), memory of the lost paradise becomes also memory of the lost territory of love:

[74] Darwīsh 1992, pp. 15–16.
[75] Darwīsh 1987, p. 51.
[76] Darwīsh 1987a, p. 45. For a translation of the entire poem, see Darwīsh 2003, p. 23. For a German translation, see Darwisch 1996, p. 47.

الكَمَنجاتُ تَبْكي معَ الغَجَرِ الذَّاهِبِينَ إلى الأنْدَلسْ
الكَمَنجاتُ تَبْكي على العَرَبِ الْخَارِجِينَ مِنَ الأنْدلُسْ

الكَمَنجاتُ تَبْكي على زَمَنٍ ضائعٍ لا يَعودْ
الكَمَنجاتُ تَبْكي على وَطَنٍ ضائعٍ قَدْ يَعودْ

الكَمَنجاتُ تُحْرقُ غاباتِ ذَاكَ الظّلَامِ الْبعيدِ
الكَمَنجاتُ تدْمي الْمُدى، وَتَشُمُّ دَمِى في الْوريدْ

الكَمَنجاتُ تَبْكي مَعَ الْغَجِر الذَّاهبينَ إلى الأنْدَلُسْ
الكَمَنجاتُ تَبْكي على الْعَرَب الْخارِجِينَ منَ الأَنْدَلُسْ

الكَمَنجاتُ خَيْلٌ على وَتَرٍ من سرابٍ وماءٍ يَئِنُّ
الكَمَنجاتُ حَقْلٌ مِنَ اللَّيْلكِ الْمُتوحِّش يَنْأَى وَيَدْنو

الكَمَنجاتُ وَحْشٌ يُعَذِّبُهُ ظُفْرُ امرأة مَسَّهُ، وابْتَعَدْ
الكَمَنجاتُ جَيْشٌ يُعَمِّرُ مَقْبَرَةً منْ رُخامٍ ومنْ نَهَوَنْدْ

الكَمَنجاتُ فَوْضى قُلوب تُجنِّنُها الرِّيحُ في قَدَمِ الرَّاقِصَةْ
الكَمَنجاتُ أسْرابُ طيْرٍ تفرُّ منَ الرَّايَة النَّاقِصَةْ

الكَمَنجاتُ شَكْوى الْحَرير المُجَعّد في لَيْلَةِ الْعاشقَةْ
الكَمَنجاتُ صَوْتُ النّبيذ الْبعيدِ على رغْبَةٍ سابِقَةْ

الكَمَنجاتُ تَتْبعُني ههُنا وهناكَ لتثأر مَنِّي
الكَمَنجاتُ تَبْحَثُ عنِّى لتقتلني، أَيْنما وَجَدتْني

الكَمَنجاتُ تَبْكي على الْعَربِ الْخارجينَ مِنَ الأندلُسْ
الكَمَنجاتُ تبكي مع الغجر الذَّاهبينَ إلى الأنْدَلُسْ

Violins are weeping seeing the gypsies coming to al-Andalus
Violins are weeping over the Arabs leaving al-Andalus

Violins are weeping over lost time which will never come back
Violins are weeping over a homeland that could return

Violins are burning the forests of that very far darkness
Violins are causing knives to bleed and smelling my blood in the veins

Violins are weeping seeing the gypsies coming to al-Andalus
Violins are weeping over the Arabs leaving al-Andalus

Violins are horses on the string of a mirage, and weeping water
Violins are a field of wild lilacs toing and froing

Violins are a wild animal tortured by a woman's finger nail
Violins are an army building a cemetery of marble and music

Violins are a chaos of hearts maddened by the wind blowing at the dancer's foot
Violins are groups of birds escaping the missed flag

Violins are the complaint of the curled silk during the beloved night
Violins are the voice of distant wine on a former desire

Violins are walking after me, here and there, to take revenge on me
Violins are looking for me to kill me, wherever they can find me

Violins are weeping over the Arabs leaving al-Andalus
Violins are weeping seeing the gypsies coming to al-Andalus.[77]

In another poem, Darwīsh asks his friend to "tear the arteries of my ancient heart with the poem of the gypsies who are going to al-Andalus / and sing to my departure from the sands and the ancient poets."[78] In Darwīsh's poetry, as in the poetry of many other Arab poets, al-Andalus has been turned into a poetic homeland as illustrated by Darwīsh himself:

وسنسأل أنفسنا في النّهاية: هل كانت الأندلس
ها هنا أم هناك؟ على الأرض، أم في القصيدة؟

And at last we will ask ourselves: Was Al-Andalus here or there?
On the earth, or in the poem?[79]

5. CONCLUSION

Used in Arabic literature as a vehicle to face the decline of the Arabs' self-image in order to challenge Western hegemony, al-Andalus survives also as a living memory to this today. In North Africa, there are many exiles that still "bear Andalusian names and keep the keys of their houses in Cordova and Seville hanging on their walls in Marrakesh and in Casablanca."[80] Side by side with such "physical" memories, the Arab national consciousness preserves memories of a cultural, spiritual, and intellectual nature. I have tried to show how the use and remembrance of al-Andalus in Arabic poetry can be placed in a developmental and historical context. For the Arab poet, the image of al-Andalus followed a twofold track: spatial, that is, from the modern Arab world into the regions of Spain; and temporal, that is, from the painful present into a medieval golden age. The Andalusian theme ranges from direct allusions to al-Andalus as the glory and splendor of the Arab past,

77 Darwīsh 1992, pp. 29–31. The poem is structured like a classical *qaṣīda*, consisting of ten stanzas each in a kind of couplet: a pair of lines that are the same length and rhyme, and form a complete thought. The first couplet imitates the *bukā' 'alā al-aṭlāl* (weeping over the ruins) of the beloved homeland, and it is repeated in the fourth stanza and again in a different order in the lines in the tenth stanza. The meter of the poem is *mutadārak* (— U —) and the rhyming scheme is AA/BB/CC/AA/DD/EE/FF/FF/GG/AA.

78 Darwīsh 1985, p. 23.

79 Darwīsh 1992, p. 10. Cf. Fernández-Parrilla 2018, p. 239.

80 Lewis 1970, p. 130. Cf. Roskies 1984, p. 1.

through al-Andalus as the lost paradise, to Andalusian figures and sites being used to express sensuous impressions and also to evoke other complicated experiences. Among the links that connect the Andalusian past with the Arab present and future is the twentieth-century Spanish poet Federico Lorca. Between the lines of poetry alluding to al-Andalus we find the hope that one day, in the not-too-distant future, there will emerge in the West a prominent intellectual figure who, like Blessed Álvaro of Córdoba (*c.* 1350–*c.* 1430), will be able to say that many of his friends

> read the poetry and tales of the Arabs, study the writings of Muhammadan theologians and philosophers, not in order to refute them, but to learn how to express themselves in Arabic with greater correctness and elegance ... All the young Christians noted for their gifts know only the language and literature of the Arabs, read and study with zeal Arabic books, building up great libraries of them at enormous cost and loudly proclaiming everywhere that this literature is worthy of admiration.[81]

Last but not least, al-Andalus was also a temporal and spatial territory shared by Muslims, Christians, and Jews, and characterized by cooperation. Before the escalation of the national conflict in Palestine, Arab nationalists at their earliest phases considered the Arab Jews as part of the Arab "race" and spoke about the Andalusian experience as a new vision for the Middle East.[82] However, since the 1930s, given a political reality in which one culture seeks to maintain its dominance over the other, this image of al-Andalus rarely occurs in modern Arabic literature. Here and there, we can find Arabic allusions to Muslim–Christian cooperation, such as by the Egyptian Fārūq Shūsha (1936–2016), who after participating in the second Muslim–Christian Conference in Cordova, in March 1977, wrote a poem titled "God's Sun in Cordova."[83] The poem joins the ancient glory of the Arabs in al-Andalus with sensuous descriptions of the Arab monuments in order to open a new road for Muslims and Christians:

أقسمت: هذه بداية الطّريق، بادروا مختتمه
عيسى وأحمد عليه يغرسان في القلوب أنجمه
تعانقا هديا إلهيّ السنا، متوّجا بالمكرمة
ونحن حاملوه في أعماقنا،
لن نسلّمه!

[81] Lewis 1970, p. 123.

[82] See, for example, a manifesto of Arab nationalists disseminated from Cairo by the Arab Revolutionary Committee at the beginning of the First World War: al-A'ẓamī 1932, IV, p. 116 (English translation: Haim 1962, pp. 87–8).

[83] Shūsha 1980, pp. 129–35.

I swear: this is the start of the road, take the initiative to finish it
On this road Jesus and Muḥammad are implanting stars in the hearts
They are embracing each other by a divine guidance, crowned with generosity
We bear it in our hearts,
We will never hand it over!

As a radiant image of tripartite religious coexistence, al-Andalus appears in the works of Jewish authors writing in Arabic,[84] where we can find allusion to the lines of the Andalusian Ṣūfī Muḥyī al-Dīn ibn ʻArabī (1164–1240) in *Tarjumān al-Ashwāq* (*The Translator of Desires*):

لقد صار قلبي قابلا كلّ صورة — فمرعى لغزلان ودير لرهبان
وبيت لأوثان وكعبة طائف — وألواح توراة ومصحف قرآن
أدين بدين الحبّ أنّى توجّهت — ركائبه فالحبّ ديني وإيماني

My heart is capable of every form,
  a pasture for gazelles, and a cloister for monks,
A place for idols, and the pilgrim's *Ka'ba,*
  the Tables of the Torah, and the Koran.
Love is the faith I hold wherever turn its
  camels, love is my belief and faith.[85]

These famous lines, which express above all the oneness of the mystical experiences of all religions, have evoked other interpretations that find here "the 'tolerance' of the mystic,"[86] but Jewish writers in Arabic as well as Arab-Israeli poets who have gone through the formal Israeli educational system generally view them as calling for cooperation between the three monotheistic religions.[87] Prince al-Ḥasan ibn Ṭalāl of Jordan (b. 1947), a strong promoter of dialogue between East and West, used these verses when he presented the Andalusian Golden Age as a way out of the conflict in the Middle East.[88] When Yael Lerer (b. 1967), an Israeli born in Tel Aviv to a

84 For example, see Sha'shū'a 1979.
85 Ibn ʻArabī 1966, pp. 43–4 (English translation according to Schimmel 1982, pp. 38–9, with some modifications. For another translation of these lines as well as for their poetic context, see Sells 1997, pp. 188–96. See also Ibn ʻArabī 1966, pp. 39–41). On these verses as part of the Christian images in Sufi poetry, see Abou-Bakr 1997, p. 99. On the understanding of these verses in the light of Ibn ʻArabī's entire teaching, see Taji-Farouki 2007, p. 189, and the notes on pp. 372–3.
86 Schimmel 1982, p. 38.
87 See, for example, Khalīl 1967, pp. 75–6; *Mifgash* 3 (May 1968), p. 287. Cf. the use of these verses in Egypt: the Arabic journal *Adab Wa-Naqd* published an article by ʻAlī al-Alfī titled "Egypt: Jews, Christians and Muslims—The Dawn of Consciousness." The author considers Egypt as "the cross-road of intellectual trends and civilizations" (p. 39)—on the back cover of the issue appear the aforementioned verses of Ibn ʻArabī (*Adab Wa-Naqd* 234 [February 2005], pp. 32–9—the quotation is from p. 39).
88 *BBC, Talking Point*, September 7, 2003.

European-Jewish family, decided in 2000 to found a publishing house to put out Hebrew translations of Arabic literature, the name al-Andalus was only natural:

> The Andalusian period was the golden age of coexistence between the Arab and Hebrew cultures. It was a period in which a great deal of literature was translated and both cultures enriched each other with ideas. When I was thinking of a name for the publishing house, it seemed only natural to me to call it Al-Andalus.[89]

Justin Stearns recently returns to the historical texts written during and immediately following the Muslim presence in the Iberian Peninsula in order to elucidate the conceptual place al-Andalus occupied in them. These narratives convey little in the way of nostalgia and frame al-Andalus instead as a place of wonders, *jihād*, and eschatological events. He concludes his article with a brief consideration of when the understanding of al-Andalus as a "lost paradise" emerged and how this understanding may now itself be changing:

> As widespread as nostalgia is for al-Andalus today, its nature may well be changing. In recent essays ... the reader encounters al-Andalus not as a past to be lamented, the memory of which should be elegized, but as a call for political and social action in the present. To what extent these revisions of Andalusian nostalgia will be effective is uncertain; yet it is possible that the long century in which al-Andalus was considered a lost paradise is beginning to end, though what precisely will replace it is not yet clear.[90]

89 See at: www.qantara.de (last accessed December 2, 2004).

90 Stearns 2009, pp. 355–74. The quotation is from p. 370.

Chapter 3

Glory: Baghdad in Verse[1]

Where are you, my first years,
The years of streets and cafés,
The years of days and long walks,
In the course of revolts with no pricking of conscience?
Where are you, my first years?
Oh my city, feverish with floods of memory,
Where are you in that drawn stream?
– ʿAbd al-Qādir al-Janābī

1. INTRODUCTION

"Poetry and Baghdad are indivisible, flowing together. One reflects, then feeds the other and so on," writes contemporary Baghdadi poet ʿAbd al-Qādir al-Janābī (b. 1944). "The very nature of Baghdad strikes the match that ignites the poetic imagination of the Iraqis, and in a sense of poets in the Arab world."[2] About ninety years ago, the historian Reuben Levy (1891–1966) wrote that even in the storied East there are few cities that hold the imagination like Baghdad "whose annals should be sought not in the humdrum narratives of the scribe but in the unfettered imagery of poet or painter."[3] As expressed in a truism by English poet William Cowper (1731–1800), "God made the country, and man made the town."[4] Indeed, cities are "living processes" rather than "products" or "formalistic shells for living,"[5] but Baghdad has been shaped also by the numerous poets who have written about the city during the more than 1,200 years since its foundation.

[1] This chapter uses material that first appeared in Snir 2013; Snir 2021, pp. 4–40.
[2] Snir 2013, p. 309.
[3] Levy 1977 [1929], p. 1.
[4] Johnston 1984, p. xv.
[5] Abu-Lughod 1987, pp. 172–3.

Surely, there are not many cities in the world about which so many verses have been written over such a span of time.

There were, of course, variations in the volume and nature of the productive creativity of Baghdad's poets. In the first few centuries after the city was founded, both the Arab and the international gaze witnessed Baghdad's great cultural and artistic achievements and the inspiration of its so very many poets and writers. In other periods, such as the 1920s–1930s and 1960s, Baghdad became known for its remarkable religious tolerance, multicultural cosmopolitan atmosphere, and peaceful cohabitation between all components of local society. There were also periods when Baghdad claimed attention because of its dramatic decline and disintegration, for example, after the thirteenth-century Mongol destruction; during Saddam Hussein's ill-reputed regime; and, for being a theater for bloody wars—such as the Iran–Iraq War of the 1980s and, in the following decades, the Gulf War and the American-led occupation. However, even during periods when Baghdad seemed to be in the process of collapse and disintegration, the image of an alternative, utopian Baghdad, as metaphor, remained immune to the vicissitudes of time and the dreary reality of the earthly city. The sway of Baghdad, the fabled city of Caliph Hārūn al-Rashīd (763–809), and the enchanted land of *A Thousand and One Nights*, will probably continue to capture the imagination of successive generations of poets, writers, and artists the world over. Neither East nor West seems immune to its irresistible charm.

Baghdad was founded at a time when Arabic poetry was at its peak. The development of the city thus coincided with, and was inspired by, the creative imagination of the poets who were associated with what was a cultural urban center during the Golden Age of medieval Arabic culture. The glorious image of the city perched on both banks of the Tigris ignited the imagination of subsequent generations of poets to depict it in verse and enshrine it in the mantle of universal myth.

2. "METROPOLIS OF THE WORLD"

Soon after the founding of the city, it became obvious that a specific identity, with the distinct characteristics of Baghdad and its residents, was coming into being. The Bedouin nomadic ideology, which retained influence even in urban centers of the Islamic Empire, placed genealogy (*nasab*) far higher on its meritorious scale than homeland (*waṭan*)—the implication being that "place" was, at best, only secondary, and perhaps even incidental, to the constitution of identity.[6] Thus, biographical dictionaries were organized

[6] On the term *waṭan*, see Lewis 1968, pp. 75–8; Noorani 2016, pp. 16–42; Günther and Milich 2016.

according to profession, legal school, or generation, and only rarely according to city; it is no wonder that one of the outstanding examples of the latter type of dictionary was *Ta'rīkh Baghdad* (*The History of Baghdad*). With the city of Baghdad, the relationship of a person to a place had acquired new meaning and became a formative constituent of individual identity—place and self became mutually interdependent, the one a reflection of the other. Abū 'Abd Allāh al-Shāfi'ī (767–820), for example, illustrates the change in the attitude toward place when he writes: "I have never stayed in a place which I did not consider a mere stage in a journey, until I came to Baghdad. As soon as I entered the city, I, at once, considered it was my very homeland."[7] Not only did the city of Baghdad begin to serve as a source of identity for Arab and Muslim alike, but the Tigris and major icons of the city, such as various quarters, mosques, and palaces, became anchors of personal identity. Baghdad became not only one of the most impressive cities in the Islamic Empire, but also a place where people literally defined their identity in relation to it.[8]

Like people, cities often have multiple layers of identity. Reflection on the subject of identity generally proceeds along one of two major premises: primordialist and non-primordialist. The first assumes that there is an essential content to any identity, which is defined by common origin or common structure of experience. The second argues that identities are constructed through an interplay of cultural reproduction, everyday reinforcements, as well as institutional indoctrination.[9] In the present case, it seems that Baghdad's identity has been acquired through its natural location, rulers, residents, historians, writers, and, of course, its poets. However, since cities, especially major ones like Baghdad, are more evolving "processes" than finished "products," they inevitably embody, express, and prioritize specific values. And this is how a city comes to acquire its particular "ethos" or "soul." "Ethos" can be defined as the characteristic spirit of a culture, era, community, or place as manifested in its beliefs and aspirations; in other words, "ethos" is "the set of values and outlooks that are generally acknowledged by people living in any specific city." Cities not only reflect but also "shape their inhabitants' values and outlooks in various ways."[10] In the case of Baghdad, from its inception the city was more than the sum total of its parts. From its Golden Age, its image has been shaped by the poetic creativity of its residents, visitors, and those who identified with it.

[7] Ibn al-Fuwaṭī 2008, p. 72.

[8] On place as an image of self in classical Arabic literature, see Hämeen-Anttila 2008, pp. 25–38.

[9] On the theoretical conceptions of identity, see Snir 2015, pp. 10–32.

[10] Bell and de-Shalit 2011, p. 2.

Daniel Bell (b. 1964) and Avner de-Shalit (b. 1957) studied the identity and "spirit" of nine contemporary cities. They concluded that Jerusalem, for example, is the city of religion; Montreal, the city of language; Oxford, the city of learning; Berlin, the city of (in)tolerance; Paris, the city of romance; and New York, the city of ambition.[11] What might we say about Baghdad's spirit? Or, should we refrain from any such attempt, lest, by reducing it to a single ethos, we end up being guilty of reductionism and simplification? And what might we add if we tried not only to judge Baghdad in "our global age," as Bell and de-Shalit have done with the aforementioned cities, but also to delve into this city's history from a diachronic perspective—that is, since its foundation in the eighth century? Does Baghdad actually have any particular ethos? If we should attempt to designate an ethos for the city, and ignore the controversy about the essence of Baghdad as an "Islamic city,"[12] there is no doubt that, from the time of its founding, and in contradistinction to the aforementioned cities, Baghdad cannot be reduced to a single universal ethos that may serve as a recognizable core identity shared in common by its inhabitants. Baghdad has been the city of Islam and Arabism *par excellence*—the center of the Islamic Empire and the Arab world in reality and certainly metaphorically. Baghdad was at times a metaphor even for the entire East. It was the city of the *Arabian Nights*, the city of the Golden Age of Islamic and Arab culture. Its destruction in 1258 reflected what erroneously was seen as the decline of Arabism and Islam (see below). For various Arab religious communities during the late nineteenth century and the first half of the twentieth century, it was the city of tolerance. By contrast, during most of the second half of the twentieth century, it was the city of Arab-Muslim dictatorship, or, during the last decades of that century, the city that illustrated the total submission of the Arab world and Islamic religion to the West.

Classical Arabic sources are full of sayings in reference to the glory of Baghdad as the capital of Islam and Arabism in the Middle Ages. "Baghdad is the mother of this world and the queen of the provinces,"[13] and "it is the

[11] It seems that the British statesman Benjamin Disraeli (1804–1881) tried to define the ethos of some cities when he said that "a great city, whose image dwells in the memory of man, is the type of some great idea. Rome represents conquest; Faith hovers over the towers of Jerusalem; and Athens embodies the pre-eminent quality of the antique world, Art" (Disraeli 1844, p. 52).

[12] On this controversy, see Lapidus 1969; Hourani and Stern 1970 (mainly the introduction on pp. 9–24); Eickelman 1974, pp. 274–94; Serjeant 1980; Abu-Lughod 1987, pp. 155–76; Raymond 1994, pp. 3–18 (Raymond quotes as well a lecture given by Eugen Wirth in 1982 where he suggested that we renounce the term "Islamic city" and instead use the more general "Oriental city," since "Islam seems to be more inhabitant or occupant of Middle Eastern urban systems than the architect" [p. 12]); Khan 2008, pp. 1035–62.

[13] Yāqūt 1990, I, p. 541.

navel of the globe, the treasure of the earth, the source of sciences and the spring of wisdom."[14] When one person declared that he had never been to Baghdad, the answer was crystal clear: "In that case, you have seen nothing on the earth."[15] "Nothing is equal to Baghdad," said another, "for the sublimity of its rank, for the splendor of its authority, for the great number of its scholars and prominent personalities, and for its glorious poets."[16]

After he founded the city in 762, the Caliph al-Manṣūr (714–775; r. 754–775)[17] called the new city *Madīnat al-Salām* (The City of Peace); this became the official name of the city on government documents and coins.[18] Later, a shorter form of the name became popular, *Dār al-Salām* (The Abode of Peace), a name that hints at the Qur'ānic description of paradise: "And God summons to the Abode of Peace, and He guides whomsoever He will to a straight path; to the good-doers the reward most fair and a surplus; neither dust nor abasement shall overspread their faces. Those are the inhabitants of Paradise, therein dwelling forever."[19] By the eleventh century, *Baghdad* had become the almost exclusive name for this world-renowned metropolis.[20] Despite the name "Baghdad" being pre-Islamic in origin, most Arabic scholars have assumed it to be derived from Middle Persian, a compound of "Bag" (god) and "dad" (given), meaning "God-given" or "God's gift." However, the name *Bagdadu* was in use from the time of Hammurabi (1800 BC), which means that the name was current before any possible Persian influence. The city was also known as *Madīnat al-Manṣūr* (The City of al-Manṣūr); *al-Zawrā'* (The Bent or The Crooked);[21] and *al-Madīna al-Mudawwara* (The Round City), since the old city was

[14] Khāliṣ 2005, p. 8.

[15] Al-Khaṭīb al-Baghdādī 1931, p. 45; al-Ālūsī 1987, p. 18; Yāqūt 1990, I, p. 548; Khāliṣ 2005, p. 7; Ibn al-Fuwaṭī 2008, p. 74.

[16] Al-Khaṭīb al-Baghdādī 1931, p. 119; Khāliṣ 2005, pp. 8–9.

[17] According to historical sources, al-Mansur laid the first brick for the city and recited the following Qur'ānic text: "Surely the earth is God's and He bequeaths it to whom He will among his servants. The issue ultimate is to the godfearing" (*al-A'raf* [*The Battlements*], 127; English translation according to Arberry 1979 [1964], pp. 157–8. See Yāqūt 1990, I, p. 543). For English references on the foundation of Baghdad and its development, see Coke 1935 [1927], pp. 34–47; El-Ali 1970, pp. 87–101; Lassner 1970, pp. 103–18; Lassner 1970a; Duri 1980, pp. 52–65; Duri 2012.

[18] According to some sources, the city was called "The City of Peace" because one of the ninety-nine names of God is *al-Salām* and the intended meaning was "The City of God." According to another suggestion, the Tigris Valley was called *Wādī al-Salām* (The Valley of Peace) (Yāqūt 1990, I, pp. 541–2).

[19] *Yūnus* (Jonah), 25–26 (English translation according to Arberry 1979 [1964], p. 200).

[20] There are additional versions of the name, such as *Baghdādh, Baghdān, Maghdād, Maghdādh*, and *Maghdān* (Yāqūt 1990, I, p. 541).

[21] One explanation is that the city took the name from the Tigris, which was bent as it passed by the city (Le Strange 1900, p. 11).

built as a circle with an approximate diameter of between 2 and 3 km. The city was planned so that within it there would be many parks, gardens, villas, and promenades, and at its center would lie the mosque and headquarters for guards. The four surrounding walls of Baghdad were named Kufa, Basra, Khurasan, and Damascus after the direction of the city gates, which faced these destinations.

After its founding, the city was developed rapidly. "Never had there been a Middle Eastern city so large," Ira M. Lapidus (b. 1937) writes; "Baghdad was not a single city, but a metropolitan center, made up of a conglomeration of districts on both sides of the Tigris River. In the ninth century it measured about 25 square miles, and had a population of between 300,000 and 500,000. It was ten times the size of Sasanian Ctesiphon."[22] Baghdad was larger than Constantinople or any other Middle Eastern city until Istanbul in the sixteenth century. In its time, Baghdad was the largest city in the world outside China.[23] With the founding of Baghdad, the Islamic Empire established an effective governing system, such as had never existed before; it had political, military, and juridical powers; a talented bureaucratic staff; and improved administrative practices. For example, the office of the vizier was further developed at the time and his power, as chief of the administration, functioned in direct connection to the wishes or, one could say, the strength of the caliph—for example, the Barmakid viziers were very powerful at the time, but Hārūn al-Rashīd did not hesitate to execute prominent members of this family.

Many sayings in classical literary sources, prose and poetry, testify to the unique nature of Baghdad. A short while after its founding, Abu 'Uthmān 'Amr ibn Baḥr al-Jāḥiẓ (776–869), one of the greatest classical Arab authors, gave the following testimony: "I have seen the greatest of cities that are known for their perfection and refinement, in the lands of Syria and the Greeks and other countries, but I have never seen a city like Baghdad whose roofs are so high, a city which is so round or more noble, the gates of which are wider and the walls better. It is as if the city were cast into a mould and poured out."[24] When referring to the three great cities in the territories known today as Iraq, al-Jāḥiẓ made the observation that "industry is in Basra, eloquence in Kufa, but goodness in Baghdad."[25] Abū al-Qāsim ibn al-Ḥasan al-Daylamī related: "I have travelled throughout the lands, visited countries from the borders of Samarkand to Qayrawān, from Sri Lanka to the lands of the Greeks, but I have never found a place better than or superior to Baghdad."[26]

[22] Lapidus 2002, p. 56.
[23] Lapidus 2002, p. 56.
[24] Al-Ālūsī 1987, p. 13; Ibn al-Fuwaṭī 2008, p. 73.
[25] Al-Ālūsī 1987, p. 13.
[26] Al-Ālūsī 1987, p. 13; Ibn al-Fuwaṭī 2008, p. 74.

Baghdad acquired acceptance as the urban center of the Arab world and Islamic Empire, to the degree that people regarded all other places outside it as rural:[27] "Baghdad is the metropolis of the world," Abū Isḥāq al-Zajjāj (d. 923) said. "Outside it, there is only desert."[28] When a visitor returned from Baghdad, he was asked about the city and replied: "Baghdad among the lands is like a master among slaves."[29] The traveler al-Muqaddasī al-Bashshārī (947–990) described Baghdad as having "a nature and elegance peculiar to her, excellent faculties and tenderness; the air is soft; the science is precise; everything is good. Everything nice is there; every wise man comes from there. Every heart longs for this city. Every war is declared against her. Her fame defies description; her goodness cannot be depicted. Praise cannot reach her heights."[30]

As the capital of the Islamic Empire, it is no wonder that Baghdad has been praised as a religious center. Abū al-Faraj al-Babbagha (925–1008) wrote:

هي مدينة السّلام بل مدينة الإسلام، فإن الدّولة النّبويّة والخلافة الإسلاميّة بها عشّشتا وفرختا وضربتا بعروقهما وبسقتا بفروعهما، وإن هواءها أغذى من كلّ هواء وماءها أعذب من كلّ ماء، وإنّ نسيمها أرقّ من كلّ نسيم.

[Baghdad] is the City of Peace; indeed she is the city of Islam. The Prophetic State and the Caliphate of Islam nested there, hatched and struck its roots into the earth, and made its branches tall. Her air is more pleasant than any other air, and her water sweeter than any other water, and her breeze is softer than any other breeze.[31]

It was said that whenever the name of Baghdad was raised in any conversation, people quoted the following Qur'ānic verse: "A good land, and a Lord All-forgiving."[32] An interpreter explained that Baghdad was enriched with the fruits of a refreshing breeze.[33] We read also in the sources:

بغداد جنّة الأرض ومدينة السّلام وقبّة الإسلام ومجمع الرّافدين وغرّة البلاد وعين العراق ودار الخلافة ومجمع المحاسن والطيّبات ومعدن الظّرائف واللّطائف، وبها أرباب الغايات في كلّ فنّ، وآحاد الدّهر في كل نوع.

Baghdad is a paradise on earth, the City of Peace; the dome of Islam; the union of two rivers; the head of the land; the eye of Iraq; the house of the caliphate; the ingathering of good deeds and actions; the source of uncommon qualities

27 Al-Ālūsī 1987, p. 13.
28 Al-Ālūsī 1987, p. 22; Yāqūt 1990, I, p. 547; Ibn al-Fuwaṭī 2008, p. 72.
29 Al-Ālūsī 1987, p. 22; Yāqūt 1990, I, p. 547.
30 Al-Ālūsī 1987, p. 22.
31 Al-Ālūsī 1987, p. 22; Yāqūt 1990, I, p. 547.
32 Saba' (Sheba), p. 15 (English translation according to Arberry 1979 [1964], p. 439).
33 Al-Ālūsī 1987, p. 14.

and niceties. There can be found experts in any of the arts and extraordinary people in every field.[34]

Also, we read: "From the merits of Islam—Friday in Baghdad, the prayer performed during the nights of Ramadan in Mecca, and religious festivals in Tarsus."[35]

Moreover, Baghdad enjoyed a pluralistic, cosmopolitan, and multiconfessional atmosphere with multicultural ethnic and religious gatherings of Muslims, Christians, Jews, Zoroastrians, pagans, Arabs, Persians, as well as various Asian populations. This atmosphere was initially inspired by the leadership of the Caliph al-Manṣūr (754–775), who propagated, from Baghdad, an open and multicultural policy toward religious minorities. The political, religious, and cultural supremacy of Baghdad as the center of the flowering of the Islamic Empire encouraged such an atmosphere not only in Baghdad itself, but throughout other close and even remote cities. A contemporary text describing a gathering in the southern city of Basra in the year 156H (772/773 AD) may serve to illustrate this policy of multiculturalism:

كان يجتمع بالبصرة عشرة في مجلس لا يعرف مثلهم في تضادّ أديانهم ونحلهم: الخليل بن أحمد سنّي، والسّيّد بن محمّد الحميريّ رافضيّ، وصالح بن عبد القدّوس ثنويّ، وسفيان بن مجاشع صفريّ، وبشّار بن برد خليع ماجن، وحمّاد عجرد زنديق، وابن رأس الجالوت يهوديّ، وابن ابن نظيرا متكلّم النّصارى، وعمرو ابن أخت المؤيّد المجوسيّ، وروح بن سنان الحرانيّ صابئيّ، فيتناشدالجماعة أشعارًا، فكان بشّار يقول: أبياتك هذه يا فلان، أحسن من سورة كذا وكذا، وبهذا المزاح ونحوه كفّروا بشّارًا.

Ten persons used to meet regularly. There was no equivalent to this gathering for the diversity of the religions and sects of its members: al-Khalīl ibn Aḥmad—a Sunni, and al-Sayyid ibn Muḥammad al-Ḥimyarī—Shiite, and Ṣāliḥ ibn 'Abd al-Qaddūs—dualist, and Sufyān ibn Mujāshi'—Khariji, and Bashshār ibn Burd—morally depraved and impudent, and Ḥammad 'Ajrad—heretic, and the exilarch's son—a Jew, and Ibn Naẓīra—a Christian theologian, and 'Amrū the nephew of al-Mu'ayyad—Zoroastrian, and Rawḥ ibn Sinān al-Harranī—Gnostic. At these gatherings, they used to recite poems, and Bashshār used to say "Your verses, Oh so-and-so, are better than *sūra* this or that [of the Qur'ān]," and from that kind of joking and similar things they declared Bashhār to be a disbeliever.[36]

34 Al-Ālūsī 1987, p. 21; Yāqūt 1990, I, p. 547.

35 Khāliṣ 2005, p. 7.

36 Al-Dhahabī 1988, p. 383. For another version of this episode, see Ibn Taghribirdī 1930, II, p. 29; Ibn Taghribirdī 1992, II, 36–7. On that liberal cultural atmosphere, see also Yāqūt 1990, III, pp. 242–4.

3. THE GOLDEN AGE

The glorious and multicultural cosmopolitan image of Baghdad, in the imagination of Arab culture, concealed a day-to-day reality of a city that suffered from all kinds of difficulties and troubles, just like any other medieval city. An example is the Caliph Hārūn al-Rashīd (763–809), whose name and fame have been associated with Baghdad as the legendary capital of the Islamic Empire. It was under him that Baghdad flourished and became the most splendid city of its period. Taxes paid by rulers were used to finance activities in fine art, the construction of buildings with a high standard of architecture, and also a luxurious and even decadent way of life at court. Due to the *A Thousand and One Nights* tales, Hārūn al-Rashīd and particularly his activities in Baghdad became legendary, but his true historic personality was thus obscured.

Hārūn al-Rashīd was virtually responsible for dismembering the empire when he apportioned Baghdad between his two sons, al-Amīn (787–813; r. 809–813) and al-Ma'mūn (786–833; r. 813–833). After his death, a civil war (*fitna*) broke out between them (811–813). Contemporary poets described the events of the civil war and, between their poetic lines, the high status of Baghdad is apparent. 'Amr ibn 'Abd al-Malik al-Warrāq (d. 815) wrote:

مَن ذا أَصابَكِ يا بَغدادُ بِالعَينِ   أَلَم تَكوني زَمانًا قُرَّةَ العَينِ

Oh Baghdad, who afflicted you with an evil eye?!
Were not you the eye's delight?![37]

Another anonymous poet said:

بكيت دما على بغداد لمّا   فقدت غضارة العيش الأنيق
تبدّلنا هموما من سرور   ومن سعة تبدّلنا بضيق

I weep blood over Baghdad,
I lost the comfort of an elegant life.
Anxiety has replaced happiness,
Instead of prosperity, there is only misery.[38]

And Isḥāq al-Khuraymī (d. 829) described a *mundus inversus* situation:

وخطّم العبد أنف سيّده   بالرّغم واستعبدت حرائرها
وصار ربّ الجيران فاسقهم   وابتزّ أمر الدّروب ذاعرها

The slave has put a mark of disgrace upon his master,
[Baghdad's] noblewomen have been enslaved.

[37] Al-Nawrasī 2009, p. 72.
[38] Snir 2013, p. 68.

Among neighbors the noble have become the most evil,
He who had been afraid of roads has become their master.[39]

This is a description of a world upside down reminiscent of the aforementioned *Carmina Burana*: the Fathers Gregory, Jerome, Augustine, and Benedict are to be found in the alehouse, in court, or in the meat market; Mary no longer delights in the contemplative life, and Lucretia has turned into a whore.[40] No restraints were enforced in that cruel war between al-Rashīd's sons. A graphic account is given in the verses of al-Ḥusayn ibn al-Ḍaḥḥāk (778–870) when, addressing al-Amīn, he says:

هتكوا بحرمتك الّتي هتكت   حرم الرّسول ودونها السّجف
ونبت أقاربك الّتي خذلت   وجميعها بالذّل معترف
أبدت مخلخلها على دهش   أبكارهنّ ورنت النّصف
سلبت معاجزهن واختلست   ذات النّقاب ونوزع الشّنف
فكأنّهنّ خلال منتهب   درّ تكشّف دونه الصّدف

Among the violations of your sanctity they abused,
Behind curtains, the honor of the Prophet's female descendants.
Your relatives remained in their places and failed to help,
All of them admitted humiliation.
Their virgin females showed their ankles
In grief, as they wept their demand for justice.
Garments were stolen, veiled women
Were exposed, ear-rings were removed.
While being assaulted they seemed as
Pearls emerging from oysters.

Notwithstanding all this turmoil, within a short time after its inception Baghdad evolved into a significant industrial and commercial center for international trade as well as the intellectual and cultural heart of the Arab and Islamic world. With regard to the latter, Baghdad garnered a worldwide reputation as the "Center of Learning," housing several key academic institutions, the best known being Bayt al-Ḥikma (House of Wisdom). This high point of Islamic civilization came when scholars of various religions from around the world flocked to that city, which was the unrivaled center for the study of the humanities and sciences, including mathematics, astronomy, medicine, chemistry, zoology, and geography, in addition to alchemy and astrology. Drawing on Persian, Indian, and Greek texts, Baghdad's scholars accumulated the greatest collection of learned texts in the world, and built on this knowledge through their own discoveries. In these times, there was

[39] Snir 2013, p. 84.
[40] See Snir 1994b, pp. 51–75. See above, Chapter 1.

also a market for copyists (*sūq al-warrāqīn*) where more than one hundred booksellers' shops were to be found and writers and merchants used to buy and sell manuscripts. Baghdad's libraries were renowned for their wealth even beyond the Arab world. Whereas the largest library in twelfth-century Europe housed around 2,000 volumes, there was a library in Baghdad that had 10,400 books.[41] In Umberto Eco's *Il Nome Della Rosa* (1980), the library of the abbey is praised as "the only light Christianity can oppose to the thirty-six libraries of Baghdad, to the ten thousand codices of the Vizir Ibn al-ʿAlqamī."[42] However, Baghdad's rapid development met with delays. In 836, the caliphate residence was removed to the new city of Samarra, recently constructed by the Caliph al-Muʿtaṣim (796–842; r. 833–842). The caliphate would remain there for over fifty-five years, that is, until the year 892 when it was returned to Baghdad by the Caliph al-Muʿtamid (842–892; r. 870–892). During that period, Baghdad missed the attention of the caliphs, even though it was still the center of commercial and cultural activity.

From the late tenth century, intersectarian conflicts between the Muslim Shiʿis and Sunnis were relatively frequent, but soon the population of Baghdad became international, a mixture of different religions, nations, and cultures. The Jews of Mesopotamia, for example, who for centuries spoke Aramaic, in which language they produced the Talmud, underwent a rapid process of Arabization and integration into the surrounding Arab-Muslim society, the majority of them congregating in the new metropolis of Baghdad. Facilitating their integration was their high level of achievement and resulting prosperity in commerce, education, and culture.[43] It is estimated that in the tenth century the population of Baghdad reached 1,500,000[44] and that Baghdad was therefore considered to be the largest city in the world, the likes of which had not been known before in the Middle East. Very sophisticated services were installed to meet the requirements of its residents. This is illustrated, for example, by the health system. We know

[41] Coke 1935 [1927], p. 63; Toorawa 2005, pp. 13–15; Ali 2010, p. 221.

[42] Eco 1984, p. 35. In Eco's novel, the historical background of fourteenth-century Christian Europe is reconstructed, but Baghdad's libraries, at least according to some Arabic chronicles and literary texts, had already been destroyed in 1258 and Baghdad lost its cultural dominance in the Arab world before the events of the novel took place. However, the destruction of the Baghdadi libraries, which was a powerful image connected to the Mongol conquest, often claimed to have precipitated the decline of Muslim civilization, has been recently challenged by some studies that reconstruct the state of libraries in Ilkhanid Baghdad, revealing a thriving intellectual community (e.g., Hirschler 2012, pp. 129–30; Biran 2019, pp. 464–502. See also below).

[43] Wasserstrom 1995, pp. 19–20.

[44] On this number and the various calculations that enable scholars to reach it, see Micheau 2008, pp. 234–5.

of hospitals in Baghdad from the ninth century. At the beginning of the tenth century, the chief court physician, Sinān ibn Thābit (880–943), was appointed director of the city's hospitals; he subsequently founded three additional hospitals.[45]

Many poems reflect various levels of life in Baghdad throughout the first centuries after its founding and in a sense may be read as an alternative history of the city. "Literature is a frail vehicle for documentation," James Dougherty writes, "but it can become powerful when understood as the imaginative review of experience, a review that both discovers and imparts those spiritual expectations against which the city's appearance must be measured."[46] Moreover, the history of Baghdad during its formative classical period cannot be fully documented without poetry. This is all the more obvious since, until the second half of the twentieth century, poetry was the principal channel of literary creativity and served as the chronicle and public register of the Arabs as illustrated in the aforementioned saying, *al-Shi'r Dīwān al-'Arab*. No other genres could challenge the supremacy of poetry in the field of *belles lettres* across more than 1,500 years of Arabic literary history. This high status that poetry enjoyed in Arab society as a whole is reflected in a passage by the eleventh-century scholar Ibn Rashīq al-Qayrawānī (d. 1063 or 1071):

> كانت القبيلة من العرب إذا نبغ فيها شاعر أتت القبائل فهنّأتها بذلك وصنعت الأطعمة واجتمع النّساء يلعبن بالمزاهر كما يصنعن في الأعراس وتتباشر الرجال والولدان لأنّه حماية لأعراضهم وذبّ عن أحسابهم وتخليد لمآثرهم وإشادة لذكرهم وكانوا لا يهنّئون إلّا بغلام يولد أو شاعر ينبغ فيهم أو فرس تنتج.

> When a poet appeared in a family of the Arabs, the adjacent tribes would gather together and wish that family the joy of their good luck. Feasts would be got ready, the women of the tribe would join together in bands, playing upon lutes, as they were wont to do at bridals, and the men and boys would congratulate one another; for a poet was a defense of the honor of them all, a weapon to ward off insult from their good name, and a means of perpetuating their glorious deeds and of establishing their fame forever. And they used not to wish one another joy but for three things: the birth of a boy, the coming to light of a poet, and the foaling of a noble mare.[47]

Poets of the time actually referred to Baghdad as a paradise on earth; they described its beauty, its natural scenes, and the attachment they felt toward it. Manṣūr al-Namarī (d. 825) described the Baghdadi breeze:

[45] Duri 1980, p. 64.

[46] Dougherty 1980, p. x. Cf. Johnston 1984, p. xx.

[47] Ibn Rashīq al-Qayrawānī 1963, p. 65; al-Suyūṭī n.d., II, p. 473. The translation is according to Lyall 1930, with minor modifications.

تحيي الرّياح المرضى إذا تنسّمت وجوّشت بين أغصان الرّياحين

Breeze reviving the sick,
blowing between sweet basil branches.[48]

And ʻAlī ibn Jabala al-Anṣarī (known as al-ʻAkawwak) (776–828) described the city as paradise on earth:

لهفي على بغداد من بلدة كانت من الأسقام لي جُنّهْ
كأنّني عند فراقي لها آدم لمّا فارق الجَنّهْ

Truly, I grieve for Baghdad, what a town!
Midst my maladies, she has protected me.
Separating from her, I was Adam
expelled from Eden.[49]

ʻAlī ibn al-Ḥusayn al-Wāsiṭī (d. 919) asks a rhetorical question and is quick to respond to himself:

ألدار السّلام في الأرض شبه؟ معجز أن ترى لبغداد مثلا
مربع للقلوب فيه ربيع متوال إذا الرّبيع تولّى

Is there any equivalent to the City of Peace?
A miracle, you will not find for Baghdad any parallel.
A temple for the hearts, spring
There everlasting, even in summer.[50]

And ʻUmāra ibn ʻUqayl (798–853) asks another, similar question:

أعاينت في طول من الأرض أو عرض كبغداد دارًا إنّها جنّة الأرضِ
صفا العيش في بغداد واخضرّ عوده وعيش سواها غير صاف ولا غضّ
تطول بها الأعمار إنّ غذاءها مريء وبعض الأرض أمرؤ من بعض

Have you seen in any corner of the world
A tranquil abode like Baghdad?!
Here, life is pure, green, and fresh;
in other places life is neither gentle nor cool.
Life here is longer; the food is wholesome;
indeed parts of the earth are better than others.[51]

In another poem, he adds:

48 Al-Nawrasī 2009, p. 62.
49 Al-Nawrasī 2009, p. 87.
50 Al-Ālūsī 1987, p. 34.
51 Al-Ālūsī 1987, p. 21; Yāqūt 1990, I, p. 546.

ما مثل بغداد في الدّنيا ولا الدّين   على تقلّبها في كلّ ما حين

There is nothing like Baghdad, worldly-wise and religiously,
Despite Time's transitions.[52]

Ibn al-Rūmī (836–896) depicted the city as

بلدٌ صَحبْتُ به الشّبيبة والصِّبا   ولبستُ فيه العيْشَ وهو جديدُ
فإذا تمثَّل في الضّمير رأيتُه   وعليه أفنان الشّباب تميدُ

A city where I accompanied youthfulness and childhood,
Where I wore a new cloak of glory.
When she appears in the imagination, I see on her
Budding branches aflutter.[53]

The likes of Baghdad's residents are unavailable in other places, as 'Alī ibn Zurayq Abū al-Ḥasan al-Baghdādī (d. 1029) argues:

سافرت أبغي لبغداد وساكنها   مثلا قد اخترت شيئا دونه الياس
هيهات بغداد والدّنيا بأجمعها   عندي وسكّان بغداد هم النّاس

I have traveled far to find a parallel for Baghdad
And her people—my task was second to despair.
Alas, for me Baghdad is the entire world,
Her people—the only genuine ones.[54]

And al-Ṭāhir ibn al-Muẓaffar ibn Ṭāhir al-Khāzin declared:

هواء رقيق في اعتدال وصحّة   وماء له طعم ألذّ من الخمر
ودجلتها شطّان قد نظما لنا   بتاج إلى تاج وقصر إلى قصر
تراها كمسك والمياه كفضّة   وحصباؤها مثل اليواقيت والدّرّ

Tender weather, balanced and healthy,
The water—what a taste! Sweeter than wine.
Her Tigris—two banks arrayed for us like pearls in a necklace,
A crown beside a crown, a palace beside a palace.
Her soil—musk; her water—silver;
Her gravel—diamonds and jewels.[55]

On the other hand, Baghdad was also known as a hedonist city, where pleasures of all sorts were available. The pleasures, as 'Alī ibn al-Jahm (804–863) wrote, were sensual with wine parties, cupbearers, young men and women, and a *carpe diem* atmosphere: "Use your hands, carefree! Do not be afraid of the master, do whatever you want! ... / Nothing is forbidden, say whatever

52 Al-Ālūsī 1987, p. 22.
53 Al-Ālūsī 1987, p. 31.
54 Al-Ālūsī 1987, p. 21; Yāqūt 1990, I, p. 547; al-Nawrasī 2009, p. 63.
55 Al-Ālūsī 1987, p. 24.

you want! Sleep with no fear, get up without any hurry."[56] Homosexual love was widespread and accepted in Baghdad at the time, and among the upper classes in society there was always an urgent need for newly imported young, beardless boys. When Abū al-Ma'ālī (1028–1085) was suddenly seen with a bearded boy, eyebrows were raised: "Look for another! They urged. In that case I will never be pleased, I replied. / If his saliva were not honey, the bees would never have invaded his mouth."[57] The hedonism of Baghdad's wealthier residents created a need for more free time for leisure. From the start, with the Abbasid Dynasty, the caliphate's public offices were closed on Fridays so that believers could pray together in the mosques. For rest, relaxation, and leisure, the Caliph al-Mu'taḍid (857–902; r. 857–902) added another off-day—Tuesday. Every Tuesday, public employees would stay at home or head for public parks, where they would spend their time in recreation and rest. Sometimes, it seemed a shame for a man to stay in the house on Tuesday and not participate in the *majālis* (sessions) of singing and wine-drinking. Various poets wrote about that weekly day of vacation, among them Ibn al-Rūmī (836–896):

يـومُ الثّلاثـاء مـا يـومُ الثّـلاثاءُ　　في ذروة من ذُرا الأيّام عليـاءِ
كأنّما هو في الأسبوعِ واسطةٌ　　في سِمْطِ دُرٍّ مُحَلٍّ جيدَ حسناءِ

Tuesday? What is Tuesday?
　It is raised high in the pick of the days.
A center in the middle of the week,
　A pearl necklace decorating a beautiful woman.

This hedonist aspect of city living aroused opposition from ascetic and mystical circles who considered Baghdad a dangerous place because of the luxurious life it afforded people and the shamelessness and excessive pleasures that newcomers could be tempted by—all of which could cause avoidance of religious observance and duties. For example, 'Abd Allāh ibn al-Mubārak (736–797) held that if you want to be pious you should avoid Baghdad:

قل لمن أظهر التّنسّك في النّا　　س وأمسى يُعدّ في الزّهّاد
ألزم الثّغـر والتّواضـع فيـه　　ليـس بغـداد منـزل العبّاد
إنّ بغـداد للملـوك محـلّ　　ومنـاخ للفـارس الصـيّاد

Please tell those preferring abstinence,
　Tell all considered to be pious:
Stay on the frontier, be modest,
　Baghdad is not an abode for hermits.

[56] Ibn al-Jahm 1981, pp. 52–6; al-Ālūsī 1987, pp. 47–9.
[57] Al-Jazrāwī 2005, p. 184.

Baghdad is a place only for kings,
An abode solely for hunters and knights.[58]

Like any other urban center, the city suffered from negative phenomena, such as social differences between the classes. Unlike poets who described Baghdad as a city of dreams, Abū Muḥammad ʻAbd al-Wahhāb al-Mālikī (d. 1031) had no doubts that

بغداد دارٌ لأهل المال واسعةٌ   وللصّعاليك دار الضّنك والضّيق
ظللت حيران أمشي في أزقتها   كأنّني مصحف في بيت زنديق

Baghdad is a fine home for the wealthy,
But an abode of misery and distress for the poor.
I walked among them in dismay
As though I were a Qur'ān in an unbeliever's house.[59]

Muḥammad ibn Aḥmad ibn Shumayʻa al-Baghdādī (tenth century) captured the self-centered nature of this urban center's residents:

ودّ أهل الزّوراء زور فلا   تغترر بالوداد من ساكنيها
هي دار السّلام حسب، فلا   يطمع منها، إلا بما قيل فيها

Friendship of al-Zawrā's residents is falsehood,
Residents' warmth as well—don't be tempted.
Baghdad is a place for a mere "how are you?"
You will not be able to gain more.[60]

And Abū al-ʻĀliya (ninth century) has strong advice:

sترحّل فما بغداد دار إقامة   ولا عند من يرجى ببغداد طائل
محلّ ملوك سمتهم في أديمهم   فكلّهم من حلية المجد عاطل

Leave! Baghdad is not a place to stay in,
There is no benefit from her.
She is a place for kings, their wickedness seen in their faces,
All of them devoid of any glory.[61]

Many anonymous verses described the immoral and evil nature of the residents, such as the following:

أذمّ بغداد والمقام بها   من بعد ما خبرة وتجريب
ما عند أملاكهم لمختبط   خير ولا فرجة لمكروب
يحتاج باغي النّوال عندهم   إلى ثلاث من بعد تقريب
كنوز قارون أن تكون له   وعمر نوح وصبر أيّوب

[58] Al-Khaṭīb al-Baghdādī 1971, p. 36; al-Ālūsī 1987, p. 37; Yāqūt 1990, I, p. 550.
[59] Al-Ālūsī 1987, p. 37; Yāqūt 1990, I, p. 550.
[60] Al-Ālūsī 1987, p. 37; Yāqūt 1990, I, p. 550; al-Nawrasī 2009, p. 98.
[61] Yāqūt 1990, I, p. 551.

قوم مواعيدهم مطرّزة   بزخارف القول والأكاذيب
خلّوا سبيل العلى لغيرهم   ونازعوا في الفسوق والحوب

I abhor Baghdad, I abhor life there,
This is from experience, after a taste,
Baghdad's residents have no pity for the needy,
No remedy for the gloomy.
Whoever among them who wants favor
Needs mainly three things:
The treasures of Korah,
Noah's age, and Job's patience.
People whose encounters are embroidered
With ornamented rhetoric and lies.
Abandoning the path of nobility,
They rival each other instead in disobedience and sinfulness.[62]

And another adds:

بلاد ترى الأرواح فيها مريضة   وتزداد نتنًا حين تمطر أو تندى

It is a land where men's souls are sick,
The stench even more when it rains.[63]

And a third poet says:

سقيا لبغداد ورعيا لها   ولا سقى صوب الحيا أهلها
يا عجبا من سفل مثلهم   كيف أبيحوا جنّة مثلها

May God rain on Baghdad, may He protect her;
Alas, may the clouds not provide rain for her residents.
Mean as they are, amazingly so,
For goodness sake, why have they been allowed such a paradise?[64]

And a fourth anonymous poet:

كفى حزنا والحمد لله أنّني   ببغداد قد أعييت عليّ مذاهبي
أصاحب قوما لا ألذّ صحابهم   وآلف قوما لست فيهم براغب

Enough of moaning, thank God, I
Could not manage in Baghdad anymore.
I consort with people who afford me no pleasure,
I keep company with people I deem undesirable.[65]

There were also corruptive phenomena, like those of the viziers. Take, for example, the vizier Abū 'Alī Muḥammad ibn Yaḥyā. He was known as a great

62 Al-Ālūsī 1987, pp. 40–1; Yāqūt 1990, I, p. 551.
63 Al-Ālūsī 1987, p. 41; al-Nawrasī 2009, p. 94.
64 Al-Ālūsī 1987, p. 42.
65 Al-Ālūsī 1987, p. 42.

opportunist and hypocrite. When he saw people praying, he would hurry to join them; when someone asked him for help, he would beat his breast saying: "With the greatest of pleasure." However, he gave nothing. That is why the people used to call him "Beating His Breast" (*Daqqa Ṣadrahu*). He was known for his hankering for bribes. When appointing officials, he did so only in exchange for bribes. At times, he would appoint someone and then after a few days regret it and accept a higher bribe from someone else. It is said that in al-Kufa over the course of twenty days he appointed and fired no less than seven governors. An anonymous poet wrote of this vizier that:

وزير قد تكامل في الرّقاعة   يولّي ثمّ يعزل بعد ساعة
إذا أهل الرّشا اجتمعوا لديه   فخيار القوم أوفرهم بضاعة
وليس يلام في هذا بحال   لأنّ الشّيخ أفلت من مجاعة

This minister—he was perfect in stupidity,
 No sooner appointing than dismissing.
In his office, he assembles bribers and campaigners,
 The best merchandiser is the winner.
I beseech you not to reproach him,
 He barely escaped beggary.[66]

It was in the prisons of Baghdad that (so we learn from poetry) the craft of weaving waistbands became highly developed, and served as a metaphor for the deterioration of the status of the prisoners. We learn this, for example, from the poetry of Prince ʿAbd Allāh ibn al-Muʿtazz (861–909), who succeeded in ruling for a single lone day before he was strangled in a palace intrigue:

تعلّمت في السّجن نسج التّكك   وكنت امرءًا قبل حبسي ملك
وقيّدت بعد ركوب الجياد   وما ذاك إلا بدور الفلك

In Baghdad, I got lessons in weaving waistbands,
 Before imprisonment, I had been a king.
After riding noble horses, I was chained,
 This is because of changing constellations.[67]

In a letter to a friend, Ibn al-Muʿtazz complains about Baghdad:

الوسخة السّماء، الومدة الماء والهواء، جوّها غبار، وأرضها خبار، وماؤها طين، وترابها سرجين، وحيطانها نزوز، وتشرينها تمّوز، فكم من شمسها من محترق، وفي ظلّها من عرق، ضيّقة الدّيار، وسيّئة الجوار، أهلها ذئاب، وكلامه سباب، وسائلهم محروم، ومالهم مكتوم، ولا يجوز إنفاقه، ولا يحلّ خناقه، حشوشهم مسايل، وطرقهم مزابل، وحيطانهم أخصاص، وبيوتهم أقفاص.

[66] Ibn al-Athīr 1987, VI, pp. 470–1; al-ʿUmarī 2010, VI, p. 125.
[67] Al-Ālūsī 1987, pp. 40–1.

> The sky of which is dirty, her water and air are muggy, her weather dusty, her soil quagmire, her water clay, her dirt dung, her walls unstable, her October—July. Many are burned by the sun. In her shade the sweat is unbearable, her houses narrow, her neighbors evil, her citizens wolves, their speeches curses, their beggars deprived, their money hidden, never for spending, never for releasing, their gardens know no gardening, their roads rubbish, their walls poorly [built], their houses cages.[68]

And he composed the following verses:

أطـــال الهمّ في بغـداد ليـلي   وقد يشقى المسافر أو يفوز
ظللت بها على رغمي مقيمـا   كـعنّيـن تعانـقه عجــوز

In Baghdad, night made my sorrow deepen,
  If you leave her, you may win or lose.
Unwillingly, I stayed there, as if I were an
  Impotent man being squeezed by an old woman.[69]

According to historical sources, one reason for selecting the site chosen for Baghdad was because it was free of mosquitoes and had lots of fresh air; but after the city had been built, there seem to have been various opinions among those who beheld the city and breathed its air. Ṭāhir ibn al-Ḥusayn al-Khuza'ī (776–822) wrote:

زعم النّاس أنّ ليلك يا بــغ   داد ليل يطيب فيه النّســيم
ولعمري ما ذاك إلّا لان خ   الفها، بالنّهار، منك السّموم
وقليل الرّخــاء يتبع الشـدّ   ة عند الأنام، خطب عظيـم

People say: Your night, Oh Baghdad,
  Is lovely, the air cool and fresh.
By my life, your night is thus only
  Because the day is beset by hellish wind.
A slight comfort after great agony,
  And people say at once: "What a paradise!"[70]

And we have, as well, the testimony of Ādam ibn 'Abd al-'Azīz al-Umawī (ninth century):

لقد طال في بغداد ليلي ومن يبت   ببغداد يصبح ليـله غيـر راقد
بــلاد إذا ولّى النـّهار تنـــافرت   براغيثها من بين مثنّى وواحد
ديازجــة شهــب البطــون كأنّـها   بغال بريـد أرســلت في مذاود

My night in Baghdad became longer, whoever spends a night in
  Baghdad will stay awake, deprived of sleep.

[68] Al-Ālūsī 1987, pp. 38–9; Yāqūt 1990, I, p. 550.
[69] Al-Ālūsī 1987, p. 39; Yāqūt 1990, I, pp. 550–1.
[70] Al-Ālūsī 1987, pp. 43–4; Yāqūt 1990, I, p. 550.

As soon as day escapes, it becomes a land where mosquitoes
  Swarm, couples and lone.
Humming, their bellies white as if they were
  Pack mules repelled by spears.[71]

In any event, Baghdad could not have achieved its supremacy without having been an industrial urban center from its earliest times. Its residents were known for their brilliance in building splendid boats and ships, some in special shapes, such as domes, lions, and eagles. According to extant statistics, there were 30,000 of these ornate boats and ships; the Caliph al-Amīn owned a number of them. In his verses, Abū Nuwās (d. 815) describes the ships:

سَخّرَ الله للأمِينِ مطـايا   لم تسـخّر لصـاحب المحـرابِ
فإذا ما رِكابُهُ سِرْنَ بَرًّا   سار في الماءِ راكبًا ليثَ غابِ

God made mounted beasts submissive to al-Amīn,
  He had never made them obedient even for the king.[72]
While the king's mounted beasts stride on the ground,
  Al-Amīn passes on water, riding a forest lion.[73]

Many verses refer to the rain, as do those by Abū 'Abd Allah Ibrahim ibn Muḥammad Niftawayhi (858–935):

سقى الله أربع الكرخ الغوادي بديمة   وكلّ ملث دائم الهطـل مسـبل
منـازل فيـها كـلّ حسـن وبهجـة   وتلك لها فضل على كلّ منزل

Clouds water al-Karkh[74] with perpetual rain,
  Unceasingly falling, never stopping.
These abodes possess beauty and joy,
  They have advantages over any other abode.

Because the climate in Baghdad is dry, poems blessing or cursing the city and its dwellers frequently open with such verses as "may God rain on Baghdad," "may the rain water the surface of your earth," "may He not rain on Baghdad," or "may clouds never rain upon you."

Poetry also chronicles spells when Baghdad was covered in snow, and these climatic events inspired poets. Ibn al-Mu'tazz (861–909) describes a sudden flurry of snow: "The clouds' eyes were bathed in water, / all at once they poured down snow, spreading it like white roses." Unlike Ibn al-Mu'tazz, al-Sharīf al-Rāḍī (930–977) had a different impression and makes

71 Al-Ālūsī 1987, p. 41; Yāqūt 1990, I, p. 551; al-Nawrasī 2009, p. 95.
72 Literally, "the owner of the *miḥrāb*" (= a throne room in a palace).
73 Al-Nawrasī 2009, p. 45.
74 A quarter on the western shore of the Tigris that runs through Baghdad.

an analogy between the damage caused by snow and people's wickedness and evil-doing:

أرَى بَغدادَ قَدْ أخنـَى عَلَيهـَا	وصبحـها بغـارته الجليـد
كـان ذرى معالـمها قـلاص	نَوَاءٍ كُشّـطَتْ عَنْـهَا الجُلـُودُ
كَأنّ بِـهِ لُغَـامَ العِيـسِ بَاتَـتْ	تُسـَاقِطُهُ عِجَـالُ الرّجعِ قُـودُ
غَطّى قِمَمَ النّـجادِ، فكـلٌّ وَادٍ	على نشـراته سبّ جديـد
كمَا تَعرَى بهِ الغِيطانُ مَحْلًا	وَتَغْبـَرُّ التّـهَايِـمُ وَالنّـجُودُ
فَمَهما شِئْتَ تَنظُرُ مِنْ رُبَاهَا	إلـى بِيـضٍ عَوَاقِبُـهُنّ سُـودُ
أقـول لـه وقـد أمسـى مكبًا	عَلَى الأقطَارِ يَضْعُفُ أوْ يَزِيدُ
وراءك فالخواطر بـاردات	على الإحسان والأيدي جمود
وأنـّك لو تروم مزيـد بـرد	إلـى بـرد لاعـوزك المزيـد

I see Baghdad, hit by snow,
    Attacking early in the morning.
As if the tips of her landmarks were burdened she-camels
    With their skins removed.
As if the snow were camels' saliva poured
    Like a torrent, shot from a water wheel.
It covered uplands, every valley,
    Upon its elevated spots a new white veil.
All valleys were smitten by snow,
    All planes and uplands became dust-colored.
Wherever you look from the hills,
    You see only white; the consequence is only dark.
I say to the snow, as it is hitting
    Lands, more strongly or less:
Beware, human minds are ice for any
    Generosity, favors are chilly.
If you want to pile up more miseries on the already
    Existing ones, you will never succeed.

Such an analogy is not unusual: for example, a rare snow storm that hit my own city, Haifa, in February 1950, inspired different narratives by Jews and Palestinians in the political and cultural contexts of the city in the aftermath of the War of 1948.[75]

Floods have been one of the most frequently chronicled natural catastrophes to strike Baghdad, as recorded by historians[76] and poets from the first centuries after its founding—the floods generally resulting from the city's neglect of its irrigation system. For example, a flood in the year 883 ruined 7,000 houses in al-Karkh. In 1243, 1248, 1255, and 1256, a series of floods ruined some of the city quarters and in one case floods even entered

75 See Rabinowitz and Mansour 2011, pp. 119–48.
76 See Micheau 2008, pp. 240–1.

the markets of eastern Baghdad. The city suffered from floods until the twentieth century as Maʿrūf al-Ruṣāfī (1875–1945) describes in one of his poems:

زحفت جيوش السّيل حتّى أصبحت   بالكرخ نازلة لها ضوضاة
فسقت بيوت الكرخ شرّ مُقيء   منها فقاءت أهلها الابيات

Flood's armies kept advancing,
They fell upon al-Karkh with a mighty uproar.
As they streamed onto houses with nauseous fluids,
The houses spat out their residents.[77]

Some decades later, Nāzik al-Malā'ika (1923–2007) wrote:

إنّه الآن إلهُ
أولم تَغْسِل مبانينا عليه قَدَمَيْها؟
إنّه يعلو ويُلْقي كنزَهُ بين يَدَيها
إنّه يمنحُنا الطّينَ وموتًا لا نراهُ
من لنا الآنَ سواهُ؟

Now the river has become a god.
Haven't our buildings washed their feet in its water?
It rises and pours its treasures in front of them,
It grants us mud and invisible death.
And now what is left for us?[78]

As with any other urban center, Baghdad had bustling squares, and poets had both a negative and positive view of them. According to Muṭīʿ ibn Iyās (704–785):

زاد هذَا الزّمان شرّا وعسرا   عندنا إذ أحلّنا بغداذا[79]
بلدة تمطر التّراب عَلَى النَّاس   كما تمطر السّماء الرّذاذا

This time has increased evil and hardness—
It made us settle in Baghdad.
A town raining dust on people
As the sky was drizzling.[80]

And another anonymous poet asked:

هل الله من بغداد يا صاح مخرجي   فأصبح لا تبدو لعيني قصورها
وميدانها المذري علينا ترابها   إذا شحجت أبغالها وحميرها

Tell me, my friend, will God let me get out of Baghdad,
Never again to set eyes on her palaces?

77 Al-Ruṣāfī 1986, I, pp. 304–15. The quotation is from pp. 308–9.
78 Al-Malā'ika 1981, II, pp. 531–4.
79 Baghdādh = Baghdād (see Yāqūt 1990, I, p. 541).
80 Al-Ālūsī 1987, pp. 37–8; al-Nawrasī 2009, p. 93.

Never again to behold her square-raising dust
  Whenever voices of mules and donkeys are heard?[81]

Unlike these poets, Muḥammad ibn ʿAbd Allāh al-Salāmī (947–1002) was inspired by the busy activities of the square:

وميدان تجول به خيول   تقود الدّارعين ولا تقادُ
ركبت به الى اَللّذات طرفًا   له جسم وليس له فؤاد
جرى فظننت أنّ الأرض وجه   ودجلة ناظر وهو السّواد

I see a busy square, galloping horses
  Leading armored fighters, nobody leading them.
Once I was riding for pleasure on a noble horse,
  With a body but no heart.
Galloping on, I imagined the ground was a lady's face;
  The Tigris was the eye, the horse the eyeball.[82]

In the early centuries after Baghdad's founding, scenes of the Tigris were frequently depicted in poems. One favorite image was the moon upon the river. Ibn al-Tammār al-Wāsiṭī (tenth century) writes:

والبدر في الأفق الغربيّ تحسبه   قد مدّ جسرا، على الشطّين، من ذهب

Full moon sits in the western horizon as though
  A golden bridge stretching between the two banks.[83]

Or as ʿAlī ibn Muḥammad al-Tanūkhī (d. 953) writes:

أحسن بدجلة والدّجى متصوب   والبدر في أفق السّماء مغرّب
فكأنّها فيه بساط أزرق   وكأنّها فيها طراز مذهب

What a beautiful river when night falls!
  The moon stirs westwards toward the horizon;
The Tigris on the moon—a blue carpet,
  The moon over the river—a golden veil.[84]

Sometimes the image of the moon shifts or blurs into other images; and this is the case with the face of the young cupbearer at a wine party, in Manṣūr ibn Kayghlagh's (d. 960) verses:

كم ليلة سامرت فيها بدرها   من فوق دجلة قبل أن يتغيّبا
قام الغلام يديرها في كفّه   فحسبت بدر التم يحمل كوكبا
والبدر يجنح للغروب كأنّه   قد سلّ فوق الماء سيفا مذهّبا

[81] Al-Ālūsī 1987, p. 40; Yāqūt 1990, I, p. 551.
[82] Al-Ālūsī 1987, p. 36.
[83] Yāqūt 1990, II, p. 504.
[84] Al-Ālūsī 1987, p. 36 ;Yāqūt 1990, II, p. 504.

Many a night did I spend with her full moon
  Hovering over the Tigris before it disappeared.
The cupbearer passed around the wine,
  I imagined he was a full moon bearing a star.
When the moon is about to set, it is
  A golden sword unsheathed over the water.[85]

Another oft-used image was a bridge over the Tigris; thus ʿAlī ibn al-Faraj al-Shāfiʿī (tenth century?) writes:

أيا حبّذا جسر على متن دجلة   بإتقان تأسيس وحسـن ورونـق
جمال وفخر للعراق ونزهـة   وسلوة من أضناه فرط التّشـوق
تراه إذا مـا جئتـه متأمّـلا   كشطر عبير خطّ في وسط مفـرق
أو العاج فيه الآبنوس مرقّش   مثال فيول تحتها أرض زئبـق

What a wonderful bridge stretching over the Tigris,
  Great in perfection, saturated with glamor and beauty.
Glory and honor to Iraq, consolation
  And solace for gloomy lovers.
Curiously, when approaching it and fixing your eyes on it,
  You see a perfumed line written on parchment.
Or an ivory with ebony decorations—
  Elephants stepping on soil of mercury.[86]

Almost a thousand years later, Maʿrūf al-Ruṣāfī wrote:

كأنّما الرّصافة اشتـاقت إلى الـ   كرخ فمدّت لاعتناقه يدا
فَلَو رأى ابن الجهم منه ما نرى   لكان يعنيه بما قد أنشـد

As if al-Ruṣāfa longed for al-Karkh,
  Extending a hand to touch it.
If Ibn al-Jahm had seen what we see,
  He would have worried about what he sang.[87]

In these verses, al-Ruṣāfī alludes to Ibn Jahm's famous poem, whose opening verse is:

عيون المها بين الرّصافة والجسر   جلبن الهوى من حيث أدري ولا أدري

Does' eyes between Ruṣāfa and the bridge
  carried desire from places I know or know not.[88]

[85] Al-Ālūsī 1987, pp. 36–7.
[86] Al-Ālūsī 1987, pp. 26–7.
[87] See at: https://www.alghadeer.tv/notes/876 (last accessed May 11, 2020).
[88] Ibn al-Jahm n.d., p. 143; Ibn al-Jahm 1981, pp. 141–8; al-Ālūsī 1987, pp. 50–2. The translation of *ʿuyūn al-mahā* as "does' eyes" is based on Stetkevych 1993, p. 108; Ali 2010, p. 92 (who translated in the singular "doe's eyes"). Al-Ruṣāfa is a quarter on the eastern shore of the Tigris in Baghdad.

Reading the aforementioned verses about the Tigris and the bridges upon the river, one may recall William Wordsworth's lines in "Composed upon Westminster Bridge, September 3, 1802":

> Earth has not anything to show more fair:
> Dull would he be of soul who could pass by
> A sight so touching in its majesty:
> This City now doth, like a garment, wear
> The beauty of the morning; silent, bare.[89]

Baghdad was the city of lovers; it was worldly and divine. As it was the greatest urban center of the Islamic Empire, this comes as no surprise! Certain parts of the city provided opportunities for the intermingling of the sexes, and had much more to offer than other less prominent, smaller places in affording space for this. An agonized earthly anonymous lover wondered:

ألا يا غراب البين ما لك واقفا　　ببغدان[90] لا تجلو وأنت صحيح
فقال غراب البين وانهلّ دمعه　　نقضي لبانات لنا ونروح
الا إنّما بغدان سجن إقامة　　أراحك من سجن العذاب مريح

> Oh crow of separation,[91] why have you landed
> 　In Baghdad to settle and never leave, are you so salubrious?
> Tears fell from the crow's eyes, while replying:
> 　We fulfill our desires and then leave.
> Baghdad, you know, is a house of calamity,
> 　May God save us from this very prison.[92]

On the other hand, it is noteworthy that, contrary to traditional thought, whereas mystical phenomena thrive in isolated places like deserts, mountains, and the countryside, Baghdad was one of the greatest centers of Muslim mysticism (i.e., Sufism). Scholars even refer to a Baghdadi Ṣūfī tendency, which places heavy stress on *zuhd* (asceticism) as opposed to the Khurasanian ecstatic tendency. Al-Ḥusayn ibn Manṣūr al-Ḥallāj (858–922), whose mysticism was Khurasanian, spent his last period in Baghdad, where he was executed for having declared "*anā al-ḥaqq*" ("I am the Absolute Truth," i.e., God). His divine love poems were inspired by Baghdadi scenes:

يا نسيم الرّوح قولي للرّشا　　لم يزدني الوِرْد إلّا عطشا
لي حبيبٌ حبّه وسط الحشا　　إن يشا يمشي على خدّي مشا
روحه روحي وروحي روحه　　إن يشا شئتُ وإن شئتُ يشا

[89] Wordsworth 1965, p. 170.
[90] Baghdān = Baghdād (see Yāqūt 1990, I, p. 541).
[91] The black crow, the "crow of separation" (*ghurāb al-bayn*), is a frequent motif in classical Arabic poetry.
[92] Al-Khaṭīb al-Baghdādī 1971, p. 82; Yāqūt 1990, I, p. 552.

Oh breeze of the soul, please tell the gazelle:
  Water only increases thirst.
I have a lover, his love is ever inside me,
  If He wishes to walk, He can do it on my cheeks.
His soul is mine—mine His;
  If He wishes, I too wish; if I wish, He does too.[93]

Another lover of the divine, Muḥyī al-Dīn ibn ʻArabī (1165–1240), wrote:

ألا يا بَانَة الوَادِي بِشاطي نَهْرِ بَغْدَادِ
شجاني فيكِ ميّادٌ طروبٌ فوقَ ميَّادِ

Oh you, the ben-tree of the valley[94]
  On Baghdad river's bank.
A melancholic dove on a swaying bough
  Filled me with grief.[95]

There were poets who compared Baghdad to other cities, as did Abū Isḥāq al-Ṣābī (925–994):

لهف نفسي على المقام ببغداد وشربي من مـــاء كوز بثلج
نحن بالبصرة الذّميمة نسقي شرّ سقيا، من مائها الأترنجي
أصفر منكر ثقيل غليـــظ خاثر مثل حقنـــة القولنـج
كيف نرضى بمائها، وبخير منه في كنف أرضنا نستنجي؟!

Alas, I deeply miss Baghdad,
  I miss her snowy water.
Here, in ugly Basra, we are watered
  With only sickly, yellowish drinks.
How could we be satisfied drinking it, while in our own land,
  We clean our asses with purer water?![96]

This particular "tradition of comparison" has lasted throughout Baghdad's history. While staying in Tabriz, Rāḍī al-Qazwīnī (1819–1868) wrote:

أحبّتنـا بـزوراء العـــراق لقد طال النّـوى فمتى التّلاقـي
وما تبريز للفصحاء مأوى وأين التّرك من عرب العراق

My beloved people in Zawrā' of Iraq,
  We have been apart for too long, when will we meet?
Tabriz is not a refuge for eloquent Arabic speakers,
  Could you ever compare Turks to the Arabs of Iraq?

93 Al-Ḥallāj 1974, p. 41.
94 The ben-tree (*ban*), according to the poet, is the tree of light.
95 Ibn ʻArabī 1966, p. 197 (for another English translation, see Ibn ʻArabī 1978 [1911], p. 46).
96 Al-Ālūsī 1987, p. 30.

And Aḥmad Shawqī (1868–1932) urged his readers:

دع عنك روما وأثينا وما حوتا   كلّ اليواقيــت في بغـداد والتّؤم

— — — — — — —

دار الشّرائع روما كلّما ذكرت   دار السّــلام لها القت يد السّــلم
ما ضارعتها بيانا عند ملتــأم   ولا حكتها قضاء عند مختصـم

Forget Rome and Athens and all that they contain,
All jewels are only in Baghdad.
— — — — — — — — — — — —
At the mention of the House of Peace, the House of Law, Rome,
Hastens to congratulate her.
When they meet, Rome cannot equal her in eloquence,
In a court of law, she cannot challenge her rival.[97]

Apart from poetry, Baghdad was a center of other literary genres, such as the *Maqāmāt* (literally, "Assemblies"), a rhymed prose with intervals of poetry in which rhetorical extravagance is noticeable. All great writers of that genre wrote assemblies set in Baghdad: Badīʿ al-Zamān al-Hamadhānī's (969–1007) twelfth *maqāma* is called *al-Maqāma al-Baghdādiyya* ("The Baghdadi Assembly") and his thirtieth *maqāma* is called *al-Ruṣāfiyya* ("The Ruṣāfiyya Assembly"),[98] and Abū Muḥammad al-Ḥarīrī's (1054–1122) thirteenth *maqāma* is called *al-Maqāma al-Baghdādiyya* ("The Baghdadi Assembly").[99] Unlike most writers of the *māqamāt*, Ibn al-Kazarūnī (d. 1298) wrote a Baghdadi *maqāma* that was not only set in Baghdad, but also included descriptions of the city before its destruction by the Mongols with many *ubi sunt* exclamations ("Where are those who were before us?") to indicate nostalgia for the bygone wondrous city of Baghdad.[100]

Because of its reputation among the Arabs, Baghdad was frequently mentioned in poems of *mufākharah* (boasting) of other cities, such as Qayrawān, as we can see in the *nūniyya* by Ibn Rashīq al-Qayrawānī (d. 1063 or 1071):

وزَهَتْ على مصر وحقّ لها، كما   تَزْهو بِهِمْ، وعَدَتْ على بَغْدانِ

[Qayrawān] outshone Cairo, as it truly deserved, as
It boasted of [its scholars], it prevailed over Baghdad.[101]

97 Shawqī 1964, p. 205.

98 Al-Hamadhānī 1973, pp. 61–4, 122–8; al-Hamadhānī 1983, pp. 55–9, 157–65; al-Hamadhānī 2005, pp. 71–4, 181–9. *Baghdādh* in the first line of the *maqāma*, as previously mentioned, is another version of the name of Baghdad. It appears as such in order to rhyme with *azādh* (dates).

99 Al-Ḥarīrī 1969 [1867], pp. 176–81; al-Ḥarīrī 1980, pp. 54–7; al-Ḥarīrī 1985, pp. 105–11.

100 Al-Ālūsī 1987, pp. 150–3; Hämeen-Anttila 2002, pp. 329–30.

101 On this poem, see Hermes 2017, pp. 270–97, where a translation of the entire poem is quoted (this specific verse is translated in two versions on pp. 282 and 295).

4. 1258 AND BEYOND

And this leads us to the major event that poets chronicled in detail—the destruction of Baghdad in 1258. Hulagu (1217–1265), the Mongol conqueror and founder of the Il-Khanid Dynasty of Persia, launched a wave of conquests throughout the Islamic world. After direct control of much of the Islamic world south of the Oxus had slipped from the hands of the Mongols, Hulagu was entrusted by the Möngke Khan (1209–1259) with the task of recovering and consolidating the Mongol conquests in western Asia. He overcame the resistance of the Isma'ilis of northern Persia, routed a caliphal army in Iraq, captured Baghdad, and murdered the Caliph al-Musta'ṣim (1213–1258; r. 1242–1258). His army sacked the city, and the killing, looting, and burning lasted for several days. The numbers killed during the fifty-day siege were estimated to be between 800,000 and 1,300,000. According to some accounts, the Tigris and Euphrates ran red with the blood of scholars.[102] Most of the city's monuments were wrecked and burned, and the famous libraries of Baghdad, including the House of Wisdom, were eradicated. Poems and chronicles describe how copies of the Qur'ān "became cattle's fodder." Books were used to make a passage across the Tigris: "The water of the river became black because of the ink of the books." Books were also pillaged from Baghdad's famous libraries and transported to a new library that Hulagu built near Lake Urmiya.[103]

As a result of these events, Baghdad remained depopulated and in ruins for several centuries, and the event is conventionally regarded as the end of the Islamic Golden Age. The destruction of Baghdad inspired many poets in the following centuries and in the years up to our own times, with Hulagu being taken as the figure of the archetypal cruel dictator. The poetry of the times was a faithful mirror of those events. Taqī al-Dīn ibn Abī al-Yusr wrote:

يا زائـــرين إلى الزّوراء لا تفــدوا   فما بذاك الحمى والدّار ديّار
تاج الخلافة والرّبع الّذي شرفت به   المعالـم قد عفـــــاه إقفار

Oh visitors to al-Zawrā', please do not come here.
In this refuge and abode, no one is here anymore.

[102] Muir 1924, pp. 591–2; Bosworth 1967, pp. 149–51; Boyle 1968, pp. 348–9.

[103] Hitti 1946, p. 378; Sedillot 1877, p. 293. As previously indicated, according to recent scholarship, the laments on the destruction of the Baghdadi libraries under Mongol rule have been vastly exaggerated. By the end of the thirteenth century, the Baghdadi libraries had regained their reputation, housed a wide selection of books on multiple subjects, and continued to contribute significantly to the development of Arabo-Islamic culture (Biran 2019, pp. 464–502. On the topos of the Mongol destruction of Baghdadi libraries, see also below).

The crown of the Caliphate, the great monuments,
    All have been burned to ashes.[104]

Al-Majd al-Nashābī (d. 1259?) complains that:

الكفر أضرم في الإسلام جذوته   وليس يرجى لنار الكفر إخماد
واضيعَة المُلك والدّين الحنيف   وما تلقاه من حادثات الدّهر بغداد
أين المنيّة منّي كي تساورني   فللمنيّة إصدار وإيراد
من قبل واقعة شنعاء مظلمة   يشيب من هولها طفل وأكباد

Heresy fanned a fire, Islam was burned,
    No hope of the fire being quenched.
Oh grief, what a loss for the kingdom, for the true religion,
    What a loss—Baghdad struck with misery.
Death is touching me,
    Death is doing what it wants.
The threat of a dark cruel catastrophe
    Turns a child, even livers, gray-haired.[105]

Standing in Abadan, Sa'dī Shirāzī (1219–1294) looked into the water of the Tigris, and, seeing "red blood flowing to the sea," he started weeping:

حبست بجفني المدامع لا تجري   فلما طغى الماء استطال على السّكر
نسيم صبا بغداد بعد خرابها   تمنّيت لو كانت تمرّ على قبري

I kept closed my eyelids to prevent tears from flowing;
    When they overflowed, the intoxication could not stop them.
If only after the destruction, Baghdad's eastern breeze
    Had blown over my grave!

Shīrazī describes how women's honor in captivity was violated by the Mongols and how

عدون حفايا سبسبا بعد سبسب   رخائم لا يسطعن مشيا على الحبر
لعمرك لو عاينت ليلة نفرهم   كأنّ العذاري في الدّجي شهب تسري
وإنّ صباح الاسر يوم قيامة   على أمم شعث تساق إلى الحشر
ومستصرخ يا للمروؤة فانصروا   ومن يصرخ العصفور بين يدي صقر
يساقون سوق المعز في كبد الفلا   عزائز قوم لم يعودن بالزّجر
جلبن سبايا سافرات وجوهها   كواعب لم يبرزن من خلل الخدر

They ran barefoot from desert to desert,
    They were so tender; thus they could not walk on ink.
By your life, had you seen them on the night of their flight;
    It was as if virgins were stars falling into darkness.

104 Al-Nawrasī 2009, p. 82.
105 al-'Azzāwī 1996, I, p. 286.

The morning of the day on when they were chained, as on Judgment Day
Coming to disheveled nations led for resurrection.
A cry is heard: Oh lost sense of honor, help!
But who would help a bird in a falcon's grip?
They were led like sheep in the desert's midst,
Noble women unused to being chided.
They were dragged away, their breasts raised, their faces unveiled,
Driven out from their private abodes.[106]

As with the civil war following the death of Hārūn al-Rashīd, the events of 1258 were described as a *mundus inversus*, such as in a poem by Shams al-Din Muḥammad ibn 'Abd Allāh al-Kūfī:

يا نكبة ما نجا من صرفها أحد   من الورى فاستوى المملوك والملك

Oh, what a catastrophe, no one saved himself from its
Calamities; kings and slaves are equal.[107]

Shams al-Dīn Maḥmūd ibn Aḥmad al-Hāshimī al-Ḥanafī addresses the destroyed abode:

يا دار أيـن السّـاكنون وأيـن   ذيّاك البهـاء وذلـك الإعـظـام
يا دار أين زمان ربعك مونقًا   وشعـارك الإجـلال والإكـرام
يا دار مذ أفلـت نجومـك عنـا   والله من بعـد الضّيـاء ظـلام

Oh house, where are your dwellers? Where
Reside the glory and honor?
Oh house, where are the days of your elegance and kindness,
Days when your slogans were greatness and respectfulness?
Oh house, by God, since your stars have set,
Darkness has covered us following light.[108]

On the whole, all that was written about the destruction of Baghdad, both at the time and in the succeeding decades and centuries, reflects the paradigm that sees political changes as pivotal in their effects on religious and cultural life. Hulagu has been engraved on the Arabs' memory as the fundamental reason for the destruction of their great medieval civilization and the cause for what has been seen as the cultural stagnation of the Arab world until the Arabic *Nahḍa* in the nineteenth century.[109] Arabs have placed emphasis,

[106] Snir 2013, pp. 156–8.
[107] al-'Azzāwī 1996, I, p. 287; al-Nawrasī 2009, p. 82.
[108] See al-Kutubī 1951, I, pp. 580–1.
[109] Referring to the term *Nahḍa*, the French scholar Nada Tomiche (1923–2019) wrote the following: "It has often been translated by 'Renaissance', a problematic translation since it refers implicitly to 16th century Europe and to the movement of return to the Greco-Roman past. In an attempt to avoid the 'Euro-centrist' approach, an attitude for which Arabists are frequently criticised, a translation such as 'Awakening', although less often used, would be

prompted by European Orientalists, on the descriptions of the aforementioned destruction of cultural institutions and libraries, the burning of books by the Mongol army, the latter's throwing of books into the Tigris and using them as a bridge to cross the river, and the killing of many of the scholars and men of letters in Baghdad.[110] We find this not only in modern historical books, but also in literary histories, and even in all kinds of works of poetry and prose. Not a few modern Arab officials have used the Hulagu myth for their own aims, as did, for example, the late Egyptian president Jamāl ʿAbd al-Nāṣir (1918–1970). A well-known Swiss writer on Middle Eastern affairs even quotes "a high Syrian government official" as saying "in deadly earnest": "If the Mongols had not burnt the libraries of Baghdad in the thirteenth century, we Arabs would have had so much science, that we would long since have invented the atomic bomb. The plundering of Baghdad put us back centuries."[111]

Bernard Lewis (1916–2018) explains that this is an extreme, even a grotesque formulation, but the thesis that it embodies was developed by European scholars, who saw in the Mongol invasions "the final catastrophe which overwhelmed and ended the great Muslim civilization of the Middle Ages." This judgment of the Mongols "was gratefully, if sometimes surreptitiously, borrowed by romantic and apologetic historians in Middle Eastern countries as an explanation both of the ending of their golden age, and of their recent backwardness."[112] Yet scholars now argue that this thesis is definitely unjustified, as the signs of the stagnation were apparent long before Hulagu appeared in Baghdad. The successive "blows by which the Mongols hewed their way across western Asia, culminating in the sacking of Baghdad and the tragic extinction of the independent Caliphate in 1258," as H. A. R. Gibb writes, "scarcely did more than give finality to a situation that had long been developing."[113] Even some modern Arab intellectuals and historians feel that the descriptions of the sacking of Baghdad as regards the cultural losses were much exaggerated. The Syrian intellectual Constantin Zurayk (Zureiq) (1909–2000) comments that "some of us still believe that the attacks of the Turks and the Mongols are what destroyed the Abbasid Caliphate and Arab power in general. But here also the fact is that the Arabs

closer to the sense of the root and therefore more satisfactory." Available at: https://referenceworks.brillonline.com/browse/encyclopaedia-of-islam-2/alpha/n?s.start=80 (last accessed March 3, 2021).

110 See, for example, D'Ohsson 1834–1835, I, p. 387 as quoted by Browne 1951, II, p. 427; Nicholson 1956, p. 129; Goldziher 1966, p. 141. Cf. Browne 1951, II, p. 463.

111 Hottinger 1957 (as quoted by Lewis 1973, p. 179).

112 Lewis 1973, p. 179.

113 Gibb 1962a, p. 141. Cf. Smith 1963, p. 40; Wiet 1966, p. 243; Lewis 1968, p. 12; Lewis 1973, pp. 179–98.

had been defeated internally before the Mongols defeated them and that, had those attacks been launched against them when they were in the period of growth and enlightenment, the Mongols would not have overcome them. On the contrary the attacks might have revitalized and re-energized them."[114]

In any event, since the destruction of Baghdad, Hulagu and the year 1258 have become a metaphor for the aforementioned so-called "decline" of Arab-Muslim civilization, and even modern Arab poets have used his figure in order to allude to other catastrophes that have struck the Arab world. On one occasion the figure of Hulagu is described in Arabic poetry positively, and that was to serve a specific aim. While spending a sabbatical year in the United States, the Palestinian poet Mīshīl Ḥaddād (1919–1997) missed his homeland and his hometown of Nazareth. In his exile, he was surrounded by books he perceived to be in opposition to the natural order of things. After returning to his natural environment in his homeland, he wrote the poem "al-Kutub" ("The Books") alluding to the descriptions of the destruction of Baghdad's cultural institutions and libraries. The books are used here as a metonym for the disasters that science and rational thinking have brought to mankind:

يأتي هولاكو ويحرق الكتب
قبل أن تكلّ العيون
وتختلط الأفكار
قبل أن تعلّمنا لغاتها المزدحمة
الاطمئنان
قبلها يأتي.

Hulagu will come and burn the books,
Before eyes grow feeble,
Before ideas are muddled,
Before their crowded languages teach us
Tranquility,
Before that,
He will come.[115]

It seems that Ḥaddād was inspired by William Wordsworth's romantic dictum from "The Tables Turned":

Up! Up! my Friend, and quit your books;
Or surely you'll grow double:
Up! Up! my Friend, and clear your looks;
Why all this toil and trouble?[116]

114 Zurayk 1956, p. 48. Cf. von Grunebaum 1962, p. 255; Lewis 1973, p. 182.
115 The poem was first published in *al-Sharq* (*Shfaram*), January–April 1985, p. 3; incorporated in Ḥaddād 1985, p. 9. On the poem, see Snir 1988, pp. 9–16.
116 Wordsworth 1965, p. 107.

Another possible inspiration is *Zorba the Greek*[117] by the Greek writer Nikos Kazantzakis (1883–1957), in which the boisterous and mysterious Alexis Zorba calls on the narrator to "make a heap of all [his] books and set light to them" (p. 94), "you've been contaminated by those blasted books of yours" (p. 78), "Aren't you ashamed? Man is a wild beast, and wild beasts don't read" (p. 152), and "all those damned books you read—what good are they?" (p. 269).

Hulagu's destruction is described in terms of the demonic; his forces are "barbaric" and are similar to those forces that brought about the destruction of the Roman Empire—that is, the Hulagu story has been united with the myth of the "anti-civilization barbarians." In most modern poems written about the destruction of Baghdad by the Mongols, there are intertextual dialogues with modern non-Arabic literary works that refer to the myth of the barbarians, the most famous of which are "Waiting for the Barbarians" (1904) by the Greek poet Constantine P. Cavafy (1863–1933) and the novel *Waiting for the Barbarians* (1983) by J. M. Coetzee (b. 1940).[118] The Egyptian poet Ṣalāḥ ʿAbd al-Ṣabūr (1931–1981) concluded his poem "The Tatars Have Attacked"[119] with the following lines:

بالحقد أقسمنا سنهتف في الضّحى بدم التّتار
أمّاه! قولي للصّغار
أيا صغار...
سنجوس بين بيوتنا الدّكناء إن طلع النّهار
ونشيد ما هدم التّتار...

We swear in hatred that tomorrow we will rejoice in the blood of the Tatars
O Mother, please tell the children:
Dear children ...
We will walk amongst our grey houses, when day rises
And build again what the Tatars destroyed.

Sarkūn (Sargon) Būluṣ (1944–2007) used the metaphor of Hulagu in two poems; the first is titled "Hulagu Praises Himself":

أنا هولاكو
بحر من الأعشاب
تقطعه الخيول/ بصمت
سيف يكره الانتظار في غمده
تحت أسوار تحلم بالغربان

117 Kazantzakis 1996 [1946].

118 On this myth and the intertextual dialogue of these two literary works with a poem by the Palestinian Maḥmūd Darwīsh (1941–2008) dealing with the same myth, see Snir 2008, pp. 123–66.

119 ʿAbd al-Ṣabūr 1972, pp. 14–17.

أسوار، أسوار يراني اللّاجئون
في أحلامهم بين الخرائب
ويشحذ الأسرى قشّة صغيرة من حصاني.

I am Hulagu!
A sea of grass
Crossed by horses / in silence.
A sword hates having to wait in its sheath.
Beneath walls that dream of crows
Walls, walls, the refugees see me
In their dreams amid the ruins
And prisoners sharpen a small straw from my horse.[120]

The second, "Hulagu (New Series)," conducts a dialogue with the former:

والحتف يتكلّم باسمي
فأنا هولاكو:

سيف في غمده لا يستريح.

ظلّه أينما ارتمى
يستنسل غيمة من العقبان الجائعة
تطفو فوق البيوت

حيث يراني
اللّاجئون في
كوابيسهم بين الخرائب

ويشحذ الأسرى
حفنة قشّ من حصاني

And death speaks in my name
I am Hulagu:

A sword in its sheath, never resting.

Its shadow, wherever it throws itself
Begets a cloud of hungry eagles
Hovering over the houses.

Where the refugees
See me in their
Nightmares between the ruins.

And the prisoners sharpen
A handful of straw from my horse.[121]

120 Būluṣ 1985, p. 62; Būluṣ 1997, p. 94; Būluṣ 2003, p. 80.
121 Būluṣ 2008, pp. 119–20.

It is interesting to see how Hulagu's destruction of Baghdad appears also in comics for children, such as in the comic-book series *al-Tis'a wa-l-Tis'ūn* or *al-99* (*The Ninety-Nine* or *The 99*), which was created by Nāyif al-Muṭawwaʿ (b. 1971) (on the series, see below), where the first episode begins in 1258, with the siege of Baghdad, but unlike the usual narrative where the Mongols invaded and destroyed the Grand Library, in this episode its countless precious books are saved from being dumped into the River Tigris.[122]

In the centuries after the city fell to the Mongols, Baghdad was pushed to the margins of the Arab and Islamic world. The Mamluk capital Cairo replaced her as the capital of the Muslim world, and for centuries the name of Baghdad was lost in Europe or confused with Babylon. After the invasion by Tamerlane (1401), al-Maqrīzī wrote in 1437 that "Baghdad is but a heap of ruins; there is neither mosque, nor congregation, nor market place. Most of its waterways are dry, and we can hardly call it a town."[123] In 1534, Baghdad was captured by the Ottoman Turks and under their rule Baghdad fell into a period of further decline. European travelers visiting the city during the sixteenth and seventeenth centuries reported that Baghdad was a center of commerce with a cosmopolitan and international atmosphere where three main languages (Arabic, Persian, and Turkish) were spoken—at the same time mentioning neglected quarters where many of the houses were in ruins. Sir Thomas Roe, the British ambassador at Constantinople from 1621 to 1628, confused Baghdad with Babylon. The French traveler Jean-Baptiste Tavernier (1605–1689), describing his journey down the Tigris in 1651, related that he arrived at "Baghdad, qu'on appele d'ordinaire Babylon."[124] Only after the French Orientalist Antoine Galland (1646–1715) translated the *Arabian Nights* into French[125] did Europeans again take an interest in Baghdad. In

[122] Akbar 2015.

[123] Raymond 2002, p. 18.

[124] Le Strange 1900, p. 348; Levy 1977 [1929], p. 9.

[125] On the translations of that popular literary work, see Huart 1966, pp. 402–3; Ḥamāda 1992, II, pp. 201–4; Classe 2000, pp. 1390–2. Even Antoine Galland (1646–1715), who first introduced this work to European readers at the beginning of the eighteenth century, did not consider it to be of high literary importance (MacDonald 1932, p. 398. On Galland and his translation, see Knipp 1974, pp. 44–54; Kabbani 1986, pp. 23–9; Hopwood 1999, pp. 13–14. On Galland's *Arabian Nights* in the traditions of English literature, see Mack 2008, pp. 51–81). On the changing value of *Alf Layla wa-Layla* for nineteenth-century Arabic, Persian, and English readerships, see Rastegar 2005, pp. 269–87. On its being among children's leisure reading during the *Nahḍah*, despite the danger that it could "poison [the child's] soul and spoil his morals," see Ayalon 2021, pp. 272–93 (the quotation is from p. 387). Cf. Snir 2017, pp. 92–4. One of the contributors to Galland's *Arabian Nights* was Ḥanna Diyāb (*c.* 1688–after 1763), a Maronite Christian who served as a guide and interpreter for the French naturalist and antiquarian Paul Lucas (1664–1737). Between 1706 and 1716, Diyāb and Lucas traveled through Syria, Cyprus, Egypt, Tripolitania, Tunisia, Italy, and France. In Paris, Ḥannā Diyāb met Galland, who added to his wildly

1774, we find a report that "this is the grand mart for the produce of India and Persia, Constantinople, Aleppo and Damascus; in short it is the grand oriental depository." However, in the overall picture, Baghdad was in constant decline; in one report, its population was at a low of 15,000. Only think that during the tenth century its population was around 1,500,000 people! 'Abd al-Ghanī al-Jamīl (1780–1863) expressed that very same comparison in his verse:

لهفي على بغداد من بلدة   قد عشعش العزّ بها ثم طار
كانت عروسًا مثل شمس الضّحى   لمستعير حليها لا يعار
كانت لآساد الوغى منزلًا   والخائف الجاني بها يستجار
واليوم لا مأوى لذي فاقة   فيها ولا في أهلها مستجار

My condolences for Baghdad, what a town!
  Once glory nested here; now, it has flown away.
She was a bride like the morning's sun,
  Her jewels were not to be lent.
An abode for warrior lions,
  A sanctuary for frightened fugitives.
Alas, no refuge now for the needy,
  Her people offer no shelter.[126]

In 1816, Dawūd Pasha arrived on the scene and brought a degree of prosperity. He maintained control over the tribes and restored order and security. He took care of the irrigation system, established factories, encouraged local industry, built bridges and mosques, founded three *madrasa*s, and organized an army of about 20,000 and had a French officer train it. However, he imposed heavy taxes, and, after his fall along with floods and plagues, Baghdad still suffered from marginality. From 1831 to the end of the Ottoman period, Baghdad was directly under Constantinople, and some governors tried to introduce administrative reforms.[127]

Under Midhat Pasha (1869–1872), the leading advocate of Ottoman *tanzimat* reforms, a modern *wilayet* system was introduced, each divided into seven *sanjak*s headed by *mutasarrif*s, Baghdad being one of them. In 1869, under his influence, the first publishing house, the Wilayet Printing Press, was established in Baghdad. The same year, he founded *al-Zawrā'*, the first newspaper to appear in Iraq as the official organ of the provincial government; it

popular translation of *Arabian Nights* several tales related by Diyāb, including "Aladdin" and "Ali Baba and the Forty Thieves." On Diyāb's remarkable first-person account of his travels and his communication with Galland, see Diyāb 2021; Diyāb 2021a.

126 See at: http://alshajara.org/poemPage.do;jsessionid=44E5C8C07FBC108E46C7C7016A441F73?poemId=611159 (last accessed January 7, 2021).

127 Duri 2012.

was a weekly that lasted until March 1917. In 1870, he founded a tramway linking Baghdad with Kazimayn.[128] With the exception of a few French missionary schools, there were no modern schools in Baghdad, but between 1869 and 1871 Midhat Pasha established modern schools, a technical school, junior (*rushdī*) and secondary (*iʿdādī*) military schools, and junior and secondary civil (*mulkī*) schools.

Minorities in Baghdad enjoyed a rare tolerance for the times.[129] In 1846, Rabbi Israel-Joseph Benjamin II said that "nowhere else as in Baghdad have I found my co-religionists so completely free of that black anxiety, of that somber and taciturn mood that is the fruit of intolerance and persecution."[130] The Christian and Jewish communities became the pioneers in modern education in Baghdad. In 1864, the Alliance Israelite Universelle (AIU),[131] a Jewish School in Baghdad, was founded; it offered a predominantly secular education and had a Western cultural orientation. It was to play a major role in the modernization of the local educational system. Visiting Baghdad in 1878, Grattan Geary, editor of the *Times of India*, wrote that instruction in the AIU School was of the best modern kind: "Arabic is the mother tongue of the Baghdad Jews," but many of them "spoke and read English with wonderful fluency," and, also, "they speak French with singular purity of accent and expression."[132]

This was also the time when Baghdad started to regain its position as one of the great urban centers in the Middle East. The *Gazetteer of Baghdad* (compiled in 1889) mentioned in its chapter on the ethnography of the city that "the present population is now estimated at about 116,000 souls, or 26,000 families divided thus: Turks, or of Turkish descent, 30,000 souls; Persians 1,600; Jews 40,000; Christians 5,000; Kurds 4,000; Arabs 25,000; Nomad Arabs 10,000."[133] The population of the city was gradually increasing and, in 1904, the population was estimated at about 140,000. In 1914, Baghdad was, numerically, a greater Jewish than a Muslim city with its law-abiding, Arabic-speaking Jewish community.[134] According to the last official yearbook of Baghdad as a *wilayet* (1917), the population figures for

128 Unlike with most historians, there are Iraqi scholars who argue that Midhat Pasha's projects in Iraq did not have a positive outcome; see, for example, al-Wardī 1971, II, pp. 235–65.

129 Batatu 1978, p. 257, and the references in n. 184.

130 Benjamin II 1856, p. 84.

131 On the role that the AIU played in the field of Jewish education in the Middle East, see Cohen 1973, pp. 105–56.

132 Geary 1878, I, pp. 132–3.

133 *Gazetteer of Baghdad, Compiled (under the Orders of the Quarter Master General in India) for Political and Military Reference, 1889, by J. A. Barlow, A. Howlett, S. H. Godfrey,* reprint by the General Staff, India, 1915, p. 3.

134 Longrigg and Stoakes 1958, p. 29.

the city were as follows: Arabs, Turks, and other Muslims except Persians and Kurds: 101,400; Persians 800; Kurds 8,000; Jews 80,000; and Christians 12,000.[135] By 1918, the population was estimated at 200,000.

Baghdad remained under Ottoman rule until 1917, when it was taken by the British during the First World War. The aim of Fayṣal, who became King of Iraq on August 23, 1921, was to create "an independent, strong Arab state, which will be a cornerstone for Arab unity."[136] Thus, the Iraqi constitution of March 21, 1925 stated that "there is no difference between the Iraqi people in rights before the law, even if they belong to different nationalities, religions and languages."[137] Expressions overtly inclusive of all citizens are not surprising, since Arab nationalists from their earliest phases had considered non-Muslims living among the Arabs as part of the Arab "race." Travelers were impressed with the great admixture of ethnicities, the diversity of speech, the rare freedom enjoyed by non-Muslims, and the great tolerance among the masses. The free intermingling of peoples left its imprint on the dialects of Baghdad.

The British Mandate from the League of Nations operated behind the façade of a native government in which every Iraqi minister had a British advisor. This was despite the fact that the entire Iraqi educational system at the time was harnessed to the ideas of Arabness and Arabization.[138] Sāṭiʿ al-Ḥuṣrī (1880–1968), Director General of Education in Iraq (1921–1927), and Arab nationalism's first true ideologue, argued that "every person who is related to the Arab lands and speaks Arabic is an Arab."[139] With the aim of making the mixed population of the new nation-state homogeneous and cohesive, he looked upon schools as the means by which to indoctrinate the young in the tenets of pan-Arabism, seeking the "assimilation of diverse elements of the population into a homogeneous whole tied by the bonds of a specific language, history, and culture to a comprehensive but still exclusive ideology of Arabism."[140] The eloquent secularist dictum *al-dīnu li-llāhi wa-l-waṭanu li-l-jamīʿ* ("Religion is for God, the Fatherland is for everyone") was in popular circulation; it was probably coined in the Coptic Congress in

[135] Quoted in the *Arab Bulletin*, No. 66, October 21, 1917.

[136] Al-ʿAfif 2008, p. 65.

[137] For the text of the constitution, see al-Ḥusnī 1974, I, pp. 319–34; the quotation is from p. 319.

[138] Tibawi 1972, pp. 94–5.

[139] See al-Ḥuṣrī 1965 [1955], p. 12. Cf. Chejne 1969, pp. 19–22; Cleveland 1971, p. 127; Esposito 1995, I, pp. 113–16. On the role of al-Ḥuṣrī in using Iraqi schools to inculcate nationalism, see Simon 1986, pp. 75–114. On the Iraqi education system in the interwar period, see Bashkin 2006, pp. 346–66. On Arabic language and identity, see the studies in Bassiouney and Walters 2021, and the insights in Walters 2021, pp. 3–10.

[140] Cleveland 1971, p. 63.

Asyut (1911) by Tawfīq Dūs (1882–1950), a Coptic politician and later the Egyptian Minister of Transportation.[141] Qur'ānic verses fostering religious tolerance and cultural pluralism, such as "There is no compulsion in religion"[142] and "You have your path and I have mine"[143] were often quoted. The Iraqi writer 'Azīz al-Ḥājj (1926–2020), who worked in the education system, saw the composition of his own class (1944–1947) in the Department of English at the High School for Teachers in Baghdad (Dār al-Mu'allimīn al-'Āliya) as a significant and symbolic representation of the harmony among the religious communities of Baghdad: out of eight students, four were Jewish, including one female student, two were Christian, and two were Muslim. He wrote: "The coexistence and intermixing between the different communities and religious sects in Baghdad is exemplary."[144]

As an offspring of a family who emigrated from Baghdad to Israel at the beginning of the 1950s, I will take as an example the Jewish residents of Baghdad, who played a major role in the life of the city during the first half of the twentieth century. The Civil Administration of Mesopotamia, in its annual review for the year 1920, stated that the Jews were "a very important section of the community, outnumbering the Sunnis or Shias."[145] According to Elie Kedourie (1926–1992), "Baghdad at the time could be said to be as much a Jewish city as an Islamic one."[146] Jewish poets wrote about Baghdad

141 See Carter 1986, pp. 290, 304, n. 2. The first part of the slogan appeared (also as *al-dīn li-l-dayyān*) in several writings, such as an elegy by Aḥmad Shawqī (1868–1932) for the assassinated Egyptian Coptic prime minister Buṭrus Ghālī (1846–1910) (Shawqī 1964, III, pp. 144–5) and an elegy for the leader of Egypt's nationalist Wafd Party Sa'd Zaghlūl (1859–1927), which was written in 1927 by Naṣr Lūzā al-Asyūṭī (1887–1965) (Kaylānī 1962, p. 167). It also appeared in the aforementioned manifesto of Arab nationalists (al-A'ẓamī 1932, pp. 113–14. Cf. Haim 1962, p. 86. See also al-Bishrī 1988, p. 62; Qilāda 1993, p. 239; Bāsīlī 1999, pp. 165, 277, 281–4). The same slogan was also used by Egyptian-Jewish Communists, such as Yūsuf Darwīsh (1910–2006) (*Al-Ahram Weekly*, December 2–8, 2004) and Marcel (Marsīl) Israel (Ceresi, Shīrīzī) (1913–2002), the leader of Taḥrīr al-Sh'ab (The People's Liberation) (Shīrīzī 2002, pp. 46–7). Also the Egyptian-Jewish journalist Albert Mizrāḥī (1916–1988) used it in his newspaper *al-Tas'īra* (*The Price List*) when Shaykh Aḥmad Ṭāhir insulted the Jews of Egypt on state radio (*al-Tas'īra*, March 22, 1954, p. 4; quoted in Beinin 1998, pp. 78–9). The same slogan has even been used in recent years—for example, Usāma al-Bāz, the presidential political advisor, was quoted by the Egyptian State Information Service on January 31, 2000; *Al-Ahram Weekly*, January 9–15, 2003. In April 2004, President Mubārak himself used this slogan in a celebration on the occasion of the birth of the Prophet (*al-Ahrām*, April 21, 2005, p. 1). See also the slogan *al-waṭaniyya dīnunā wa-l-istiqlāl ḥayātunā* ("patriotism is our faith and independence is our life"), which is found in Coptic texts (Baḥr 1979, pp. 94–5, 100).

142 *Al-Baqara* 256.

143 *Al-Kāfirūn* 6.

144 Al-Ḥājj 1999, pp. 125–31.

145 Rejwan 1985, p. 210.

146 Kedourie 1989, p. 21.

from the 1920s onward, even after the mass immigration of Jews to Israel after its independence. The most famous of these Iraqi-Jewish poets was Anwar Sha'ul (1904–1984), who started to publish under the pseudonym of Ibn al-Samaw'al (the son of al-Samaw'al), referring to the pre-Islamic Jewish poet al-Samaw'al ibn 'Adiyā', who was proverbial in the ancient Arabic heritage for his loyalty. According to the ancient sources, al-Samaw'al refused to hand over weapons that had been entrusted to him. As a consequence, he would witness the murder of his own son by the Bedouin chieftain who laid siege to his fortress al-Ablaq in Taymā', north of al-Madīna. He is commemorated in Arab history by the well-known saying "as faithful as al-Samaw'al." In one of his poems, Sha'ul said:

سأظلّ ذيّاك السّموأل في الوفا أسَعُدْتُ في بغداد أم لم أسعد

Faithful I will stay like al-Samaw'al
Whether happy in Baghdad or miserable.[147]

And in another poem, he said:

فعلى الفرات طفولتي قد أزهرت وبدجلة نهل الشّباب الرّيق

My childhood blossomed by the waters of the Euphrates.
The days of my youth drank of the Tigris.[148]

Another prominent Iraqi-Jewish poet, Mīr Baṣrī (1911–2006), feeling that, because of his Jewish faith, there were doubts regarding his loyalty to his Iraqi homeland and the Arab nation, wrote:

يا رفاق العمر إن يدن حمامي فادفنوني في حمى الأرض الرّحيبة
جنب آبائي الألى ناموا دهورا في ثرى بغداد – ذي الأم الحبيبة

Oh friends of life, even as my death draws near,
Please bury me in the safety of the wide land.[149]
Near my ancestors who slept for ages
In Baghdad's soil—this is the beloved mother.

And Murād Mīkhā'īl (1906–1986), when he was only sixteen, wrote a poem titled "Oh My Fatherland," which included the following verses:

روحي فداؤك يا وطن فاسلم ولا تخشى الفتن
اليوم ربعك لي سكن وغدا ثراك يضمّني
يا وطني يا وطني

My soul is your ransom, Oh My Fatherland!
Be at peace, do not be afraid of any trials!

147 Shā'ul 1983, p. 69.
148 Shā'ul 1980, p. 336.
149 Baṣrī 1991, p. 140.

Today, your soil is my abode;
  Tomorrow your soil will embrace my corpse.
Oh My Fatherland! Oh My Fatherland![150]

Likewise, another Jewish poet, Ibrāhīm Obadyā (1924–2006), even when he suffered from the attitude of the Iraqi authorities, never hesitated to declare:

أنا ابن بغداد حين تعرفني   أنا ابن بغداد حيث تلقاني

I am the son of Baghdad, whenever you meet me,
  I am the son of Baghdad, wherever you see me.[151]

Moreover, more than sixty years after their departure from Baghdad, this city is still alive in the minds and hearts of the Iraqi-Jewish immigrants now in Israel. The poets among them write about Baghdad in both Arabic and Hebrew. When Iraqi missiles hit various parts of Israel in 1991, the Iraqi-born Israeli-Hebrew poet Ronny Someck (b. 1951) wrote a poem titled "Baghdad, February 1991":

בָּרְחוֹבוֹת הַמּוּפְגָּזִים הָאֵלֶּה נִדְחֲפָה עֶגְלַת הַתִּינוֹק שֶׁלִּי.
נְעָרוֹת בַּבֶּל צָבְטוּ בִּלְחָיַי וְנוֹפְפוּ כַּפּוֹת תְּמָרִים
מֵעַל פְּלוּמַת שַׂעֲרִי הַבְּלוֹנְדִּינִי.
מָה שֶׁנִּשְׁאַר מֵאָז הִשְׁחִיר מְאוֹד,
כְּמוֹ בַּגְדָּד וּכְמוֹ עֶגְלַת הַתִּינוֹק שֶׁפִּנִּינוּ מִן הַמִּקְלָט
בִּימֵי הַהַמְתָּנָה שֶׁלִּפְנֵי מִלְחָמָה אַחֶרֶת.
הוֹ חִידֶּקֶל הוֹ פְּרָת, נַחֲשֵׁי הַתַּפְנוּקִים בַּמַּפָּה הָרִאשׁוֹנָה שֶׁל חַיַּי,
אֵיךְ הִשַּׁלְתֶּם עוֹר וַהֲיִיתֶם לִצְפָעִים?

Along these bombed-out streets my baby carriage was pushed.
Babylonian girls pinched my cheeks and waved palm fronds
Over my fine blond hair.
What's left from them became very black.
Like Baghdad and
Like the baby carriage we moved from the shelter
During the days of waiting for another war.
Oh Tigris, Oh Euphrates—pet snakes in the first map of my life,
How did you shed your skin and become vipers?

With the recognition of Iraq as an independent state, Baghdad had gradually regained some of its former prominence as a significant center of Arabic culture. This was a time when, on the political level, the relationship between the authorities in Baghdad and the West became a major issue, as also reflected in poetry. For example, in a celebration held in 1929 by

150 The poem was published in the newspaper *Dijla* on April 11, 1922. It was republished in Mīkhā'īl 1988, pp. 181–2.

151 Obadyā 2003, p. 75.

the National Party on the occasion of a visit to Baghdad of the wealthy American businessman and Arabist Charles Richard Crane (1858–1939), Maʿrūf al-Ruṣāfī recited a poem in which he says:

جئت يا مستر كراين   فانظر الشّرق وعاين
فهو للغرب أسير   أسر مديون لدائن
إن هذا الشّرق والغر   ب لمغبون وغابن
— — — — — — — — — —
وإذا تسأل عمّا   هو في بغداد كائن
فهو حكم مشرقيّ الـ   ضرع غربيّ الملابن
عربيّ أعجميّ   معرب اللهجة راطن
فيه للإيعاز من لن   دن بالأمر مكامن
هو ذو وجهين وجه   ظاهر يتبع باطن
قد ملكنا كلّ شيء   نحن في المظاهر لكن
نحن في الباطن لا نم   لك تحريكًا لساكن
أفهذا جائز في الـ   غرب يا مستر كراين؟

You have come, Mr. Crane,
  So please see the East and explore,
It is a prisoner of the West,
  In a prison of a debtor to a creditor.
East and West—
  Like a deceived and a deceiver.
— — — — — — — — — — — —
And if you ask about
  What happens in Baghdad,
It is an Eastern udder,
  But the milk is Western
Arab but dumb,
  Arabized language but gibberish.
The advice coming from London,
  Full of secrets,
There are two faces,
  One external, the other is internal.
We are the owners, but this
  Is only the visible,
In fact, we
  Own nothing.
Is it possible in the West,
  O, Mr. Crane?[152]

All major modern Arabic poets referred to Baghdad in their poetry, and the emergence of modernist Arabic poetry, from the 1950s, accompanied the

[152] Al-Ruṣāfī 1986, II, pp. 344–8.

transformation of Baghdad as a physical and spatial entity into what al-Janābī considers to be "an easy metaphor for revival and eclipse—for what disintegrates into a lulling daylight!"[153] This was also the time when different poetic forms dictated changes in the ways Baghdad was imagined and described. Until the mid-twentieth century, the basic poetic form of the poems written about Baghdad was the classical *qaṣīda*. This was the same poetic form that was developed in pre-Islamic Arabia and perpetuated throughout Arabic literary history. The *qaṣīda* is a structured ode maintaining a single end rhyme that runs through the entire piece; the same rhyme also occurs at the end of the first hemistich (half-line) of the first verse. The central poetic conception of the so-called "neoclassical" poets emerging from the late nineteenth century was basically the same: although "there is nothing specifically religious about it,"[154] the *qaṣīda* is the sacred form for poetry, and the relationship between the poet and his readers was like that between an orator and his audience. It is when we come to the late 1940s and the rise of the aforementioned *al-shi'r al-ḥurr*, the Arabic development of "free verse," that we encounter significant deviation from classical metrics. As the new free verse succeeded in gaining some measure of canonical status, traditional poets and critics felt that this new poetry was in opposition to the accepted and ancient form of Arabic poetry they were used to. Based upon earlier experiments of Arab poets and inspired by English poetry, the essential concept of this poetic form entails reliance on the free repetition of the basic unit of conventional prosody—the use of an irregular number of a single foot (*taf'īla*) instead of a fixed number of feet. The poet varies the number of feet in a single line according to need. The new form was closely associated with the names of two Baghdadi poets, Nāzik al-Malā'ika (1923–2007) and Badr Shākir al-Sayyāb (1926–1964). More recent developments in Arabic poetry, especially the type of prose poem known as *qaṣīdat al-nathr*, as well as its variant types and forms, have already gradually pushed free verse to the margins. The change in the poetry written about Baghdad since the 1960s demonstrates that modernity has taken hold and that Arabic modernist poets are, to a certain extent, mainstream poets. The poets born of this decade—that is, those whose creativity became evident in the 1960s—are called the "generation of the sixties."[155] Instead of tribal membership, writes al-Janābī, "poets now felt that they belonged to a worldwide avant-garde. Baghdad figured as a metropolis, a state of mind, an explosive consonant." They no longer wrote "poetry about Baghdad; they wrote poetry of Baghdad. In the first instance, poets tinkled their bells in order

[153] Snir 2013, p. 310.
[154] Irwin 2011 (Introduction), p. 3.
[155] See al-'Azzāwī 1997.

that nostalgia be remembered, while in the second instance, poets nibbled the sun's black teat in order to set the limpid substance of the city ablaze and wave to the magnet of time!"[156]

During the last three decades, Baghdad has suffered severe infrastructural damage, particularly following the First and Second Gulf Wars, the American-led occupation in 2003, sectarian violence, and terrorist attacks. Nevertheless, the present population of Baghdad is now over 7,000,000, making it the second-largest city in the Arab world after Cairo. Almost all poems written about Baghdad during the last decades are melancholic and reflect the political and moral collapse in the reality of existence in the city, though the ethos of the city as a metaphor for Arabism and Islam still remains, and poets combine the reality of immediate history with the city's ethos. There are also dialogues between modern and medieval poets. 'Abd al-Wahhāb al-Bayyātī (1926–1999) referred to al-'Abbās ibn al-Aḥnaf's (750–809) life and poetry in this way:

أظلمت حانات بغداد
فلا جدوى
فعبّاس من الحبّ يموت

Baghdad's taverns have darkened.
There is no use
'Abbās is dying of love.[157]

Similarly, Sarkūn (Sargon) Būluṣ (1944–2007) revived the figure of Sa'dī Shīrāzī in his poem "In the Garden of Sa'dī Shīrāzī When He Was in Prison." Buland al-Ḥaydarī (1926–1996), for example, who spent thirty years of his life in exile,[158] wrote about the dictatorship in Baghdad at the time of Saddām Ḥusayn. In his poem "al-Madīna al-latī Ahlakahā al-Ṣamt" ("The City that the Silence Killed"), he uses the myth of Troy:

طروادة ماتت من جرح فينا، من جرح فيها
من خرس أعمى شلّ لسان بنيها
طروادة أهلكها الصّمت

[156] Snir 2013, pp. 310–11.
[157] See at: https://nesasysy.wordpress.com/2006/05/08/1140/5.
[158] On his tombstone in London, we find the following words:

في المنفى، إن متّ غدًا، فسيحمل شاهد قبري: هذا وطني، هذا من أجلك يا وطني إن متّ هنا في الغربة،

"If I die here in exile, if I die tomorrow, my tombstone will bear the following: This is my homeland, this is for you my homeland."

These words are the final line of the poem "They Were Four," which was published before his death and dedicated to his Baghdadi friend, the Jewish writer Nissīm Rajwān (Rejwan) (1924–2017) (*Mashārif* [Haifa] 7 [1996], pp. 14–15).

فليس لنا فيها، فليس لها فينا، إلّا الموت
وإلّا الجثّة والمسمار.

Troy died because of a wound inside us, because of a wound inside her,
Because of a blind silence that tied her children's tongue,
Troy, the silence killed her,
We have nothing inside her, she has nothing inside us save death,
Nothing but the corpse and the nail.[159]

In a later version, the poet substituted Troy with Baghdad throughout the poem.[160] And Sarkūn (Sargon) Būluṣ (1944–2007) follows this with:

أيّها الجلّاد
عد إلى قريتك الصّغيرة
لقد طردناك وألغينا هذه الوظيفة.

Oh Hangman,
Return to your small village.
We have expelled you today and canceled your job.[161]

In another poem, "I Have Come to You from There," Būluṣ described a chilling encounter with one of the victims who revisited him after death. One of the major contemporary Arabic poets whose work about Baghdad reflects the new form-related change in Arabic poetry and at the same time expresses the influence of that change on the new attitude toward Baghdad is not Baghdadi. He is not even Iraqi; moreover, he visited Baghdad only once. This is the Syrian poet Adūnīs (Adonis) (b. 1930), whose poetry has been accompanying the city of Baghdad throughout the last fifty years. In 1961, Adūnīs, who at the time thought of himself as the new prophet of the utopian Baghdad, published his poem "Elegy for al-Ḥallāj," in which he orchestrates a dialogue with the poet-mystic al-Ḥusayn ibn Manṣūr al-Ḥallāj (who lived in Baghdad more than 1,000 years before him). The speaker in the poem, which will be fully discussed in the next chapter, addresses al-Ḥallāj as a "star rising from Baghdad, / Loaded with poetry and birth." Baghdad, the place where al-Ḥallāj was executed in 922, symbolizes the glories of ancient Arab and Muslim civilization. Moreover, the star is rising from, and not over, Baghdad—that is, there is an allusion to a possible universal message. The use

159 Al-Ḥaydarī 1990, pp. 45–9.

160 Al-Ḥaydarī 1993, pp. 723–8. The Syrian poet Nūrī al-Jarrāḥ (b. 1956) also uses the myth of Troy to express the suffering of the citizens during the civil war in Syria during the second decade of our century—his poetry collection bears the ironic title *Lā Ḥarba fī Ṭurwāda: Kalimāt Hūmīrūs al-Akhīra* (*There Is No War in Troy: Homer's Last Words*) (al-Jarrāḥ 2019). The book was included in the long list of the literature branch eligible for the Sheikh Zayed Book Award for 2021–2022.

161 Būluṣ 1997, p. 96; Būluṣ 2003, p. 121.

of the active participle stresses the present relevance of the poem: the star *is rising now*, which is to say, the beginning of the 1960s. The very choice of the figure of al-Ḥallāj as the symbol of death and rebirth indicates the intention of the poet to stress the Arab and Islamic context of the poem as well as that of the entire collection in which it appears. Supposedly, according to its title, a lamentation for a personage who died more than 1,000 years earlier, "Elegy for al-Ḥallāj" is ironically transformed in the process of reading the poem into a vision of the Arab nation's rebirth. Since the star is rising now, from Baghdad, the death of al-Ḥallāj is the bridge that Arab-Islamic civilization crosses to reach a more perfect existence.

Soon, however, hopes and expectations for Baghdad as a symbol of Arab rebirth had completely collapsed. Perhaps the most famous text with this message was written in 1969 but published only in May 2003—the title being "Please, Look How the Dictator's Sword Is Sharpened, How Necks are Prepared to Be Cut."[162] It was published again in 2008 with the new title "Poetry Presses Her Lips to Baghdad's Breast."[163] Adūnīs had written these verses after visiting Baghdad in 1969, his only visit to the city. He went as a member of the Lebanese Association of Writers' delegation, and stayed in Baghdad for several days, where he wrote these verses describing Baghdad's cultural and political atmosphere of fear and death. At the beginning of the text, this atmosphere is presented plainly:

تحدّثْ همسًا. كلّ نَجْم هنا يخطّط لقتل جاره.
همسًا؟ تعْني كما لو أنّني اتحدثُ مع الموت؟

Whisper, please! Every star here plans to kill his neighbor
Whisper? You mean as if I'm talking with death?

Adūnīs walks in the streets of Baghdad of the *Arabian Nights* but sees men as mere "shapes without faces. Shapes like holes in the page of space"—men walking in the streets "as if digging them. It seems to me their steps have the forms of graves."

These lines and others may call to mind sections from *Istanbul* by the Turkish novelist Orhan Pamuk (b. 1952), where he describes the empty city as mirroring the empty souls, the "living dead," the corpse "that still breathes," and the feeling that expresses "the sadness that a century of defeat and poverty would bring to the people of Istanbul."[164] Like Pamuk, Adūnīs describes the "sewage systems, in open air, facing stores. Bad smells plunder the empty space ... embracing even the birds that revolt against him." But the

162 See *al-Ḥayāt*, May 10, 2003, p. 12.
163 Adūnīs 2008a, pp. 140–56; Adūnīs 2012–2015, pp. 136–52.
164 Pamuk 2006, pp. 253, 317.

resemblance is only superficial because Pamuk's sadness is in essence melancholic and the romantic sadness of a lover, "The Melancholy of Autumn,"[165] while Adūnīs' feeling is the sadness of a terrorized people.

Adūnīs describes the fear among people when informants could be anyone—a neighbor, a friend, a relative or family member, or just a passerby. It is the atmosphere of an "upside-down society." The poet does not see any difference between the Baghdad of 1258, the year Hulagu destroyed it, and the Baghdad of 1969, the year of his own visit:

- الأولى فتَكَ بها التَّتار،
والثانية يفتك بها أبناؤها.

The first, the Mongols destroyed,
And the second, her children do the same.

The speaker addresses Gilgamesh and accuses him of deluding the people that life in Baghdad has a secret to be revealed, while in reality "life here is nothing but continuous death. Please, look how the dictator's sword is sharpened, how necks are prepared to be cut." Against the background of the sayings (some of which are quoted above) that Baghdad is paradise, Adūnīs does not have any hesitation:

- بغداد جنَّة!
- الإنسانُ هو الجنَّة، لا المكان.

- Baghdad is a paradise!
- Man is a paradise, not the place.

He concludes the text with the following:

وكنتُ، حتَّى تلك اللحظة من السنة 1969، أتعبُ كثيرًا في التمييز بين البشر والشياطين والآلهة عندما أنظر إلى "أهل السلطة في العراق". ربَّما لهذا لم أشعر في بغداد إلا بالبرد، حتَّى وأنا في حضن الشَّمس!
لَكِنْ، لَكِن،
ضَعْ، أيُّها الشِّعر، شفتيكَ على ثدي بغداد.

Until that moment in 1969, I had tried hard to distinguish between human beings, demons, and gods, while watching "the men of power in Iraq." Perhaps, that is why in Baghdad, when I was in the arms of the sun, I didn't feel anything other than absolute cold.
But, but,
Oh poetry, please press your lips to Baghdad's breast!

Some days before the American invasion of Baghdad in April 2003, Adūnīs wrote "Salute to Baghdad," which he opens with the following:

[165] The title of a chapter in Pamuk's *The Museum of Innocence* (Pamuk 2009, pp. 197–204).

ضَعْ قهوتكَ جانبًا واشربْ شيئًا آخر،
مُصغيًا إلى ما يقوله الغُزاة:
بتوفيقٍ من السّماء
نُديرُ حربًا وقائيّة
حاملينَ ماءَ الحياة
من ضفاف الهدسون والتّايمز
لكي تتدفّق في دجلة والفرات.

Put your coffee aside and drink something else.
Listening to what the invaders are declaring:
With the help of God,
We are conducting a preventive war,
Transporting the water of life
From the banks of the Hudson and Thames
To flow in the Tigris and Euphrates.

And the poem is concluded thus:

وطنٌ يُوشكُ أن يَنْسيَ اسْمَهُ.
ولماذا،
عَلّمتْني وردةٌ جوريّةٌ كيف أنَامْ
بين أَحضْانِ الشّآمْ؟
أكَلَ القاتلُ خُبزَ الأغنيْة،
لاَ تَسَلْ، يا أيّها الشّاعِرُ، لن يُوقظَ هذي الأرض
غيرُ المعَصِيةْ.

A homeland almost forgets its name.
And why
A red flower teaches me how to sleep
In the laps of Damascus?
The fighter eats the bread of the song,
Don't ask, Oh poet, for nothing but disobedience
Will awake this land.

In another poem, "Time Crushes into Baghdad's Body," written in 2005, Adūnīs contemplates the history of Baghdad against the background of her tragic present: "But, behold the river of history, how it flows into the language plain, emerging from / Baghdad's wounds. A history which flies in my imagination as though it were a black crocodile."[166] In his poem "Baghdad, Feel No Pain," the Egyptian poet Fārūq Juwayda (b. 1946) illustrates the tragedy through the eyes of Baghdad's children:

أطفال بغداد الحزينة يسألون
عن أيّ ذنب يقتلون! يترنحون على شظايا الجوع
يقتسمون خبز الموت ثم يودّعون

[166] Adūnīs 2008b, pp. 334–5.

Children in grieved Baghdad wonder
For what crime they are being killed, staggering on the splinters of hunger,
They share death's bread, then they bid farewell.[167]

Juwayda's poem was set to music and performed by the Iraqi singer Kāẓim al-Sāhir (b. 1957) and became very popular. Bushrā al-Bustānī (b. 1949), in her "A Sorrowful Melody," describes the horrors of the occupation:

دبّابات الحقد تدور
منكفئٌ مثل حصان مهجور
جرحي
تلفحه الشّمسُ العربيّة
ينخره الدّود
بيكاسو يرسم جرنيكا أخرى
يرسم بغداد طريحةً أقدام الغوغاءْ

The tanks of malice wander.
My wound
Is turned away like an abandoned horse
Scorched by the Arabian sun,
Chewed by worms
Picasso paints another Guernica,
Painting Baghdad under the feet of boors.[168]

And there is the nostalgic Baghdad following the destruction: Sarkūn (Sargon) Būluṣ (1944–2007) wrote "An Elegy for al-Sindbād Cinema,"[169] and Sinān Anṭūn (Antoon) (b. 1967) wrote "A Letter to al-Mutanabbī (Street)"—this street was the cultural heart of the city. On March 5, 2007, after a suicide bombing had destroyed many bookshops and killed twenty-six people, he wrote:

إنّه فصل آخر
ملحمة الحبر والدم

This is another chapter
In the saga of blood and ink.[170]

5. CONCLUSION

A study of poems and epigrams included in the *Palatine Anthology* about Greek cities reaches the conclusion that the vast majority of them "are

[167] See at: http://m.iraq-amsi.net/view.php?id=12025.
[168] See at: https://pulpit.alwatanvoice.com/content/print/96645.html.
[169] See at: https://soundcloud.com/iahmedmansour/sargon-boulus-3.
[170] Anṭūn 2010, pp. 49–51.

laments for a fallen city, destroyed by war, by nature, or the ravages of time. Others celebrate [the] mythology of a site."[171] Retrospectively, readers of the present chapter might well arrive at similar conclusions in regard to Baghdad! The utopian city of Hārūn al-Rashīd, the realm of the *A Thousand and One Nights*, was, in the end, a fallen city destroyed by wars and the calamities of time. As in the case of Greek cities, immediately after its founding, many poems celebrated the mythical city and its ethos as an Arab and Islamic city. Even before the ravages of the second half of the twentieth century, events had made reality more prominent than the romance, and people "brought reports eloquent of disillusionment," as Reuben Levy testified in his *A Baghdad Chronicle* (1929).[172]

Thus, as seen above, the history of Baghdad may be divided roughly into three periods: from its founding to its destruction by the Mongols (762–1258)—the city as the prestigious capital of the Islamic Empire; from then to the establishment of the modern Iraq (1258–1921)—and continuous decline and decay; and, finally, the present period with its glimpses of flowering and thriving (such as those seen during the 1920s, 1930s, and 1960s), which have been buried under the ruins of decades of dictatorship and internal and external devastation. In the beginning of his book *Baghdad: The City of Peace*, Richard Coke writes that the story of Baghdad is largely the story of continuous war and "where there is not war, there is pestilence, famine and civil disturbance. Such is the paradox which cynical history has written across the high aims implied in the name bestowed upon the city by her founder."[173] More than eighty-five years later, one cannot maintain that Coke was wrong in his historical judgment of Baghdad. In other words, the glorious Baghdad is only an image and memory of the remote past; Baghdad of the present evokes only sadness, distress, and nostalgia for bygone days.

The writer and journalist Ḥusayn al-Mūzānī (Hussain al-Mozany) (1954–2016), who lived in Berlin, wrote about the contrast between the Baghdad he left and the one he found after thirty years of absence, which "has become a non-place, represented by concrete walls." Al-Rashīd Street, which "some used to call Iraq's aorta, has committed suicide, and now all that is left is its long corpse stretched out along the scattered, blackened shops that mourn a street which bid its people farewell and then killed itself."[174] The poem "In Baghdad, Where My Past Generation Would Be"

171 Hartigan 1979, p. 102. *The Palatine Anthology* is a collection of Greek poems and epigrams composed from 300 BC to 600 AD.
172 Levy 1977 [1929], p. 1.
173 Coke 1935 [1927], p. 15.
174 Al-Mozany 2010, pp. 6–19; Duclos 2012, pp. 399–400.

by ʿAbd al-Qādir al-Janābī (b. 1944) encapsulates all that lovers of Baghdad must feel nowadays:

أين أنت يا سنواتي الأولى
سنوات الشّارع والمقهى
سنوات النّهار والمشي الطّويل
في مجرى التّمرّدات دون وخز ضمير
أين أنت يا سنواتي الأولى
يا مدينتي المحمومة في فيضانات الذّكرى
أين أنت في هذا الجدول المرسوم

Where are you, my first years,
The years of streets and cafés,
The years of days and long walks,
In the course of the revolts with no pricking of conscience?
Where are you, my first years?
Oh my city, feverish with floods of memory,
Where are you in that drawn stream?[175]

[175] See al-Janābī 2012, p. 68.

Chapter 4

Religion: "I Saw My God"[1]

Death embraces us into its breast
Venturing and abstaining
It bears us as a secret upon its secret
Making our multitude one
– Adūnīs

1. INTRODUCTION

Early mystic Arabic poetry arose along with the development of Ṣūfī theory at the beginning of the ninth century AD and flourished during the next several centuries. Its origins were in the spontaneous utterances of the early Ṣūfī mystics, who poetically expressed their love of God and at the same time their rejection of worldly pleasures. They were inspired by the profane secular Arabic love poetry in its both erotic (*ḥissī*) and Platonic (*'udhrī*) trends, which emerged out of the pre-Islamic period and the early Islamic era. Noteworthy medieval Ṣūfī poets include Rābi'a al-'Adawiyya (d. 801), although there is no clear evidence that she actually composed all the verses attributed to her; al-Ḥusayn ibn Manṣūr al-Ḥallāj (858–922); 'Umar ibn al-Fāriḍ (1181–1234); and Muḥyī al-Dīn ibn 'Arabī (1164–1240). Ṣūfī poetry also developed in other languages, such as Persian, Turkish, and Urdu.[2] From the thirteenth century AD, a new genre of Ṣūfī poetry emerged, the panegyric poems for the Prophet Muḥammad (*al-madā'iḥ al-nabawiyya*), the most famous being "al-Burda" ("The Mantle Ode") by the Egyptian poet Sharaf al-Dīn al-Būṣīrī (d. 1295). This poem, in memory of the poet's miraculous recovery from paralysis through a vision in which the Prophet cast his

[1] This chapter uses material that appeared in various previous publications, such as Snir 1986; Snir 2002; Snir 2006.
[2] On Ṣūfī poetry in general, see Schimmel 1982.

mantle over him, is thought to have special powers against illness and misfortune and has had over forty interpretations and even more imitations.[3] Gradually losing the spontaneity and enthusiasm that had characterized its early stages, Arabic mystic poetry underwent the same process experienced by medieval Arabic canonical poetry, which was integral to it from the standpoint of poetics. Only a very few poets stood out against the background of their era, such as ʻAbd al-Ghanī al-Nābulusī (1640–1731), who also wrote a commentary on Ibn al-Fāriḍ's poetry. In our times, traditional Ṣūfī poetry has been primarily written within the circles of Ṣūfī orders and published by magazines, such as *Majallat al-Taṣawwuf al-Islāmī* (*The Magazine of Islamic Sufism*), the organ of the High Council of the Ṣūfī Orders in Egypt, as well as in special religious collections. Needless to say, the discourse that such poetry supports and of which it is an integral part is the Islamist discourse, which is of marginal status in the contemporary secular literary system.[4]

The birth of modern Arabic secular poetry in the second half of the nineteenth century paved the way for the appearance of mystic dimensions in non-religious poetry. Neoclassical poets, such as the Egyptians Maḥmūd Sāmī al-Bārūdī (1839–1904), Aḥmad Shawqī (1868–1932), and Ḥāfiẓ Ibrāhīm (1871–1932); and the Iraqis Jamīl Ṣidqī al-Zahāwī (1863–1936), Maʻrūf al-Ruṣāfī (1875–1945), and Muḥammad Mahdī al-Jawāhirī (1900–1997), turned to the poetic medieval heritage in trying to achieve similar qualities by means of *muʻāraḍa* (a contestatory emulation), that is, composing a poem according to the rhyme and meter of a well-known poem. Among the classical poems that served as models were Ṣūfī poems, such as the aforementioned "al-Burda." Dealing only marginally with mystic essential or ecstatic topics, these poets concentrated primarily on stylistic imitation of the early Ṣūfī and panegyric poems for the Prophet. Consequently, their poems—prompted by the attempt to exhibit a high degree of technical ability—generally seem insincere in their expressions of divine love. An important shift became apparent in the poetry written especially after the First World War. Poets started to emphasize personal experiences and feelings, a desire to be absorbed by nature, and numerous pantheistic revelations and mythological elements. Among them were Muslim poets, such as the Egyptians Aḥmad Zakī Abū Shādī (1892–1955), Ibrāhīm Nājī (1893–1953), and ʻAlī Maḥmūd Ṭāhā (1902–1949); the Tunisian Abū al-Qāsim al-Shābbī (1909–1934); and the Sudanese al-Tījānī Yūsuf Bashīr (1910–1937); as well as Christian poets, such as the Mahjari poets active mainly in New York—Jubrān Khalīl

3 Mubārak 1935, pp. 148, 161–70.

4 On the Islamist discourse, see Snir 2006.

Jubrān (Gibran) (1883–1931), Mīkhā'īl Nu'ayma (1889–1988), Nasīb 'Arīḍa (1887–1946), Īliyā Abū Māḍī (1889–1957), and Rashīd Ayyūb (1872–1941).

Following the Second World War, which undermined the belief that technology and science would be able to bring about human salvation, one senses a strong tendency to return to the early, pure values of Muslim mysticism. This appeared first in the works of Muslim poets who had previously been Communist or leftists. Trying to heal their spiritual malaise and to express their sense of alienation in modern civilization, they found refuge in Sufism. The spread of classical Ṣūfī literature among the intellectuals, as part of the disappointment from material civilization and Westernization, has reinforced the mystical tendency in Arab poetry. It was also prompted by the great impact of the "irrational" schools in modern Western literature—Romanticism, Surrealism, and Symbolism. This trend, which we may call the "neo-Ṣūfī trend" in contemporary Arabic poetry, has since the late 1950s been a part of the canonical secular discourse. The neo-Ṣūfī poets have employed mystical concepts, figures, and motifs, particularly Islamic, for the expression of contemporary experiences, philosophies, and ideologies.[5] Mystical dimensions in contemporary Arabic poetry reflect nearly all aspects of mysticism, beginning with asceticism, that is, the *via purgativa* (the purifying path), and ending in the supreme mystical stage, or the *via unitiva* (the unifying path). However, contrary to the medieval Ṣūfī poets, contemporary Arab poets do not practicably follow a mystic or Ṣūfī way of life. Three of the major canonical poets since the 1950s have been at the center of the neo-Ṣūfī[6] canonical trend: the Iraqi 'Abd al-Wahhāb al-Bayyātī (1926–1999), the Egyptian Ṣalāḥ 'Abd al-Ṣabūr (1931–1981), and the Syrian 'Alī Aḥmad Sa'īd, Adūnīs (b. 1930). Modern Arabic fiction also includes conspicuous mystic dimensions requiring a separate comprehensive study—suffice it to mention the Nobel laureate Najīb Maḥfūẓ (1911-2006), whose works are loaded not only with many Qur'ānic allusions,[7] but also with mystical Ṣūfī terminology

[5] On this subject, see Semaan 1979, pp. 517–31; Haddāra 1981, pp. 107–22; Schimmel 1983, pp. 216–28; Snir 1984, pp. 12–13; Snir 1986; Snir 1992, pp. 24–6; Snir 1993, pp. 74–88; Snir 1994–1995, pp. 165–175; Snir 1995, pp. 23–7; al-Mūsawī 2006a, pp. 115–17, 142–3, 260–3; Snir 2006; Ayachi 2012.

[6] The use of the term "neo-Sufism" in the present study has no relevance to the concept of neo-Sufism in Sufi Studies. There, it is part of a discussion on the concept of an early Enlightenment movement in the Muslim world that predated, and was independent of, the European models. See O'Fahey and Radtke 1993, pp. 52–87; Radtke 1996, pp. 326–64; Lawrence 2011, pp. 355–84.

[7] 'Abd al-Ḥalīm 2014, pp. 104–26. See also the insights of the critic Muḥammad Ḥasan 'Abd Allāh (b. 1935) in *al-Ahrām*, November 6, 2020.

and insights, especially from the 1960s onward.[8] However, Maḥfūẓ's mystical tendency never came at the expense of man's concern with the world and the life of people:

> *Sufism* is a form of aristocracy, but my way is the people's way. The hierarchy of *sufism* consists in repentance, renunciation, piety, surrender to Divine will etc., but my way consists in freedom, culture, science, industry, agriculture, technology, democracy and faith. *Sufism* sees the Devil as the true enemy of mankind, whereas my enemies include poverty, ignorance, disease, exploitation, despotism, falsity and fear.[9]

2. POETRY AND MYSTICISM

The poetic experience and the most intense religious experience—the mystical experience—share several similarities.[10] For example, both of them are emotional experiences that are given verbal expression. At the same time, it is claimed, especially in mysticism, both in general[11] and within the context of Islam,[12] that it is impossible to convey an emotional experience in its entirety through the medium of words—the experience is beyond the power of language, even if there is a desire to speak about it. The ineffable is by definition inexpressible, and no small number of poets and mystics have fallen into deep silence or at least expressed their craving for it (besides, of course, those unknown poets and mystics who chose silence from the start). But, paradoxically, the difficulties in expression have not prevented mystics and poets from attempting to communicate these experiences, for otherwise no one would know of their existence. Furthermore, a cursory survey of the massive corpus of literary and religious writings reveals that those difficulties would seem to have only prompted such attempts to convey these experiences.

Another similarity between both experiences when expressed verbally is the intense use of poetic means of expression—the evident fact that the most successful attempts to give verbal vent to mystical experiences have been through the medium of poetry. The extensive employment of symbols, similes, metaphors, synesthesia, and oxymorons, in addition to a distinct tendency toward opaqueness and ambiguousness, is shared by both poets and mystics in trying to describe their experiences. Surrealism had a

[8] On Sufism in modern Arabic fiction, see Snir 1986, pp. 178–82; El-Enany 1993, pp. 14–16, 60, 102–10, 157–64; Kropp 2004–2005, pp. 61–9; Elmarsafy 2012.

[9] See al-Enany 1993, pp. 230–1.

[10] Korteling 1928, pp. 163–4.

[11] See Knox 1951, p. 249; Scholem 1954, pp. 4–5; Heiler 1958, pp. 139–42, 147, 190; Eliade 1959, p. 10.

[12] See al-Ghazālī 1956, p. 96.

powerful impact on such poetry, for example, in automatic writing. A major characteristic common to poetry and mysticism is the leap beyond recognized reality to a world always in need of revelation. In order to provide this, the ancient image of the poet as a prophet was revived. This image was also common in Romantic poetry and is still used by post-Romantic poets.[13] In addition, the vision (*ru'yā*) has a prominent place, according to contemporary poets, in both mystical and poetic experiences. The vision reconstructs the world beyond ordinary perception, and things in everyday reality are seen in a different light as being distinct from their external appearances.[14]

Both mysticism and poetry are described as being inspired by supernatural forces. The mystical experience is referred to as a divine gift, as illustrated by the first part of the Ṣūfī saying *al-aḥwāl mawāhib wa-l-maqāmāt makāsib* ("the mystical states are divine gifts, while the stations can be attained by human efforts").[15] The poet is compared with *majnūn*, or a madman,[16] as long ago it was common in Arab society to treat the poet as an individual in touch with devils and spirits (*jinn*), a conception whose roots may be attributed to the pre-Islamic period.[17] This was also common in Romantic poetry in general,[18] being an echo of the same view familiar to ancient Greek culture,[19] such as found in the teachings of Plato.[20] Significantly, madness, or the psychotic state, is sometimes considered a special mode of consciousness parallel to the mystical experience.[21] Poetry and mysticism are also united in their rejection of rational thought, which, according to the Ṣūfī mystics, is an obstacle on the path to true experience. Contact with the divine essence, according to Ṣūfī theory, can be achieved only through the heart.[22]

13 See, for example, 'Abd al-Ṣabūr 1982, p. 70.

14 See al-Bayyātī 1968, pp. 109–10; Adūnīs 1974, p. 97.

15 See al-Qushayrī n.d., p. 54. Cf. Surūr 1957, pp. 111–12; Trimingham 1971, p. 201 n. 2; Snir 1999, pp. 6–7.

16 See al-Bayyātī 1979, III, p. 155.

17 For example, see Imru' al-Qays 1964, p. 322. Cf. Majali 1988, ch. 1. Jan Retsö rejects the usual rendering of the terms *shā'ir* and *shu'arā'* in the Qur'ān as "poet" and "poets," arguing that this is an example of how later concepts distort the original text and its meaning. Instead, he sees the two words *shā'ir* and *kāhin* as designating "different kinds of soothsayers or diviners, that is, people who were in contact with the divine world" (Retsö 2010, p. 290. Cf. Haq 2011, pp. 643–4; Zekavat 2015, pp. 50–1). See also the discussion between Irfan Shahīd (1926–2016) and Michael J. Zwettler (1940–2010) on the Sūra of the Poets (xxvi) (Shahīd 1965, pp. 563–80; Zwettler 1978; Shahīd 1983, pp. 1–21; Zwettler 1990, pp. 75–119, 205–31; Shahīd 2004, pp. 175–220; Zwettler 2007, pp. 111–66).

18 Adams 1971, p. 511.

19 See Homer 1984, p. 337.

20 Plato 1937 [1892], I, pp. 249–50, 288–90.

21 See James 1945, p. 26; Tart 1969, pp. 23–43; Dols 1992, pp. 388–410.

22 See Stoddart 1976, pp. 45–6; al-Ḥifnī 1980, pp. 35, 218.

Arab poets also find parallels between the stages of mystical experience and the poetic creative process, sometimes even stating that they are identical. Ṣalāḥ ʿAbd al-Ṣabūr goes so far as to make some very unusual interpretations of early Ṣūfī texts, which actually constitute a unique independent theory of the creative process. Since poetry is not the fruit of a simple combination of inspiration and craftsmanship, ʿAbd al-Ṣabūr introduces new ideas and incorporates them into his own theory of the creative poetic process.[23] Poetry is a kind of *nashwa* (ecstasy), and art in general is "the moments of ecstasy of human beings." ʿAbd al-Ṣabūr borrows the image of the Ṣūfī progressing on the path toward the divine essence: poetry is a path with many obstacles and risks, and he who chooses it takes his life into his own hands, just like the mystic who takes the path to God. This path is full of dangers, about which various mystical traditions warn, among them being madness. The severance of all connections with the commonplace reality—a fundamental condition of the mystical experience and, according to ʿAbd al-Ṣabūr, also of the creative experience—and the propinquity to the absolute essence are likely to cost one his sanity:

> يتاح لكثير من الشّعراء والفنّانين أن يقتربوا من دائرة النّار مرّة أو مرّات في حياتهم، وهم حينئذ يذهلون عن ذواتهم ليقتربوا من هذه الذّات اللّافحة. ولكنّ هذا الاقتراب محفوف بالمخاطر، إذ أنّهم حين يعودون إلى عالمهم العاديّ بعد هذا الاغتراب المخيف تظلّ هذه الأقباس الّتي حازوها مشتعلة في نفوسهم، فتنعكس بعد ذلك على رؤيتهم للحياة، وعلى تصرّفاتهم اليوميّة العاديّة. فلن يستطيع شاعر وصل إلى قلب دائرة اليأس العميق أن يبتسم بعد ذلك. ولن يستطيع قصّاص لمس قلب الجنون أن يتعقّل، ولنذكر عندئذ جي دي موباسان، فهو أحد الّذين كتبهم ما كتبوه.

Many a poet and artist, once or several times in their life, have the opportunity to be close to the circle of fire, and at the same time to be absent from themselves in order to be close to this burning essence. However, moving close to it has its dangers, as when they return to their normal world after that frightening estrangement, the firebrands they have acquired remain burning in their souls, to be reflected afterward in their vision of life, and in their daily normal behavior. After reaching the heart of the circle of deep despair, a poet will never be able to smile. And a writer, after touching the heart of madness, will never be able to be sane. Let us mention Guy de Maupassant, who was one of those who were written by what they had written.[24]

[23] ʿAbd al-Ṣabūr 1969, pp. 5–18.

[24] ʿAbd al-Ṣabūr 1983, p. 11. The French writer Guy de Maupassant (1850–1893) had suffered since his twenties from syphilis, which later caused his mental disorder. He attempted suicide (December 1891) and spent the last eighteen months of his life in a mental home in Paris, as described by his valet François Tassart in *Maupassant* (1883–1893) (1911) (Reid 1976, pp. 395, 609).

In these words 'Abd al-Ṣabūr alludes as well to Nikos Kazantzakis' aforementioned novel *Zorba the Greek* (1946) where the dangers of the poetic creative process are presented in a dialogue between the narrator and Zorba:

> I felt deep within me that the highest point a man can attain is not Knowledge, or Virtue, or Goodness, or Victory, but something even greater, more heroic and more despairing: Sacred Awe! "Can't you answer?" asked Zorba anxiously. I tried to make my companion understand what I meant by Sacred Awe. "We are little grubs, Zorba, minute grubs on the small leaf of a tremendous tree. This small leaf is the earth. The other leaves are the stars that you see moving at night. We make our way on this little leaf examining it anxiously and carefully. We smell it; it smells good or bad to us. We taste it and find it eatable. We beat on it and it cries out like a living thing. Some men—the more intrepid ones—reach the edge of the leaf. From there we stretch out, gazing into chaos. We tremble. We guess what a frightening abyss lies beneath us. In the distance we can hear the noise of the other leaves of the tremendous tree, we feel the sap rising from the roots to our leaf and our hearts swell. Bent thus over the awe-inspiring abyss, with all our bodies and all our souls, we tremble with terror. From that moment begins ..." I stopped. I wanted to say "from that moment begins poetry", but Zorba would not have understood. I stopped. "What begins?" asked Zorba's anxious voice. "Why did you stop?" "... begins the great danger, Zorba. Some grow dizzy and delirious, others are afraid; they try to find an answer to strengthen their hearts, and they say: 'God!'. Others again, from the edge of the leaf, look over the precipice calmly and bravely and say: 'I like it.'"[25]

Particularly for those who undertake the journey without the necessary preparation, the dangers of the true poetic and mystical experience are great. 'Abd al-Ṣabūr mentions ancient traditions that maintain that it even can lead to death, as in the case of Abū al-Ḥusayn al-Nūrī (d. 908), whose soul expired after achieving a mystical ecstasy.[26] Also, it is reminiscent of the view that poetry is a type of madness, as we find in Plato's writings, in which his political and moral philosophy dominate any artistic conceptions. For example, in *Phaedrus* he absolutely rejects the possibility that valuable works of art can be created without some form of madness:

> He who, having no touch of the Muses' madness in his soul, comes to the door and thinks that he will get into the temple by the halo of art—he, I say, and his poetry are not admitted; the sane man disappears and is nowhere when he enters into rivalry with the madman.[27]

25 Kazantzakis 1996 [1946], pp. 269–70.

26 See al-Ṭūsī 1960, p. 363. Cf. the Kabbalistic perception of Ben Azai's death (Talmud Bavli, Ḥagiga 14b). See Scholem 1954, pp. 52, 361; Scholem 1972, p. 57.

27 Plato 1937 [1892], I, pp. 249–50. On madness and poetry in Arabic literary history, see Van Gelder 2017, pp. 150–75. On "Oriental madness" and civilization, see Abi-Rached 2020, ch. 1.

The view that, possessed by a madness, the poet is not in control of himself when he writes was a popular belief in the Renaissance. The question of whether or not there is a scientific basis for the idea of poetic madness is beyond the scope of the present study; however, history has shown that poets, such as Sappho (*c.* 630 BC), Lucretius (*c.* 99–*c.* 55 BC), François Villon (1431–1489?), William Collins (1721–1759), Christopher Smart (1722–1771), Gerard de Nerval (1808–1855), and Ezra Pound (1885–1972) all exhibited personality disturbances. The Romantic theory of the artist as tormented outcast was subsumed by Sigmund Freud, who says that the artist is neurotic and that his work is a by-product and often symbolic statement of his disturbance.[28]

The parallel between the poet, the mystic, and the madman is also expressed in 'Abd al-Ṣabūr's poetry.[29] In his poetics, he focused his attention on the similarities and parallels between the mystical experience and the poetic creative process. Both of them take place in the soul, but they also receive verbal expression, although the claim is frequently made that it is impossible to convey the experience in its entirety through the medium of words. Out of a deep belief in the basic correspondence between the mystical experience and the poetic creative one, together with studying Western theories 'Abd al-Ṣabūr searched through the classical Ṣūfī literature, and particularly *al-Risāla fī 'Ilm al-Taṣawwuf* by Abū al-Qāsim 'Abd al-Karīm ibn Hawāzin al-Qushayrī (986–1072) and *Kitāb al-Luma'* by Abū Naṣr al-Sarrāj al-Ṭūsī (d. 988/989).[30] The process of creating a poem comprises, according to 'Abd al-Ṣabūr, three stages, the first being the original idea for the writing of the poem. This idea is somewhat obscure and totally lacking context, and under no circumstances is it to be subjected to the authority of the intellect—if it is subordinated to the intellect, then it will be dry and barren of fruit. The intellect must remove its censor from the gate and let the ideas flash unimpeded through the mind. These flashing ideas are characteristic of both dreams and the creative process, but 'Abd al-Ṣabūr maintains that this is also the link between the poetic process and mystical experience: the first stage of the poetic creative process is similar to the *wārid* (lit. "something which comes"), a Ṣūfī term denoting one of the preliminary stages of mystical experience.[31] 'Abd al-Ṣabūr chooses this term because of the condition accompanying it in Ṣūfī sources:

أن يستغرق القلب وأن يكون له فعل.

It must occupy the heart and entail some activity.

[28] Preminger 1974, p. 635.
[29] For example, see 'Abd al-Ṣabūr 1972, I, p. 79.
[30] For example, see 'Abd al-Ṣabūr 1969, pp. 7–12.
[31] On its meaning in the Ṣūfī tradition, see al-Qushayrī n.d., p. 74.

The advantage of the *wārid* is that it is completely divorced from rational thought, and for this reason it more appropriately describes the initial idea for the creation of a poem than does the term "intuition," which was coined by the French philosopher Henri Louis Bergson (1859–1941).[32] "Intuition," says 'Abd al-Ṣabūr, while by nature very different from rational thought, is not entirely separate from it, whereas in the *wārid* there is no rational element whatsoever. It is evident from the short passage in which 'Abd al-Ṣabūr comments on the Bergsonian "intuition" that he closely read Bergson's writings. Considering "intuition" to be the decisive philosophical act, Bergson applied his contrast between dynamic reality and static appearance to the activities of the mind, seeing "intuition"—the direct apprehension of process—as the discoverer of truth, whereas the intellect, the analytic faculty, was only the servant of the will. "Intuition," according to Bergson, is the state of mind in which we are aware of the quality and flow of inner consciousness. In "Introduction to Metaphysics" from his *The Creative Mind*, he writes:

> If we compare the various ways of defining metaphysics and of conceiving the absolute, we shall find, despite apparent discrepancies, that philosophers agree in making a deep distinction between two ways of knowing a thing. The first implies going all around it, the second entering into it. The first depends on the viewpoint chosen and the symbols employed, while the second is taken from no viewpoint and rests on no symbol. Of the first kind of knowledge we shall say that it stops at the relative; of the second that, wherever possible, it attains the absolute ... An absolute can only be given in an intuition, while all the rest has to do with analysis. We call intuition here the sympathy by which one is transported into the interior of an object in order to coincide with what there is unique and consequently inexpressible in it.[33]

Bergson says that intelligence and instinct are turned in opposite directions, the former toward inert matter, the latter toward life. Intelligence, by means of science, which is its handmaiden, will deliver up to us more and more completely the secret of physical operations; of life, it brings us—moreover only claims to bring us—a translation that is inert. Intelligence goes all around life, taking from outside the greatest possible number of views of it, drawing it into itself instead of entering into it. But it is to the very inwardness of life that "intuition" leads us. In his *Creative Evolution*, Bergson states that by intuition he means

> instinct that has become disinterested, self-conscious, capable of reflecting upon its object and of enlarging it indefinitely. That an effort of this kind is not

[32] 'Abd al-Ṣabūr translates it into Arabic as *ḥads*. Another frequent translation is *ru'yā* (e.g., Wahba 1974, pp. 167–8, 211).

[33] Bergson 1968, pp. 187–90.

> impossible, is proved by the existence in man of an aesthetic faculty along with normal perception. Our eye perceives the features of the living being, merely as assembled, not as mutually organized. The intention of life, the simple movement that runs through the lines, that binds them together and gives them significance, escapes it. This intention is just what the artist tries to regain, in placing himself back within the object by the kind of sympathy, in breaking down, by an effort of intuition, the barrier that puts up between him and his model ... Intuition may enable us to grasp what it is that intelligence fails to give us, and indicate the means of supplementing it.[34]

Hence, "intuition" is compared with the inner excitement that enables a writer to fuse his mass of materials into a unity, which he cannot do unless he has first gathered the materials by intellectual effort.[35] As ʿAbd al-Ṣabūr rightly indicates, Bergson does not present "intuition" as something apart from the intellect, although he does describe both of them as if they were polar opposites. Conceiving the initial idea for composing a poem as something like "intuition," ʿAbd al-Ṣabūr is fond of Bergson's analysis but at the same time refuses to let the intellect play any role at this stage of the creative poetic process. He prefers the Ṣūfī term *wārid* to signify the initial stage in which the poet is suddenly seized by the idea for a poem: it could be a sentence whose meaning is obscure at first, or a new verse whose words suddenly leap into the poet's consciousness. This could happen anywhere or at any time—when the poet is alone or in society, at work or lying in bed at night—without needing to perform any activity so as to hasten its arrival.

Based upon the first stage of the *wārid*, and following a period of incubation of this initial idea, now begins the second stage of the creative process, which is also grounded in the Ṣūfī tradition. According to the Ṣūfī mystics, the *wārid* must be followed by an act, and this act in the creative process, according to ʿAbd al-Ṣabūr, is *al-talwīn wa-l-tamkīn* (lit. "the change and consolidation"), that is, the transition of the Ṣūfī mystic from one ecstatic state to another along the path of union with God.[36] The term *talwīn* means perpetual change from one state to another, while *tamkīn* means consolidation in a certain state, or, as described by Ibn ʿArabī, *ḥāl ahl al-wuṣūl* (the state in which are found those who are on their way to the highest mystical level).[37] Using this Ṣūfī term to describe the second stage of the creative process, ʿAbd al-Ṣabūr maintains that it is here that the poet actually creates the poem. In order

34 Bergson 1954, pp. 186–7.

35 Cf. Flew 1979, p. 65; Urmson and Rée, 1989, p. 44.

36 On its meaning in the Ṣūfī tradition, see al-Qushayrī n.d., pp. 69–70; Ibn ʿArabī 1938, pp. 239–40.

37 Ibn ʿArabī 1938, p. 240.

to explain this term, he quotes the following sentence from al-Qushayrī's *al-Risāla fī ʿIlm al-Taṣawwuf*:

واعلم أن التّغيّر بما يرد على العبد يكون لأحد أمرين: إما لقوّة الوارد أو لضعف صاحبه والسّكون من صاحبه لأحد أمرين إما لقوّته أو لضعف الوارد عليه.

> Know that the change by means of the *wārid* is caused by one of the following two conditions: either because of the power of the *wārid* or the weakness of the man smitten by it. In contrast, lack of change is either the result of the strength of the man or the weakness of the *wārid*.[38]

Illustrative of the reason for the failure of some of the mystics to arrive at the stage of *al-talwīn wa-l-tamkīn*, ʿAbd al-Ṣabūr also states that it can explain the failure of certain poets to complete a poem they have started. A reading of the entire section from al-Qushayrī's *al-Risāla* shows, however, that ʿAbd al-Ṣabūr interprets the text, knowingly or unknowingly, in a way that is inconsistent with Ṣūfī terminology. Prior to the sentence quoted above, al-Qushayrī writes[39] that *talwīn* is the stage of change, of ascent from state to state until the mystic arrives at the state of consolidation (*tamkīn*) in an ecstatic state. He uses concepts borrowed from the nomadic life: *talwīn* is compared with wandering in the desert, while *tamkīn* is arrival at the base camp. Al-Qushayrī cites a number of examples: Moses was in a state of *talwīn*, that is, of change, and when he heard the voice of God he had to cover his face. It is found in the Qur'ān:

فلما تجلّى ربّه للجبل جعله دكّا وخرّ موسى صعقا.

> And when his Lord revealed Him to the mountain He made it crumble to dust, and Moses fell down swooning.[40]

All this because of the dreadful thing that he saw, for the contact with the divine essence had a deep impact upon him.[41] In contrast, the Prophet Muḥammad was in a state of *tamkīn* and therefore, as al-Qushayrī says, "he returned as he had gone, for what he saw on that night did not affect him." This is similar to the story of Joseph: when the women saw him, in their amazement at his beauty, they wounded their hands with their knives, which were meant for cutting food, and cried:

حاش لله ما هذا بشرا إن هذا إلا ملك كريم.

> God save us! This is no mortal, he is no other but a noble angel.[42]

38 Al-Qushayrī n.d., p. 70.
39 Al-Qushayrī n.d., p. 69.
40 *Al-Aʿrāf* 143.
41 Cf. "for man shall not see me and live" (Exodus 33:20).
42 *Yūsuf* 31.

By contrast, Zulaykhā was "stronger than them in terms of her ability to withstand Joseph's charm." In other words, she was in the state of consolidation, *tamkīn*, and therefore she remained untouched.[43] Only after adducing these examples does al-Qushayrī cite the sentence quoted by ʻAbd al-Ṣabūr. Hence, unlike the explanation given by ʻAbd al-Ṣabūr, this sentence was not intended, in its original Ṣūfī context, to clarify the reason for the failure of the mystic to arrive at the stage of *al-talwīn wa-l-tamkīn*. Instead, it describes when both states, *talwīn* and *tamkīn*, separately, are possible. ʻAbd al-Ṣabūr's eagerness to draw a parallel between the ecstatic state of the mystic and the state of the poet during the creative process led him to project onto the early Ṣūfī text new meanings. This enthusiasm is also expressed in the purpose of the creative process found, according to ʻAbd al-Ṣabūr, in the stage of *al-talwīn wa-l-tamkīn*, a purpose that is summarized in a sentence that he quotes without reference:

إنتهى سفر الطّالبين إلى الظّفر بنفوسهم فإذا ظفروا بنفوسهم فقد وصلوا.

This sentence, says ʻAbd al-Ṣabūr, states the purpose of the poetic experience as well as that of the mystical experience, namely, *al-ẓafar bi-l-nafs*. Introducing two concepts from the philosophy of art, he asserts that mimesis (imitation) for the artist and catharsis (purgation) for the receptor composed the axis of Aristotle's view on art: "Both are two sides of *al-ẓafar bi-l-nafs*."

According to Plato's pragmatic theory, poetry, like art in general, is a harmful lie and poets are dangerous to society, since their activity leads men away from the truth. This view is based upon metaphysical, ethical, and psychological considerations. Locating reality in what he calls "Ideas," or "Forms," rather than in the world of "appearances" as experienced through the senses, Plato maintains that there is an intelligible world of Ideas and that knowing them is the first possible kind of knowledge. In fact, it is the only kind of knowledge, for, strictly speaking, only the immutable can be known and only the Ideas are immutable. Our rational powers acquaint us with the Ideas and with the truth, while the objects perceived through the senses are merely copies of the Ideas—the concrete reality is nothing but a kind of mimesis, an imitation of eternal ideas. Hence, the poet is comparable

[43] See al-Kalābādhī 1980, p. 151. The story of Joseph and Zulaykhā (her name is mentioned only in later traditions) is frequently mentioned in *Adab* books so as to illustrate such love predicaments as women's trickery (e.g., al-Washshā' 1965, p. 172). The story is also widespread in mystical contexts, where it is used, for example, to illustrate the stage of *fanā*' based upon the Qur'ān's words: "And when they saw him, they so admired him that they cut their hands" (*Yūsuf* 31). See al-Iskandarī 1954, pp. 163–4, 214. Cf. Davidson 1972, I, pp. 44–5; Mughulṭāy 1997, p. 37. On the story, see also Dols 1992, pp. 340–5.

with someone holding up a mirror to the physical world,[44] making copies of copies, his creation twice removed from reality. Being a secondary imitation of true reality, poetry can thus be of no use to us in educating the community and consequently has no place in the ideal city. Poetry can also have a detrimental effect on the human soul, creating an illusion that can foment unnecessary emotions and lead to emotional imbalance, thus indirectly turning citizens into negative social factors. In the ideal state, the Kallipolis, ruled by the philosopher, art is a lie and only the philosopher possesses absolute knowledge. The only good government, according to Plato, is by those who have entry into the pure realm of Ideas—philosophers should be kings, and the ideal city should be a "philosophocracy." In the Cave Parable in *Politeia* (= *Republic*), which is essentially a combination of the Sun Parable and the Divided Line Parable,[45] the philosopher is morally obligated to descend into the cave—in which the only perceptions are of shadowy images of the outside world—in order to guide people out into the light. As for the poets, they must be banished from the state or limited by strict censorship on the composition of songs offering innocuous praise to the state, propagating myths, and praising the gods and the leaders. For perhaps the first time in human history, Plato has decreed a harsh and thorough censorship of the arts. Art must serve the state and be purified of any elements that might corrupt the youth.[46]

In his later dialogues, Plato hints at the possibility of a true mimesis that would reproduce real nature and even present the universe as a work of art, an image of the world of Ideas made by a divine craftsman. From here, it is only a small step to conceiving visual arts, and then poetry, as a sensuous embodiment of the ideal. Plato never took this step, but the Neoplatonists did and in Plotinus' system he assigns art a higher place. He believes that the beauty of the artist's creation lies not in any physical object that it may copy, but in what the artist imposes on his materials, turning them into something other than what they were and giving them a new form; this attainment comes from within the artist, who is capable of adding where nature is lacking. In the tractate *On Intellectual Beauty*, he opines that there exists a struggle between the artist and his materials and that in any successful

[44] Plato 1937 [1892], I, pp. 852–6.
[45] Plato 1937 [1892], I, pp. 769–76.
[46] Plato's views on poetry are very similar to those of early Islam, especially the absence of a distinction between ethics and aesthetics and the judging of art by standards of morality. For a comparison between the poetics of Plato and his attack on poetry and poets, and the attitude of the Prophet Muḥammad and the Qur'ān to poetry and poets, see Kawar 1954, pp. 61–9; Zekavat 2015, pp. 39–58. On the attitude of the religious establishment toward poets and poetry in the first centuries of Islam, see Yosefi 2017, pp. 49–82.

work of art these materials are partly subdued—the form in the artist's mind, which is derived from the intellect and ultimately from the unknowable "One," is given visible expression:

> The arts are not to be slighted on the ground that they create by imitation of natural objects; for, to begin with, these natural objects are themselves imitations; then, we must recognize that they give no bare reproduction of the thing seen but go back to the Reason-Principles from which Nature itself derives, and, furthermore, that much of their work is all their own; they are holders of beauty and add where nature is lacking. Thus Pheidias wrought the *Zeus* upon no model among things of sense but by apprehending what form Zeus must take if he chose to become manifest to sight.[47]

Replying to Plato's criticism of the poet as a mere imitator of appearances, Aristotle states in his *Poetics* that the world of appearances is not merely an ephemeral copy of that changeless heaven of Ideas. He believes that change is a fundamental process of nature, which he regards as a creative force with a direction. Reality is the process by which a form manifests itself through the concrete and by which the concrete takes on meaning working in accordance with ordered principles. The poet's imitation is an analogue of this process; he takes a form from nature and reshapes it in a different matter or medium. This medium, which the form does not inhabit in nature, is the source of each work's inward principle of order and consequently of its independence from slavish mimicry. The poet is thus an imitator and a creator. It is through his peculiar form of imitation that the poet discovers the ultimate form of actions. Art is a sort of improvement on nature, in that the poet has brought to completion what nature, operating with different principles of order, is still endeavoring to complete. In contrast to Plato, Aristotle thought that the concepts of truth and falsehood did not apply to art. Moreover, he believed that the artist had a higher degree of intellectual understanding than the craftsman, since he did not deal with facts but with possibilities. Aristotle did not see in mimesis an act of mechanical imitation of what was in nature and life, but a description of what was typical in them, the creation of a new reality that was not a mere copy of concrete reality.[48] Artistic imitation embodied general truths, but not in the sense of metaphysical entities like the Platonic Ideas but rather in the sense of the possibilities inherent in human nature.

As for catharsis (purgation), its meaning has been the subject of much debate in the philosophy of art.[49] Aristotle used this term within the general

[47] Plotinus 1956 [1917–1930], pp. 422–3.
[48] Aristotle 1968, p. 15; Aristotle 1967, pp. 32–3.
[49] For example, see Preminger 1974, pp. 106–8.

framework of his pragmatic poetic theory, but did not sufficiently define it. In his *Poetics,* he writes:

> Tragedy, then, is a process of imitating an action which has serious implication, is complete, and possesses magnitude; by means of language which has been made sensuously attractive, with each of its varieties found separately in the parts; enacted by the persons themselves and not presented through narrative; through a course of pity and fear completing the purification [catharsis] of tragic acts which have those emotional characteristics.[50]

Opposing his concept of catharsis to Plato's view of art as fanning dangerous emotions, Aristotle considers art to be beneficial: it cleanses and purifies the soul. Anarchy in the soul is most effectively prevented by giving the emotions expression in a wisely regulated manner, and tragedy is the chief instrument of such wise regulation, for it works by first exciting the emotions of pity and fear and then allaying them, thereby effecting an emotional cure.

'Abd al-Ṣabūr attempted to reconcile the philosophical and aesthetic background of mimesis and catharsis—both concepts being aspects of the *al-ẓafar bi-l-nafs* achieved in the Ṣūfī stage of *al-talwīn wa-l-tamkīn.* Through mimesis, the artist fulfills himself, and this is the great *ẓafar* of his personality. As regards the receptor, he is granted a certain intellectual pleasure. 'Abd al-Ṣabūr rejects Plato's theory of mimesis and instead embraces Aristotle's. As regards the pragmatic aspects of poetry, he also rejects Plato's theory, but does not fully accept Aristotle's. Indicating that it is unclear who is undergoing the cathartic process, the artist or the receptor, 'Abd al-Ṣabūr posits a new interpretation, which is that Aristotle, when writing of catharsis, was referring as much to the artist as to the receptor. Catharsis is, in 'Abd al-Ṣabūr's opinion, *ẓafar akhlāqī bi-l-nafs*, that is, the achievement of spiritual satisfaction, thus raising the soul to a higher level, to one of refinement or simply victory, as though what was being spoken of was *ẓafar al-nafs* without the preposition *bi.*[51]

In his play *Ba'da an Yamūta al-Malik* (*After the King Dies*) (1973),[52] 'Abd al-Ṣabūr introduces yet another interpretation of catharsis. One of the women who opens the play says that its subject is gratification of one's thirst for revenge (*tashaffin*), then another woman says: "Aristotle did not speak of this passion when he spoke of the function of drama as arousing

[50] Aristotle 1967, p. 25; Aristotle 1968, p. 10. Aristotle's understanding of catharsis acquires its overtones from a double linguistic heritage that is in part medical and in part religious (Preminger 1974, pp. 106–7).

[51] 'Abd al-Ṣabūr 1969, pp. 15–17.

[52] This is one of the first examples in modern Arabic literature where the medium turns back on itself and art becomes its own mirror, or, as it is commonly said to do, it becomes narcissistic art; see Alter 1975; Hofstadter 1979; Thiher 1984.

the emotions of pity and fear, thereby forgetting the most beautiful and soft human passion which abides within his soul like a fresh flower—the passion of revenge."[53] 'Abd al-Ṣabūr indicates here that art also cleanses the soul of the emotion of revenge, which is intrinsic to every human being. His interpretation of mimesis and catharsis and his attempt to bring them into harmony with one another and with the Ṣūfī theory of *al-talwīn wa-l-tamkīn* are not in accordance with classical sources. However, his arguments reflect a belief that both mimesis and catharsis are two sides of the same coin of *al-ẓafar bi-l-nafs*, and that they prove the essentially similar features of both poetic and Ṣūfī experiences.

Eager to show the harmony between poetry and Sufism, 'Abd al-Ṣabūr's selective reading of the classical sources is most manifest in his understanding of the Aristotelian definition of catharsis. Although the meaning of catharsis is a subject of debate, no one to my knowledge has argued that catharsis, according to Aristotle, takes place within the artist himself. The debate focuses on whether the catharsis takes place within the soul of the actor if we are speaking of a play or, according to the more generally accepted view, in the spectator. What is more, to say that Aristotle meant that catharsis takes place within the artist is to completely ignore the fact that Aristotle's whole theory of catharsis was framed as an answer to Plato's charge that poetic drama encourages anarchy in the soul by feeding the passions instead of starving them. In addition, Aristotle does not speak of catharsis as taking place at the time of the artistic creative process, but rather as taking effect following completion of the artistic work and its presentation before an audience.[54]

As regards the Ṣūfī sources, the sentence that 'Abd al-Ṣabūr quotes is taken from the *al-Risāla* of al-Qushayrī and from the same chapter dealing with *al-talwīn wa-l-tamkīn*.[55] It is not intended to present the aim of the mystical experience, but rather to clarify the transition of the Ṣūfī from the state of *talwīn*, in which his human traits still exist, to the state of *tamkīn*, which is a divine state. The Ṣūfī must free himself from those desires and other earthly aspects of his existence, which are known in Ṣūfī literature as *nafs*.[56] Thus, the battle against the desires of the body is called *mujāhada* or *jihād*

[53] 'Abd al-Ṣabūr 1983 [1973], p. 10. For an English translation of the play, titled *Now the King Is Dead*, see Abdul Saboor 1986.

[54] Philosophy of art has produced theories maintaining that poetry is a catharsis for the author himself (e.g., Edmund Wilson's *The Wound and the Bow* [Wilson 1941], where "wound" refers to the artist's neurosis and "bow" to the art that is its compensation); however, Aristotle himself does not deal with the catharsis of the poet.

[55] Al-Qushayrī n.d., p. 70.

[56] Afīfī 1963, p. 143; Nicholson 1975, p. 39.

al-nafs—al-jihād al-akbar (the greater *jihād*)—as opposed to the *jihād* on the field of battle—*al-jihād al-aṣghar* (the smaller *jihād*). The term is based on the Qur'ānic verse:

والّذين جاهدوا فينا لَنَهْدِيَنَّهُمْ سُبُلَنا.

But those who struggle in Our cause, surely we shall guide them in Our ways.[57]

Returning from his military campaign in Tabūk, the Prophet said, according to one tradition: "We have returned from the smaller *jihād* to the greater *jihād*." When asked what the greater *jihād* was, he replied: "the battle against the desires."[58] *Jihād al-nafs*, which is one of the principles of Muslim asceticism and which appears in early traditions,[59] is based upon verses in the Qur'ān[60] and is a central issue in Ṣūfī and non-Ṣūfī sources.[61] It is also one of the *maqāmāt* (stations) along the Ṣūfī path.[62] Hence, according to the Ṣūfī theory, the sentence quoted by 'Abd al-Ṣabūr should be translated as follows: "The Ṣūfī mystics' journey has concluded in overcoming their souls—if they have overcome their souls, they have arrived [at contact with God]." In other words, *ẓafar bi-l-nafs* in the original context means "overcoming the soul," and this is indeed the early definition of the verb *ẓafira*[63] still used today (*ẓafira 'alayhi = ẓafira bihi*).[64] This meaning is in agreement with the Ṣūfī outlook concerning the suppression of earthly desires as a prerequisite for mystical experience.

Significantly, 'Abd al-Ṣabūr's eagerness to prove the parallel between the mystical experience and the poetic creative process is so great that he reads the ancient texts, be they Ṣūfī or aesthetic, in an untraditional way. His belief in the identity of both experiences was also expressed in a lecture that he gave in the fall of 1979 at the American University in Cairo, in which he stated that the poetic experience "is close to the mystical experience in the common attempt of both to arrive at the truth and the essence of things, without paying any heed to their external qualities."[65] In the stage parallel to *al-talwīn wa-l-tamkīn*, the poem is written, and afterward it arrives at

57 *Al-'Ankabūt* 69.

58 See al-Jīlānī 1331H, I, p. 71; al-Hujwīrī 1926, p. 251; al-Yāfi'ī 1961, p. 103. Cf. Tayan 1965, II, pp. 538–40.

59 For example, see al-Mu'āfā ibn 'Imrān, *Kitāb al-Zuhd* (MS) (Damascus: al-Ẓāhiriyya), 264; Ibn al-Mubārak 1966, pp. 284–5.

60 For example, see *al-'Ankabūt* 6 and 69; *al-Ḥajj* 78; *al-Nāzi'āt* 40.

61 For example, see al-Munāwī 1321H, I, p. 43; al-Tirmidhī 1947, p. 100; al-Tirmidhī 1947a, p. 42; al-Muḥāsibī 1964, p. 59; Ibn Ḥanbal 1969, VI, p. 22.

62 Al-Qushayrī n.d., p. 81; Arberry 1979 [1950], p. 75.

63 Ibn Manẓūr n.d., IV, p. 519; Lane 1968 [1863–1893]), V, p. 1912.

64 Wehr 1976, p. 581.

65 'Abd al-Ṣabūr 1981a, p. 18.

the third stage, that is, the return of the poet to his ordinary state prior to the arrival of the *wārid* and prior to his entrance into the stage of *al-talwīn wa-l-tamkīn*:

> الشّاعر عندئذ يقطع الحوار ليبدأ المحاكمة، فتتجلّى عندئذ حاسّته النّقديّة حين يعيد قراءة قصيدته ليتلمس ما أخطأ من نفسه وما أصاب.

> The poet breaks off the dialogue so that he can pronounce judgment, and then his sense of criticism is revealed when he returns to read the poem which he wrote in order to check where he succeeded and where he failed.[66]

Breaking off from the ecstatic state, the poet returns to his normal psychic condition. Now, he must separate himself from the experience so that his critical faculty can polish the work, correcting deviations in meter and rhyme, changing inappropriate words and the like, before the poem is showcased to the public. In this final stage of the creative process, according to ʻAbd al-Ṣabūr, we sense the spirit of T. S. Eliot (1888–1965), who felt that "the more perfect the artist, the more completely separate in him will be the man who suffers and the mind which creates."[67] It is reminiscent also of William Wordsworth's (1770–1850) words in the preface to the second edition of his *Lyrical Ballads* (1800): "Poetry is the spontaneous overflow of powerful feelings: it takes its origin from emotion recollected in tranquillity."[68] The source of poetry is emotion, but the final poem is not created at the time of the emotion itself but only after it has passed. This idea is widely held among contemporary poets—the Hebrew poet Nathan Zach (1930–2020) says in "The Right Poem," from the collection *All the Milk and Honey* (1966):

> כְּשֶׁהָרֶגֶשׁ דּוֹעֵךְ, הַשִּׁיר הַנָּכוֹן מְדַבֵּר.
> עַד אָז דִּבֵּר הָרֶגֶשׁ, הַשִּׁיר הָאַחֵר.
> עַכְשָׁו הִגִּיעַ הַזְּמַן לַשִּׁיר הַנָּכוֹן לְדַבֵּר.

> When the emotion subsides, the right poem speaks.
> Till then the emotion, the other poem, spoke.
> Now the time has arrived for the right poem to speak.[69]

There is a difference, then, between the "right poem," written in poetic and rhythmic language and employing other poetic methods, and the emotional experience that was the source of that poem. Even the Surrealists, who claimed that the creative process was pure psychic automatism, detached from the bonds of thought, did sometimes endeavor to polish and even

66 ʻAbd al-Ṣabūr 1969, p. 18.
67 Eliot 1960 [1932], pp. 7–8, 358.
68 Wordsworth 1965, p. 460. Cf. Eliot 1960 [1932], p. 10.
69 Zach 1983, p. 68.

rewrite those works originally created by automatic writing.[70] Testifying to his own experience, ʿAbd al-Ṣabūr said: "I have never written when I am at the height of emotion."[71] And in another place: "The poet does not reveal his emotions immediately upon their eruption within him."[72] A generally similar conception we find expressed by ʿAbd al-Wahhāb al-Bayyātī, who states that emotions are nothing but the means for artistic creation in its final form.[73] Al-Bayyātī means not only the temporal difference between the emotional experience and the final poem, but the qualitative difference as well: the poem cannot encompass the whole experience, for there will always remain something of it which is inexpressible.[74] This is an allusion to the argument that the mystical experience cannot be expressed through human language,[75] which is something also found in Ṣūfī sources.[76]

The role of the intellect as opposed to the role of the emotions in the poetic creative process now leads us to the way ʿAbd al-Ṣabūr was inspired by Friedrich Nietzsche. He became acquainted with Nietzsche through the aforementioned Lebanese-American poet and artist Jubrān Khalīl Jubrān (1883–1931), who "enslaved me throughout my youth ... and thus I entered, in my fifteenth year, the strange and frightening world of Nietzsche."[77] After reading works by Jubrān and the book by Mīkhāʾīl Nuʿayma (1889–1988) on Jubrān,[78] ʿAbd al-Ṣabūr read Nietzsche's book *Also sprach Zarathustra* (*Thus Spoke Zarathustra*) (1883–1884), which shook his soul: "Few are the philosophers who can influence the human conscience like Nietzsche; these are the philosophers of the soul, whose philosophy is immersed in poetry, and who dip their quills in the blood of the heart."[79] This book left its imprint on the young poet, as it influenced many other poets and writers of the twentieth

70 Mendelson 1986, p. 17.
71 See al-Miṣrī 1983, p. 41.
72 ʿAbd al-Ṣabūr 1982 [1968], p. 18.
73 Al-Bayyātī 1968, p. 33.
74 *Al-Ahrām*, August 30, 1984, p. 11.
75 Scholem 1954, pp. 4–5; Heiler 1958, pp. 139–42, 147, 190; Eliade 1959, p. 10.
76 Ibn al-ʿArīf 1933, p. 91 (French translation: pp. 51–2); al-Iskandarī 1954, pp. 153–4; al-Ghazālī 1956, p. 96; Ibn al-ʿArīf 1980, pp. 68–9. Cf. Jurji 1938, p. 47; Ḥusayn 1964, p. 77; Waugh 1989, p. 21. See also Scharfstein 1993. On the psychological aspects of ineffability, see Tart 1969, p. 16: "Most often, because of the uniqueness of the subjective experience associated with certain ASC [Altered States of Consciousness] (e.g., transcendental, aesthetic, creative, psychotic, and mystical states), persons claim a certain ineptness or inability to communicate the nature or essence of the experience to someone who has not undergone a similar experience." On ineffability in poetry, see Cariou 2014, pp. 27–58.
77 ʿAbd al-Ṣabūr 1969, p. 40.
78 Nuʿayma 1934; Naimy 1950.
79 ʿAbd al-Ṣabūr 1969, p. 40.

century.[80] From the day ʻAbd al-Ṣabūr read this book, Nietzsche remained close to his heart; for this reason, he was greatly pained when he heard that Nietzsche was considered the spiritual father of Nazism; and he rejoiced when, after many years, he read an article that "purified" Nietzsche of this guilt.[81] Relying on Nietzsche, especially on his Apollonian–Dionysian antinomy, ʻAbd al-Ṣabūr tried to prove that there is a certain rational element in the determination of the structure of a poem. Nietzsche uses this antinomy in his *Die Geburt der Tragödie* (*The Birth of Tragedy*) (1872) in order to distinguish the rational from the emotional and the irrational: "The continuous development of art is bound up with the Apollonian and Dionysian duality—just as procreation depends on the duality of the sexes, involving perpetual strife with only periodically intervening reconciliations."[82] The Apollonian pole in this antinomy, named for Apollo, the god of poetry, medicine, youth, truth, and harmony, represents the rational basis of life and art and can lead to the tyranny of the intellect. By contrast, the Dionysian pole, named for Dionysos, the god of vegetation, wine, and ecstasy, who dies and comes back to life, is the voice of the instincts and desires. It is assumed that the ritual festivities in honor of Dionysos, who was seen by the Greeks as identical to the Egyptian god Osiris, were the beginning of Greek tragedy, namely, the drama of the god's suffering and his return to life. As Greek tragedy developed, one impulse came to balance the other, irrational Dionysian ecstasy being ordered by Apollonian form and repose.

In artistic creation, the Apollonian factor symbolizes the poet's dream of form, the impulse that compels him to create an understandable and beautiful world, to crystallize and establish harmony and a symmetrical and meaningful structure. The Dionysian element is the voice of instincts, suffering, ecstasy, and the yearning for death. This Apollonian–Dionysian duality represents, according to some views, not only the dichotomy between the intellect and the heart, logic and instinct, but also, when projected onto broader systems, the dichotomy between culture and the primitive, classicism and romanticism, Hebraism and Hellenism, and (before it was strongly affirmed that "the evidence to support [any] hypothesis of 'innate difference' [between men and women] turns out to be quite slim"),[83] it had been even

[80] Cf. the similarity between *Also sprach Zarathustra*'s influence on ʻAbd al-Ṣabūr and its influence on the Hebrew author Pinḥas Sadeh (1929–1994), who, after reading the book at the age of fourteen, states: "Suddenly I ceased to be alone in the world. I was like a man who found, after long days of sadness and obscure yearnings, the love of which he had dreamed" (Sadeh 1974 [1958], p. 71).

[81] ʻAbd al-Ṣabūr 1969, p. 41.

[82] Nietzsche 1955, p. 47; Nietzsche 1967, p. 33.

[83] Editorial, *Nature Neuroscience* 8.3 (March 2005), p. 253.

argued that this duality represented the dichotomy between the rational male and emotional female; in music, it was argued that this dichotomy was embodied in Ludwig van Beethoven's eighth and seventh symphonies.[84] It was also used to reflect the paradox of different "patterns of culture"—a pattern encouraging emotional abandonment in social responses on the one hand and another producing order and control on the other.[85]

Speaking about the third stage of the poetic process, in which the poet separates himself from the ecstatic experience, 'Abd al-Ṣabūr adopts Nietzsche's dichotomy and declares that great art is that which can "serve both these masters [Apollo and Dionysos] at one and the same time."[86] After the Dionysian phase has passed, the Apollonian phase determines the relationship between the parts of the poem and its internal harmony. This dichotomy becomes an instrument with which 'Abd al-Ṣabūr analyzes artistic works. If we take the Parable of the Chariot and the Two Horses from *Phaedrus*,[87] the intellect is not the driver but rather one of the two horses, alongside which is the other horse, which represents the instincts—the driver is the poet. This, in fact, is the pairing of art and craft, which are combined in the creative process without distinction. Art relates to the emotional source, while craft relates to technique and the medium. In broader terms, this is the pairing of content and form.

'Abd al-Ṣabūr sees in Nikos Kazantzakis' aforementioned novel *Zorba the Greek* (1946) the embodiment of the Apollonian and Dionysian antinomy: Zorba, who loves life and lives in the moment, does not think of the absolute; on the other hand, there is his rational friend, the narrator who behaves according to the intellect. The essay written by 'Abd al-Ṣabūr on this work concludes with the following words:

> The question which hovers over this work is: who is more worthy of being our master and teacher—or holy Sheikh, in the language of the Muslim mystics? He who studies books, acquires knowledge, and spends his nights by the light of the pale lamp, while he struggles with questions for which confusion is the only answer? Or perhaps he who loves life, the earth, and the people, and who tries and experiences everything? Or in the language of the ancient Greeks: are we to live our lives as rational and wise human beings like the followers of Apollo, or spend our lives in the Dionysian camp of those possessed by madness? Have we come into the world in order to tremble on the frozen heights of thought, or to excite ourselves in the burning depths of drunkenness?[88]

84 Cf. Cuddon 1986, pp. 51–2.
85 Benedict 1934.
86 'Abd al-Ṣabūr 1969, p. 20.
87 Plato 1937 [1892], I, pp. 250–1.
88 'Abd al-Ṣabūr 1982a, p. 199.

3. SILENCE AND SPEECH

Early Muslim asceticism (*zuhd*) is the historical basis of Sufism, and many of its principles were later assimilated into the theories of Muslim mysticism. Three primary dimensions of the early *zuhd* are reflected in contemporary Arabic poetry:

(a). *The philosophical dimension*: the dualism between the soul and the body is a fundamental aspect of Muslim asceticism and mysticism, as is the yearning of the soul to escape from the bodily prison and to merge with its divine source.[89] References in contemporary Arabic poetry to the body as despised and to the soul as a divine essence are generally an expression of the search for meaning by human beings. The alienation of man in modern civilization is often compared with the alienation of the soul in its bodily prison.[90] Quite a few poets describe their sense of alienation in terms of the shock experienced by the naïve poet on coming from the sleepy village into the bustling city.[91]

(b). *The existentialist dimension*: like early ascetics (*zuhhād*) and Ṣūfī mystics (who were also called *al-ghurabā'*—"the strangers"), contemporary poets reject materialist reality and express their existentialist alienation from it. They wonder about the meaning and purpose of life, taking imaginary trips to reveal the secret of existence and frequently becoming immersed in a deep depression over the nature of human existence, from which there is no escape. In order to concretize these ideas they use Ṣūfī, folkloristic, and mythological images, such as that of Bishr ibn al-Ḥārith al-Ḥāfī (d. 841),[92] Sindbād (Sinbād),[93] and Sisyphus.[94] As in existentialist philosophy, the conviction of the worthlessness of human existence is often described as an inescapable loss of bearings.[95] Human existence is considered tragic and absurd—alienation, strangeness, spiritual confusion, and sadness are imprinted on the character of man by the very nature his humanness. Expressions of these feelings are found, for example, in 'Abd al-Ṣabūr's play *Musāfir Layl* (*Night*

89 See Al-Ghazālī 1933, III, p. 51; al-Suhrawardī 1957, pp. 9, 39–40; al-Ḥallāj 1974, p. 40.
90 See, for example, 'Abd al-Ṣabūr 1981, pp. 25–7.
91 See, for example, al-Bayyātī 1968, pp. 11–12; Ḥijāzī 1982, 106–12, 188–9, 221–30, 439–46.
92 See, for example, 'Abd al-Ṣabūr 1972, I, pp. 261–9.
93 See, for example, 'Abd al-Ṣabūr 1972, I, pp. 7–13. Cf. Khoury 2016, pp. 95–122, 145–65.
94 See, for example, al-Bayyātī 1984 [1979], pp. 105–10.
95 See, for example, 'Abd al-Ṣabūr 1972, I, pp. 7–13; 'Abd al-Ṣabūr 1981, pp. 19–22, 55–7.

Traveler),[96] which was profoundly inspired by his reading of *Les Mots* by the French existentialist philosopher Jean-Paul Sartre (1905–1980).[97]

(c). *The dimension of self-discipline*: The negation of worldly life is illustrated in Ṣūfī theory in the denial of bodily desires and the striving for death. Likewise, contemporary poets express their loathing of this world and its vanities, encouraging an abstinence from its pleasures and a craving for death, which is, in their eyes, the gate of true life. However, whereas among early Muslim ascetics and Ṣūfī mystics the negation of worldly desires was particularly conspicuous while the yearning for death rather limited—at least in the texts they produced, since Prophetic traditions had forbidden such—contemporary poets frequently express their desire for death. Apart from that, they do not speak out against life in this world but rather against life in modern civilization, yearning for the purity and simplicity of the past, which was free of enslavement to technology and science. Also, unlike the ascetics and early Ṣūfī mystics, contemporary poets generally do not put their ascetic views into daily practice.

At the heart of every form of mysticism, however, lies the yearning for contact with the divine, which assumes the form of love. The expression of this love in contemporary poetry is nearly always linked with Ṣūfī tradition and distinguished by the extensive use of erotic[98] and wine symbolism.[99] As in early Ṣūfī tradition, this love is a secret between the lovers—the mystic-poet and God—and it cannot continue at the same level of intensity once revealed. Also, this love cannot be but reciprocal: Abū al-Qāsim ʿAbd al-Karīm ibn Hawāzin al-Qushayrī (986–1072) defines Ṣūfī love as follows:

> المحبّة حالة شريفة شهد الحقّ سبحانه بها للعبد وأخبر عن محبّته للعبد فالحقّ سبحانه يوصف بأنّه يحبّ العبد والعبد يوصف بأنّه يحبّ الحقّ سبحانه.

> Love is a noble state that God has confirmed as existing in the servant, and He has informed [the servant] of His love for him. So God—Glorious and

[96] ʿAbd al-Ṣabūr 1981 [1969]a.

[97] See especially Sartre 1964, pp. 89–90; Arabic translation: Sartre 1983, pp. 81–2. On Arab existentialism and the impact of Jean-Paul Sartre on Arab intellectuals, see Di-Capua 2012, pp. 1061–91; Di-Capua 2018. See also below, Chapter 6. On how Ṭāhā Ḥusayn (1889–1973) took serious issue with how Sartre reconfigured the relationship between the writer, the text, and society at large, as well as the exclusion of poetry and other non-representational arts like music and the visual arts from the list of committed modes of expression and the engaged arts, see Di-Capua 2012, pp. 89–104.

[98] See, for example, ʿAbd al-Ṣabūr 1981, pp. 43–8; ʿAbd al-Ṣabūr 1986, pp. 13–19.

[99] See, for example, ʿAbd al-Ṣabūr 1981, pp. 69, 85.

> Majestic—is characterized as loving the servant, and the servant is characterized[100] as loving God.[101]

Through this definition, al-Qushayrī states the reciprocity in love that exists between God and the Ṣūfi mystic, but without in any way diminishing the high status of God in that relationship. When depicting the gap between the two agents of love, al-Qushayrī uses the same terms that are employed by the canonical law of Islam: God is *al-Ḥaqq* (The Truth) and the human being is *al-ʿabd* (the servant).[102] Thus, not only does God love His servant, it is He who makes His servant love Him. As for the love of the servant:

> أمّا محبّة العبد لله تعالى فحالة يجدها من قلبه تلطف عن العبارة وقد تحمله تلك الحالة على التّعظيم له وإيثار رضاه وقلّة الصّبر عنه والاهتياج إليه وعدم القرار من دونه ووجود الاستئناس بدوام ذكره له بقلبه وليست محبّة العبد له سبحانه متضمّنة ميلا ولا اختطاطا كيف وحقيقة الصّمديّة مقدّسة عن اللّحوق والدّرك والإحاطة والمحبّ بوصف الاستهلاك في المحبوب أولى منه بأنّ يوصف بالاختطاط ولا توصف المحبّة بوصف ولا تحدّ بحدّ أوضح ولا أقرب إلى الفهم من المحبّة والاستقصاء في المقال عند حصول الإشكال فإذا زال الاستعجام والاستبهام سقطت الحاجة إلى الاستغراق في شرح الكلام.
>
> As for the servant's love for God, it is a state experienced in his heart, too subtle to express it in words. This state may bring him to glorify God, to try to gain His satisfaction, to have little patience in separation from Him, to feel an excitement for him, to find no comfort in anything other than Him, and to experience delight by making continual remembrance of Him in his heart. The servant's love for God does not imply affection or enjoyment. How could this be when the essence of God's eternal subsistence is exalted beyond all attainment, perception, and comprehension? Describing the lover as annihilated in the Beloved is more fitting than describing him as having enjoyment. There is no clearer or more understanding description of love than "love." One should engage in lengthy discussions of any matter only when difficulties appear, but once obscurity and ambiguity depart, there is no need to plunge into the interpretation of words.[103]

The title of one of the poems by Ṣalāḥ ʿAbd al-Ṣabūr, "Tajrīdāt" ("Strippings"),[104] alludes to the Ṣūfi term *tajrīd*, which describes the mystical state of being devoid of everything except for God.[105] The poem, which is divided into three parts, is the last poem in his last collection, *al-Ibḥār*

[100] That is, has the *ṣifa* (quality, attribute, either of the individual or of God) of loving.
[101] Al-Qushayrī 1940, pp. 156–7.
[102] That gap is also emphasized by the phrases used normally in Islamic texts about God (e.g., *Allāh ʿazza wa-jalla*; *al-ḥaqq subḥānahu*; *Allāh taʿālā*).
[103] Al-Qushayrī 1940, p. 158.
[104] ʿAbd al-Ṣabūr 1981, pp. 79–85.
[105] See Ibn ʿArabī 1938, p. 238; al-Ḥifnī 1980, p. 41; al-Kalābādhī 1980, pp. 133–4; al-Ḥakīm 1981, pp. 878–80.

fī al-Dhākira (*Sailing in Memory*). It is loaded with Ṣūfī terms, such as *ḥāl* (a mystical "state"),[106] *yaqīn* (certitude),[107] *ṣaḥw* (sobriety),[108] *maḥw* (effacement),[109] *ṣamt* (silence),[110] and *sirr* (secret—the innermost part of the heart in which the divine revelation is experienced).[111] The first part of the poem describes an ecstatic state that the poet has experienced, while the second part is very rational and refers only indirectly to the mystic refuge. The last part alludes to the radical Ṣūfī *tawakkul* (trust in God);[112] moreover, the speaker considers the yearning for God and the unitive state—the attainment of the absolute, according to the mystics—as the only refuge from the hopelessness of worldly desires. Referring to the ineffable, which is inevitable in the highest mystical state, and employing wine symbolism, he says in the concluding lines of the poem:

يا ربّ! يا ربّ!
أسقيتني حتّى إذا ما مشت
كأسك في موطن إسراري
ألزمتني الصّمت، وهذا أنا
أغصّ مخنوقا بأسراري

Oh Lord! Oh Lord!
You have given me drink so that whenever
Your wine penetrates into my spot of intoxication
You force me to keep silent, and so I am
Choked with my secrets.

The fact that these lines allude to the following two wine verses attributed to the libertine medieval poet Abū Nuwās (*c.* 755–*c.* 813) is not a surprise due to the close relationship of Ṣūfī poetry with classical wine and erotic love poetry:

ولمّا شربناها ودبّ دبيبها   إلى موضع الأسرار قلت لها قفي
مخافة أن يسطو عليّ شعاعها   فتطلع ندماني على سرّي الخفيّ

106 See al-Qushayrī n.d., p. 54; al-Ṭūsī 1960, pp. 66–7; Gardet 1971, pp. 83–5; Trimingham 1971, p. 200; al-Ḥifnī 1980, p. 73; Schimmel 1983, pp. 99–100.

107 See al-Qushayrī n.d., pp. 140–3; al-Ṭūsī 1960, pp. 102–4; al-Ḥakīm 1981, pp. 1247–52.

108 The antithesis of *sukr* (intoxication); see al-Qushayrī n.d., pp. 64–5; Ibn ʿArabī 1938, p. 236; Nicholson 1975, p. 59; al-Kalābādhī 1980, pp. 138–40; al-Ḥakīm 1981, pp. 1205–7; al-Ḥifnī 1980, pp. 131–2, 149; Schimmel 1983, pp. 58, 129.

109 The antithesis of *ithbāt* (assertion); see al-Qushayrī n.d., p. 66; al-Ḥifnī 1980, pp. 10, 239–40; al-Ḥakīm 1981, pp. 1016–17.

110 See al-Qushayrī n.d., pp. 96–100; al-Ḥifnī 1980, pp. 155–6; al-Ḥakīm 1981, pp. 699–702.

111 See al-Ḥifnī 1980, pp. 129–30; Schimmel 1983, p. 192.

112 See al-Qushayrī n.d., pp. 129–37; al-Tirmidhī 1947, p. 100; al-Ṭūsī 1960, pp. 78–9; al-Yāfiʿī 1961, p. 170; al-Kalābādhī 1980, pp. 120–1; Hujwīrī 1999 [1926], p. 146; al-Jīlānī 1331H, II, p. 129; Nicholson 1975, p. 41; Arberry 1979 [1950], p. 76; Schimmel 1983, pp. 117–20.

And when we drank it, its flow crept
Into the spot of the secrets, I command it: stop!
For fear that its rays would assail me so as
My companions would know my hidden secret.[113]

Such wine verses were the background against which the mystical Arab poets composed their poetry alluding to the highest illuminative, ecstatic, and pantheistic stages, including *unio mystica,* in which all distinctions vanish and the mystic and God become one entity.[114]

Some poems by neo-Ṣūfī poets describe the highest illuminative, ecstatic, and pantheistic stages, including *unio mystica.*[115] One of the most outstanding works in this regard is Adūnīs' *Kitāb al-Taḥawwulāt wa-l-Hijra fī Aqālīm al-Nahār wa-l-Layl* (*The Book of Metamorphoses and Migration in the Regions of Night and Day*).[116] This ecstatic and pantheistic work combines alchemical metamorphoses and transformations. Much of the book pretends to be a Surrealist psychogram of the unconscious in accordance with Adūnīs' outlook on the close similarity between Muslim mysticism and Surrealism.[117]

Alongside the expression of personal experiences, since the beginning of the 1960s there has been a tendency among Arabic poets to combine

[113] See al-ʿAbbāsī 1947, III, p. 46; al-Thaʿālibī 1983, p. 147; al-Ṣafadī 2000, I, p. 144.

[114] Ṣūfī poets adopted the poetic themes of Abbasid poetry and refashioned them for mystical rituals in which believers were supposed to find rapture through the recollection (*dhikr*) of God. They also adapted themes of court poetry, such as standing at the ruins of the beloved's campsite, recalling the journey of a poet through the desert, and love poetry (*ġazal*), demonstrating the ways that court performance profoundly influenced modes of mystical experience (Orfali 2017, pp. 196–214). Also, in *Tarjumān al-ašwāq* (*The Translator of Desires*), by the Andalusian Ṣūfī Muḥyī al-Dīn ibn ʿArabī (1164–1240), a flesh-and-blood young woman whom Ibn ʿArabī met in Mecca becomes a figure for higher spiritual truths (see Ibn ʿArabī 1978 [1911], pp. 10–15). Ibn ʿArabī also states that the rhythm and rhyme of poetry echoes the structure of the cosmos; the arrangement of letters into words is something akin to a divine creative command; and his theory of imagery is tied up with cosmology: poetic images belong in the world of imagination, a sort of twilight zone in which spiritual truths take on the appearance of sensible forms (McAuley 2012, pp. 19–20, 44–5, 194–7).

[115] See, for example, ʿAbd al-Ṣabūr 1957, pp. 95–6 (= ʿAbd al-Ṣabūr 1972, I, pp. 47–9). Cf. Snir 1985, pp. 129–46.

[116] Adūnīs 1965; Adūnīs 1988 [1983], pp. 431–597; Adūnīs 2012, II, pp. 7–166.

[117] See Adūnīs 1992; Adonis 2005a. For a sharp critical approach to Adūnīs' mystical and Surrealist poetics, see *Risāla Maftūḥa ilā Adūnīs* (*An Open Letter to Adūnīs*) by ʿAbd al-Qādir al-Janābī (b. 1944) (al-Janābī 1994), published as the first work in a series titled *Faḍḥ al-Sāʾid* (*The Disgrace of the Prevailing Situation*) (later it proved to be the only work published within the series, a fact which may be interpreted as having been planned from the start in order to magnify the critical attitude of the author to Adūnīs). See also the first issue of the Arabic Surrealist magazine *al-Ghurfa* (*The Room*) (January 2020) edited by Muḥsin al-Billāsī, available at: https://drive.google.com/file/d/16iQocozIPVVvo4v4FM8LvIBuO5nJOYfp/view. (last accessed December 19, 2020).

figures and concepts from the Ṣūfī tradition with their own social and political views. By conjoining their views with their mystical outlooks, contemporary poets have succeeded in expressing their ideas in a most innovative and original way. Prominent among them are the aforementioned Ṣalāḥ ʻAbd al-Ṣabūr,[118] ʻAbd al-Wahhāb al-Bayyātī,[119] and Adūnīs.[120] To this purpose, they have delved into early Ṣūfī sources in search of appropriate figures through whom they could express their views and to whom they could add new and modern dimensions. The central idea is that the striving for contact with God cannot be realized without a concomitant enforcement of social justice. The words are not tools for mere amusement but means by which the poet should contribute to society. A Ṣūfī tradition attributed to Bishr ibn al-Ḥārith al-Ḥāfī ("The Barefooted") (d. 841) reads:

إذا أعجبك الكلام فاصمت وإذا أعجبك الصمت فتكلّم

If speaking delights you—keep silent! And if silence pleases you—speak![121]

A similar worldview combining mystical vision with a striving for absolute social justice became apparent, as indicated above, in such prose as in the works of Najīb Maḥfūẓ. The timing of the appearance of this type of social-mystical worldview in both poetry and prose is apparently connected with the disappointment felt by Arab intellectuals with leftist worldviews in the wake of the Arab political events and the revelation of Stalinist crimes in the mid-1950s.

The East–West or the spiritual–materialistic dialectic is another dimension of the neo-Ṣūfī trend in Arabic poetry. For Adūnīs, for example, creative ability (*ibdāʻ*) is an intrinsic part of the East. In contrast, Western ability is substantially technical, and the origins of any creative progress in the West are in fact Eastern.[122] We find an echo of Adūnīs' worldview in his poem "Marthiyat al-Ḥallāj" ("Elegy for al-Ḥallāj"), which was published in his collection *Aghānī Mihyār al-Dimashqī* (*Songs of Mihyār of Damascus*)

118 For example, see ʻAbd al-Ṣabūr 1965 [1964]; ʻAbd al-Ṣabūr 1972.
119 For example, see al-Bayyātī 1979, II, pp. 143–56.
120 For example, see Adūnīs 1971 [1961], pp. 190–1.
121 See al-Qushayrī 1940, p. 63; al-Qushayri 1990, p. 50.
122 Adūnīs 1980, pp. 330–1; *Mawāqif* 36 (Winter 1980), pp. 150–1. For a critical response to Adūnīs' argument, see al-ʻAẓm 1992, pp. 109–19. See also Darrāj 2005; Darrāj considers Adūnīs' conceptions as part of the retreat in Arab modernism: "His dialogue was with the texts, in which he locked himself." Unlike Adūnīs, Darrāj sees Ṭāhā Ḥusayn as the most outstanding figure in the modern Arab idea of enlightenment, because he derived his questions "from the actual concrete needs of society" (p. 12). Cf. Ahmed 2021, p. 214. See also below, Chapter 5.

(1961),[123] and was later incorporated in his *Complete Works* in all subsequent editions.[124] The poem appeared in the section "al-Mawt al-Muʻād" ("The Recurring Death"), in which all the titles of the nine poems contain the word *marthiya*.[125] "Marthiyat al-Ḥallāj" deals with the martyrdom of the previously mentioned mystic al-Ḥusayn ibn Manṣūr al-Ḥallāj, whose name has become a symbol for suffering love and unitive mystical experience. The following applied study of the poem is an example of the multilayered creativity of the neo-Ṣūfī Arabic poets (the numbers given to the lines do not exist in the original).[126]

4. "ELEGY FOR AL-ḤALLĀJ"

4.1 Text

0. مرثية الحلاج
1. ريشتُك المسمومة الخضراءْ
2. ريشتُك المنفوخةُ الأوداج باللّهيبْ
3. بالكوكب الطّالع من بغدادْ،
4. تاريخنا وبعثنا القريبْ
5. في أرضنا — في موتِنا المُعادْ.

6. الزّمنُ استلقى على يديكْ
7. والنّار في عينيكْ
8. مجتاحة تمتدّ للسّماء

9. يا كوكبا يطلع من بغدادْ
10. محمّلا بالشّعر والميلادْ،
11. يا ريشةً مسمومةً خضراء.
12. لم يبق للآتين من بعيدْ
13. مع الصّدى والموت والجليدْ

123 Adūnīs 1971 [1961], pp. 190–1. The poem was published in the updated version of the poet's *Complete Works* without any change (Adūnīs 2012–2015, I, pp. 419–20). German translation: Schimmel 1975, p. 154.

124 For example, see Adūnīs 1971, I, pp. 506–7; Adūnīs 1988 [1983], I, pp. 426–7. For earlier readings of the poem, see Snir 1994d, pp. 245–56; Snir 2000c, pp. 171–2; Snir 2004, pp. 177–9; Snir 2006, pp. 117–30.

125 The titles are, successively, "Marthiya bi-lā Mawt," "Marthiyat ʻUmar ibn al-Khaṭṭāb," "Marthiyat Abī Nuwās," "Marthiyat al-Ḥallāj," "Marthiyat Bashshār," "Marthiya," "Marthiya," "Marthiyat al-Ayyām al-Ḥāḍira," and "Marthiyat al-Qarn al-Awwal." The last two long poems were omitted from the collection in the 1988 [1983] edition of Adūnīs' *Complete Works* and appear elsewhere (Adūnīs 1988 [1983], I, pp. 220–35; Adūnīs 2012, I, pp. 211–26).

126 On al-Ḥallāj in modern Arabic poetry, see also Snir 1992a, pp. 7–54; Snir 1993b, pp. 49–93; Snir 1994d, pp. 245–56; Snir 2002; Snir 2004, pp. 177–9; Snir 2006; Na'āmneh 2022, pp. 59–67.

14. في هذه الأرض النّشوريّهْ —
15. لم يبقَ إلا أنتَ والحضورْ
16. يا لغة الرّعد الجليليّة
17. في هذه الأرض القشوريّهْ18
18. يا شاعر الأسرار والجذورْ.

4.2. Translation

0. Elegy for al-Ḥallāj
1. Your green poisonous quill.
2. Your quill whose veins swelled with flame
3. With the star rising from Baghdad
4. Is our history and our immediate resurrection
5. In our land—in our recurring death.

6. Time lied down on your hands
7. And fire is in your eyes
8. Sweeping away and spreading up to the sky

9. O star rising from Baghdad
10. Loaded with poetry and birth,
11. O green poisonous quill.

12. Nothing is left for those who come from afar
13. With thirst, death and ice.
14. In this land of resurrection—
15. Nothing is left but you and the Presence.
16. O Galilean language of thunder
17. In this land of peels
18. O poet of secrets and roots.[127]

4.3. Interpretation

The following is a line-by-line analysis based upon the poetic diction, connotations, and associations of the words—that is, the possible responses that the words dispose a native reader to make, apart from his or her response to their denotative meanings. They may be any sensory, emotional, or cognitive responses that are a consequence of suggestion, association, or inference, or even of the look, spelling, or sound of a word. These connotations and associations are the means by which the poetic language achieves its depth, density, and richness.

[127] For other English translations, see *Banipal* 1 (February 1998), p. 6; Snir 2006, pp. 119–20; Adonis 2008, pp. 112–13.

Line 0: The title alludes to the martyrdom of a famous mystic, but unlike other early Ṣūfī mystics the reader should bear in mind that al-Ḥallāj was also known for his involvement in the surrounding society without giving up his mystical aspirations. He was described as being very sensitive to the social gaps existing between the poor and rich classes, and he used to distribute money among the miserable people. He advised people that they should, instead of performing the pilgrimage to Mecca, feed orphans, dress them, and make them happy.[128] Involved politically as well, he expressed his support for the chamberlain Naṣr al-Qushūrī, who favored better administration and fairer taxation—dangerous ideas at a time when the caliph was almost powerless and the viziers changed frequently. The political and social elite feared that al-Ḥallāj's ideas might have repercussions in terms of social and political organization and structure.[129] Al-Ḥallāj also participated in an attempt to overthrow the regime and was subsequently arrested and executed. Contrary to popular legend, it was not so much his aforementioned utterance "*anā al-ḥaqq*" ("I am the Absolute Truth," i.e., God) that brought about his execution, but rather his religious and social theories, which were viewed as subversive.[130] Since the 1950s, there has been great interest in the figure of al-Ḥallāj throughout the Islamic world. In Arab lands—where he was less renowned than in those areas influenced by the Persian mystical tradition—he has gained fame and recognition, especially among poets, who have seized upon his social message.[131]

Line 1: *rīsha* signifies both a quill of a bird's wing and a quill pen, as well as being associated with an arrow.[132] Hence, the first line may be understood as:

I. The *poet* al-Ḥallāj uses his *pen* in favor of the oppressed and against the oppressors.

II. The *mystic* al-Ḥallāj is presented as a *bird*, alluding to al-Ḥallāj's own verse:

وطار قلبي بريش شوق   مركّب في جناح العزم

And my heart flew with quills of longing fixed on a wing of determination.[133]

[128] *Akhbār al-Ḥallāj*, p. 36.
[129] Schimmel 1983, p. 68.
[130] See Massignon 1971, III, pp. 99–104; Massignon 1982, I, pp. 271–337.
[131] Prominent among them Ṣalāḥ ʿAbd al-Ṣabūr (e.g., ʿAbd al-Ṣabūr 1965 [1964] [English translation: ʿAbd al-Ṣabūr 1972a]); ʿAbd al-Wahhāb al-Bayyātī (al-Bayyātī 1979, II, pp. 143–56 [English translation: *Journal of Arabic Literature* 10 [1979], pp. 65–9. German translation: Schimmel 1975, pp. 78–83. For a study of the poem, see Snir 1992a, pp. 7–54; Snir 2002, pp. 83–156).
[132] For example, see Ibn Manẓūr n.d., VI, pp. 308–9 (s.v. *RYSH*).
[133] Al-Ḥallāj 1974, p. 53.

At the same time, it may be an allusion to the popular equation of soul = bird, which frequently occurs in mystical imagery and is found also in the writings of Muslim authors, such as Ibn Sīnā (Avicenna) (970–1037), Abū Ḥāmid al-Ghazālī (1057–1111), Jalāl al-Dīn Rūmī (1207–1273), and Farīd al-Dīn ʻAṭṭār (d. 1230).[134]

III. The *committed rebel* al-Ḥallāj struggles with his arrow for the implementation of his ideas. *Masmūma* connotes *sahm masmūm* (poisonous arrow), while *khadrā'* connotes not only fertility, green herbs, hope, and love,[135] but also the Qur'ānic "green garments of silk" in Paradise.[136] It may also allude to the death–rebirth cycle embodied in the *rīsha*, be it a pen, a quill, or an arrow, as well as alluding to al-Ḥallāj's sacrifice: what is poisonous and deadly for him signifies rebirth for his community.

Line 2: *wadaj* is the jugular vein. The expression *intafakhat awdājuhu* (lit. "his jugular vein swelled") means he flew into a rage. The jugular vein swelled with flame instead of with blood—al-Ḥallāj's rage is metaphorically compared with a flame burning in his veins. Since the words *intafakhat awdājuhu* are usually applied to human beings, the *rīsha* undergoes a sort of personification, which heralds a subsequent development in the poem. *Lahīb* appeared in al-Ḥallāj's poetry as the ecstatic flame that was ignited in the innermost heart of the Ṣūfī.[137] The combination of the *rīsha* and *lahīb* is associated with the idea of death and rebirth as illustrated by the Myth of the Phoenix: the fabulous Egyptian bird that, after living hundreds of years in the Arabian desert, burned itself on a funeral pyre and rose from the ashes reborn to live another cycle of life and death.[138] This association is reinforced in the mind of the reader if he or she is acquainted with Adūnīs' previous collection, *Awrāq fī al-Rīḥ* (*Leaves in the Wind*) (1958) and with the poem "Tartīlat al-Baʻth" ("Hymn to Resurrection").[139]

134 Schimmel 1983, pp. 306–7.

135 Cf. The poem "Ughniyya Khaḍrā'" ("Green Song") by Ṣalāḥ ʻAbd al-Ṣabūr (ʻAbd al-Ṣabūr 1972, I, pp. 123–8).

136 *Al-Insān* 21.

137 Al-Ḥallāj 1974, p. 34.

138 On the Myth of the Phoenix, see Broek 1972; Nigg 2016. Referring to ʻAnqā', the fantastic bird that incorporates human and bestial features, he mentions qualities reminiscent of mythical birds of other cultures, such as the Phoenix (al-Qazwīnī 1849, pp. 419–20). In a recent article, Guy Ron-Gilboa indicates that the ʻAnqā' "is a mirror of the cultures that fashioned it and of the literary traditions that gave it life. As an 'image in the soul,' it offers a way of searching for the boundaries of meaning and signification—from the absence of being to its utmost fullness. As a creature of literature, it is a synecdoche for the imagination itself" (Ron-Gilboa 2021, pp. 75–103).

139 Adūnīs 1988 [1983], I, pp. 165–73; Adūnīs 2012, I, pp. 152–60. Apart from the death–rebirth cycle embodied in the Myth of the Phoenix, the similarity in the poetic diction is striking (e.g., *rīsha*, *lahīb*, *kawkab*, *huḍūr*, *judhūr*).

Line 3: Aside from the flame, alluding to the burning rage, the quill also contains the star, connoting hope for the future. Baghdad—the place where al-Ḥallāj was executed—symbolizes the glories of ancient Arab and Muslim civilization. The star is rising *from*, and not *over*, Baghdad, which is an allusion to a possible universal message. The use of the active participle *ṭāliʿ* stresses the present relevance of the poem: the star is rising *now*.

Line 4: *baʿth* is associated with *yawm al-baʿth*, the Day of Resurrection, when those who are in their graves shall rise up again. The preposition "with" (*bi*) added to both the "flame" (*bi-l-lahīb*) and the "star" (*bi-l-kawkab*), is not attached to the words *ta'rīkh* and *baʿth*. Hence, this line may be conceived in both ways: the *rīsha* is our history and immediate resurrection, or, assuming that *bi* was omitted for reasons of prosody,[140] the *rīsha* is swelled not only with the flame and the star but also with the grandeur of the past and hope for the future. Both readings refer to the power of the *rīsha* as a guarantee for the future based upon the past.

Line 5: While the previous line alludes to resurrection in the hereafter, the enjambment with the words *fī arḍinā* may imply a hope for rebirth in this world. As for *fī mawtinā al-muʿādi*, God is alluded to in the Qur'ān several times as *yabda'u al-khalq thumma yuʿīduhu*, as, for example, in the following verse:

إليه مرجعكم جميعا وعد الله حقّا إنّه يبدأ الخلق ثمّ يعيده.

> To Him shall you return, all together—God's promise, in truth. He originates creation, then He brings it back again.[141]

Tafsīr al-Jalālayn comments on *thumma yuʿīduhu* by saying: *bi-l-baʿth* (by resurrection). Additionally, the look, spelling, and sound of the word *muʿād*, voweled by the poet himself, connotes the words *maʿād al-khalq*—Paradise, or whither one goes on the Day of Resurrection. This allusion emphasizes the rebirth against the background of recurring death in this world. The manner in which *mawt* is combined with *muʿād* is reminiscent of the translation of Job's words to God in the Bible:

أعلم أنّك إلى موتي تعيدني وإلى بيتي ميعاد كلّ حيّ.

> Yea, I know that thou wilt bring me to death, and to the house appointed for all living.[142]

140 Adding the preposition (*bi-ta'rīkhinā wa-baʿthinā*), the line would have become the only one in the poem not starting with one of the variations of *mustafʿilun*.

141 *Yūnus* 4.

142 Job 30:23.

This allusion is reinforced by the title "al-Mawt al-Mu'ād," which was given to the section in the collection in which the poem appeared.

Line 6: al-Ḥallāj is described as a Ṣūfī saint capable of performing *karāmāt*—various kinds of miracles. Claiming gifts of grace and miraculous powers, al-Ḥallāj produced sweetmeats from Yemen and brought down heavenly food in the middle of the desert.[143] One of the miracles attributed to Ṣūfī saints is the ability to control time: *ṭayy al-zamān*—folding up time, that is, accelerating time—and *nashr al-zamān*—unfolding time, that is, retarding time.[144] Though not attributed in the Ṣūfī sources to al-Ḥallāj, Adūnīs probably refers here to that *karāma* presumably in order to demonstrate the link between past and present.

Line 7: Fire in the eyes is usually an allusion to the fighter's zeal. Alluding to his elevated mystical state, in one of his poems al-Ḥallāj says: "*al-nār fī kabidī*" ("fire is in my liver").[145] The fire at the depth of the poet's soul is also a frequent romantic motif.

Line 8: The spreading of the fire up to the sky is associated with the spreading of al-Ḥallāj's message. The use of the active participle and the imperfect form of the verbs contributes to the relevance of the text to our time.

Line 9: Addressing the star planted in the quill, the worldly personage of al-Ḥallāj has passed through a sort of metamorphosis in which he has been transformed into an abstract meaning. It is reminiscent of the alchemic and spiritual transmutations in mysticism,[146] of which Adūnīs' poems abound, fluctuating between the dark regions of the body and the light regions of the spirit.[147]

Line 10: The star into which al-Ḥallāj is transformed is suffused with poetry. *Mīlād* may be associated with the connections found between al-Ḥallāj and Christian theology and with the assumption that the dogma of Incarnation influenced him.[148]

Line 11: al-Ḥallāj becomes himself the quill—a complete identification between the figure and its message: al-Ḥallāj is nothing more than his mysticism, poetry, and commitment to his nation and society.

Line 12: *ba'īd* alludes to several Qur'ānic verses associated with disbelievers, as, for example, "But those who believe not, in their ears is a heaviness, and to them it is a blindness; those—they are called from a far place [*min*

143 Schimmel 1983, p. 67.
144 See al-Nabhānī 1984, I, p. 50.
145 Al-Ḥallāj 1974, p. 38.
146 Cf. al-Ghazālī 1936, pp. 3–4; Underhill 1961, pp. 140–8.
147 For example, see Adūnīs 1965; Adūnīs 1988 [1983], pp. 431–597; Adūnīs 2012, II, pp. 7–166.
148 Schimmel 1983, pp. 64, 72.

makān ba'īd]," [149] or "But those who believe not in the hereafter are in chastisement and far error [*fi ḍalāl ba'īd*]," [150] or "And those that are at variance regarding the Book are in wide schism [*fi shiqāq ba'īd*]." [151] Since the poem is not religious, at least not in the traditional sense, disloyalty to God is rendered as political and social faithlessness. It could be supported by the allusion to the biblical allegory of the sisters Oholah and Oholibah, in which the Arabic translation says "*ilā rijāl ātīn min ba'īd*" ("for men to come from afar"). [152]

Line 13: *ma'a* should be understood as "with" and not as "despite"; *ṣadā* denotes an echo as well, but it is more plausible to understand it as "thirst." Those mentioned in line 12 come *with* thirst, death, and ice—that is, they are thirsty, dead, and cold. This meaning is strengthened by the allusion to the Prophetic tradition: *la-taridunna yawm al-qiyāma ṣawādiya* ("you will come on the Day of Resurrection thirsty"). [153] Conceiving *ma'a* as "despite" and *ṣadā* as "echo" is not consistent with the following lines describing the rebirth and resurrection symbolized by al-Ḥallāj. Those who come from afar seem to allude to the dead men on the Day of Resurrection.

Line 14: *al-arḍ al-nushūriyya* could be associated with the Qur'ān: "God is He that looses the winds that stir up the clouds, then We drive them to a dead land and therewith revive the earth [*al-arḍ*], after it is dead. Even so is the Uprising [*nushūr*]." [154] The resurrection will not occur in the hereafter but here in the Arab world, the land of resurrection.

Line 15: *lam yabqa* is reminiscent of the Ṣūfī terms *fanā'* and *baqā'*, that is, annihilation in God and everlasting life in Him. [155] Appearing in this context the word *anta* could be associated with one of al-Ḥallāj's poems, all ten verses of which conclude with this word. The first verse is as follows:

رأيت ربّي بعين قلبي   فقلت: من أنت؟ قال: أنت

I saw my God in the heart of my eye;
I asked: who are you? He replied: You! [156]

Ḥuḍūr means (as plural of *ḥāḍir*) "those present" and also alludes to the Ṣūfī terms *ḥuḍūr wa-ghayba*, that is, presence in God and absence from oneself. [157] Al-Ḥallāj himself says in one of his poems:

149 *Saba'* 52–53.
150 *Saba'* 8.
151 *Al-Baqara* 176.
152 Ezekiel 23:40.
153 Ibn Manẓūr n.d., XV, 453 (s.v. *ṢDY*).
154 *Fāṭir* 9.
155 See al-Qushayrī n.d., pp. 61–3; al-Ḥakīm 1981, pp. 201–5.
156 Al-Ḥallāj 1974, p. 26.
157 See al-Qushayrī n.d., pp. 63–4.

واتّصل الوصل بافتراق فصار في غيبتي حضوري

And the union was connected with a separation,
And my presence existed in my absence.[158]

The allusion of *ḥuḍūr* to *al-ḥaḍra al-ilāhiyya* (the divine presence) also cannot be overlooked. Based upon the Ṣūfī connotations of the words, this line may refer to the high mystical experience attained by al-Ḥallāj, but compounded with the previous lines, and particularly lines 12–14, it asserts al-Ḥallāj's message as the only hope of salvation for the Arab nation.

Line 16: *ra'd* is associated in the Bible with the voice of God, who is often described as speaking with the voice of thunder, for example, *ra'd jabarūtihi* (the thunder of his power)[159] or *ra'd ṣawtihi* (the thunder of his voice).[160] Thus, this allusion reinforces al-Ḥallāj's divine nature; however, this line also contains an ironic allusion to the thunder in the last part of T. S. Eliot's "The Waste Land" (1922), titled "What the Thunder Said."[161] Eliot refers there to the arrest of Jesus and his preliminary trial in the palace of the high priest of the Jews before he was taken before Pontius Pilate, the Roman governor in Jerusalem. According to the account in the New Testament, at the death of Jesus the earth shook and a sudden darkness occurred. Eliot speaks about "dry sterile thunder without rain" and "Then spoke the thunder / Da."[162] The allusion to Jesus is strengthened by the word *al-jalīliyya*, which is associated

158 Al-Ḥallāj 1974, p. 36.
159 Job 26:14.
160 Job 37:2.
161 Eliot 1969, pp. 72–5. On the impact "The Waste Land" had on Arabic poetry, see El-Azma 1968, pp. 671–8; Moreh 1969, pp. 1–50; Semaan 1969, pp. 472–89; Moreh 1976, pp. 216–66; El-Azma 1980, pp. 215–31; Brugman 1984, p. 204; Moreh 1984, p. 168; Faddul 1992; Allen 1998, p. 211; DeYoung 1998, pp. 65–95; DeYoung 2000, pp. 3–21; Azouqa 2001, pp. 167–211; al-Musawi 2020, pp. 172, 179; Nsiri 2020, pp. 215–37; Iskander 2021, ch. 2. There are at least nine translations of the poem into Arabic (on some of them, see al-Sulṭānī 2021). In one of the latest original poetic expressions of the inspiration Arabic poetry drew from Eliot's poem, the Lebanese poet 'Aql al-'Awīṭ (b. 1952) published a poem in memory of the devastating explosion in Beirut's port on August 4, 2020 that killed 218 people and injured thousands. The title of the poem consists of the first words of Eliot's poem in Arabic translation (see al-'Awīṭ 2021).
162 In his notes to the poem, Eliot mentions a fable from the Brihadaranyaka Upanishad, India's holy book, about Prajapati, the Creator, who has three groups of offspring: gods, men, and demons; they each seek his wisdom. To each, he utters the syllable "Da" (the Sanskrit root of words relating to "give" and an imitation of the sound of thunder) and asks if they understand. The gods think that he says: "Damyata" ("Restrain yourselves") and he agrees. The men think that he says "Datta" ("Give") and he agrees. The demons think that he says "Dayadhvam" ("Be compassionate") and he agrees. The thunder, the divine voice, repeats: "Da! Da! Da!" (i.e., "Restrain yourselves! Give! Be compassionate!"). The words "Da Dayadhvam Damyata" appear also at the end of the poem before the word "Shantih," which marks the formal ending of an Upanishad.

with Jesus the Galilean. This association is supported by addressing al-Ḥallāj as *lugha*: language. Jesus was referred to as *al-Kalima* (The Word) based upon the New Testament and Ṣūfī sources.[163]

Line 17: *al-arḍ al-qushūriyya* is the antithesis of *al-arḍ al-nushūriyya* (line 14): the Arab land is capable of being a land of resurrection, but it is now a land of *qushūr* (peels). This meaning is associated also with Eliot's "The Waste Land" in its title and vision.

Line 18: *asrār* alludes to al-Ḥallāj's greatest sin, according to the Ṣūfī mystics: the disclosure of his secret love for God.[164] Apart from that, after he left Baghdad for Khurasan, al-Ḥallāj was surnamed *Ḥallāj al-Asrār*—the Cotton Carder of the Innermost Hearts—since he knew all things concealed in the human heart.[165] The word *asrār* also alludes to the unknown future, whereas *judhūr* indicates the past. The word *asrār,* which appears in the aforementioned short poem by Ṣalāḥ 'Abd al-Ṣabūr as the means by which the mystic is forced to keep silent, is also the title of one of Adūnīs' earlier poems:

يضمّنا الموت إلى صدره
مغامرًا، زاهدًا
يحملنا سرًّا على سرّه
يجعل من كثرتنا واحدا.

Death embraces us into its breast
Venturing and abstaining
It bears us as a secret upon its secret
Making our multitude one.[166]

Presenting al-Ḥallāj as a contemporary figure, the last line of the poem may be conceived as the link between the past and the future of the Arab nation. *Judhūr* also comes as al-Ḥallāj's response to the *qushūr* in the previous line, that is, beneath the peels there exist roots.

4.4. Interpretation

Divided into four strophes, the poem has a peculiar thematic structure:

I. The persona addresses al-Ḥallāj, whose quill might be a bird's quill, a pen, or an arrow. Being presented as a mystic, poet, and committed rebel, his image alludes to the resurrection of the Arab nation (lines 1–5).

[163] John 1:1; al-Ḥakīm 1981, pp. 974–81. Cf. Zadādiqa 2008, p. 462.
[164] Al-Ḥallāj 1974, p. 41.
[165] Schimmel 1983, pp. 66–7.
[166] Adūnīs 1988 [1983], I, p. 37; Adūnīs 2012, I, p. 32.

II. Gifted by divine power and by his native enthusiasm, al-Ḥallāj performs miracles (lines 6–8).
III. Transformed into a star and a quill, al-Ḥallāj's message traverses the mystical path from poetry to social commitment (lines 9–11).
IV. Al-Ḥallāj—the figure and his message—is the only hope for the rebirth of the Arab nation (lines 12–18).

The first three strophes (lines 1–11) are united by a rhetorical frame: closing the circle opened in the first line, line 11 introduces al-Ḥallāj's metamorphosis and his transformation into the message he desires to bear. This idea is reinforced by the parallel between lines 2 and 10, and between lines 3 and 9. In an attempt to achieve harmony between poetic form and content, the second strophe is the only one in the poem that does not end with a full stop: thanks to his contact with the divine, al-Ḥallāj has the ability to perform unlimited miracles. The last strophe (lines 12–18) defines the relevant context, pointing out the current desperate condition of the Arab nation. This thematic division of the poem is expressed also in the structure of the rhymes:

I. ABCBC.
II. DDA.
III. CCA.
IV. EEFGFFG.

Joining together all the levels in which al-Ḥallāj was historically active—poetry, mysticism, and social and political commitment—the text has become a zone in which they all intersect: poetry (lines 1, 2, 10, 11, 16, 18), mysticism (lines 6, 15, 18), and ideological commitment (lines 2, 4, 5, 7, 9). The allusions to the Old and New Testaments, especially to Jesus (lines 10, 16) add to the poem's universal dimension.

Sketching an equilateral triangle consisting of art, mysticism, and reality, elsewhere Adūnīs sees the aforementioned poet and artist Jubrān Khalīl Jubrān (1883–1931) as uniting these three levels.[167] According to Adūnīs, this Mahjari poet, who combined the voice of the prophet and the voice of the committed rebel, was the first in modern Arabic poetry to present a vision that strived to change the world. To illustrate the relation between art and freedom—which he regards as one of the ideas that modern Arab poets have borrowed from the Ṣūfī heritage[168]—he quotes from Jubrān's letter to

[167] Adūnīs 1978, pp. 164–5.
[168] Adūnīs 1971a, p. 132.

Mary Haskell on May 16, 1913 concerning the international exhibition of modern art:

> [It] is a revolt, a declaration of independence. The pictures, individually, are not great; in fact, few are beautiful. But the spirit of the exhibition as a whole is both beautiful and great. Cubism, Omissionism, Post-Impressionism and Futurism will pass away. The world will forget them. But the spirit of the movement will never pass away, for it is as real as the human hunger for freedom. Turner,[169] seventy years ago, was the only free soul among the artists. Today we have hundreds of free souls whose only desire is to be and not to follow. These free artists may not be as great as Turner, but they are as independent as he was. We can not [sic] measure freedom as we measure greatness. A man can be free without being great, but no man can be great without being free.[170]

Adūnīs, who considers himself as the inheritor of Jubrān and the Mahjar group whom he considered as "the true trailblazers of twentieth-century Arabic literature,"[171] declares that this passage illustrates how Jubrān is striving for the future, for freedom, and for a new world.[172]

The Palestinian writer and critic Jabrā Ibrāhīm Jabrā (1919–1994) argues that Adūnīs' sensibility is marred by an egocentric attitude in which the "narcissistic self, enlarged by mystical ecstasy, becomes the whole universe."[173] His compatriot Salmā al-Khadrā' al-Jayyūsī (b. 1928) posits that, in the poetry he published in the 1960s, Adūnīs showed an increasing preoccupation with the past, which afforded him a constant voyage of discovery. It was seen in his continuous attempts at discovering the possible effectiveness in a poetic medium of such personages from the Islamic past as al-Ḥallāj, Muḥammad ibn 'Abd al-Jabbār al-Niffarī (d. 965), Abū Ḥāmid al-Ghazzālī (1057–1111), the Andalusian Emir of Cordova 'Abd al-Raḥmān al-Dākhil (731–788), and others. In this preoccupation, says Jayyūsī, he "tends sometimes to forget about the present and to lose touch with his own age."[174]

In "Marthiyat al-Ḥallāj," however, the egocentric and narcissistic attitude and the preoccupation with the past are modes of self-expression; they inhere in a kind of *qaṣīdat qināʿ* (mask poem), in which the poet, to use words by 'Abd al-Wahhāb al-Bayyātī, reconciles through an artistic mask "the mortal with the eternal, the finite with the infinite, the present with

[169] Joseph Mallord William Turner (1775–1851), English landscape painter.

[170] Adūnīs 1971a, p. 82. The original text of the letter can be found in Hilu 1976, p. 129. Otto 1970, p. 260, reads "Impressionism" instead of "Omissionism."

[171] Creswell 2019, p. 27.

[172] Adūnīs 1971a, pp. 79–85.

[173] Jabrā 1968, p. 119.

[174] Jayyusi 1977, p. 746.

what transcends the present."[175] In the poem, al-Ḥallāj demonstrates the continuous progression from the past to present and future in which "all man's experience throughout history is unified, proving the endless capacity of human experience for reproducing itself."[176]

This meaning may be reinforced in the reader's mind through the process of reading as he moves between the poles winter/death and spring/rebirth; and, of course, there is also the poet's pen name, Adūnīs, associated with the idea of death and rebirth. After the death of the old, there is a new and powerful renewal as represented by the mythological figures of Adonis, Tammuz, Osiris, the Phoenix, and the Christ, all of whom rise from the dead.[177] In this regard, Adūnīs' poem can be conjugated with the aforementioned "The Waste Land," in which Eliot is preoccupied with the myths associated with these deities, which have been seen by successive civilizations in the Eastern Mediterranean and the Middle East as the powers of nature. Eliot's poem indicates the contribution of the dead to the replenishing and perpetuation of life as indicated in the first lines of the poem:

> April is the cruellest month, breeding
> Lilacs out of the dead land, mixing
> Memory and desire, stirring
> Dull roots with spring rain.

In Christian terms, the sacrificial death of Jesus Christ, the God-man, is essential to the spiritual salubrity of the world. Al-Ḥallāj's death and rebirth is, according to Adūnīs, an allegory of the dying Arab nation and its future resurrection.

The spatial and temporal context of the poem is evident not only from the fact that the poem was published in the early 1960s, in Arabic, and for Arab readers, but also from the "star rising from Baghdad" (lines 3, 9), "this land" (lines 14, 17), "our land" (line 5), "our history" (line 4), "our recurring death" (line 5), and "our immediate resurrection" (line 4). Furthermore, the very choice of the figure of al-Ḥallāj as the symbol of death and rebirth—although this use of his figure was rare in the ancient Islamic Arabic sources[178]—indicates the intention of the poet to stress the Arab and Islamic context of the poem as well as that of the entire collection in which it appears. The meaning of rebirth and revival, associated with the figures of al-Ḥallāj, who was executed more than 1,000 years before the poem was written, and Jesus,

175 Al-Bayyātī 1968, p. 134.
176 Jayyusi 1977, p. 745.
177 See Adūnīs' article in *Adab* (Beirut) 1.4 (1962), pp. 73–84.
178 Abū al-ʿAlāʾ al-Maʿarrī (973–1057) indicates that in his day people stood on the banks of the Tigris awaiting al-Ḥallāj's rebirth (al-Maʿarrī 1975, p. 228).

who was executed about 1,000 years before al-Ḥallāj's execution, emphasizes the relevance of the poem to both the present and the future. But this relevance also stirs up in the reader's mind the image of Adūnīs himself, specifically in view of the parallels that the poet sees between himself and al-Ḥallāj, who is presented as a new Jesus. Adūnīs is not only a poet but, from the start of his career, also inclined toward mysticism, especially Sufism, and he is convinced that he has proved his commitment to both his society and nation.

Before he left Syria in 1956, Adūnīs had been engaged in hectic political activity in connection with the Syrian Social Nationalist Party (SSNP; al-Ḥizb al-Sūrī al-Qawmī al-Ijtimāʿī)—which was founded by Anṭūn Saʿāda (1904–1949).[179] This activity landed him in jail, prompting the writing of poetry of social and political protest in condemnation of Arabic authorities and society.[180] Saʿāda—who, it is said, even chose Adūnīs' pen name—stressed the national Syrian identity and the Western features of Syrian civilization in an attempt to separate the Syrians from the other Arab nations and cultures. Adūnīs' poems from the 1950s are replete with direct allusions to the earth, which is longing for salvation, and for a new cultural dawn to fructify the wasteland of the senile, collapsing Arab-Islamic culture, using myths, such as Tammuz, the Phoenix, and the Christ. Joseph Zeidan argues that Adūnīs' political convictions underwent a drastic change only in the aftermath of the 1967 War and that his interest in real Arab conditions overshadowed his Syrian Nationalist affiliation.[181] But it seems that this change was manifested earlier in *Aghānī Mihyār al-Dimashqī*, where his poetry became not only more obscure and complicated but also less committed to SSNP ideology.[182]

[179] For a critical study of Saʿāda's ideas and their impact on the history of ideas and literature in the Middle East, see Maʿtūq 1992; Bawārdī 1998; Maʿtūq 2013.

[180] Cf. Hazo 1971, p. xiv; Badawi 1975, pp. 231–2.

[181] Zeidan 1979, p. 85.

[182] Only during the 1960s did Adūnīs distance himself from the views that he held as a member in the SSNP; most of the poems written under the influence of the party were excluded from his *Complete Works* in subsequent editions (1971, 1983, and 1996), and he even claims that his pen name was not given to him by Saʿāda (Zeidan 1979, p. 86). On how Adūnīs got his pen name and its affinities to James Frazer's *The Golden Bough* and to Surrealism, see Irwin 2000, pp. 14–15. For some observations relating to Irwin's references to the contributions that Adūnīs made to Arab Surrealism, see my letter to *The Times Literary Supplement*, September 22, 2000, p. 17. On the importance of *Aghānī Mihyār al-Dimashqī* in Adūnīs' poetic development, see Creswell 2019, esp. pp. 94–120, 172–4. See also Adūnīs' recent book *Dafātir Mihyār al-Dimashqī* (*Mihyār al-Dimashqī's Notebooks*) (Adūnīs 2020), whose motto, in Adūnīs' handwriting, is the following:

لا يؤرّخ الضّوء لأشعّته، ما مضى يتسلسل في ما يحضر وفيما وراءه. لما يحضر جذور تتمدّد في حقول ما يأتي:
تلك هي "دفاتر مهيار الدمشقيّ" أمس الآن غدا

Intended to be, according to its title, a lamentation for a personage who died more than 1,000 years ago, "Elegy for al-Ḥallāj" is ironically transformed in the process of reading into a vision of the Arab nation's rebirth. Since the star is rising now *from* Baghdad, the death of al-Ḥallāj, as al-Bayyātī says, "is the bridge which civilization and mankind cross to reach a more perfect existence."[183] This is the Adūnīsian vision in which poetry, mysticism, and reality coexist: none of these is blind or excludes the other.[184] Adūnīs' disappointment in recent years with the passivity and inflexibility of Arab culture[185] only emphasizes, in his view, the need to see this vision come true. As for 2020, Adūnīs by no means sees any hope:

عرف الغرب ويعرف
كيف يتفنّن في صناعة الطّبول
الّتي تعرف عصيّ العرب
كيف تتفنّن في قرعها

The West knew and knows
How to be versatile in designing drums
On which the Arabs' beaters know
How to be versatile in beating them.[186]

5. CONCLUSION

Neo-Ṣūfī secular contemporary poetry is similar to classical Ṣūfī poetry, especially from the point of view of its spontaneity and the expression of intimate and unmediated contact with the divine. Contemporary secular Arab poets close a circle originally opened by the first Ṣūfī religious poets twelve centuries ago. The simplicity and spontaneity that characterized the early Muslim works of mysticism are revived in contemporary poetic expressions of mystical love. One need only compare the poetry of the Egyptian Wafā'

183 Al-Bayyātī 1968, p. 41.

184 Cf. Allen 1987, pp. 31–2. For the relationship between Adūnīs' conceptions and Ṣūfī discourse, see Adūnīs 1992; Balqāsim 2000.

185 For example, Adūnīs 2005, pp. 70–1, 94–5, 239–41, 382–3, 393–4, 505–6, 566, 582–3. On October 31, 2003, Adūnīs delivered a presentation in Beirut titled "Bayrūt, Ahiya Ḥaqqan Madīna Am Mujarrad Ism Ta'rīkhī" ("Beirut, Is It Really a City or Just a Historical Name?"), in which he severely criticized the Arabs, such as in the following rhetorical questions: "Where is the mastership of the Lebanese people shown, in rebirthing or in killing? In celebrating life or in digging graves, lamenting the dead and celebrating death? In establishing life or, alternatively, in establishing death?" The Lebanese poet Paul Shaul (Būl Shā'ūl) (b. 1942) reacted by launching a fierce personal attack on Adūnīs in an article titled "Ḍaw' Bayrūt" ("The Light of Beirut") (*al-Mustaqbal*, November 8, 2003). Both texts were published in *Adūnīs Yastabīḥu Bayrūt* (Beirut: Riyāḍ al-Rayyis, 2003).

186 Adūnīs 2020, p. 113. On Adūnīs' attitude to the West in earlier stages of his literary work, see Natour 2019, pp. 77–87.

Wajdī (1945–2011)[187] with that of Rābiʿa al-ʿAdawiyya to realize the close similarity in the expression of mystic feelings—despite the interval of time dividing them and the barrier of religious piety.

As secular poets, contemporary Arab poets who make frequent use of early Ṣūfī terms and figures rarely concern themselves with the precise original meanings of the ancient terms, concentrating rather on the expression of their experiences and feelings as well as their social views. They load the classical terms with new meanings, each according to his own experiences and cultural horizons. Unlike the early Ṣūfī poets, they, of course, are not solely committed to Ṣūfī themes, and Sufism is not a way of life for them. Prominent poets of the neo-Ṣūfī school belong geographically to various parts of the Arab world, including poets who are not Muslims, like the Christians Yūsuf al-Khāl (1917–1987) and Khalīl Ḥāwī (1925–1982), the Iraqi-Jewish poet Murād Mīkhā'īl (1906–1986), who was nicknamed "the Ṣūfī poet," and the Bahai Mu'ayyad Ibrāhīm al-Īrānī (1910–1987). However, it goes without saying that this trend includes primarily Muslim poets for whom the Ṣūfī tradition is both their religious and cultural heritage.

All poets of this trend are united in their sensitivity to the dialectical tension between language and silence, and all of them occupy themselves with the alchemical metamorphoses and transformation of the despised body into the pure divine essence. That is why they adopt the metaphor of the poet as a mystic constantly advancing on the path toward the divine essence. Poetry for them is a *safar* (journey) that only takes you into a new *safar*. The first lines of one of Adūnīs' poems, "Zahrat al-Kīmyā'" ("The Flower of Chemistry"), published in his *Kitāb al-Taḥawwulāt wa-l-Hijra fī Aqālīm al-Layl wa-l-Nahār*, are as follows:

ينبغي أن أسافر في جنّة الرمادْ
بين أشجارها الخفيّهْ
في الرماد الخواتيمُ والماسُ والجزّةُ الذهبيّهْ.

I must travel in the paradise of the ashes
Between its hidden trees.
In the ashes are the rings, the diamonds, and the Golden Fleece.[188]

[187] See, for example, her poems in Wajdī 1980; Wajdī 1985. On her, see Zaydān 1986, p. 300; Campbell 1996, pp. 1368–70.

[188] Adūnīs 1965, p. 11. In a subsequent edition, Adūnīs changed the word "al-Khwātīm" to "al-Asāṭīr" ("the myths") (see Adūnīs 2012, II, p. 9).

PART II

East, West, and World Literature

نحن في دور من رقيّنا الأدبيّ والاجتماعيّ قد تنبّهت فيه حاجات روحيّة كثيرة لم نكن نشعر بها من قبل احتكاكنا الحديث بالغرب. وليس عندنا من الأقلام والأدمغة ما يفي بسدّ هذه الحاجات. فلنترجم! ولنجلّ مقام المترجم لأنّه واسطة تعارف بيننا وبين العائلة البشريّة العظمى.

– ميخائيل نعيمة

We are at a stage of our literary and social evolution in which many spiritual needs have awakened which we did not know before our new contact with the West. As we have no pens and brains that can fulfill those needs, let us then translate! Let us honor the status of the translator because he is an agent of acquaintance between us and the larger human family.

– Mīkhā'īl Nu'ayma

I will discuss in this part of the book four cases of one-sided interference from Western culture into Arab culture, relying on the theoretical conceptions formulated during the 1980s and 1990s.[1] Interference can be defined as "a relation(ship) between literatures, whereby a certain literature A (a source literature) may become a source of direct or indirect loans for another literature B (a target literature)."[2] What may move, be borrowed, taken over from one culture to another is not just an item of repertoire, but also a host of other features and items:

> The role and function of literature, the rules of the game of the literary institution, the nature of literary criticism and scholarship, the relations between religious, political, and other activities within culture and literary production—all may be modelled in a given culture in relation to some other system. It would therefore be inadequate to reduce interference to just the seemingly more visible level of the text or even of the model(s) behind it. I say "seemingly" because in many specific cases of interference in the history of literatures, once one looks elsewhere, other pertinent phenomena become no less "visible."[3]

As for the channels of interference, they are multiple and various, depending chiefly on whether interference is direct or indirect:

> In the case of direct interference, a source literature is available to, and accessed by, agents of the target literature without intermediaries. They know the language of the source literature and may have better access to its resources than in the case of the second type. In this second type, interference is intermediated through some channel, such as translation. Though in both cases translation may be a major channel for *actual* transfer, it is obvious that in the latter case its role is more crucial ... In the case of minority groups physically living among majority groups, being exposed daily to the culture of the majority, interference may be much more powerful than in those cases when the target can to some degree avoid the source. In other words, massive exposure can significantly support the impact of interference. But this exposure *per se* is neither a sufficient nor a necessary condition for interference to take place.[4]

Itamar Even-Zohar (b. 1939) mentions ten laws of interference; all of them in some way or another are relevant to the cases discussed in the following chapters. Among these laws[5] is the argument that literatures are never in non-interference and that interference is mostly unilateral. And it is important to note the following:

[1] See especially Even-Zohar 1990a, pp. 53–72.
[2] Even-Zohar 1990a, p. 54.
[3] Even-Zohar 1990a, pp. 54–5.
[4] Even-Zohar 1990a, pp. 57–8.
[5] According to Even-Zohar 1990a, pp. 58–72. Pages of later quotations appear immediately afterward in the text.

> There is no symmetry in literary interference. A target literature is, more often than not, interfered with by a source literature which completely ignores it. There are also cases when there may be some minor interference in one direction and a major one in another. For instance, Russian literature did have some impact upon French literature toward the late nineteenth century, but this impact can in no way be compared with the role played by French for Russian.[6]

Also, literary interference is not necessarily linked with interference on other levels between communities; contacts will sooner or later generate interference if no resisting conditions arise, or contacts will not generate interference unless favorable conditions arise;[7] a source literature is selected by prestige,[8] which means that "political and/or economic power may play a role in establishing such prestige, but not necessarily. What counts most is the cultural power of the source system."[9] Additionally:

> The perpetuation of cultural power in spite of political decline is well attested. Conquered people often transmitted their culture to their conquerors by virtue of this ineradicable prestige. Thus, the conquering Germanic tribes adopted the most fundamental components of their official culture from the conquered Gaelic and Italic peoples. Colonizers may also behave like such conquerors, as is probably the case with the Akkadians, who adopted the culture of the Sumerians and cherished the formers' language and heritage for ages. Hellenistic culture was respectfully treated by the Romans, and the Roman cultures of Italy and Gaul by their respective Germanic invaders.[10]

Among the other laws, we can find that a source literature is selected by dominance. Interference occurs when a system is in need of items unavailable within itself; contacts may take place with only one part of the target literature; they may then proceed to other parts; an appropriated repertoire does not necessarily maintain source literature functions; and appropriation tends to be simplified, regularized, and schematized. I will discuss here three cases of interference from Western culture, all of them responding, in one way or another, to the aforementioned laws of interference. The first chapter in this part will refer to the cultural circumstances that had prepared the ground for the emergence of these cases.

[6] Even-Zohar 1990a, p. 62.

[7] On the literary activities of Palestinians in Hebrew, see Snir 1991a, pp. 245–53; Snir 1992, pp. 6–9; Snir 1995, pp. 163–83; Snir 1997, pp. 141–53; Snir 2001a, pp. 197–224. On the Arabic literary activities of Jews, see Snir 2005; Snir 2015; Snir 2019a.

[8] See, for example, below, Chapter 6, on the impact of Franz Kafka (1883–1924) on Arabic literary writing.

[9] Even-Zohar 1990a, p. 66.

[10] Even-Zohar 1990a, p. 67.

Chapter 5, "Self-Image: Between 'Decadence' and Renaissance," concentrates on the self-image of Arabic literature against the background of its relationship with the West. Examining the repeated lamentations by Arab intellectuals and writers about the status of Arab culture and literature throughout the last two centuries, the nuances and wording of each of them enable the student of Arabic literature to understand the complicated attitude toward the West in light of the decline of the Arabs' cultural self-image and the huge gap between the august status enjoyed by Arab culture in the Middle Ages and its feeble modern counterpart. The chapter deals as well with the relationship between modern and classical Arabic literature, which is essential to our understanding of the nature of the contemporary Arabic literary system. The question is whether modern Arabic literature is an extension of classical Arabic literature, or whether it is a new creation that has hardly any relationship at all with its medieval predecessor. It is no coincidence that Arab, especially Muslim, scholars tend to adopt the former view, whereas Western scholars tend to adopt the latter. Considering the modern Arabic literary system as a new creation means accepting the view that Arabic literature prior to the nineteenth century had somehow collapsed and been abandoned by its own community, as though the Arabs during the eighteenth and nineteenth centuries had in one way or another exchanged all or parts of their culture for another. Although it is autonomous, the Arabic literary system, like any other literary system, retains various relationships with other literary systems by means of interference. Arabic literature may become a source for direct or indirect loans to another literature and vice versa. Besides being a target for other literatures and cultures, Arabic and Islamic literature and culture were also important sources of inspiration for certain cultures. Two major examples of reciprocal interference between Arabic and Western literatures in the twentieth century and at the start of the twenty-first century are Arabic and English, and Arabic and French.

Chapter 6, "Existentialism: The Frightened Mouse," discusses the significant impact of Franz Kafka on Arabic literary writing, not least because his work is torn between his conviction that the tragic fate of human existence is determined and his frustrated desire to change it. We can look at Kafka's world from two points of view: (1) the outlook that the human being should not lose his hope till his last moment; and (2) the metaphysical outlook that does not see any refuge for human beings in this world. Here between the lines, we meet the nostalgia for a lost paradise, or the concept of God, even if this God is not the same God for which "religious" people yearn. Kafka and many Arab writers share the feeling of hope, since it is not contradictory for fundamentally existentialist writing to find cause for hope. The major impact of Kafka on Arab writers has been in the area of fiction as is illustrated, for example, in the writing of Najīb Maḥfūẓ (1911–2006)[11] and Ṣunʿ Allāh Ibrāhīm (b. 1937),[12] but here I will explore his impact on Arabic poetry, discussing the inspiration that the Egyptian poet Ṣalāḥ ʿAbd al-Ṣabūr drew from Kafka. Both of them meet within the context of twentieth-century existentialism, sharing some kind of vision of the condition and existence of man, his place and function in the world, and his relation to God. They seem to present contradictory views on human existence: Kafka presents a desperate world with no recourse left, whereas ʿAbd al-Ṣabūr presents a hope to escape by means of mystic ecstasy. But it is only an illusionary contradiction, since there is more in the writings of Kafka than the pessimism that dominates the surface. In different ways, both of them offer a salvation in which death could be the gate to the true life. ʿAbd al-Ṣabūr offers the yearning for God as the only refuge from the hopelessness of the material (and materialistic) world, while Kafka offers us a similar refuge with a spiritual dimension. If there is a refuge and if there is an agent of mercy, it can only be the unknowable and ineffable God or any absolute essence. Here, despite the differences between the two writers, we find the common yearning.

Chapter 7, "Reception: Stream of Consciousness," deals with the process of reception of Western authors in Arabic literature as a process of indirect interference—that is, their writings were not accessed directly by agents of Arabic literature but by intermediaries, especially by translators. There is a good deal of research in both Arabic and English on the formative stage of modern Arabic literature—that is, the second half of the nineteenth century, when the Arab world set about creating responses to the growing impact and domination, cultural as well political, of the West. The case of *Robinson Crusoe* (1719) by Daniel Defoe (1660–1731) is highly instructive in this respect, as its translation into Arabic in the nineteenth century was one of the factors that helped to shape the norms of the emerging Arabic novel. It was then that such European literary models as the novel and the short story were "imported" into Arabic literature, although one can hardly agree that it was only import that brought about the rise of Arabic fiction. There is surprisingly limited research on the contemporary Arab literary scene as to Western borrowings or interference. "Stream of consciousness" is a salient example—it is clearly present in Arabic literature by the 1960s, but no one (to my mind) has so far followed its trajectory from West to East. In this chapter, I will discuss the reception of Virginia Woolf (1882–1941) in Arabic literature, which later opened the way for Arab authors to write original fiction in her spirit. The major impact of Woolf on Arabic literature did

[11] See, for example, Myers 1986, pp. 82–96.

[12] See, for example, the novel *al-Lajna* (*The Committee*) (Ṣunʿ Allāh 1981).

not come as a direct interference—that is, her writings were not in general accessed directly by writers but by intermediaries, especially by translators. This chapter will be a preliminary survey of the presence of Virginia Woolf in Arabic literature.

Chapter 8, "Import: Science Fiction," deals with the genre of science fiction (SF) as a new emerging imported genre in Arabic literature, first, through translations and adaptations, and afterward by the rising of original Arabic SF progressing toward canonization. The emergence of SF in Arabic literature is the most evident illustration of an imported genre, and, at least from the point of view of the beginnings of the genre, it grew by borrowing the relevant Western pattern, though at a later stage the genre would pass through a process of Arabization and even Islamization. SF in Arabic has been around since the 1970s; however, as with most genres of popular non-canonical Arabic prose, the scholarly academic research has paid little or no attention to it. This chapter attempts to partly fill that gap, approaching the topic within the aforementioned proposed theoretical framework for the study of Arabic literature. Though the bulk of Arabic SF literature is still generally referred to in the Arab world as stories for children and adventures of young men, Arabic SF has already taken its first steps on the road toward canonization. Its emergence is mostly due to the impact of Western popular culture and the advent of modern technology, but the contribution that SF can make to Arab society goes far beyond literature: it can accustom readers, in the words of Isaac Asimov (1920–1992), to the thought of "the inevitability of continuing change and the necessity of directing and shaping that change rather than opposing it blindly or blindly permitting it to overwhelm us."[13] At the same time, as in the efforts toward the decolonization of African literature, Arab authors and critics in this field might also stop being mesmerized by the West and improve the quality of their writing.

[13] Quoted in Knight 1977, p. 61

Chapter 5

Self-image: Between "Decadence" and Renaissance[1]

The Arabs in our time are very satisfied with the matter of culture. They are satisfied with the minimum of it, considering themselves having arrived at the highest levels of science, although they have never even knocked on its door.
– Buṭrus al-Bustānī

1. INTRODUCTION

In 1923, the Lebanese-Christian Mahjari poet Mīkhā'īl Nu'ayma (1889–1988) called on Arab authors to concentrate on translating Western literary masterpieces into Arabic as a necessary step toward bringing Arabic literature into the ambit of world literature and the universal human spirit.[2] Alluding to the urgent need for Arab culture to benefit from its contacts with the West, Nu'ayma wrote the following in his "Fa-l-Nutarjim" ("Let Us Translate"), which was published in his book *al-Ghirbāl* (*The Sieve*):

> نحن في دور من رقيّنا الأدبيّ والاجتماعيّ قد تنبّهت فيه حاجات روحيّة كثيرة لم نكن نشعر بها من قبل احتكاكنا الحديث بالغرب. وليس عندنا من الأقلام والأدمغة ما يفي بسدّ هذه الحاجات. فلنترجم! ولنجلّ مقام المترجم لأنه واسطة تعارف بيننا وبين العائلة البشريّة العظمى.

We are at a stage of our literary and social evolution in which many spiritual needs have awakened which we did not feel before our new contact with the West. As we have no pens and brains that can fulfill those needs, let us then

[1] This chapter uses material that first appeared in Snir 2000a, pp. 53–71; Snir 2017.

[2] The fact that Mīkhā'īl Nu'ayma was inspired by Russian literature and even wrote poetry in Russian sheds light on his vision regarding the role of multilingualism in generating literary identities and in shaping literary form. Furthermore, "the multilingual poetry of Nu'ayma can be used as the basis for a deeper study of *nahḍah* multilingualism, including its role in shaping Arabic modernism" (Swanson and Gould 2021, pp. 170–201; the quotation is from p. 201).

> translate! Let us honor the status of the translator because he is an agent of acquaintance between us and the larger human family.[3]

Nu'ayma's call did not emerge in the Arab world or on the international scene *ex nihilo*. We can see similar calls in other societies, especially during the nineteenth century, when writers and scholars felt that their local culture should benefit from Western culture. For example, in *A House of Gentlefolk* by Ivan Sergeyevich Turgenev (1818–1883),[4] we find the following at the beginning of chapter 33:

> Panshin was the only guest. He was stimulated by the beauty of the evening, and conscious of a flood of artistic sensations, but he did not care to sing before Lavretsky, so he fell to reading poetry; he read aloud well, but too self-consciously and with unnecessary refinements, a few poems of Lermontov (Pushkin had not then come into fashion again). Then suddenly, as though ashamed of his enthusiasm, [he] began, à propos of the well-known poem, "A Reverie," to attack and fall foul of the younger generation. While doing so, he did not lose the opportunity of expounding how he would change everything after his own fashion, if the power were in his hands. "Russia," he said, "has fallen behind Europe; we must catch her up. It is maintained that we are young—that's nonsense. Moreover, we have no inventiveness: Homakov himself admits that we have not even invented mouse-traps. Consequently, whether we will or no, we must borrow from others. We are sick, Lermontov says—I agree with him. But we are sick from having only half become Europeans, we must take a hair of the dog that bit us ("*le cadastre*," thought Lavretsky). "The best heads, *les meilleures tâtes*," he continued, "among us have long been convinced of it. All peoples are essentially alike; only introduce among them good institutions, and the thing is done. Of course there may be adaptation to the existing national life; that is our affair—the affair of the official (he almost said 'governing') class. But in case of need, don't be uneasy. The institutions will transform the life itself."

When Nu'ayma published his own call, translations had already been the primary channel of interaction between Arabic literature and Western culture for several decades. Already in 1890, we find the Egyptian philologist Aḥmad Zakī (1867–1934), known as the "Dean of Arabism" (*Shaykh al-'Urūba*), saying that "we are at a time in which composing (*taṣnīf*) is

[3] Nu'ayma 1964 [1923], p. 126. Cf. Badawi 1975, p. 182; Ostle 1991, p. 42. See also the introduction to Nu'ayma's play *al-Ābā' wa-l-Banūn* (*Fathers and Sons*) (Nu'ayma 1989 [1917], pp. 11–19). The title of the play evokes a novel with the same title (1862) by I. S. Turgenev. The introduction was also published in al-Khaṭīb 1994, pp. 443–9. Twelve years after the publication of Nu'ayma's article, his compatriot Sa'īd 'Aql (1911–2014), in the course of a review of several works of Lebanese poets in French, issued a similar *cri de coeur* ('Aql 1935, especially pp. 381–4). There have been many similar calls, and even sixty years later we find such a call in 'Abd al-Wahhāb 1995, pp. 10–12. See also Snir 2017, pp. 108–10.

[4] Turgenev 1951 [1917].

decreasing and translation (*ta'rīb*) is increasing; how often an Arabic book is described as being composed while it is nothing but a translation or a summary of a European book."[5] In retrospect, then, "Fa-l-Nutarjim" seems less an attempt to boost the process of cultural borrowing from the West—at the time in full progress and in no need for such a call—and more a kind of a persistent lament over the state of Arab culture. Although "nobody seems to know when the term *inḥiṭāṭ* was first used to denote 'decadence' as [the] self-view of intellectuals of the Ottoman Empire,"[6] we can hardly find anyone who has denied the collapse of the Arabs' cultural self-image and the significant decline in their self-esteem in modern times. The movement that sought to translate Western classics into Arabic, which began in the nineteenth century, reflected the state of Arab culture and the frustration of its agents.[7] Emphasizing the intellectual backwardness of the Arab world, forty-five years after Nu'ayma published his essay, the Egyptian critic Ghālī Shukrī (1935–1998) still finds no comfort in the state of Arab culture. Furthermore, unlike Nu'ayma, he seems to have no hope for the near future:

> No cultural unity connects the Arab poet with his counterpart in Western or Eastern Europe. We are living under the influence of an undeveloped civilization compared to Western civilization ... The modern Arab poet stands on the mouth of a volcano boiling for about a hundred years with strange and complex interactions. No less than four centuries, the temporal distance between the European Renaissance and that of the Arabs, separate the Arabic poet from the caravan of human civilization at the peak of its artistic expression in Europe.[8]

Considering Nu'ayma and Shukrī's comments about the decline of the Arabs' cultural self-esteem and the change in the self-image of the very culture they are part of, it is no accident that both writers are not Muslim. They are part of a long list of Christian intellectuals and men of letters for whom the high reverence accorded to Arabic not only as the language of the Qur'ān but also as the language of their own literary heritage[9] did not prevent them, as it prevented Muslim intellectuals, from voicing dissatisfaction at the state and status of their own culture. The lecture "Khuṭba fī Ādāb al-'Arab" ("A Lecture on the Culture of the Arabs"), delivered on February 15, 1859 by the

[5] *Al-Muqtaṭaf* 15 (October 1890), p. 269.
[6] Wild 1996, p. 386.
[7] Cf. Lefevere 1990, p. 27.
[8] Shukrī 1978, pp. 18–19.
[9] In his introduction to a collection of articles dealing with the Arab Christians, the Lebanese writer and critic Ilyās Khūrī (Elias Khoury) (b. 1948) argues that "Arab Christianity is an integral part of the Arab and Islamic social and cultural reality; it cannot separate itself of that reality; otherwise, it will lose its identity and distinctiveness" (Khūrī 1981, p. 9). Khūrī even refers to himself as Christian-Muslim (*Masāhārif* [Haifa] 17 [2002], pp. 253–4).

Christian scholar Buṭrus al-Bustānī (1819–1883), one of the most prominent figures of the *Nahḍa* (often called the "Father of the *Nahḍa*" or *al-Muʿallim* ["The Educator"]),[10] seems to be one of the first sharp statements reflecting that essential change in the Arabs' self-esteem. Concentrating on the culture of the Arabs in his time, at the beginning of the third chapter of his screed, al-Bustānī complains in metaphorical language that the contemporary Arabs in his time are satisfied with the low state of their literature and, at the same time, falsely consider themselves as having obtained the highest levels of science:

> إنّ العرب في أيّامنا هذه قنعون جدّا في أمر الآداب. فإنّهم يكتفون بأقلّها، ويحسبون أنفسهم أنّهم قد وصلوا إلى أعلى طبقات العلم، مع أنّهم لم يقرعوا بابه. ومن تعلّم منهم كتاب الزّبور، والقرآن، يقال إنّه قد ختم علمه، وإذا تعلّم شيئا من أصول الصّرف والنّحو يقال فيه إنّه قد صار علاّمة زمانه وإذا نطق بالشّعر فلا يبقى عندهم لقب يصفونه به. وما ذلك إلاّ لأنّ ظهور نور قليل في العاقل كاف لأن يغشى على عيني الجاهل، لأنّهم إلى الآن لم يقفوا على شاطئ أوقيانوس العلوم ويروا عظمته واتّساعه. ومع أنّنا نعتقد بأنّ عرب هذه الأيّام هم من نسل العرب القدماء، لا نرى فيهم ما رأيناه في أولائك المجاهدين من الثّبات والجهاد في ميدان العلوم، ولا نقدر أن نسلّم بأنّ النّسل قد فسد، وذلك لأنّ جودة عقول العرب، وحسن استعدادها في هذه الأيّام لتحصيل العلوم، ببرهان النّقيض. ولكنّ ذلك ناتج من أحوال كثيرة وأسباب متنوّعة نودّ لو سمحت لنا الأوقات لبيانها لكي نخفّف عمّن هم من لحمنا ودمنا اللّوم الواقع عليهم من الأجانب الّذين لا نشكّ بأنّهم كانوا وصلوا إلى حالة أردأ من حالتنا لو ألقاهم الدهر في ظروف كظروفنا. ولكنّ مهما كانت الأسباب فلا سبيل إلى إنكار كساد بضاعة العلم عند العرب، وعدم رواج سوقها بين جماهيرهم، وعلى الخصوص أكابرهم.

> The Arabs in our time are very satisfied with the matter of culture. They are satisfied with the minimum of it, considering themselves having arrived at the highest levels of science, although they have never even knocked on its door. It is said that any one of them who studies the *Book of Psalms* and the Qur'ān has finished his study, and if he studies something from the principles of *ʿilm al-ṣarf* [morphology] and *ʿilm al-naḥw* [grammar], it is said of him that he has become the scholar of his time, and if he composes poetry, they find a difficulty in finding a suitable phrase to describe his greatness. We cannot explain this but for the fact that a small light for the intelligent man is sufficient to cause blindness in the eyes of the ignorant; that because they have not stood on the shore of the ocean of sciences they cannot know its greatness and wideness. Although we think that the Arabs of our time are the offspring of the ancient Arabs, we do not see in them the firmness and struggle in the field of sciences that we have seen in those ancient fighters. We cannot agree that the progeny has become spoiled, because the quality of the brains of the Arabs and their good ability to acquire sciences bear witness to the opposite. However, this is due to many circumstances and various reasons we wish we had enough time to explain in order to ease the blame laid upon those who are of our flesh and blood by the foreigners who would have been in worse shape than us if fate had decreed to

[10] On Buṭrus al-Bustānī and his family and relevant references, see Zachs 2018.

> them circumstances such as ours. However, whatever the reasons, we cannot deny the dullness of the Arab science market and the absence of its popularity among their masses, especially their senior members.[11]

Viewing al-Bustānī's complaint about the attitude toward the Other that prevailed among the Arabs several centuries before his time illuminates the abysmal collapse of the Arabs' cultural self-image. For example, in his *Kitāb al-I'tibār* (*The Book of Esteem*), Usāma ibn Munqidh (1095–1188) refers to the Franks as follows:

> سبحان الخالق البارئ إذا خبر الإنسان أمور الإفرنج سبّح الله تعالى وقدّسه ورأى بهائم فيهم فضيلة الشّجاعة والقتال لا غير، كما في البهائم فضيلة القوّة والحمل. وسأذكر شيئا من أمورهم وعجائب عقولهم. كان في عسكر الملك فلك بن فلك فارس محتشم إفرنجي قد وصل من بلادهم يحجّ ويعود. فأنس بي وصار ملازمي يدعوني «أخي» وبيننا المودّة والمعاشرة. فلمّا عزم على التّوجّه في البحر إلى بلاده قال لي: «يا أخي، أنا سائر إلى بلادي. وأريدك تنفّذ معي ابنك، وكان ابني معي وهو ابن أربع عشرة سنة، إلى بلادي يبصر الفرسان ويتعلّم العقل والفروسيّة. وإذا رجع كان مثل رجل عاقل». فطرق سمعي كلام ما يسمع من رأس عاقل. فإنّ ابني لو أُسر ما بلغ به الأسر أكثر من رواحه إلى بلاد الإفرنج. فقلت «وحياتك، هذا الّذي كان في نفسي، لكن منعني من ذلك أن جدّته تحبّه وما تركته يخرج معي حتّى استحلفتني أنّي أردّه إليها». قال «وأمّك تعيش؟» قلت «نعم». قال «لا تخالفها».

> Mysterious are the works of the Creator, the author of all things! When one comes to recount cases regarding the Franks, he cannot but glorify Allah (exalted is he!) and sanctify him, for he sees them as animals possessing the virtues of courage and fighting, but nothing else; just as animals have only the virtues of strength and carrying loads. I shall now give some instances of their doings and their curious mentality. In the army of King Fulk, son of Fulk, was a Frankish reverend knight who had just arrived from their land in order to make the holy pilgrimage and then return home. He was of my intimate fel-

[11] Al-Bustānī 1859, p. 31; al-Bustānī 1990, pp. 113–14. Cf. Sheehi 2004, pp. 19–45; Zachs 2005, pp. 145–8; Allen 2006, pp. 13–17; Zachs and Halevi 2015, pp. 1–4; Bellino 2020, pp. 152–3. Sixty-three years after al-Bustānī delivered his lecture, the Lebanese-American Christian author Amīn al-Rīḥānī (1876–1940), in his poem "Anā al-Sharq" ("I am the East"), published in *al-Ahrām* in 1922, expressed the same views—he concluded the poem with the following lines:

> "أنا الشّرق عندي فلسفات وعندي ديانات،
> فمن يبيعني بها طيّارات؟"

(republished in al-Rīḥānī 1955, pp. 84–91. The quotation is from p. 91). In another place he wrote:

> "حبذا الشّرقيّون والغربيّون لو أخذ بعضهم عن بعض ممّا هو جميل في أديانهم، صحيح في عاداتهم، سام في فنونهم، عادل في أحكامهم وشرائعهم، سليم في أخلاقهم. إن خلاصة الصّحيح السّليم من ثقافة الشّرق والغرب ممزوجة موحّدة إنّما هي الدّواء الوحيد لأمراض هذا الزّمان الدّينيّة والاجتماعيّة والسّياسيّة. فالغربيّ عندئذ يعود إلى الله. والشّرقيّ يرفع عن الله بعض أثقاله."

(al-Rīḥānī 1955, I, p. 292. For more on al-Rīḥānī's views toward East and West, see El-Enany 2006, pp. 154–8).

> lowship and kept such constant company with me that he began to call me "my brother." Between us were mutual bonds of amity and friendship. When he resolved to return by sea to his homeland, he said to me: "My brother, I am leaving for my country and I want thee to send with me thy son (my son, who was then fourteen years old, was at that time in my company) to our country, where he can see the knights and learn wisdom and chivalry. When he returns, he will be like a wise man." Thus there fell upon my ears words which would never come out of the head of a sensible man; for even if my son were to be taken captive, his captivity could not bring him worse misfortune than carrying him into the lands of the Franks. However, I said to the man: "By thy life, this has exactly been my idea. But the only thing that prevented me from carrying it out was the fact that his grandmother, my mother, is so fond of him and did not this time let him come out with me until she exacted an oath from me to the effect that I would return him to her." Thereupon he asked, "Is thy mother still alive?" "Yes." I replied. "Well," said he, "disobey her not."[12]

In the next century, the geographer Zakariyyā ibn Muḥammad al-Qazwīnī (1203–1283) mentions a city on the Atlantic called "Shlashwīq" (Schleswig, a town located in northeastern Schleswig-Holstein, Germany) which was visited by someone who said: "I have never heard singing more terrible than that of the people of Shlashwīq. It is a sound that emerges from their mouths like the barking of dogs or much worse than that."[13]

Against this background, it is highly instructive to find that none other than "The Prince of Poets," Aḥmad Shawqī (1868–1932), described in the introduction to the first edition of his *Dīwān* the expeditions sent out in the nineteenth century to "the lands of the Franks" to benefit from the achievements of Western civilization as "learning wisdom,"[14] precisely from those whom Usāma ibn Munqidh described above as "animals possessing the virtues of courage and fighting, but nothing else; just as animals have only the virtues of strength and carrying loads." Bernard Lewis (1916–2018) writes that it is difficult for a Westerner to appreciate the magnitude of such a change in a society accustomed to despise the infidel barbarians beyond the frontiers of civilization because "even traveling abroad was suspect; the

12 Ibn Munqidh 1930, p. 132 (English translation according to Ibn Munqidh 1987, p. 161). Cf. Hitti 1962, pp. 184–7; Ayyad and Witherspoon 1999, pp. 3–18. On Ibn Munqidh, see DeYoung and Germain 2011, pp. 364–71 (by Terri DeYoung). The term "Franks" (*al-Ifranj*) was used by earlier Arabic authors to refer to all Western Europeans (Hermes 2012, pp. 48–9).

13 Al-Qazwīnī 1960, p. 602. Cf. Abdullah 1997, pp. 78–9. On the European "other" in medieval Arabic literature and culture, see Hermes 2012.

14 Mandūr 1970, p. 43.

idea of studying under infidel teachers was inconceivable."[15] No sooner had the first expeditions returned, than the change was noticed on the level of literature as well. For example, *'Alam al-Dīn* (*The Sign of Religion*) (1882) by 'Alī Mubārak (1824–1893), described as *ḥikāya laṭīfa* (fine story) and as belonging to the literature of travel (*adab al-riḥla*),[16] was written in a narrative structure that did not entirely follow the usual Arabic literary norms of the time. From a thematic point of view, the West in that work proves to be far superior to the East, insofar as the author produces an almost degrading image of an East which is yet unaware of its inferior position.[17]

Significantly enough, even one hundred years later that awareness was still deeply rooted in the minds of Arab intellectuals. Pointing out the build-up of literary criticism in the 1980s, the Egyptian poet and critic Yusrī al-'Azab (1947–2020) finds no way forward but to benefit from the West. Emphasizing the contributions that medieval Arab culture made to universal civilization compared with its present, gloomy state, he indicates that "since we became petty states, splinters, we have been moving in circles in the ideological and cultural orbit of others. There is no other way but to benefit from their estates, even in the field of literature and criticism."[18] Even in 2006, the Libyan writer Ibrāhīm al-Kawnī (al-Koni) (b. 1948) argues that the real crisis facing Arab culture is that Arabs have not yet admitted their weakness:

> أزمتنا قبل أن تكون سياسيّة أو ثقافيّة أم غيرها هي أزمة أخلاقيّة [...] من المستحيل أن يستشفي إنسان من مرض ما دام هذا الإنسان يرفض أن يعترف بمرضه. أزمتنا لهذا السّبب أخلاقيّة لأنّنا أمّة لا تريد أن تعترف بعلّتها المميتة ما دامت تصرّ أنها خير أمّة أخرجت للنّاس وتتجاهل الوصيّة الإلهيّة [...] الّتي كانت سرّ قيام، بل واستمرار الحضارة الأوروبيّة، والمنقولة على لسان سقراط "إعرف نفسك!" [...] المحنة الأخلاقيّة (هي) المتمثّلة في اليقين المسبق بتميّز موهوم (أو فلنقل غابر) [...] هذا في حين تسلّح المخاطب (أو الآخر) بيقين بسيط كان سرّ سلطانه دائما ألا وهو "إعرف نفسك!"

> Our crisis, before it is a political or cultural or other, is a moral crisis ... man cannot find a cure for his malady as long as he does not admit it. Our crisis thus is moral because we are a nation which does not want to admit its fatal malady as long as it insists it has been the best nation emerged to human beings and ignores the divine command ... that was the secret of the emergence, moreover, of the continuation of European civilization that was transmitted by Socrates: "Know yourself!" ... the moral ordeal is that which is expressed in the premature certitude of imagined advantage (or, in fact, let us say bygone [advantage]) ... while in the meantime the addressee (or the Other) has armed himself with

15 Lewis 2003, p. 43.
16 Mubārak 1882, p. 7.
17 Cf. Hopwood 1999, pp. 248–9.
18 Al-Rāwī 1982, pp. 249–50.

> a simple certitude, which was always the secret of his power, namely, "know yourself!"[19]

More than thirty-five years earlier, the Egyptian poet Ṣalāḥ ʿAbd al-Ṣabūr (1931–1981) had alluded to the same position by considering Socrates' aforementioned saying as the turning point in the history of humanity—it was the first time that a human being turned his attention to himself:

> لأنّ الإنسان هو الموجود الوحيد الّذي يستطيع أن يعي ذاته، فهو إذن وعي الكون فالكون قوّة عمياء، أو جسم عملاقيّ فائر. الإنسان هو عقله ووعيه وعظمة ذلك العقل أنّه يستطيع أن يعقل ذاته، وجلال الإنسان أنّه يقدر أن يواجه نفسه، أن يجعل من نفسه ذاتا وموضوعا في نفس الآونة، ناظرا ومنظورا إليه ومرآة، أن ينقسم ويلتئم في لحظة واحدة.

> Because the human being is the sole creature who is able to become aware of himself, he is thus the consciousness of the universe. The universe is a blind force, or a giant boiling body whose mind and consciousness is the human being. The greatness of this mind is that it is able to realize itself and the greatness of the human being is that he is able to confront himself and make himself the subject and the object at the same time, the observer and the observed as well as a mirror, to be split up and combined in the same moment.[20]

Examining the repeated lamentations by Arab intellectuals and writers about the status of Arab culture and literature throughout the last two centuries, the nuances and wording of each of them enable the student of Arabic literature to understand the complicated attitude toward the West in light of the decline of the Arabs' cultural self-image and the huge gap between the august status enjoyed by Arab culture in the Middle Ages and its feeble modern counterpart. And here, and against the background of the aforementioned lamentations, it is necessary to mention that there are different views and opinions regarding the relationship and connections between premodern Arab culture, before the encounter with the West, and modern Arab culture, including the role of modernist Arab intellectuals in that encounter.

2. EXTENSION OR BREAK?

As I have already pointed out, the way we view the relationship between modern and classical Arabic literature is essential to our understanding of the nature of the contemporary literary system. The question is whether modern literature is an extension of classical literature or whether it is a new creation that has hardly any relationship at all with its medieval predecessor. It is no coincidence that Arab, especially Muslim, scholars tend to adopt the former

[19] Quoted on www.elaph.com, August 1, 2006.
[20] ʿAbd al-Ṣabūr 1969, p. 6. Cf. Snir 2006, p. 93.

view, whereas Western scholars tend to adopt the latter. For example, in his aforementioned article "al-Adab al-'Arabī Bayna Amsihi wa-Ghadihi" ("Arabic Literature between Its Past and Future"),[21] which in October 1945 led the first issue of his journal *al-Kātib al-Miṣrī*, Ṭāhā Ḥusayn asserts the continuity of Arabic literature. Unlike Greek and Latin literatures, which have no direct contemporary extension, modern Arabic literature, according to Ḥusayn, is a direct linear extension of classical Arabic literature. "The historical existence of Arabic literature has never been cut off, and it seems that it will never be cut off," he writes. "Arabic literature is very traditional and at the same time very modern. Its ancient past has been directly mingled with its modern present without any break or bend ... Our Arabic literature is a living being and resembles, more than anything else, a huge tree the roots of which have been consolidated and extended into the depths of the earth, while its branches have risen and spread out in space, breaking the connection between it and the new time as well as deterring it from the road of the continuous life of the living literatures into the road of cut-off life which the Greek and Latin literatures took."[22] This direct extension of classical into modern literature has been guaranteed, according to Ḥusayn, by the continuous equilibrium that Arabic literature maintained until modern times between aspects of continuity and change. By preserving some traditional principles to ensure its distinctive identity and, at the same time, incorporating a variety of innovations both in form and content, Arabic literature, according to Ḥusayn, has proven its vitality down through the ages.[23]

The contrary view we find neatly summarized by Hamilton Gibb, one of the first Western scholars to systematically study modern Arabic literature,[24] in an article published in 1928:

> It may be asked ... by what right Arabic literature is called a young literature. To all appearances, it is entitled to claim a history of thirteen centuries, a longer period of continuous literary activity than any living European language can boast. But beneath the apparent linguistic continuity, Arabic literature is undergoing an evolution comparable, in some respects, to the substitution of Patristic for Classical Greek literature and idiom. Neo-Arabic literature is only to a limited extent the heir of the old "classical" Arabic literature, and *even shows a tendency to repudiate its inheritance entirely*. Its leaders are, for the most part,

[21] Ḥusayn 1945, pp. 4–27. The article was also incorporated into Ḥusayn n.d. [1958], pp. 5–32.
[22] Ḥusayn 1945, pp. 10–11; Ḥusayn n.d. [1958], pp. 11–13.
[23] Cf. Semah 1974, p. 122.
[24] See "Studies in Contemporary Arabic Literature," in Gibb 1962, pp. 245–319, which is based on a series of articles that Gibb first published in *Bulletin of the School of Oriental Studies* (*BSOAS*) (IV.4 [1928], pp. 745–60; V.2 [1929], pp. 311–22; V.3 [1929], pp. 445–66; VII.1 [1933], pp. 1–22).

> men who have drunk from other springs and look at the world with different eyes. Yet the past still plays a part in their intellectual background, and there is a section among them upon whom that past retains a hold scarcely shaken by newer influences. For many decades, the partisans of the "old" and the "new" have engaged in a struggle for the soul of the Arabic world, a struggle in which the victory of one side over the other is even yet not assured. The protagonists are (to classify them roughly for practical purposes) the European-educated classes of Egyptians and Syrians on the one hand, and those in Egypt and the less advanced Arabic lands whose education has followed traditional lines, on the other. Whatever the ultimate result may be, however, there can be no question that the conflict has torn the Arabic world from its ancient moorings, and that *the contemporary literature of Egypt and Syria breathes, in its more recent developments, a spirit foreign to the old traditions.*[25]

Regarding the modern Arabic literary system as a new creation[26] means accepting the view that Arabic literature prior to the nineteenth century had somehow collapsed and been abandoned by its own community, as though the Arabs during the eighteenth and nineteenth centuries had in one way or another exchanged all or parts of their culture for another. Of course, slippage or collapse may occur, and a given community may let go of its literature when changes in its sociocultural conditions fail to leave their mark on that literature, but long before this happens one should be able to detect certain signals, such as the literature being pushed to the periphery of the cultural system. In any event, it is an unsupported and unjustifiable assumption to refer to classical, medieval, and premodern Arabic literature as a case of collapse and abandonment, side by side with Latin, Byzantine Greek, and Church Slavonic literatures.[27] It is also an unsupported assumption to refer to Arabic literature as consisting of "two separate literary systems" or "two different periods."[28] Any student of Arabic literature familiar with literary production prior to the nineteenth century, especially with the various branches of non-canonical literary production before the encounter between Arabic literature and Western culture, would hesitate to speak of "two separate literary systems." The Moroccan scholar Abdelfattah Kilito (b. 1945) emphasizes this insight in his essay "This Is Why We Read Classic

[25] Gibb 1962, pp. 246–7 (my emphasis).

[26] ʿAfīf al-Bahnassī (1928–2017), art historian and General Director of Antiquities and Museums in Damascus, refers to this general conception as "*siyāsat al-batr*" (i.e., "the policy of amputation") (al-Bahnassī 1997, p. 62). On this issue, see also Mestyan 2016, pp. 97–118.

[27] Even-Zohar in Sebeok 1986, I, p. 461. Cf. Somekh 1983, p. 4: "[Modern Arabic literature] emerged after a period of hundreds of years of virtual isolation, during which Arabic literature suffered from stagnation and triviality."

[28] See Somekh 1991, p. 3.

Literature ..."[29] Alluding to the Italian writer Italo Calvino's (1923–1985) essay *Why Read the Classics?*[30] in which fourteen definitions of the term "classic" are introduced, Kilito refers to the same concept in Arab culture:

> في الثّقافة العربيّة، تبدو الأمور معقّدة لأوّل وهلة. أوّلا هل لكلمة كلاسيك ما يعادلها في اللّغة العربيّة؟ يتمّ استخدامها أحيانا للإشارة إلى الأدب القديم، يُنعت بالأدب الكلاسيكيّ، ولكن غالبا ما يُشار إليه بالأدب القديم تمييزا له عن الأدب الحديث. يوجد متخصّصون في هذا أو ذاك، كما لو أنّنا أمام أدبين مختلفين، أمام عالمين متباينين، لكنّ الواقع أنّه عندما يذكر أحدهما، فإنّ الآخر يتبادر إلى الذّهن على الفور. في كثير من الحالات يتمّ الحكم على الأدب العربيّ القديم من خلال ما جاء بعده، من خلال الأدب الحديث، وعلى العكس من ذلك، وكما يشير إيطالو كالفينو، فإنّ الكتاب الكلاسيكيّ يجعلنا نحدّد أنفسنا بالمقارنة معه، وربّما بمعارضته، أي يجعلنا نكتشف أنفسنا. مهما يكن، فإنّ من يدرس مؤلّفا عربيّا كلاسيكيّا يكشف حتما عن أصله ومحتده، نعرف توّا هل هو عربيّ، أو فرنسيّ، أو أمريكيّ مهما كانت اللغة المستعملة.

> As for Arab culture, matters appear complicated from the first glance. First of all, is there any Arabic word that could approximate the meaning of the word *klāsīk*? It is sometimes used to refer to ancient literature, described as classic literature. But, that said, it is usually referred to as ancient literature in order to distinguish it from modern literature. There are specialists in this or that field, as if we were confronted with two different literatures, two disparate worlds. Yet the reality is that as soon as one is mentioned, the other comes to mind at once. In many cases, ancient Arabic literature is judged in light of what came after it, in light of modern literature. And conversely, as Italo Calvino points out, the classic book compels us to identify ourselves in comparison with it, and perhaps in opposition to it. Whatever the case may be, anyone who studies a classic Arabic work inevitably reveals their own origin and lineage—we know instantly whether they are Arab, or French, or American, regardless of the language they are using.[31]

It should be noted that several years after Hamilton Gibb re-emphasized his view that Arabic literature prior to the nineteenth century had somehow collapsed and been abandoned by its own community, the Russian literary critic Isaak Moiseevich Filshtinsky (1918–2013) utterly refuted it. After describing at length the popular romances and tales of the late Middle Ages,[32] Filshtinsky concluded his *Arabic Literature* (1966) with the following passage:

> The Arab literary tradition was never totally broken. This was a favourable factor during the period of the Arab literary renaissance in the nineteenth century. The starting point of the Arab political and cultural advance is usually placed

[29] Kilito 2020, pp. 59–68.
[30] Calvino 1999, pp. 3–10.
[31] Translation by Safwan Khatib with minor modifications, available at: https://thebaffler.com/latest/why-read-the-classics-kilito (last accessed April 17, 2021).
[32] Filshtinsky 1966, pp. 205–24.

> in the early years of the nineteenth century, and is associated with the struggle of the Egyptians against the invading armies of Napoleon Bonaparte. From that moment, in the Arab countries, the long struggle for independence was launched; it was in these conditions that the new literature came into existence, closely linked with contemporaneity, yet resting upon, and adhering to, the age-old literary tradition.[33]

As the present study seeks to underline, modern Arabic literature is connected with the ancient Arabic literary heritage in all aspects of its development. Every signal innovation is based *on* or is introduced *against* that literary background. Moreover, no Arab poet, writer, or playwright has ever succeeded in gaining fame or becoming canonical without a deep knowledge of the Arabic literary heritage.[34] This makes it impossible to refer to modern Arabic poetry as lending itself "to Western modes of composition" and to claim that "it is hardly recognizable as a direct offspring of classical Arabic poetry in the output of the most representative Arab poets today."[35] Moreover, from the literary-aesthetic point of view, literary texts written since the Arab world had its first intensive cultural contacts with the West cannot be studied separately from medieval Arabic literary texts. Some phenomena and features in modern literature first appeared in medieval literature and have either remained essential components of Arabic literature throughout its history (i.e., continuity) or have disappeared only to be revived in modern

[33] Filshtinsky 1966, p. 224. On this topic, specifically on the attitude to the Mamluk period, "one of the apogees of Arabic literature," see Bauer 2005, pp. 105–32: "Mamluk literature is fascinating because it transcends boundaries: the boundaries between everyday and literary communication; between popular and high literature; between poetry and prose; between the private and the public; between theory and praxis. Colonial delusions have thus far prevented a proper appreciation of this culture" (p. 130). See also Bauer 2007, pp. 137–67.

[34] In a proposal for a seminar at the annual conference of the American Comparative Literature Association (ACLA), which was held at Harvard University, March17–20, 2016, titled "The Classical in the Modern: Specters of Arabic Literature," Muhsin al-Musawi and Yasmine Khayyat write that "contemporary debates in Arabic literary production often posit artificial borders between Classical and modern literary production such that Arabic literature allegedly stagnated for hundreds of years, until modern Arabic literature emerged with European intervention in the region. As that account of Arabic literature's history would have it, Classical Arabic's rich repertoire of poetry and prose was either put aside or rejuvenated by the ostensibly purely modern themes and forms preoccupying authors and poets since Napoleon arrived in Egypt in 1798." The proposal pushes against this sharp divide, probing the intersections of modern Arabic literature with tropes and motifs of the classical period, asking how classical Arabic poetry, storytelling, myth, and prose affected Arabic literary production in the last two centuries (according to "Arabic Lit Scholars" list, July 25, 2015).

[35] Somekh 1991, p. 4. On the issue of foreign influence on modern Arabic poetry, see the various contributions in Ṣāliḥ 1995. In his introduction to the book, Fakhrī Ṣāliḥ (b. 1957) criticizes both Arab and Western critics for the methods they have used to examine that influence (pp. 11–12).

times (i.e., renovation) under the impact of the West. A good example is the rationale that the Bahraini poet Ibrāhīm al-'Urayyiḍ (1908–2002) gives in the introduction to his *Min al-Shi'r al-Ḥadīth 1900–1950* (*From the Modern Poetry 1900–1950*) for the way he put together his anthology of modern Arabic poetry:

> كانت أمامي — في عهد صباي — لمختار الشّعر مجموعتان قديمتان، إحداهما عربيّة وهي حماسة أبي تمّام، والثّانية إنكليزيّة وهي «الذّخيرة الذّهبيّة» لمؤلّفها بالغريف، وكنت معجبا بالاثنين لمخضهما زبدة الشّعر في كلّ من اللّغتين. ولكنّي كنت أشدّ إعجابا بهما لاشتراكهما معا في ظاهرة نادرة هي سلكهما القطع المختارة كلّها — على نظام القلادة — في سلك منظّم بحيث كانت تتساوق القطعة التّالية مع الّتي تسبقها في الغرض والموضوع (...) فخطر لي أن أنتخب من الشّعر الحديث مختارا أجري فيه على نهج أبي تمّام وبالغريف وأصنع صنعهما في الاختيار والتّرتيب.

> In my youth I had before me two ancient collections of selected poetry, one of them in Arabic, that is, Abū Tammām's *Ḥamāsa*, and the second *The Golden Treasury* by Palgrave. I admired both of them since they contain the best poetry in both languages. However, I admired them more due to a common rare phenomenon, that is, the chaining of all the selected poems—as in a necklace—in an organized string. Each poem is in harmony with the preceding one as regards the purpose and theme ... Therefore, it came to me to select from modern poetry an anthology after the pattern of Abū Tammām and Palgrave, and to do as they did from the point of view of selection and arrangement.[36]

The *Ḥamāsa* by Abū Tammām Ḥabīb ibn Aws (d. 845) is the most widely known anthology of classical Arabic poetry.[37] Similarly, *The Golden Treasury* by Turner Francis Palgrave (1824–1897) compiled in 1861 is perhaps the most famous anthology of poems and lyrics in the English language,[38] and during the first half of the twentieth century it was one of the factors behind the gradual change in the poetic models of Arabic poetry.[39] But, as alluded to in al-'Urayyiḍ's aforementioned quotation, features of Western culture have most appealed to modern Arab poets when they could see them as being synonymous with features of continuity or renovation as they pertained to

36 Al-'Urayyiḍ 1958, p. 5.

37 See Abū Tammām n.d.

38 See Palgrave 1906 [1861]. The book changed with the World's Classics edition of 1907, which carried additional poems, and the 1928 edition, which included more works by contemporary poets. Further contemporary poems were included in the World's Classics edition of 1941. Finally, a complete fifth book was added to the existing four by John Press (Oxford Standard Authors, 1964), bringing the anthology up to date. The same text is used in the World's Classics edition of 1964 (on the various editions, see Palgrave 1906 [1861], pp. vii–xix; Stapleton 1985, p. 667).

39 Palgrave's anthology was a major inspiration for Arab writers, especially during the first half of the twentieth century; see Semah 1974, p. 193; Badawi 1975, pp. 88–90; Moreh 1976, p. 56; Badīr 1982, pp. 50, 152; Somekh 1991, p. 109; Badawi 1992, p. 90. On the importance of the poems included in *The Golden Treasury* to Arabic poetry in general and to Nāzik al-Malā'ika's poetry in particular, see Abdul-Razak 1989.

various aspects of the Arab heritage. Another example is Adūnīs, probably the most sophisticated of all contemporary canonical Arab poets. Because of his poetic innovations, he has been accused of betraying Arabism and Islam,[40] but all his writings are deeply rooted in ancient Arabic poetics and the classical Ṣūfī heritage.[41] Even the most avant-garde Arab poets, championing poetic iconoclasm and the abrogation of poetic values long held sacred, are deeply rooted in their traditions—if only in the way they oppose or challenge them.[42]

Modern Arabic literature has been inspired by Western literary models and concepts, but this inspiration has not changed the awareness in the Arab world that the present literary creation is a direct extension of ancient production.[43] Quite a few Arab authors, critics, and scholars regard even those genres considered to be a direct result of Western impact (such as the novel, the short story, and theater) as stemming from or inspired by the classical and medieval Arab literary tradition or as at least benefiting from early Arab and Islamic literary forms.[44] Najīb Maḥfūẓ even argued that his initial understanding of the genre of the novel was formed by the stories of the Qur'ān, which attracted him as a fine form of the art of storytelling. These stories follow the most modern principles of novel-writing:

> They do not begin, likc nineteenth-century novels, by setting the stage for the drama, then build up toward a climax, before reaching a resolution in the last pages. They are more like twentieth-century literary experiments, in which events do not follow a monotonous sequence but move according to dramatic requirements, which dictate where the different parts of the story are located.

[40] See, for example, al-Malā'ika 1983 [1962], pp. 213–27. Cf. a review of Moreh 1988 in *al-Karmil: Studies in Arabic Language and Literature* 10 (1989), pp. 161–71.

[41] Nevertheless, the Egyptian poet Muḥammad Ādām (b. 1954), who considers his poetry a continuation of the Ṣūfī heritage, contends that Adūnīs writes Arabic with "European pronunciation" (*lukna ūrūbiyya*) (*al-Ḥawādith*, April 6, 1990, p. 53).

[42] Cf. Kronholm 1993, pp. 20–2; Burt 1995, pp. 91–9; Allen 1998, pp. 203–17. See also what 'Abd al-Wahhāb al-Bayyātī (1926–1999) said before his death (*al-Ḥayāt*, August 7, 1999):

> حداثة شعر الرّوّاد جاءت من أو خرجت من معطف الشّعر العربيّ، يعني هي مولود أصيل، ولد ولادة عسيرة ولكنّه كان ابن أبيه، كما يقال.

[43] It was illustrated during the conference held at Philadelphia University in Amman, December 5–7, 1999, under the title "Modernism and Post-Modernism" (on the contributions to the conference, see the reports in *al-Ra'y*, December 6, 1999, p. 41; December 7, 1999, p. 50; December 8, 1999, p. 45).

[44] See Maḥmūd 1979; al-Ghīṭānī 1986, p. 9; al-Ghīṭānī 1986a, p. 9; al-Ghīṭānī 1986b, p. 9; al-Ghīṭānī 1986c, p. 9; al-Ḥakīm 1986, p. 9; Zaydān 1992, pp. 48–9; Badrān 2001; Wādī 2001, pp. 21–60. See also Khaldūn al-Sham'a's (b. 1941) essay in *al-Thawra* (Damascus), June 24, 1978 (according to al-Nafzāwī 1983, pp. 9–11). Cf. Snir 1993b, pp. 149–70. See also Elkhadem 1985, p. 55, about the *maqāma* that "has often been regarded as a forerunner of, if not a model for, the European picaresque novel." Cf. also Wilpert 1964, p. 406; al-Bustānī 1990, p. 125.

> In modern European novel writing, this represented a revolution, as can be seen in the works of Joyce or Proust. In the Qur'ān, the story of Mary, for example, is distributed among various *suras*. Each of these contains part of the story. For this reason, the Qur'ānic stories, with their noble content and style, were the first to provide me with a concept of the novel that I felt I could use in my writing.[45]

Naturally, Maḥfūẓ cannot but completely disagree with such decisive statements as Charles Vial's (b. 1928) on the birth and evolution of Arabic fictional literature:

> The modern *ḳiṣṣa* owes nothing to Arab tradition. It is linked neither with the folklore of the *Thousand and One Nights* nor with tales of chivalry nor with narratives of *adab*. The tradition of classical *maḳāma*, although taken up by two men of imagination and dual culture (Fāris al-Shidyāḳ for *al-Sāḳ 'alā 'l-Sāḳ*, 1855; and Muḥammad al-Muwayliḥī [for *Ḥadīth 'Īsā b. Hishām*], 1907), has left no legacy. It is from Europe that the Arabs have borrowed this literary genre totally unfamiliar to them, sc. the novel.[46]

And one does not have to look far to find scholars and intellectuals for whom the encounter between Islamic culture and European culture in al-Andalus,[47] Sicily,[48] or in other parts of Europe during the Crusades was a major factor in the renaissance of Western culture.[49] One should mention as well Miguel de Cervantes' (1547–1616) *Don Quixote* and the meta-fictional reflection on the identity of the author;[50] and some even went so far as to argue that William Shakespeare was of Arab origin and that his original name was al-Shaykh Zubayr.[51] That such an argument seems, even to the majority of Arab scholars, to have no basis in reality does not change their feeling that Islamic culture has not received sufficient credit for the development of modern

45 Mahfouz 2001, p. 66. In another place, however, Maḥfūẓ states that "there had not been any [Arabic] fictional heritage which I could use as a basis" (al-Ghīṭānī 2006, p. 149). Maḥfūẓ was probably referring to an actual modern heritage of fiction-writing.

46 Vial 1986, p. 187.

47 See, for example, Chejne 1980, pp. 110–33; Recapito 1998, pp. 55–74.

48 See, for example, Carpentieri 2018, pp. 1–18.

49 See, for example, al-Ṭawīl 1990, pp. 142–69. See also the following argument by Jabrā Ibrāhīm Jabrā (1920–1994) (Jabrā 1989, pp. 16–17. Cf. Krachkovskii 1989, p. 20):

> في القرون الوسطى، بعد اكتساح العرب للأندلس، وانتشارهم على سواحل البحر الأبيض المتوسّط وبثّ فنونهم الأدبيّة والحضاريّة في أرجاء أوربا الّتي أخذت عندها تستيقظ من ظلمات التردّي والجهل، أعطى العرب كتّاب الفرنسيّة والإيطاليّة لا المادّة فقط لملاحمهم البطوليّة، بل الكثير من أسلوبها الشعريّ بالذات. وظهرت "الروماسات" (كذا!) المطوّلة في الآداب الأوربيّة شعرا، وقد يكون بعضها في آلاف من الأبيات. وكان الفنّ الروائي عندهم فنّا شعريّا، لحمته الفروسيّة والحبّ — وكلاهما مستقى عن النموذج العربيّ أصلا — وسداه الصيغ الإيقاعيّة والقوافي الّتي تلقّنها شعراء الإفرنج عن العرب، فأضافوها إلى الصيغ اللاتينيّة القديمة لديهم، أو حوّروا بموجبها الصيغ الميسّرة في لغاتهم.

50 See Kilito 2001, pp. 91–7.

51 See al-Nāshif 1989, pp. 36–41. For more on that argument, search الشيخ زبير on the Internet.

civilization. A corollary of this is the view that it was the impact of Western culture in the nineteenth century that directly caused Arab culture to slide into a state of inferiority.[52] Adūnīs goes one step further by stating that "creative ability" (*ibdāʿ*) is an essential characteristic of the East:

> التّقنيّة «تقدّم» في إعادة إنتاج النّموذج. الإبداع ليس تقدّما تقنيّا أو نموذجيّا، إنّه انبثاق — اكتشاف للأصل لا نهاية له. إبداعيّا، أعني على مستوى الحضارة بمعناها الأكثر عمقا وإنسانيّة، ليس في «الغرب» شيء لم يأخذه من الشّرق. الدّين، الفلسفة، الشّعر (الفنّ، بعامّة) «شرقيّة» كلّها. ويمكنكم أن تستأنسوا بأسماء المبدعين في هذه الحقول، بدءا من دانتي حتى اليوم. فخصوصيّة «الغرب» هي التّقنيّة، لا الإبداع. لذلك يمكن القول إنّ الغرب، حضاريّا، هو ابن للشّرق. لكنّه، تقنيّا، «لقيط»: انحراف، استغلال، هيمنة، استعمار، إمبرياليّة، إنّه، في دلالة أخرى، تمرّد على الأب. وهو، الآن، لم يعد يكتفي بمجرّد التّمرّد، وإنّما يريد أن يقتل الأب (...) لهذا كانت الإبداعات الكبرى في الغرب، سواء أكانت دينيّة أو فنّيّة أو فلسفيّة، تجاوزا للتقنيّة، أي «شرقيّة» الينابيع. إنّها نوع من شَرْقَنَة الغرب.

> Technical ability is "progress" in the reproducing of a known pattern. Creative ability is not technical progress or progress from the point of view of reproduction according to some pattern. It is emanation—a never-ending discovery of the essence. From the point of view of creative ability, I mean on the level of culture in its deepest and most human sense, there is nothing in the "West" that was not taken from the "East." Religion, philosophy, poetry (art, in general), all of them are originally Eastern. You can include the names of the creators in those fields, from Dante until now. The obvious feature of the "West" is its technical rather than creative ability. Therefore, we could say, from the cultural point of view, that the West is the son of the East, but actually it is a "foundling": deviation, exploitation, domination, Colonialism, Imperialism; in other words, revolt against the father. Moreover, it is now no longer content with revolt, but is willing to kill the father ... That is why the great creations of the West—religious, artistic, or philosophical—traversed technicality, that is, they had "Eastern" roots. They were a sort of Easternization of the West.[53]

52 See, for example, the extreme position of Muḥammad Farīd Abū Ḥadīd (1893–1967) (Abū Ḥadīd 1935, p. 207):

> فالحقّ أنّ شعب مصر في القرن الثّامن عشر كان آخذا في سبيل نهضة حقيقيّة في كلّ جوانبه نهضة وطنيّة صرف لا تشوبها رطانة أجنبيّة ولا لوثة أعجميّة ولا سيطرة غربيّة. نهضة لو سارت في سبيلها وبلغت قصارها لكانت مصر اليوم في مستوى اليابان وإيطاليا أو فيما هو فوق ذلك. غير أنّ القرن الثّامن عشر، واحسرتاه، انتهى بنكبة شاملة وداهية فادحة بإغارة الفرنسيّين على مصر، واكتساحهم كلّ آثار تلك النّهضة الشّابّة فقضى عليها ولمّا يتمّ نموّها، وحفرت بين ماضي مصر وحاضرها هوّة عميقة تقطع تيّار الرقيّ الوطنيّ، وتقف في سبيل وصل الطّارف بالتّالد.

53 Adūnīs 1980, pp. 330–1; *Mawāqif* 36 (Winter 1980), pp. 150–1. For a critical response to Adūnīs' argument, see al-ʿAẓm 1992, pp. 109–19. Adūnīs' aforementioned argument that "the West is the son of the East" by no means reflects his great disappointment at the failure of the Arabs to regain their ancient glory. In dozens of essays that he has published under the title *Madārāt* (*Orbits*) during the last decade in the London-based newspaper *al-Ḥayāt*, he has expressed his sadness over the deterioration of the Arabs: "From what is called the 'Period of Renaissance' (*ʿAṣr al-Nahḍa*) until today, the Arabs have deteriorated on all levels, relatively and comparatively to the progress of others, in education and culture, in economic and social growth and in human rights and democratic freedom" (*al-Ḥayāt*,

It is, however, generally accepted that canonical and non canonical Arabic literary models helped guide the emergence of the new modern Arabic genres, but the marginal status of certain non-canonical models changed only after their interaction with their Western equivalents.[54] The case of *Robinson Crusoe* (1719) by Daniel Defoe (1660–1731)[55] is highly instructive in this respect, as its translation into Arabic by Buṭrus al-Bustānī as *al-Tuḥfa al-Bustāniyya fi al-Asfār al-Karūziyya* (*Bustani's Treasure on Crusoe's Travels*) (1861) was one of the factors that helped to shape the norms of the emerging Arabic novel.[56] However, it seems that *Robinson Crusoe* was not just a purely English cultural product but also the outcome of the interaction between English and Arab culture in general and between *Robinson Crusoe* and the philosophical tale *Ḥayy ibn Yaqẓān* by Abū Bakr Ibn Ṭufayl (1100–1185) in particular.[57] A comparative study by Ḥasan Maḥmūd ʿAbbās arrives at the conclusion that Defoe was highly inspired by Ibn Ṭufayl's tale.[58] It is also possible that *Ḥayy ibn Yaqẓān*, together with other classical Arabic autobiographical works[59] (though it cannot be considered an autobiography according

January 6, 2009). He also wrote: "We, the Arabs, have a strong presence throughout the world on the level of form, and, at the same time, we are absent of the world on the level of meaning" (January 7, 2016. Cf. his essays on April 24, 2014; December 11, 2014; October 1, 2015; January 7, 2016. See also Adūnīs 2022; and below in the Epilogue).

54 Cf. the argument of ʿAbd al-Raḥmān Yāghī (1924–2017) regarding the development of Arab theater (Yāghī 1980, p. 86).

55 Defoe 1906 [1719].

56 On the norms of translation for this novel, see ʿAnānī 1976, pp. 8–25; Badr 1983, pp. 57–67; Somekh 1991, pp. 75–82. It is interesting to note that even in the 1990s Arab scholars still used Buṭrus al-Bustānī's translation of the novel for their studies on *Robinson Crusoe* (e.g., al-Khaṭīb 1995, pp. 123–38). On the Arabic translations of *Robinson Crusoe,* see Hill 2015, pp. 177–201; Hill 2019, pp. 95–211. On the novel that was originally destined for an elite audience of scholars and educated readers, see Johnson 2021, pp. 66–89.

57 Ibn Ṭufayl 1940. For an English translation of this tale, see Goodman 1972, pp. 95–166. On an earlier translation by the Elder Edward Pococke (1604–1691), see Nahas 1985, pp. 88–90.

58 See ʿAbbās 1983, especially the conclusions on pp. 249–52, which end with the following:

ولم يغرب عن بالنا أنّ الأدب والفكر العربيّين كانا طيلة عهودهما عرضة للتّأثير والتّأثّر، وذلك هو شأن الأدب الإنكليزيّ وآداب الأمم الأخرى جميعا. فلا يعلي من شأن هذا الأدب أن يؤثّر ولا ينتقص من شأن ذلك الأدب أن يتأثّر، فالتّأثير والتأثّر قائمان ما دامت الصّلات الثّقافيّة قائمة بين الشّعوب.

59 Such as *al-Munqidh min al-Ḍalāl* by Abū Ḥāmid al-Ghazālī (1059–1111) (al-Ghazālī 1956 [English translation in Watt 1963]) and *Kitāb al-Iʿtibār* by Usāma ibn Munqidh (1095–1188) (Ibn Munqidh 1930 [English translation: Ibn Munqidh 1987]). On autobiography in classical Arabic literature, see al-Ghamdi 1989; Kilpatrick 1991, pp. 1–20; Kilito 1999, pp. 69–80; Cooperson 2000; Rooke 2001. See also Reynolds 2001, which is a survey of premodern Arabic autobiography. The book examines a corpus of over one hundred Arabic autobiographies from the ninth to the nineteenth centuries and includes thirteen translated selections as well as an annotated bibliography of approximately 140 pre-twentieth-century primary sources. On autobiography in Arab culture in general, see ʿAbd al-Dā'im 1975; Shuiskii 1982, pp. 111–23; Malti-Douglas 1988b; Sharaf 1992; Philipp 1993 pp. 573–604; al-Qāḍī

to Philippe Lejeune),[60] played an important role in the development of the apprenticeship novel (*Bildungsroman*) in modern Arabic literature.[61]

Although it is autonomous, the Arabic literary system, like any other system, retains various relationships with other literary systems by means of interference. Arabic literature may become a source for direct or indirect loans to another literature and vice versa. Translated texts may constitute the initial channel for interference.[62] Moreover, together with historiography, anthologizing, and criticism, translation—the main medium through which one literature influences another—prepares works for inclusion in the canon

1993, pp. 207–32; al-Hassan 1994; al-Bāridī 1997, pp. 68–80; Rooke 1997; Enderwitz 1998, pp. 1–19; Ostle et al. 1998 (for a review of the book, see *IBLA* 184 [1999], pp. 221–3); Enderwitz 1999, pp. 29–50; Machut-Mendecka 1999, pp. 510–22; Mowafy 1999; Wild 1999, pp. 349–61; Enderwitz 2000, pp. 189–99; Kattānī 2000–2001, pp. 315–63; Malti-Douglas 2001; Enderwitz 2002, pp. 49–72; Shākir 2002; Golley 2003; Reynolds 2005, pp. 261–84; Mus'id 2006; Lowry and Stewart 2009; al-Qāḍī 2009, pp. 241–51; Allen 2010; DeYoung and Germain 2011; Guth and Ramsay 2011, II, pp. 139–65 (by Christian Junge); Sheetrit 2012, pp. 102–31; Anishchenkova 2014; Abdel Nasser 2017; al-Musawi 2022. For essays in Arabic on the genre of autobiography from both critical as well as literary points of view, see the study of Iḥsān ʻAbbās (1920–2003) on the genre (Abbās n.d. [1956]) and his own autobiography (Abbās 1996). See also Robert B. Campbell's two-volume *Aʻlām al-Adab al-ʻArabī al-Muʻāṣir: Siyar wa-Siyar Dhātiyya* (*Contemporary Arab Writers: Biographies and Autobiographies*) (Campbell 1996). The autobiography in Arabic literature was also the topic of a conference held on March 10, 1997 at the University of Haifa with papers such as "Can Self-Exposure Be Considered Autobiography?" (by A. Arazi); "Autobiographical Elements in *Adab* Books" (by I. Geries); "Autobiographies in Modern Literature" (by S. Wild); and "Autobiographies of Contemporary Arab Poets" (by R. Snir). For lack of space, we cannot discuss here the relevance of the genre in Arabic literature, both modern and classical, to the various presuppositions behind the prevalent definitions of the autobiographic genre, especially the "typological" and the "dynamic" as well as to the problematic relationship between fact and fiction (e.g., Elbaz 1988, esp. pp. 1–16). For the phenomenon of autobiographical poetry, see Abū Ṭālib 2016, pp. 131–45. The adoption of the Internet has favored the proliferation of new forms of autobiographical writing and literary creativity all over the world. Blogs in particular are used by people worldwide to record and share their writing (Pepe 2015, pp. 73–91).

60 "A retrospective prose narrative produced by a real person concerning his own existence, focusing on his individual life, in particular on the development of his personality" (Lejeune 1982, p. 193). Cf. Genette 1992, p. 79. See also Lejeune 1975 (two chapters of that book [pp. 13–46, 311–41] were translated into Arabic in Lejeune 1994); Lejeune 1989. On the dilemma of literary theory with regard to Arabic literature, see R. C. Ostle's introduction to Ostle et al. 1998 (pp. 18–24). See also the roundtable "Theory and Arabic Literature in the United States" in the *International Journal of Middle East Studies* 43.4 (2011), with an introduction (Selim 2011, p. 721) and contributions of five literary scholars (Aboul-Ela 2011, pp. 725–7; Colla 2011, pp. 722–4; Omri 2011, pp. 731–3; Selim 2011a, pp. 734–6; Tageldin 2011, pp. 728–30).

61 Cf. al-Ḥakīm 1990, p. 6 (introduction). The Egyptian SF writer Nihād Sharīf (1932–2011) considered *Ḥayy ibn Yaqẓān* to be among the Arab roots of SF in the West (*al-Qāhira*, July 15, 1988, p. 41).

62 Cf. Sebeok 1986, I, pp. 462–3.

of world literature.[63] Interference normally occurs when a target literature lacks a sufficient repertoire to absorb newly needed functions, and it tends to be stronger when a body of literature is either in a state of emergence, in a vacuum, or at a turning point in its history.[64] Thus, whenever it is in need of innovation and unable to use its own repertoire to that end, a literature tends to make use of whatever repertoire is within reach. Although availability may arise as a result of physical contacts, "it is nevertheless ultimately determined by the cultural promptness ('openness,' 'readiness') of the target literature to consider a potential source as 'available.'"[65] In the following pages, attention will be turned to the way in which Arabic literature has functioned as a target literature and as a source literature for other cultures and literatures.

3. TARGET LITERATURE

Although Arabic literature during the Abbasid period came under the strong influence of Greek culture, no major Greek literary models were introduced into the Arabic literary system.[66] Indeed, works in other fields, such as agriculture, astronomy, grammar, music, philosophy, medicine, and even

63 Lefevere 1990, p. 27. On the concept of world literature, see Elster 1901, pp. 33–47; Elster 1986, pp. 7–13; Damrosch 2003; Schildgen et al. 2007; Damrosch 2009; Damrosch 2009a; D'haen et al. 2013; Ganguly 2015, pp. 272–81. One of the definitions of world literature is in agreement with the conception of the present study that excludes any evaluative judgments or hierarchies of value, namely, "all of the world's literature, without pronouncing on questions of quality and influence" (D'haen et al. 2013, p. xi). On Arabic fiction and world literature, see Rooke 2011, pp. 201–13; Rooke 2011a, pp. 27–146. On extending the paradigm of world literature beyond hegemonic global centers and attending to the trajectories that shape "literature in the world," see Helgesson 2015, pp. 253–60. On world literature and the demise of national literatures, see Clüver 1986, pp. 14–24; Clüver 1988, pp. 134–9; Clüver 1988a, pp. 143–4; Konstantinovic 1988, pp. 141–2; Steinmetz 1988, pp. 131–3; Snir 2017, pp. 160–74. On world literature and Orientalism, see Hafez 2014, pp. 1–29; Ouyang 2018, pp. 125–52. On responses to world literature from various Middle Eastern perspectives, see a special issue of *Middle Eastern Literatures* 20.1 (2017), edited by Paulo Horta. On world literature and the role of the Lebanese writer and critic Ilyās Khūrī (b. 1948), see Parr 2021, pp. 167–83.

64 Cf. Haddad 1970, p. 3; al-'Aẓm 1992, p. 159:

> لا ينجح الغزو الثّقافيّ في التّأثير الفاعل والعميق على المجتمع المغزوّ إلّا بمقدار الخواء الثّقافيّ الّذي يقع عليه الغزو. فحيثما توجد ثقافة حيّة نامية متحرّكة تتعامل مع مشكلات عصرها الكبرى وتحدّياته المصيريّة بنجاح معقول وتتفاعل مع قضاياها الوطنيّة والفكريّة والعلميّة والتّقنيّة والفنيّة بصورة خلاّقة ينكمش تأثير الغزو الثّقافيّ ويميل فعله إلى التّلاشي تلقائيّا والعكس بالعكس.

65 Sebeok 1986, I, p. 462.

66 Rajā' 'Īd's description of the great impact of Greek culture on Abbasid literature ('Īd 1993, pp. 285–90) is highly exaggerated—it does not distinguish between the Greek impact on literature and its impact on other aspects of Arab culture.

poetics and some literary genres were translated from Greek into Arabic,[67] but Greek epic poetry, represented by such works as Homer's *Iliad* and *Odyssey*, although it was translated by other Eastern cultural groups, such as the Indians, Persians, and Syrians into their own languages, was not translated into Arabic until the twentieth century.[68] Unaware of or outright ignoring the Greek models, the Arabs produced no epic poetry, unlike their Indian, Persian, (ancient) Egyptian, and Turkish counterparts.[69]

Sulaymān al-Bustānī (1856–1925), the first to translate the *Iliad* into Arabic at the beginning of the twentieth century,[70] suggested three main reasons why the Arabs had neglected Greek literature: first, there was religion (*al-dīn*), that is, the strong pagan elements depicted in the *Iliad* (e.g., gods, sacrifices, libations);[71] second, the Arab poets did not know Greek (*ighlāq fahm*

[67] On translations from Greek into Arabic, see Gutas 1998, pp. 225–31 (for the various fields, see p. 229); Gutas 1999; Mavroudi 2015, pp. 28–59. For a chronological bibliography of studies on the significance of the translation movement for Islamic civilization, see Gutas 1999, pp. 212–15. See also Gutas 2000. On the Greek impact on Arab culture, see Goodman 1983, pp. 460–82.

[68] According to Gutas 1999, pp. 194–5, "high Greek literature was not translated into Arabic. It was reported that Ḥunayn [ibn Isḥāq, (809–873)] himself could recite Homer in Greek by heart, but none of this Homeric citation survives in either Syriac or Arabic translation ... What was translated into Arabic from Greek literature was what may be loosely called 'popular' and 'paraenetic' literature." Cf. Kilito 2002, pp. 47–55, 110–14; al-Musawi 2015b, pp. 205–19.

[69] On views opposing such a statement, see Qabbish 1970, pp. 372–3; Gamal 1984, pp. 25–38; Makdisi 1990, p. 134. The Egyptian literary critic Aḥmad Ḥasan al-Zayyāt (1885–1968) considered *Sīrat 'Antara* to be the *Iliad* of the Arabs (al-Zayyāt n.d., p. 394. Cf. Elkhadem 1985, p. 55; Reynolds 1995, pp. 1–20).

[70] See al-Bustānī 1904; al-Bustānī 1996. On the nature of his translation, see Hamori 1980, pp. 15–22. This translation is considered by some Arab scholars and intellectuals to be a great triumph for the Arabic language (e.g., al-Jundī 1963, p. 159). In 1925, the Lebanese poet Ilyās Abū Shabaka (1903–1947) wrote an elegy on Sulaymān al-Bustānī (Abū Shabaka 1985, I, pp. 119–21), in which he alludes to the excellence of the *Iliad* translation. In another elegy on al-Bustānī, Abū Shabaka (1985, I, pp. 188–9) argues that the Arabic translation is more sublime than the original Greek, and that is why

وخفّ هومير بالإلياذ محرقـــــــــها أمام عينيك بخورا وقربانـــــــا
فصافحتك أثينا وهي باســـــــــمة حبّا وعانقت اليونان لبنــــــان

Homer hurried burning the *Iliad*
Before your eyes as incense and a thanks offering.
Athens is greeting you smiling
With love, Greece embracing Lebanon.

On the main aspects of literary criticism presented in al-Bustānī's introduction to his translation of the *Iliad* and in the notes appended to it, as well as on al-Bustānī's general critical conceptions, see Ṣawāyā 1960; Fanous 1980, pp. 185–227; Fanus 1986, pp. 105–19; Fahd 1993, pp. 259–66; Holmberg 2006, pp. 141–65. On al-Bustānī and his literary and critical work, see al-Hāshim 1960; Hourani 1991, pp. 174–87.

[71] Cf. "Greek poetry and drama ... seem not to have appealed to Muslim audiences, possibly because of too frequent mention of the Olympian gods" (Bulliet 2011, p. 214).

al-Yūnāniyya ʿalā al-ʿArab), that is, those Arab poets capable of translating the *Iliad* into Arabic never mastered Greek; and, third, the translators were unable to compose Arabic poetry (*ʿajz al-naqala ʿan naẓm al-shiʿr al-ʿArabī*), that is, the mainly Christian translators of Greek science were unable to write gracefully in Arabic.[72] Ṭāhā Ḥusayn (1889–1973) rejected al-Bustānī's arguments, even describing the first of them regarding the pagan elements in the *Iliad* as "highly stupid and foolish," since the Arabs did translate Greek philosophical texts, which also contained elements of ancient Greek religion.[73] Other scholars[74] have tried to explain the phenomenon by quoting al-Jāḥiẓ's (776–886) words:

الشِّعر لا يُستطاع أن يترجم ولا يجوز عليه النَّقل ومتى حُوِّل تقطَّع نظمه وبطل وزنه وذهب حسنه وسقط موضع التَّعجُّب لا كالكلام المنثور [...] لو حُوِّلت حكمة العرب بطل ذلك المعجز الَّذي هو الوزن [...] إنَّ التَّرجمان لا يؤدِّي أبدا ما قال الحكيم.

It is impossible to translate poetry and to convert it [to another language], since when it is translated the arrangement of words is disrupted and the meter is abolished and the beauty of poetry disappears and likewise its charm. Poetry is not like prose ... If the wisdom of the Arabs is translated, this miracle which is the meter disappears ... translation will never convey the meaning of what the wise man says.[75]

In a study of the translation of the *Iliad*, Yaseen Noorani writes that for al-Bustānī and many of his contemporaries, "the translation of the *Iliad* into Arabic rectifies a deficit in the history of Arabic literature." He argues that the absence of a medieval Arabic translation of the *Iliad* cannot be regarded as merely the result of any obstacles:

What was lacking was a shared framework that would have allowed Greek poetic works to have prestige and meaning for Arabic readers. The idea that great poetic works across the world, on the basis of their intrinsic value as expressions of the human spirit, constitute a universal cultural legacy that should be translated into every literary language was not present, and poetic works were seldom translated into Arabic.[76]

---

[72] See al-Bustānī 1904, pp. 65–7; al-Bustānī 1996, pp. 61–3. Cf. al-Labābīdī 1943, pp. 33–4; al-Badawī al-Mulaththam 1963, pp. 81–3; Semah 1974, pp. 115–16; Moreh 1976, p. 129, n. 19.

[73] Ḥusayn 1967 [1956], pp. 192–3.

[74] Such as ʿAbd al-Ḥayy 1977, p. 15. On the attitude of the Arabs to Greek poetry, see also ʿAbbās 1977, pp. 23–38.

[75] Cf. al-Jāḥiẓ 1938, I, pp. 75–6. On al-Jāḥiẓ's views and on whether Arabic poses unique problems that render it less translatable than other languages, see Kilito 2002; Kilito, 2008; Montgomery 2013, pp. 454–5. See also Cooperson and Hassan 2011, pp. 566–75. On Kilito's injunction "thou shalt not translate me," see Apter 2013, pp. 247–61.

[76] Noorani 2019, pp. 236–65. The quotations are from pp. 243 and 252, respectively.

As a target literature, Arabic literature in the Abbasid period, far from being in a state of emergence, stuck in a vacuum, or at some turning point or crossroads in its history, was fully capable of performing the functions that Arab society needed it to fulfill. This means that, because Arabic literature at the time saw itself as self-sufficient and regarded the outsider with contempt, other repertoires, even when available,[77] were simply ignored or rejected. If the Arabic literary system in the Abbasid period had been in need of new models, it had Greek literary models at hand and certainly would have found ways "to eliminate or neutralize any element endangering its religious foundation ... to obscure the foreign character of important borrowings and to reject what could not be thus adjusted to its style of thinking and feeling."[78]

In contrast, interference from foreign cultures from the start of the nineteenth century onward existed because most branches of Arab culture found themselves during this period without a sufficient repertoire for newly needed functions.[79] This comes most clearly to the fore when we look at concepts current in languages of other societies with which Arabs were in contact and for which they sought equivalents. An illustration of this may be found in the following statement in 1858 by a Lebanese journalist in *Ḥadīqat al-Akhbār*, one of the first privately owned Arabic newspapers:

> If anybody should find [such a definition] presumptuous and insulting to the Arab intelligence, let him take the trouble of translating a speech by a British Parliament member or, better still, render into Arabic the proceedings of a

[77] The psychological explanation alluded to by Gustave E. von Grunebaum is also relevant here (von Grunebaum 1953, pp. 258–347; von Grunebaum 1967, pp. 1–14). On von Grunebaum's approach to literary criticism and the role of history and psychology within the Western Orientalist tradition, see Riedel 1998, pp. 111–22.

[78] von Grunebaum 1953, p. 321. Cf. Abū Sa'ūd 1934, p. 968. L. E. Goodman states that "the processes by which Greek themes and modes of thought were made at home in the Islamic world of *Arabic literature*, not merely disguised, but adjusted to the Islamic experience and the Arabic idiom, is an even more fascinating and complex subject than the movement of translation itself" (Goodman 1983, pp. 481–2, my emphasis); however, as is evident from his study, he is not referring to *belles lettres*.

[79] The absence of a sufficient repertoire for newly needed functions is illustrated in Salāma Mūsā's statement in his article "al-Klasiyya Dā' al-Adab al-'Arabī" ("Classicism Is the Malady of Arabic Literature") (Mūsā 1945, p. 82). Cf. Tobi's (1995, pp. 39–42) argument concerning the development of the relationship between Hebrew poetry and Arabic poetry in the Middle Ages: during the first century of Islam, "thanks to the strength of Hebrew poetry and its distance from Arabic poetry, there was no need for defensive measures ... Arab culture and Islam, which had not yet attained a high level of development, still did not constitute a threat to the integrity of Judaism." However, during the ninth and tenth centuries, "the turn to Arabic poetry came about as a result of the marked weakness of the paytanic school of Hebrew poetry, which had exhausted itself almost entirely after an active period of close to seven centuries."

> session; an article on European theater; a political study; a commercial report; and the like. Surely, he would find himself facing an abyss with every single sentence. He might not transcend it without seriously complicating the language, leaving his readers in disconcertment and doubt.[80]

As the aforementioned examples show, translations into Arabic may tell us about the self-image of Arab culture at various periods in time and the changes which that self-image have gone through over time.[81]

Factors associated with changes in a given literature cannot be dealt with separately from those associated with changes in the culture and society in which that literature exists. However, unlike pre-functionalist doctrines, a literary system, like any literary text,[82] is not considered to be subject to external factors. The pre-functionalists assumed a unilateral and univalent subordination of literature to either social, spiritual, or economic forces in society. Modern theories of literature have hypothesized literature itself to be a social force, and have suggested conceiving of it as both an autonomous and heteronomous system "among a series of (semiotically) correlated systems operating in the 'system-of-systems' of society."[83] Literature is just one system of institutionalized symbolic interactions among many others within society.[84] From this perspective, literature becomes part of a social and cultural system, and it should be analyzed with regard to other social and cultural systems. Yet, while the need for and the rate and tempo of change may depend on the social and cultural norms adapted by the literary system, any change that is actualized is conditioned by the literary system and the specific poetic norms within it.[85]

80 *Ḥadīqat al-Akhbār*, December 22, 1858, p. 2 (quoted from Ayalon 1987, p. 5).

81 Cf. Lefevere 1990, p. 27. On the self-image of Arab culture as reflected in Arab responses to Western culture and values and on the ambivalence that characterized Arab perceptions of the West in modern times, as expressed through works of fiction and non-fiction written by Arab authors during the nineteenth and twentieth centuries, see El-Enany 2006.

82 Although a literary text might be considered to be a microcosm of a literary system, one can by no means employ any textual component in the description of the literary system, especially when referring to several types of criticism, such as historical, biographical, sociological, and psychological criticism. These types have distinctive ways of defining the relations between the text and external factors, such as trying "to suggest what is in the poem by showing what lies behind it" (Preminger 1974, p. 167). In that sense, the characteristics of the literary system are similar to the characteristics of the text as seen by those critics who argue that there is no necessary connection between an idea or experience inside a text and the same idea or experience outside it. Moreover, an idea or experience inside a text is not considered to be subject to the same idea or experience outside it.

83 Sebeok 1986, I, p. 459.

84 With regard to literary theory, cf. Navarrete 1986, pp. 123–4.

85 Sebeok 1986, I, p. 460. It seems that Idwār al-Kharrāṭ (1926–2015) alludes to these specific intra-literary circumstances by what he described as "*āliyyāt hādhā al-mujtama' al-aṣīla*

4. SOURCE LITERATURE

Besides being a target for other literatures and cultures, Arabic and Islamic literature and culture were also important sources of inspiration for certain cultures.[86] However, we must not talk about this inspiration in the sense of the polemical statement by the Syrian poet and critic Adūnīs (ʿAlī Aḥmad Saʿīd) (b. 1930) that "there is nothing in the West that the West did not take from the East,"[87] or Gustave E. von Grunebaum's (1909–1972) hyperbolic statement that "there is hardly an area of human experience where Islam has not enriched Western tradition."[88] Samuel Miklos Stern (1920–1969) argued

al-kāmina" ("the genuine inherited mechanics of this [Arab] society") (al-Kharrāṭ 2005, p. 94).

86 See, for example, Hitti 1962, pp. 48–63; Southern 1962; Hunke 1965 (Arabic translation: Hunke 1979); Conant 1966 [1908]; Watt 1972; Hilāl 1977, pp. 55–68; Metlitzki 1977; Rosenthal 1979, pp. 345–9; Bushrūʾi 1982, pp. 153–9; Menocal 1985, pp. 61–78; Kabbani 1986, pp. 23–36; al-Mūsawī 1986; Menocal 1987; Caracciolo 1988; Saad el Din and Cromer 1991; Ḥamāda 1992; Agius and Hitchcock 1993; Engels and Schreiner 1993; Sharfuddin 1994; Lewis 1995, p. 13 (and the references on pp. 83–4, n. 1); Bosworth 1996, pp. 155–64; Starkey and Starkey 1998, pp. 179–230 (contributions by M. Taymanova, M. Orr, P. Whyte, J. W. Weryho, and J. D. Ragan); Reeves 2000. Canonical Arabic literature has been a source of direct and indirect loans mainly for literature in Muslim societies since the Middle Ages, while popular Arabic literature has been a source of loans mainly for Western societies, especially since the nineteenth century. See, for example, the widespread circulation of the canonical model of the *qaṣīda* in classical and modern cultures, such as those written in Persian, Turkish, Urdu, Indonesian, Swahili, and Hausa. On various classical and modern *qaṣīda* traditions in Islamic Asia and Africa, see the articles, original poems, and translations appearing in Sperl and Shackle 1996 and Sperl and Shackle 1996a, which came about as a result of the London *Qaṣīda* Conference, which took place at SOAS, University of London, in July 1993. Also, the medieval Arabic poetic theorization of wonder and the mechanisms through which it is evoked can also inform our understanding of other literatures written in the Islamicate context, including medieval Persian, Hebrew, and even Ottoman literatures. They bear a resemblance to some Western theories of aesthetics (Harb 2020, pp. 263–4). On the traveling of the *qaṣīda* structure in Asia and Africa, see al-Musawi 2015b, pp. 34–45; Ogunnaike 2020. For popular Arabic literature as source literature for modern Western literary traditions, see the case of *Alf Layla wa-Layla* in Snir 2017, pp. 92–4, 97; al-Musawi 2021. Mention should also be made of the substantial influence that Arabo-Spanish popular strophic poetry had on emerging Romance lyrics and the troubadours (Nykl 1946; Gorton 1974, pp. 11–16). For a symbolic Islamo-European encounter in prosody between *muwashshaḥāt, azjāl,* and Catalan troubadours, see Sanaullah 2010, pp. 357–400. On Arabic poetry and the songs of the troubadours, see Jafri 2004, pp. 374–87; Nieten 2006, pp. 253–61. For a comprehensive study of the relationship and interaction between Islam and the West, see al-Azmeh 1996.

87 See Adūnīs 1980, pp. 330–1; *Mawāqif* 36 (Winter 1980), pp. 150–1. For a critical response to Adūnīs' argument, see al-ʿAẓm 1992, pp. 109–19. Cf. the argument of the Palestinian poet and critic Jabrā Ibrāhīm Jabrā (1919–1994) that the European Renaissance was nothing but the result of the translation of Arab investigation and creativity into Latin (Jabrā 1992, p. 191).

88 von Grunebaum 1953, p. 342.

that "not even the most fanatical advocate of the case for Arabic influence on the West would seek to set out a long catalogue" of literary loans after the twelfth century.[89] Among the exceptions to this, however, is Sufism, which proved to be a living tradition that shielded Islam against its assailants and at the same time stimulated cross-cultural interaction:

> This interaction cast doubt on the validity of the view that cultural transfer in modern times was unidirectional, from Europe to the Arab-Muslim world. A striking example of this phenomenon was to be found in the cultural dialogue that emerged at the end of the Ottoman era between Muslims and Christians in Cairo, Rome, and Paris. The players in this dialogue highlighted the spirituality of Islam, and advocated rapprochement between East and West at a time of growing friction. They sought to position their agenda at the forefront of the discourse of their respective communities.[90]

As for literary interaction, although the reading of Arabic literature in the original outside the Arab world is still mainly confined to a limited number of academic circles, there has been an upsurge of translations of Arabic literature into various foreign languages.[91] The impact, albeit minor, of these

[89] Stern 1974, p. 204.

[90] Hatina 2007, p. 404.

[91] On translations of Arabic literature into English, see Howarth and Shukrallah 1944; Alwan 1972, pp. 195–200; Alwan 1973, pp. 373–81; Anderson 1980, pp. 180–207; Allen and Hillmann 1989, pp. 104–16; Le Gassick 1992, pp. 47–60; Altoma 1993, pp. 160–79; Altoma 1993a; Allen 1994, pp. 165–8; Johnson-Davies 1994, pp. 272–82; Altoma 1996, pp. 137–53; Altoma 1997, pp. 131–72; Classe 2000, pp. 62–71; France 2000, pp. 139–58; Altoma 2005; Altoma 2009, pp. 307–19; Altoma 2010; Reynolds 2015, pp. 108–10 (by Shawkat M. Toorawa). On translations of Arabic literature into French, see Jacquemond 1992, pp. 139–58; Jacquemond 1992a, pp. 43–57; Nuṣayr 1992, pp. 43–7; Altoma 1993a; Tomiche 1993, pp. 152–6. On translations of Arabic literature into Spanish, see Comendador et al. 2000, pp. 115–25; Comendador and Fernández-Parrilla 2006, pp. 69–77; Amo 2010, pp. 239–57; Fernández-Parrilla 2013, pp. 88–101. On translations of Arabic literature into Italian, see Ruocco 2000, pp. 63–73; Avino 2001, pp. 53–66, 115; Camera d'Afflitto 2001, pp. 11–16, 109–10; Corrao 2001, pp. 17–21, 110–11; Giorgio 2001, pp. 23–8, 111–12; Ruocco 2001, pp. 29–37, 112. On translations of Arabic literature into Romanian, see Feodorov 2001, pp. 35–45; Feodorov 2001a, pp. 101–53; Dobrişan 2004, pp. 29–32. See also *Romano-Arabica* 4 (2004) dedicated to translation from/into Arabic. On translations of Arabic literature into Swedish, see Stagh 1999, pp. 41–6; Stagh 2000, pp. 107–14. On translations of Arabic literature into Russian, see Frolova 2004, pp. 143–9. On translations of Arabic literature into German, see 'Abbūd 1995, pp. 31–53; Trudewind 2000, pp. 49–51, as well as the review sections of *Fikr wa-Fann*, which has been published since the early 1960s by Inter Nations in Bonn, Germany. On the reception of Arabic literature in Germany in the shadow of the *Arabian Nights*, see Fähndrich 2000, pp. 95–106. On the situation of contemporary Arabic literature in German-speaking countries in general, see Fähndrich 2000a, pp. 167–80. On translations of Arabic literature into European languages in general, see Gibb and Landau 1968, pp. 317–19; Cachia 1990, pp. 222–8. On translations of Arabic literature into Hebrew, see Gibb and Landau 1970, pp. 195–7; Somekh 1973, pp. 141–52; Amit-Kochavi 1996, pp. 27–44; Amit-Kochavi 1999; Amit-Kochavi 2000, pp. 53–80;

translations[92] cannot be overlooked. In addition, the number of Arab authors writing in foreign languages is increasing.[93] Interference between the Arabic literary system and other literary systems is occurring throughout the world at an ever-increasing pace.

Two major examples of reciprocal interference between Arabic and Western literatures in the twentieth century and the start of the twenty-first century are Arabic and English,[94] and Arabic and

Amit-Kochavi 2003, pp. 39–68; Amit-Kochavi 2006, pp. 100–9. See also the special issue of *The Translator* 21 (July 2015) titled "Translating in the Arab World," edited by Richard Jacquemond and Samah Selim, as well as various issues of various issues of *Arablit & Arablit Quarterly: A Magazine of Arabic Literature in Translation*—one recent example is the glimpse of what was translated from Arabic and published in world languages in 2021, available at: https://arablit.org/2021/12/02/published-in-2021-arabic-literature-in-english-french-german-greek-italian-malayalam-portuguese-turkish-translation (last accessed December 2, 2021).

92 See, for example, Allen 1993, pp. 87–117. Maḥfūẓ is the most popular Arab writer in the West, especially after he won the Nobel Prize (on his reception in American publications, see Altoma 1993, pp. 160–79. See also El-Enany 2006, pp. 89–94). Maḥfūẓ himself considered the Nobel Prize as the world's recognition of Arab culture (Larry Luxner, "A Nobel for the Arab Nation," *Aramco World* 40.2 [March/April 1989], pp. 15–16 [according to Lawall 1993, p. 25, n. 21]). Almost all of Maḥfūẓ's novels and short story collections have been translated into English (for a list of these translations, see Cachia 1990, p. 226; Gordon 1990, pp. 141–2; Altoma 1993, pp. 169–70, 174–5; Altoma 1996, pp. 137–53. On issues related to the translation of his work, see Etman 1993, pp. 355–8). The impact of his literary works might be inferred also from the fact that scholarly study of his work is carried out even by academics who do not read Arabic and therefore use translations (e.g., Gordon 1990). However, it seems that his popularity in the West might be explained by the sociopolitical value of his work (see Lūwīs ʿAwaḍ's [1915–1990] opinion in *al-Muṣawwar*, August 11, 1989, p. 35). A different example is the popularity of *Alf Layla wa-Layla* in the West, which is mainly due to literary considerations (al-Qalamāwī 1966, p. 65). In the nineteenth century, E. W. Lane (1801–1876) considered *Alf Layla wa-Layla*'s value to lie in the "fullness and fidelity with which they describe the character, manners and customs of the Arabs" (Lane 1859 [1839–1841], III, p. 686. Cf. Kabbani 1986, pp. 37, 44). Lane, who translated *Alf Layla wa-Layla* into English (first published in parts from 1838 onward), "was primarily a scholar, not a *littérateur*" (Starkey and Starkey 1998, p. 246).

93 On this general phenomenon, see Adūnīs 1993, pp. 95–6.

94 For example, Jubrān Khalīl Jubrān's works written originally in English: *The Madman* (Gibran 1918); *The Forerunner* (Gibran 1920); *The Prophet* (Gibran 1924); *Sand and Foam* (Gibran 1926); *Jesus, the Son of Man* (Gibran 1928); *The Earth Gods* (Gibran 1931); *The Wanderer: His Parables and His Sayings* (Gibran 1932); *The Garden of the Prophet* (Gibran 1933); *Lazarus and His Beloved* (Gibran 1973; Gibran 1982); *The Blind* (Gibran 1982). Except for the last two, all of these works were translated into Arabic by Anṭūnyūs Bashīr (1898–1966) and were published in one volume under the title *al-Majmūʿa al-Kāmila li-Muʾallafāt Jubrān Khalīl Jubrān al-Muʿarraba ʿan al-Inklīziyya* (*The Complete Collection of Jubrān Khalīl Jubrān's Writings Translated into Arabic from English*) (Jubrān 1981). For Jubrān's Arabic works, see Jubrān 1985. For a list of the English translations of most of these works, see Bushrūʾi 1987, pp. 91–2. For a general bibliography on Jubrān, see Bushrūʾi 1987, pp. 93–4; Altoma 2000, pp. 255–7. On Lebanese literature in English in general (in fact, on Jubrān, as well as on Amīn al-Rīḥānī [1876–1940] and Mīkhāʾīl Nuʿayma

French.[95] Especially noteworthy is the participation of Arab writers in the French literary system, which already in the 1930s was seen as an inspiring way to enrich the Arabic poetic tradition.[96] This phenomenon, which was also criticized,[97] has begun attracting the attention of Arab writers.[98] Among the winners of France's most prestigious literary award, the *Prix Goncourt*, we find three Arab writers: the Moroccan writer Tahar Ben Jelloun (al-Ṭāhir ibn Jallūn) (b. 1944), who won in 1987 for his *La nuit sacrée*;[99] the Lebanese writer Amin Maalouf (Amīn Maʿlūf) (b. 1949), who won in 1993 for his *Le rocher de Tanois*;[100] and the Moroccan novelist Leïla Slimani (Laylā al-Sulaymānī) (b. 1981), who won in 2016 for her novel *Chanson Douce* (2016), a thriller that opens with the killing of two young children by their caretaker. Another novel by Maalouf, *Samarkand*,[101] was given the *Prix de Maison de la Presse*. Other distinguished Arab authors who wrote in French include Georges Schéhadé (1905–1989), Andrée Chedid (1920–2011), Driss

[1889–1988]), see Bushrūʾi 2000. Among the other writers in English, mention can be made of Jabrā Ibrāhīm Jabrā (1920–1994), who also translated literary works from English into Arabic (Luʾluʾa 1989, pp. 26–31). On Palestinian writers in English, see Jayyusi 1992, pp. 333–66. On the "experimental encounter" with English, see "The Smell of Writing" by ʿAbd al-Qādir al-Janābī (b. 1944) (El Janabi 1996, pp. 55–6). For the development of Arab–American culture, see, for example, the journal *Mizna*, "A Forum for Arab American Expression," which started to appear in 1999, available at: http://www.mizna.org (last accessed August 3, 2020); Kadi 1994; Akash and Mattawa 2000; Barakat 2000, pp. 304–20; Reynolds 2015, pp. 109–10 (by Shawkat M. Toorawa). An interesting phenomenon is the emergence of English poetry inspired by Arabic poetry, such as the elegy by Oludamini Ogunnaike to lament the death of George Floyd (1973–2020), the African American man killed in Minneapolis during an arrest after a white police officer knelt on his neck. After his death, protests against police brutality toward Black people quickly spread across the United States and internationally. Ogunnaike's poem, which borrows heavily from the Arabic and West African traditions of *qaṣīda* poetry and elegy, starts with the lines "Did lightning just flash from the far northern plains? / Or is it thunder crying out with their names?" available at: https://sapelosquare.com/2020/06/10/an-elegy-for-george-floyd (last accessed September 9, 2020).

95 See Déjeux 1973; Bouraoui 1980, pp. 129–44; Joyaux 1980, pp. 117–27; Accad 1990, pp. 78–90; Achour 1991; Benarab 1995; Giovannucci 2008. See also the series *Écritures Arabes*, edited by Marc Gontard (Paris: Éditions L'Harmattan), in which more than one hundred literary works (poetry, short stories, novels, and plays) of Arab writers in French were published. On the relationship between Arabic and French writing and the bilingual phenomenon, see Bamia 1992, pp. 61–88; Amanṣūr n.d., pp. 79–98. On the influence of French literature on the Arabic novel, see El Beheiry 1980.

96 See ʿAql 1935, pp. 381–93.

97 On the negative attitude of cultural circles in the Arab world toward writers and intellectuals writing in French, see the interview with Algerian writer and scholar Mālik Shibl (1953–2016) published in *al-Ḥayāt*, March 11, 1996, p. 11.

98 See, for example, Qāsim 1996.

99 Ben Jelloun 1987. For more on Ben Jelloun, see M'henni 1993; Elbaz 1996.

100 Maalouf 1993 (English translation: Maalouf 1995).

101 Maalouf 1989 (English translation: Maalouf 1994).

Chraïbi (1926–2007), Kātib Yāsīn (Kateb Yacine) (1929–1989), Assia Djebar (1936–2015), Muḥammad Barrāda (Mohammed Berrada) (b. 1938), and ʿAbd al-Kabīr al-Khaṭībī (Abdelkebir Khatibi) (1938–2009). The participation of these writers in French literature by no means came about as a result of their abandoning of their original cultural identities. In fact, most of them were appreciated at home as well as abroad. For example, Maalouf, who was formerly the director of the weekly international edition of the leading Beirut daily *al-Nahār* and editor-in-chief of *Jeune Afrique*, dedicated his novel "to the memory of the man with the broken wings"—an allusion to *al-Ajniḥa al-Mutakassira* by Jubrān Khalīl Jubrān (1883–1931),[102] who was himself successful at writing in a foreign language and "the only Arab or Arabic-speaking author who succeeded in authoring a book that has had this extensive presence in the four corners of the earth."[103] Inevitably, however, along with the role (which was sometimes even subversive)[104] that these writers have taken up in foreign literary systems came the slow decline of the high status they had once occupied in their original literary systems.[105]

In the French literary system, the participation of Arab writers is indeed quite high, but even in literary systems that see lower rates of participation when it comes to Arab writers one can still find reciprocal interference. Compared with English and French literatures (and we can add Russian literature to this list as well), German literature did not, until recently, manage to attract much attention in Arab society, and this is probably due, as the Russian Orientalist Ignaty Yulianovich Krachkovsky (Krachkovskii) (1883–1951) indicates, to the limited direct colonial influence of Germany

[102] Jubrān n.d. [1912] (English translation: Gibran 1957).

[103] Shahīd 2000, p. 321. The book is *The Prophet* (Gibran 1924), which has been translated into more than forty languages. On Jubrān Khalīl Jubrān's significance and role in Arabic and world literature and his creative reception around the world, see Michalak-Pikulska 1999, pp. 93–100.

[104] See, for example, the way Robert Elbaz interprets the Arabic words in Ben Jelloun's novels: "Ces signes arabes, c'est le surplus textuel, le supplément qui vient combler l'absence du signifiant premier. Et comme ils sont disséminés à travers tout le Texte, ils brisent la surface textuelle, démantèlent la séquence narrative, et fonctionnent comme des réservoirs virtuels dans lesquels on pourrait emmagasiner tout ce qu'incorpore l'espace discursif maghrébin. Ils s'infiltrent, se posent comme objets sur la surface du Texte, et l'empêchent d'accéder à une transcendance, étant donné que le rapport terme à terme entre le monde et le Texte est affecté. Ces signes ne s'intègrent pas dans la séquence, ils la sapent. Ils la fragmentent" (Elbaz 1996, p. 16).

[105] This was clearly illustrated by the irony with which the literary critic of one of the Arab journals described Maalouf's visit to his homeland, Lebanon (Shūmān 1994, p. 41). Maalouf's novels have been translated into Arabic and published by Manshūrāt Milaff al-ʿĀlām al-ʿArabī in Beirut.

in the Middle East.[106] Yet, we do find the writer ʻAlī Aḥmad Bākathīr's (1910–1969) subversive recasting of the Goethean tragedy of *Faust*, the aim of which was "to provoke an audience while confronting it with patterns from its own culture in the disguise of foreign settings and characters in order to criticize the Westernization of the own culture."[107] We also see striking similarities between the novels of Jurjī Zaydān (1861–1914) and the historical novels of the German Egyptologist George Ebers (1837–1898).[108] And, finally, Aḥmad Shawqī (1868–1932), in his *Riwāyat Dal wa-Taymān aw Ākhir al-Farāʻina* (*Dal and Taymān* or *The Last Pharaohs*) (1899) freely adapted Ebers' *Eine Ägyptische Königstochter* (1864), which he had read in Arabic translation.[109] Conversely, Arab participation in German culture has not traditionally been high, but one can still find important examples of literary interaction.[110] Two of the most prominent Arab writers in German are the Syrian-Christian Rafik Schami (pseudonym of Suhayl Fāḍil; b. 1946),[111] who never published in Arabic, and the Bedouin Palestinian writer Salīm

106 Primarily through its support of Istanbul as of the end of the nineteenth century. Cf. Krachkovskii 1989, p. 23. Omitted from Edward Said's *Orientalism* (Said 1985 [1978]), the influence of German scholarship in and about the Middle East remains also relatively unexplored. During the past few years, there have been some movements in that direction: *Comparative Studies of South Asia, Africa, and the Middle East* published in 2002 a call for papers on this topic. Volume 24.2 (2004) of the journal published a section on German Orientalism with only five contributions, none of them relating to literary issues. In September 2003, the Institute of Germanic Studies and SOAS, University of London, published a call for papers on the topic of "Oriental Motifs in 19th- and 20th-Century German Literature and Thought." The aim was to examine "the strengths and weaknesses of the German contribution to what was chiefly a literary and intellectual Orientalism and one comparatively unencumbered by imperialistic ambition."

107 Szyska 1997, p. 144.

108 See Elkhadem 1985, p. 18 (and n. II.4 on p. 58).

109 See Elkhadem 1985, p. 21 (and n. II.12 on p. 59).

110 On immigrant Muslim writers in Germany, see Stoll 1998, pp. 266–83; and the special file in *Fikr wa-Fann* (Bonn), issue 80 (2004) on immigrant authors writing in German. An interesting case is the inspiration that the German director Wolfgang Becker's (b. 1954) film *Good Bye, Lenin!* (2003) apparently drew from *Saʻdūn al-Majnūn* (al-Ramlī 1992) by the Egyptian dramatist Līnīn (Lenin) al-Ramlī (1945–2020). The way this inspiration reached Becker has yet to be explored.

111 See, for example, Schami 1987 (English translation: Schami 1993). On the book, see Schami 1989 (Hebrew translation: Schami 1996); Schami 1995; Amin 2000, pp. 211–33; Schami 2004 (English translation: Schami 2009). The first Arabic translation has been published in Israel (Shāmī 1997), where a few articles have been published on his literary work: *Haaretz* (weekly supplement) (Tel Aviv), February 7, 1997, pp. 30–2 (in Hebrew); *Yediot Aḥronoth*, literary supplement, March 7, 1997, p. 28 (in Hebrew); Schami 1996, pp. 237–42 (in Hebrew); Shāmī 1997, pp. 219–30. The publisher Manshūrāt al-Jamal in Cologne planned to publish an Arabic translation of Schami's *Der geheime Bericht über den Dichter Goethe* (1999) (*al-Ḥayāt*, October 27, 2004). On Schami, see Khalil 1994, pp. 217–24; Khalil 1995, pp. 521–7; *Banipal* 14 (Summer 2002), pp. 66–70.

Alafenisch (b. 1948).[112] In addition, there are numerous German translations of Arabic works,[113] many of which have been put out by the Cologne-based publisher Al-Kamel Verlag (Manshūrāt al-Jamal), which is headed by the Iraqi poet Khālid al-Maʿālī (b. 1956). Among its main activities are the publication of classical and modern literary works and poetry collections, including those of German poets,[114] and the publication, since the mid-1990s, of the magazine *ʿUyūn*. Al-Maʿālī himself translated many Arabic poems into German, some of which he translated in collaboration with his German colleagues.[115] Until recently, only a few German literary authors have been translated into Arabic[116] with the exception of J. W. von Goethe (1749–1832), whose works were not only translated into Arabic, but reprinted in multiple editions.[117] Due to the emigration of many intellectuals from the Arab world to the West, we can find Arab writers who publish in other languages as well. In general, these writers stopped writing in Arabic and started to concentrate on composing in the language of their adopted country. For example, the Iraqi poet ʿAī al-Bazzāz (Ali Albazzaz) (b. 1958), who published several poetry collections in Dutch, was the only Arab poet included in an anthology of 120 poets from the Netherlands and Belgium

[112] On him, see Khalil 1995, pp. 521–7; Berman 1998, pp. 271–83; and *Yediot Aḥronoth*, literary supplement, December 29, 2000, p. 26.

[113] See, for example, Māhir 1970; Māhir 1974.

[114] On Arab-German literature in general, see Khalil 1995, pp. 521–7. In 2001, a new bilingual Arabic-German magazine appeared with the title *Dīwān: Majalla li-l-Shiʿr al-ʿArabī wa-l-Almānī / Diwan: Zeitschrift für arabische und deutsche Poesie*, its aim being to strengthen the Arab-German cultural dialogue (the first issue came out in May 2001). The magazine has two sections: the Arabic section includes works by German writers in Arabic translation, and the German section includes works by Arab writers in German translation. The editor is the Iraqi poet Amal al-Jubbūrī (Jubouri) (b. 1968). Adūnīs, who is a member of the editorial board, says in his opening remarks to the first issue that the aim of the magazine was to traverse the dualism between East and West and get rid of the "mentality of domination" ("*ʿaqliyyat al-haymana*") (on the magazine, see also *Fikr wa-Fann* 74 [2001], pp. 68–9). See also Midad (Midād)—Deutsch-Arabisches Literaturforum, available at: https://literaturblog-duftender-doppelpunkt.at/2006/05/10/midad-deutsch-arabisches-literaturforum (last accessed December 22, 2020).

[115] See, for example, Boulus 1997, with Stefan Weidner, and the file on Arabic literature published in *Die Horen: Zeitschrift für Literatur Kunst und Kritik* 189 (1998), pp. 61–134, with Mona Naggar and Heribert Becker. On the translation of Badr Shākir al-Sayyāb's poetry into German, see *Barīd al-Janūb*, October 27, 1997, p. 17. On the cultural achievements of Arab authors in Germany, see Weidner 2012, pp. 68–74.

[116] See, for example, Benn 1997.

[117] See, for example, Goethe 1964; Goethe 1966; Goethe 1967; Goethe 1968; Goethe 1978; Goethe 1980; Goethe 1980a; Goethe 1999; Goethe 1999a. For translations of Goethe's works, see also Badrān 1972, p. 108. For a comparative study on "the fortunes of Faust in Arabic literature," see al-Mousa 1998, pp. 103–17.

writing in Dutch.[118] Of interest too is the emergence of Palestinian writers in Hebrew, especially the bilingual writers Naʿīm ʿArāyidī (1948–2015), Anton Shammās (b. 1950), and Sayyid Qashshūʿa (Sayed Kashua) (b. 1975),[119] as well as the recent Palestinian writing rooted in diasporic countries but focused in theme and content on Palestine, such as the English novels of Sūzān Abū al-Hawā (Susan Abulhawa) (b. 1970) and Sūzān Muʿādī Darrāj (Susan Muaddi Darraj) (b. 1967).[120]

5. CONCLUSION

Despite increased interest in Arabic literature, particularly since Najīb Maḥfūẓ was awarded the Nobel Prize in 1988, the negative attitude toward Arabic literature has basically remained the same.[121] Unfortunately, Maḥfūẓ's hope in his Nobel Lecture before the Swedish Academy that "writers of my nation will have the pleasure to sit with full merit amongst your international," has not yet been fulfilled. Moreover, even if another Arab writer wins the prize in the near future, the same scene will be probably repeated as Maḥfūẓ mentioned in his lecture:

> I was told by a foreign correspondent in Cairo that the moment my name was mentioned in connection with the prize silence fell, and many wondered who I was.[122]

The new interest in Arabic literature is mainly due to non-aesthetic (e.g., political, sociological) reasons, some viewing Arabic literature as a means to familiarize oneself with the Arab world and its many societies. Here, it is not hard to recognize the Orientalist attitude that has characterized so much of Western scholarship on Arab and Islamic culture in the twentieth century.[123]

118 See Enquist 2006. On Maghrebi-Dutch authors, see at: https://arablit.org/2020/08/21/three-to-read-maghrebi-women-writing-in-dutch (last accessed August 21, 2020).

119 On the Hebrew writing of Palestinian authors, see also Snir 1991a, pp. 245–53; Snir 1995, pp. 163–83; Snir 1995a, pp. 29–73; Snir 1997, pp. 141–53; Snir 2001a, pp. 197–224. On translations of Hebrew literature into Arabic, see Zipin 1980; Kayyal 2000; Kayyal 2006; Kayyal 2016.

120 On the portrayals of Palestinian exiles in the English-language novels of Susan Abulhawa and Susan Muaddi Darraj and how certain narratives can become increasingly insensitive to the diverse cultural and social settings that are developing among the Palestinian *communitas* around the globe, see Ebileeni 2019, pp. 628–41.

121 See the various contributions in Beard and Haydar 1993.

122 Maḥfūẓ's Nobel Lecture on December 8, 1988; available at: https://www.nobelprize.org/prizes/literature/1988/mahfouz/lecture (last accessed August 21, 2020); see also S. Allen 1993, p. 125.

123 We can mention here also the phenomenon of Westerners confirmedly writing about Muslim and Arab culture while hardly knowing Arabic (e.g., Hever 1987, pp. 47–76; Hever 1989, pp. 30–2; Gordon 1990; Hever 1991, pp. 129–47; Shenberg 1998, pp. 21–9; Brenner

But unlike the undifferentiated patronizing attitude toward Arabic literature that was predominant until the nineteenth century,[124] a new attitude emerged among the Orientalists with the rise of modern Arabic literature—one that saw modern Arabs culturally as an *umma bā'ida* (extinct nation), that is, a nation that has an ancient culture but no modern one.[125] This was presumably due to a classicist bias that viewed the artistic work of the late Middle Ages and early modern period as essentially decadent without any aesthetic merit and thus not deserving of scholarly attention. As I have already pointed out, until the 1960s modern Arabic literature, among all the other modern literatures of the East, received singularly little attention in the West. When Badawi (1925–2012), came to teach at Oxford in 1964, modern Arabic literature as a subject "was barely known" there:

> I found myself continually engaged in attempts to persuade some of my colleagues that Arabic literature had not really ceased, as was commonly believed, with Ibn Khaldun (who died in 1406), but that a sizable body of writing of considerable literary merit had been and was being produced by the Arab of today, and that Taha Husayn's autobiography *al-Ayyam* was not a solitary phenomenon. All too often modern Arabic literature was dismissed by scholars who did not take the trouble to read it.[126]

1999, pp. 85–108; Brenner 2003). And see what Edward W. Said wrote in his review of *God Has Ninety-Nine Names: Reporting from a Militant Middle East* by Judith Miller (Miller 1996).

124 See, for example, the speech that T. B. Macaulay (1800–1859) made before the General Committee on Public Instruction shortly after he reached India in 1834. In the speech, titled "Minute on Indian Education," he said: "I am quite ready to take the Oriental learning at the valuation of the Orientalists themselves. I have never found one among them who could deny that a single shelf of a good European library was worth the whole native literature of India and Arabia ... I certainly never met with any Orientalist who ventured to maintain that the Arabic and Sanskrit poetry could be compared to that of the great European nations" (Macaulay 1972, p. 241. Cf. Anderson 1991, pp. 90–1).

125 On the marginality assigned to modern Arabic literature in general in Oriental or Middle Eastern Studies, see Altoma 1996, p. 137. Stating that "Islamic literature has for the most part remained so unappreciated in the West," James Kritzeck does not refer only to *belles lettres* and neither does he distinguish between Western scholarly attitudes toward classical or modern literature or between various branches of Islamic literature (Kritzeck 1964, p. 5. Cf. Krachkovskii 1989, pp. 15–16). On the other hand, it seems somewhat exaggerated to argue that the negative attitude toward modern Arab culture is shared by Arab scholars as well. It is true that "when a modern Arab thinks of his cultural heritage, he is inclined to skip over the last one thousand years or so, reaching back to the glorious centuries of Islamic civilizations" (Ayyad and Witherspoon 1999, p. 1), but that is not because "the golden age of Islam ... does not seem to link up with the present" (Ayyad and Witherspoon 1999, p. 2). The Golden Age serves as a kind of lost paradise from the point of view of the relationship between Arab civilization and other civilizations; it is by no means due to a low regard for the present culture (Snir 2000, pp. 263–93. See also Martínez Lillo 2011, pp. 57–86). On the concept of "golden age," see Bauer 2007, p. 144.

126 Badawi 2000, pp. 129–30.

Roger Allen (b. 1942), who was among the very first pioneers specializing in what was then (the early 1960s) a radically new and somewhat disparaged field—that of "modern Arabic literature studies"—was in fact the first Oxford graduate student to obtain a doctorate in that subject (1968). Allen, a professor emeritus of Arabic and comparative literature at the University of Pennsylvania, indicates that modern Arabic texts were taught at Oxford before that decade, but were considered a "special subject"—something "that you might dabble in if you so desired, but only after you had studied the texts of the major canon (or, at least, the Oxonian version thereof)."[127] As late as 1971, John A. Haywood still complained in his *Modern Arabic Literature 1800–1970* that "modern Arabic literature has been largely neglected until the last few years."[128] And in 1974, Ilse Lichtenstadter (1907–1991) wrote in her *Introduction to Classical Arabic Literature* that the Arabs "have rested on their ancient laurels and so far have failed to create new masterpieces."[129]

A probable explanation, already given by Gibb, is that the small body of Europeans who read Arabic with any ease were "occupied with researches into the rich historic past of Islam and the Islamic peoples that the present holds no interest, or possibly no attraction, for them."[130] Another possible explanation is the general negative attitude in the West toward Arabic literature as a *literary* phenomenon. Gibb himself alluded to this attitude, the strongest variant of which may well be George Young's dictum that "nearly all national movements—for example, those of Turkey, Greece, Ireland, and other modern nations—begin with a renascence of the national language, legends, and literature. This, in time, leads to a political rebellion against the alien authority or *ancien régime*. But *Modern Egypt has no language, no literature, no legends of its own.*"[131]

127 Allen 2007, p. 248.
128 Haywood 1971, p. 1.
129 Lichtenstadter 1976, p. 119. Cf. Pierre Cachia's comments in Naff 1993, p. 17; Aboul-Ela 2001, pp. 42–4; Aboul-Ela 2011, pp. 725–7.
130 Gibb 1962a, p. 245.
131 Young 1927, p. x (my emphasis).

Chapter 6

Existentialism: The Frightened Mouse[1]

Oh Lord! Oh Lord!
You have given me drink so that whenever
Your wine penetrates into my spot of intoxication
You force me to keep silent, and so I am
Choked with my secrets.
– Ṣalāḥ ʻAbd al-Ṣabūr

1. INTRODUCTION

Twentieth-century literatures of different nations share an outstanding concern with individual human existence. A common thread is the existentialist doctrine derived from the writings of the Danish philosopher Søren Kierkegaard (1813–1855), such as *Fear and Trembling* (1843), *The Concept of Dread* (1844), and *Sickness Unto Death* (1848). In a violent reaction against absolute Hegelian idealism, Kierkegaard insisted on the utter distinctness of God and human beings and on the inexplicability, or even the absurdity, of their actions and the relations between them.

As we saw above, the neo-Ṣūfī trend in Arabic poetry has incorporated contemporary poets who, like early ascetics (*zuhhād*) and Ṣūfī mystics (called also *al-ghurabāʼ*—"the strangers"), reject materialist reality and express their existentialist alienation from it. However, as secular poets, they rarely concern themselves with the precise original meanings of the ancient terms, concentrating rather on the expression of their experiences and feelings as well as their social views. Unlike the early Ṣūfī poets, they are not solely committed to Ṣūfī themes, and Sufism is not a practical way of life for them. However, as previously indicated, like the classical Ṣūfī

[1] This chapter uses material that first appeared in Snir 1989a, pp. 31–43; Snir 2021a, pp. 1–24.

authors, the modernist poets of this trend are also united in their sensitivity to the dialectical tension between language and silence, and are occupying themselves with the alchemical metamorphoses and transformation of the despised body into the pure divine essence. That is why most of them adopt the metaphor of the poet as a mystic constantly advancing on the path toward the divine essence. Poetry for them is a *safar* (journey) that only takes you into a new *safar*. They wonder about the meaning and purpose of life, taking imaginary trips to reveal the secret of existence and frequently becoming immersed in a deep depression over the nature of human existence, from which there is no escape. In order to concretize these ideas, they use Ṣūfī, folkloristic, and various mythological images. As in existentialist philosophy, the conviction of the worthlessness of human existence is often described as an inescapable loss of bearings. Human existence is considered tragic and absurd—alienation, strangeness, spiritual confusion, and sadness are imprinted on the character of man by the very nature of his humanness.

In the field of fiction, one can hardly deny the inspiration that Arab authors have derived from existentialist Western writings since the 1950s, as we can see the numerous literary expressions in books, articles, and magazines. Nevertheless, by no means can one argue that it was a blind imitation: inspired by existentialist ideas that they found suitable to express their experiences, Arab authors incorporated them with Arab and Islamic conceptions. Two short fables, one by the Austrian novelist Franz Kafka (1883–1924) and the other by the Egyptian poet Ṣalāḥ ʻAbd al-Ṣabūr (1931–1981), illustrate that kind of inspiration which the Arab authors draw in order to create a new original vision. A mouse is the central figure in both of their works.

2. "A LITTLE FABLE"

Kafka's work reflects the confusion of the human being in the twentieth century, his wandering between the nihility of existence and divine salvation. A clear example is "Kleine Fabel" ("A Little Fable"), which was not published in Kafka's lifetime and first published by Max Brod (1884–1968) in *Beim Bau der Chinesischen Mauer* (1931).[2] The story is only one paragraph in length:

> "Alas," said the mouse, "the world is growing smaller every day. At the beginning it was so big that I was afraid, I kept running and running, and I was glad when at last I saw walls far away to the right and left, but these long walls have narrowed so quickly that I am in the last chamber already, and there in the

[2] In his will, Kafka instructed his executor and friend Max Brod to destroy his unfinished works, but Brod ignored these instructions.

corner stands the trap that I must run into." "You only need to change your direction," said the cat, and ate it up.[3]

Written between 1917 and 1923, likely in 1920, the story has not gained considerable attention from Kafka's commentators.[4] It consists of only three sentences:

(a) The brief declaration of the mouse that "the world is growing smaller every day."
(b) The mouse's own life story to its tragic end. The mouse tells it in quick rhythm and without a stop to his last gasp. This sentence reaches its end only with the end of the mouse's life (i.e., correspondence between the grammatical structure of the sentence and its meaning).
(c) The saying of the cat, who exploits the tragic situation of the mouse. The involvement of the narrator is restricted to "said the mouse" in the beginning and "said the cat, and ate it up" at the end.

The literary form of the fable, in which we find "the presentation of human beings as animals,"[5] acting "according to their nature, save that they have speech,"[6] leaves no doubt that the mouse represents the human being in his life course from the cradle to the grave.[7] Like the human being, the mouse is possessed by two contradictory fears: the immenseness of the world—"at the beginning it was so big that I was afraid"—and its narrowness—"these long walls have narrowed so quickly." Its life goes through two dimensions: the newborn infant begins immediately "running," distancing himself, in space and time, from the point of his birth.

It is interesting that a year before he wrote that fable, in 1919, Kafka wrote another short piece, which could be considered as dealing with the same idea, "Das nächste Dorf" ("The Next Village"):

[3] Kafka 1931, p. 59; Kafka 1946, p. 119 (English translation: Kafka 1971, p. 445).

[4] See Flores 1976, p. 170. Since the publication of Flores' work, the attention of Kafka scholars to the story has not increased.

[5] Cuddon 1986, p. 256.

[6] Shipley 1972, p. 153.

[7] In the present study, I will not consider the "funniness" in the story. In "Some Remarks on Kafka's Funniness from Which Probably Not Enough Has Been Removed," David Foster Wallace refers to the story as a case study for reading humor in Kafka and how he tried to teach his students to do this when teaching Kafka: "It's not that students don't 'get' Kafka's humor but that we've taught them to see humor as something you *get*—the same way we've taught them that a self is something you just *have*. No wonder they cannot appreciate the really central Kafka joke: that the horrific struggle to establish a human self results in a self whose humanity is inseparable from that horrific struggle. That our endless and impossible journey toward home is in fact our home" (Wallace 2006, pp. 60–5. The quotation is from pp. 64–5).

> My grandfather used to say: “Life is astoundingly short. To me, looking back over it, life seems so foreshortened that I scarcely understand, for instance, how a young man can decide to ride over to the next village without being afraid that—not to mention accidents—even the span of a normal happy life may fall far short of the time needed for such a journey.”[8]

We find some connections between the mouse’s fears about the size of the world and some of Kafka’s reflections in a letter he wrote at the beginning of 1920, almost a year before he wrote “Kleine Fabel,” to Minze Eisner (1901–1972), a young Jewish woman he met at Pension Stüdl, who was convalescing from a serious illness:

> It’s a big world and a wide one, as you write, but not a hairsbreadth bigger than people are able to make it. The immensity of the world, as you now see it, springs from both the truthfulness of a brave heart and the illusions of your nineteen years. You can easily verify that by noticing that an age of, say, forty years likewise seems immense to you, and yet, as all the people you know will demonstrate, does not have that immensity you imagine.[9]

Immenseness and narrowness are a person’s feeling about the world in different stages of his life. The newborn infant, who has been just thrown out from his mother’s narrow and warm womb, cannot help but observe the horrible cold immensity of his new dwelling place. Cut off from his fetal connection with his mother’s physiological processes, he yearns to return to this womb. This is the birth trauma, which finds its archetypal expression in yearning for death, seen as a return to the mother’s womb, or God’s lap.[10] From the moment of his birth, a human being begins running, escaping this immensity. As this fear fades, a new threat bursts forth—the narrowing of man’s life. We can present this situation in the following manner:

(1) The womb—absolute safety without any fear.
(2) Birth and youth—fear of immensity.
(3) Maturity and old age—fear of narrowness.
(4) Death—absolute safety without any fear.

The mouse’s running corresponds to the movements that we find in this fable, or short story, between several poles: existence–nothing; birth–death; and immenseness–narrowness. The first time the mouse watches his entire life is also the last time. That is the minute of revelation, like Poseidon in

8 Kafka 1948, p. 158.
9 Kafka 1958, pp. 258–9 (English translation: Kafka 1977, pp. 222–3).
10 See, for example, Ferenczi 1924, pp. 112–15; Schachtel 1963, p. 49.

Kafka's *Poseidon*,[11] who postponed the crossing of the ocean he was responsible for to the last minute:

> He used to say that he was postponing this until the end of the world, for then there might come a quiet moment when, just before the end and having gone through the last account, he could still make a quick little tour.

A similar situation can be found in the fable "Die Brucke" ("The Bridge").[12] The bridge knows that "without falling, no bridge, once spanned, can cease to be a bridge." And, indeed, realization of life entails annihilation: when the bridge turns around to get a comprehensive look on the ravine—one step outside the reality of life—he ceased to be a bridge, since it is not natural for

> a bridge to turn around! I had not yet turned quite around when I already began to fall, I fell and in a moment I was torn and transpierced by the sharp rocks which had always gazed up at me so peacefully from the rushing water.[13]

The mouse in "Kleine Fabel" is running toward its end. There is no reason to wait because, as in *Heimkehr* (*Homecoming*),[14] "the longer one hesitates before the door, the more estranged one becomes."

The strangeness and alienation of the human being in this world force him to run away, like the mouse in "Kleine Fabel," toward his end. The mouse's conviction that "the world is growing smaller every day" does not result from its birth but from its attempt to escape the world's immensity. Its original conviction, that the world is immense, fades out and is replaced by another conviction or another fear that the world is narrow. Man in this world, like the mouse in our story, cannot be free; he is always possessed by some fear, no matter what kind it may be. His whole life is spent running away from one fear to another until his end.

Why does the mouse keep on running when he is fully conscious that his running adds to his fear? Why does he not stop when he realizes that "these long walls have narrowed so quickly"? Maybe it is because he cannot stop running, just like man, who has no choice but to march toward his death.

In fables, "the outlook is realistic and ironical,"[15] so when the mouse comes "in the last chamber," face to face with death, he undergoes an ironic experience: being aware of his running into the trap, he agrees with the cat's advice, which brings upon him his inevitable death. He escapes one

11 Kafka 1946, pp. 97–8 (English translation: Kafka 1971, pp. 434–5).
12 Kafka 1946, pp. 111–12 (English translation: Kafka 1971, pp. 411–12).
13 Cf. Binder 1966, pp. 196–7; Binder 1977, pp. 193, 245.
14 Kafka 1946, p. 139 (English translation: Kafka 1971, pp. 445–6).
15 Shipley 1972, p. 153.

inevitable trap to fall into another. The ironic relation between the mouse and the cat in "Kleine Fabel" becomes clearer if we read one of the fragments that Kafka left:

> A cat had caught a mouse. "What are you going to do now?" the mouse asked. "You have terrible eyes." "Oh," the cat said, "my eyes are always like that. You'll get used to it." "I think I'll go away, if you don't mind," the mouse said, "my children are waiting for me." "Your children are waiting?" the cat said. "Then go along as quickly as you can. I was only just going to ask you something." "Then please ask, it's really very late indeed."[16]

Kafka's existentialism, according to "Kleine Fabel," is an atheistic one, of which Jean-Paul Sartre (1905–1980) is the chief exponent: man is a self-creating being who is not initially endowed with a character and goals, but who chooses them by acts of pure decision. Being born into a kind of void (*le neant*) and mud (*le visqueux*)—like the mouse, in our fable, who was born into this vast and horrible world—man has the liberty to remain in this mud, within which he is totally responsible for the choices he makes. As a temporal being, conscious, through his will, of a future whose only certainty is his own death, rejecting passivity and trying to become aware of himself, man experiences a metaphysical and moral anguish (*angoisse*) and a sense of absurdity, alienation, and despair—like the mouse who began escaping from the first moment of his life. "If so, he would then have a sense of the absurdity of his predicament and suffer despair"[17]—like the mouse who "saw walls far away to the right and left," which "have narrowed so quickly." The energy deriving from this awareness would enable him to drag himself out of the mud and begin to exist. By exercising his power of choice, "he can give meaning to existence and the universe"[18]—like the mouse who, standing face to face with death, gives meaning to his existence by exercising his liberty to choose, no matter what choices stand before him.

3. "STRIPPINGS"

The mouse is also the hero of Ṣalāḥ ʻAbd al-Ṣabūr's last poem in his last collection *al-Ibḥār fi al-Dhākira* (*The Sailing in the Memory*) (1979). The poem is the previously mentioned "Tajrīdāt" ("Strippings")[19] and is divided into three parts. It is one of the outstanding mystical poems of this Egyptian poet, who has stood out, since the late 1950s, as one of the leaders of the new

[16] Kafka 1953, p. 294 (English translation: Kafka 1954, p. 262).
[17] Cuddon 1986, p. 252.
[18] Cuddon 1986, p. 252.
[19] ʻAbd al-Ṣabūr 1981, pp. 79–85.

mystical, or neo-Ṣūfī, trend in modern Arabic poetry.[20] I am referring to the tendency of Arab poets, since the late 1950s, themselves espousing secular worldviews, to utilize mystical, and primarily Ṣūfī, concepts, figures, and motifs to express the philosophies and experiences of contemporary human beings. Not only do they mention concepts and figures from the ancient Ṣūfī tradition; they also express spiritual experiences and ascetic and mystical outlooks of the same type that exist in early Sufism or in mysticism in general, and they also sometimes combine Ṣūfī motifs with modern philosophies and ideologies, loading them with new meanings.[21]

The first and the third parts of ʻAbd al-Ṣabūr's poem describe mystical and ecstatic states that the persona experienced, using Ṣūfī terms like the aforementioned *ḥāl* (a mystical "state"), *yaqīn* (certitude), *ṣaḥw* (sobriety), *maḥw* (effacement), *ṣamt* (silence), and *sirr* (secret; the innermost part of the heart in which the divine revelation is experienced). The emotional and spiritual states of the persona in the poem are based upon the Ṣūfī saying "*al-aḥwāl mawāhib wa-l-maqāmāt makāsib*" ("the mystical states are divine gifts, while the stations can be attained by human efforts").[22] Here is the first part of the poem:

حال قد كنت رقيت إليها أمس
لا تأتيني اليوم
هي حال أعطتني نعمى النّوم
ويقين الصّحو
حال الهابط من سطح الإعياء إلى قاع الغفو
أو حال الصّاعد من قاع الغفو إلى سطح الإعياء
لم أسمع فيها الأصداء
لكنّ الأصداء استمعتني
لم ألمس فيها الأشياء
لكنّ الأشياء
لمستني واعتصرتني
حتّى أصبحت هواء
يتسرّب في المحو

***

آه... ما أثقل جسمي اللّيلة
ما أثقل جسمي اللّيلة

[20] See Snir 2006, pp. 91–116.

[21] On this trend, see Snir 1986. See also Snir 1984, pp. 12–13; Snir 1985, pp. 129–46; Snir 1986a; Snir 2002; Snir 2006.

[22] See al-Qushayrī 1940, p. 34. Cf. Trimingham 1971, p. 201 n. 2; Nicholson 1975, p. 29; al-Suhrawardī 1993, p. 66. See also Surūr 1957, pp. 111–12; Schimmel 1983, p. 99.

A state to which I had been elevated yesterday,
Does not reach me today
It is a state which provided me with the happiness of sleep
And the certitude of sobriety
The state of that who drops from the surface of fatigue into the bottom of slumber
Or that who climbs from the bottom of slumber into the surface of fatigue
I did not hear there the echoes
But the echoes listened to me
I did not touch objects
But objects
Touched and squeezed me
Till I became air flowing in the effacement

***

Oh, what a heavy body I carry this night
What a heavy body I carry this night

As a divine gift, the *ḥāl* cannot be acquired by human efforts but comes to the heart without any deliberate intention. It can be compared with a flash of lightning: the moment it is there is also the moment it is gone again. As Hujwīrī states, it is "something that descends from God into man's heart, without his being able to repel it when it comes, or to attract it when it goes, by his own effort."[23] Contrary to the *ḥāl*, the *maqām* is an enduring stage, which man can reach, to a certain extent, by his own striving. It belongs to the category of acts, whereas the *ḥāl* is always a gift of grace.[24]

Al-Qushayrī says that while the *ḥāl* is like lightning in that it disappears the moment it strikes in the heart of the believer, it leaves traces that ensure his ascent along the mystical path.[25] Jalāl al-Dīn Rūmī (1207–1273) puts it as follows: "The *ḥāl* is like the unveiling of the beauteous bride, while the *maqām* is [the king's] being alone with the bride."[26] There are Ṣūfī mystics who claim that the *ḥāl* does not disappear as soon as it arrives but that it is a lasting phenomenon. According to them, the term *waqt* (lit. "time") designates the "present moment," that is, the moment the gift of *ḥāl* is granted to the Ṣūfī mystic. *Waqt*, says the Ṣūfī mystic, is like a cutting sword: it cuts whatever is before and after, leaving man in absolute nakedness in the presence of God.[27] That is why the Ṣūfī mystic has been called "*ibn al-waqt*"—he

23 Hujwīrī 1959, p. 181.
24 Schimmel 1983, pp. 99–100. Cf. Arberry 1979 [1950], p. 75.
25 Al-Qushayrī 1940, p. 34.
26 Rūmī 1925, I, p. 88; Rūmī 1968, II, p. 79.
27 Cf. Meister Eckhart's concept of time: "The person who lives in the light of God is conscious neither of time past nor of time to come but only of one eternity ... Therefore he gets

gives himself completely over to the present moment and receives what God sends down to him without a single thought about present, past, and future.[28] For the Ṣūfī mystics, the Prophet's expression "*lī maʿa Allāh waqt*" ("I have a time with God") pointed to their own mystical experience when, as the German Orientalist and scholar of Sufism Annemarie Schimmel (1922–2003) puts it, "they break through created time and reach the Eternal Now in God," when everything created is annihilated. Similarly, for the Indian poet and philosopher Muḥammad Iqbāl (1873–1938) this Prophetic tradition signifies the moment at which "the infidel's girdle," namely, "serial" time is torn and "the mystic establishes direct contact with God in a person-to-person encounter."[29]

Mystic and Ṣūfī motifs are combined in the poem, as is frequently found in the new mystical trend in modern Arabic poetry. They include the strangeness of the soul in the despised bodily prison and the death of the passions;[30] ecstatic and pantheistic states;[31] the symbolism of the wine;[32] and, finally, the issue of the ineffable and the silence,[33] which is inevitable in the highest mystical state, as expressed in the third part, which also comprises the concluding lines of the poem. These lines were mentioned above, but it is important to quote them again as an organic part of ʿAbd al-Ṣabūr's poem:

يا ربّ! يا ربّ!
أسقيتني حتّى إذا ما مشت
كأسك في موطن إسراري
ألزمتني الصّمت، وهذا أنا
أغصّ مخنوقا بأسراري

Oh Lord! Oh Lord!
You have given me drink so that whenever
Your wine penetrates into my spot of intoxication
You force me to keep silent, and so I am
Choked with my secrets.

Referring to the symbolism of the wine and the ineffable, and due to the close relationship of Ṣūfī poetry with the classical wine and erotic love poetry, it comes as no surprise that these lines allude to the aforementioned two wine

nothing new of future events, nor from chance, for he lives in the Now-moment that is, unfailingly, 'in verdure newly clad'" (Scharfstein 1973, p. 151).

28 Schimmel 1983, pp. 129–30. Cf. al-Suhrawardī 1993, pp. 79–80.

29 Schimmel 1983, p. 220.

30 See Snir 1986, pp. 114–220.

31 Snir 1986, pp. 258–314.

32 Snir 1986, pp. 235–43.

33 Snir 1986, pp. 405–20.

verses attributed to the libertine medieval poet Abū Nuwās (*c.* 755–*c.* 813).[34] Unlike the first and the third parts, the second part of 'Abd al-Ṣabūr's poem is totally different: it does not have direct allusion to any mystical states. On the contrary, it is very much rationalistic and based upon intellectualism:

سيف اللّاجدوى
يهوي ما بين الرّغبة والعقل
صحراء اللّافعل
تتمدّد ما بين الرّغبة والجدوى
ماذا في طوق الفأر المذعور
ما بين السّيف وبين الصّحراء؟
فرض أوّل:
يهرب من سيف اللّاجدوى للفعل اللّامجدي
فرض ثان:
يهرب من صحراء اللّافعل إلى قاع اللّارغبة
فيداهمه سيف اللّاجدوى
فرض ثالث:
يثوى في جحر اللّاجدوى
واللّارغبة
واللّافعل
ويموت ...!!

The sword of futility
Falls between the desire and the intellect
The desert of inactivity
Spreads between the desire and the utility
What can the frightened mouse do
Between the sword and the desert?
First assumption:
Escape the sword of futility to the useless activity
Second assumption:
Escape the desert of inactivity to the depths of desirelessness
Where the sword of futility will surprise him
Third assumption:
Stay in the hole of futility
And desirelessness
And inactivity
And die.

[34] See al-'Abbāsī 1947, III, p. 46; al-Tha'ālibī 1983, p. 147; al-Ṣafadī 2000, I, p. 144.

Since we assume that the poet had known Kafka's aforementioned "A Little Fable," I provide here its Arabic translation[35] in order to show the connections between the texts:

> "واحسرتاه" قال الفأر، "العالم يصغر يومًا بعد يوم. في البدء كان كبيرًا جدًا لدرجة أنّي ارتعبت منه، وأخذت أجري وأجري وسررت جدًا حين رأيت الحوائط أخيرًا – على البعد إلى اليمين وإلى اليسار، لكنّ تلك الحوائط العالية الواسعة سريعًا جدًا ما ضاقت حتّى إنّني أصبحت في الحجرة الأخيرة بالفعل، وهناك في الرّكن فخٌّ عليّ السّقوط بداخله". "ما عليك سوى تغيير اتّجاهك" قالت القطّة وابتلعته في لمحة

This rationalistic part of the poem, coming between the two mystical and ecstatic parts, describes the mouse's effort to escape his fate. The frightened mouse—the frightened human being in this world—stands confused between two threats:

(a) The sword of futility—a symbol of the metaphysical futility of all man's actions in this world—falls between the desire and the intellect: man's actions are futile whether their source is the desire or the intellect. The contrast between the desire and the intellect reminds us of the distinction that Friedrich Nietzsche (1844–1900) made in his first philosophical work, *Die Geburt der Tragödie* (*The Birth of Tragedy*) (1872), between the Apollonian and Dionysian dimensions, to contrast reason with instinct, culture with primitive nature.[36]
(b) The desert of inactivity—worldly life—spreads between the desire and the utility: between the desire and its realization, there is a desert that man must pass through in order to put his desire into effect.

Three options face the mouse seeking to escape his fate, two of which are familiar to man in this world:

(a) To run away from the sword of futility to useless activity: trying to escape his futile life, he explores all kinds of actions to find meaning, but everything proves to be useless.
(b) To run away from the desert of inactivity to the depths of undesire, where the sword of futility will surprise him: even the condition of inactivity and undesire in this world is futile.

35 The translation is according to http://www.menalmuheetlelkhaleej.com/archive/index.php?t-54007.html (last accessed August 5, 2019). For another translation, see Kafka 2014, p. 46.
36 See Nietzsche 1955, p. 47 (English translation: Nietzsche 1967, p. 33); Preminger 1974, p. 41; Cuddon 1986, pp. 51–2.

These two options, which are based upon sticking to the worldly life, cannot save man from his distress. But there is a third option, a quietist one:

(c) To stay in the hole of futility and undesire and inactivity and to die.

The conclusion of this part of the poem is so radical that it reminds us of the Quietism and Hesychasm of the Christian Church[37] and of the aforementioned Ṣūfī *tawakkul* (trust in God): any active action is useless, including writing poetry—death is the only refuge for a human being in this world, even from a rational and intellectual point of view. One may identify in this part of the poem some echoes of the quietistic atmosphere in Samuel Beckett's (1906–1989) writings,[38] which introduce the need to conduct a comparative study between ʿAbd al-Ṣabūr and Beckett—two writers whose existential and humanist approaches deserve a deeper investigation.

4. "FOR THINE IS THE KINGDOM"

As "existentialism is often regarded as a reflection of the spiritual and moral disarray caused by two world wars,"[39] we can regard ʿAbd al-Ṣabūr's religious existentialist inclinations as a reflection of the disappointment from the spiritual poverty of the modern era and as a lament for twentieth-century civilization. The disappointment in logical thinking and science, which led humanity to two horrible world wars, is one of the characteristic themes of modern Arabic poetry.[40] This is one of the important causes of the neo-Ṣūfī trend in modern Arabic poetry: the Arab poets tried to fill the spiritual emptiness that they felt, and to express the sense of alienation and strangeness of man in modern civilization, and they found refuge in religion and mysticism.

The disappointment in logical thinking and science is also one of the reasons for the great popularity, among modern Arab poets, of the poet and the critic T. S. Eliot (1888–1965), who laments, particularly in "The Waste Land," the spiritual poverty of Western civilization.[41] ʿAbd al-Ṣabūr himself was very strongly affected by Eliot,[42] and translated from his poetry.[43] Even

[37] See Krivoshein 1938–1939, IV, pp. 193–214; Knox 1951, pp. 231–87.
[38] See, for example, Wimbush 2016, pp. 439–55.
[39] Reid 1976, p. 220.
[40] Mīkhāʾīl 1968, p. 191; Moreh 1976, p. 313; Moreh 1984, p. 175.
[41] Badawi 1975, p. 224; Moreh 1976, pp. 216–66; Brugman 1984, p. 204; Moreh 1984, p. 168; Snir 2002, pp. 28–30. For a different opinion on the influence of Eliot on Arabic poetry, see Shukrī 1978, p. 215.
[42] See ʿAbd al-Ṣabūr 1969, pp. 49, 90–2; ʿAbd al-Ṣabūr 1982a, pp. 143–54; ʿAbd al-Ṣabūr 1983, pp. 81–4.
[43] See *Fuṣūl* 2.1 (October 1981), pp. 282, 317; Badīr 1982, p. 180.

the second part of the poem quoted above betrays, in its very first lines, the inspiration of Eliot's last lines in "The Hollow Men" (1925):

Between the desire
And the spasm
Between the potency
And the existence
Between the essence
And the descent
Falls the Shadow
For Thine is the Kingdom

For Thine is
Life is
For Thine is the

This is the way the world ends
This is the way the world ends
This is the way the world ends
Not with a bang but a whimper.[44]

'Abd al-Ṣabūr's existentialism reminds us of Kierkegaard, the pioneer of modern Christian existentialism, who believed "that through God and in God man may find freedom from tension and discontent and therefore find peace of mind and spiritual serenity."[45] A mystic refuge, according to 'Abd al-Ṣabūr, is the only solution to human distress: the dualism between the soul and the body, and the soul's yearning to escape the despised bodily prison and to merge with its divine source;[46] the rejection of reality and the feeling of alienation in this tragic and absurd human existence;[47] the negation of worldly desires and striving for death:[48] all these elements, revealed in 'Abd al-Ṣabūr's poetry, make the mystic refuge by means of illuminative and ecstatic states the only solution.[49] Even his social poetry is imbued with mystical and Ṣūfī elements.[50]

'Abd al-Ṣabūr, like his famous compatriot novelist Najīb Maḥfūẓ,[51] meets Kafka within the context of twentieth-century existentialism. Both of them share some kind of "vision of the condition and existence of man, his place

44 Eliot 1969, pp. 85–6.
45 Cuddon 1986, p. 251.
46 Snir 1986, pp. 125–6.
47 Snir 1986, pp. 141–50.
48 Snir 1986, pp. 196–201.
49 Snir 1986, pp. 269–76.
50 Snir 1986, pp. 337–70.
51 Cf. Myers 1986, pp. 82–96.

and function in the world, and his relation to God."[52] Kafka inspired 'Abd al-Ṣabūr,[53] as he inspired other prominent Arab writers, one of which is Najīb Maḥfūẓ,[54] who resembles Kafka especially in the intensive use of his works to convey universal messages.[55]

[52] Cuddon 1986, p. 251.

[53] See 'Abd al-Ṣabūr 1971, pp. 63–6; 'Uthmān 1981, p. 197. The issue of inspiration discussed in the present chapter should by no means blur the major differences between the two authors (or between Kafka and other Arab creative writers and artists) due to the fundamental distinction of each culture within which each of them was active. Suffice it to take, for example, the attitude to the specific religious heritage—Kafka's Jewish roots and 'Abd al-Ṣabūr's Islamic background, not to speak about other issues that had a major impact on their writings encapsulating existential worldviews. For example, reading Kafka's "Letter to His Father" ("Brief a den Vater") (Kafka 1966) and the poem "Abī" ("My Father") ('Abd al-Ṣabūr 1972, pp. 23–8) may reflect the separate intellectual and cultural contexts in which each of them was active. Only recently may we find more complicated Arab literary and artistic interactions with Kafka's worldview such as the works, both literary and artistic, by the Lebanese writer and artist Shadhā Sharaf al-Dīn (b. 1964), her exhibition "Letter to the Father" being one example: reminiscent of Islamic manuscript layout design and in an attempt to write to her own father, she subverts the original German letter, copies it in Arabic and reveals an interest in appropriating visual elements from the past. The exhibition was held in Beirut between November 10 and December 10, 2021, see at: https://www.minaimagecentre.org/letter-to-the-father, last accessed November 21, 2021. See also the novel *Kafka fī Ṭanja* (*Kafka in Tanjier*) by the Moroccan writer Muḥammad Sa'īd Aḥjayūj (Mohammed Said Hjiouj) (b. 1982) (Aḥjayūj 2019). For an excerpt from the novel translated by Phoebe Bay Carter, see *Arablit & Arablit Quarterly: A Magazine of Arabic Literature in Translation*, available at: https://arablit.org/2021/12/20/new-an-excerpt-of-mohammed-said-hjiouijs-kafka-in-tangier, last accessed December 19, 2021.

[54] See Duwāra 1963, pp. 8, 11; Duwāra 1965, pp. 270, 275; *Mawāqif*, I (October–November 1968), p. 87; Somekh 1973a, p. 45; Hafez 1975, p. 111; al-Ghīṭānī 1980, p. 42; Ballas 1980, p. 179; Shukrī 1982, p. 389. It should be noted that Maḥfūẓ, probably inspired by Kafka, published a short story whose protagonist is also a mouse: "al-Fa'r al-Nurwīǧī" ("Rattus Norvegicus") published in *Ibdā'*, May 1983, pp. 4–6; the story was incorporated later into his collection *al-Tanẓīm al-Sirrī* (Cairo: Dār al-Shurūq, 2006 [1984]), pp. 107–14. For a study of the story, see Snir 1989, pp. 120–53.

[55] Somekh 1973a, pp. 195–6; Sakkout 1975, p. 122; 'Aṭiyya 1977, pp. 99–112; Myers 1986, pp. 82–96. One can argue, however, that Mahfuz's message in his works, at the time he wrote them, was sometimes a response to specific circumstances (such as the 1950s and 1960s), and then argue that Kafka usually emphasizes universal and philosophical issues. However, in retrospect, all Mahfuz's works seem now to carry universal messages. In an essay on the American painter Charles Sheeler (1883–1965), the American poet William Carlos Williams (1883–1963) says: "The local is the universal. It was a banana to Cezanne. Look! That's where painting begins. A bird, up above, flying, may be the essence of it—but a dead canary, with glazed eye, has no less an eye for that, well seen becomes sight and song itself. It is in things that for the artist the power lies, not beyond them. Only where the eye hits does sight occur. Take a cross-eyed child at birth. For him to see at all one of the eyes must go blind, he cannot focus it. But let him look past the object to 'abstraction' long enough and soon the other eye will follow" (Sheeler 1939, pp. 8–9). And the Indian writer from Odisha Jagannath Prasad Das (J. P.) (b. 1936) adds: "In literature the local is the universal. A picture of a locality can have a universal appeal" (*The Tribune*, April 18, 2010). On Kafka and the Arabs in general, see Hanssen 2012, pp. 167–97. It would

Kafka and ʿAbd al-Ṣabūr seem to present contradictory views on human existence: Kafka presents a desperate world with no recourse left, whereas ʿAbd al-Ṣabūr presents a hope of escape by means of mystic ecstasy. But it is an illusionary contradiction: is the mouse in "Kleine Fabel" without hope? There is more in this fable than the pessimism that dominates the surface. In spite of the mouse's desperate running away, from its first day it does not lose hope in every minute of its life. It does not give up when the world seems so immense. It tries to escape this immensity, and when the "long walls have narrowed" it does not stop running away. Even in its last moment, when it is running into the trap, it tries the last hope of salvation: it accepts the advice of the cat, knowing that nothing will come of it, as the crazy man who was fishing in a bathtub in the essay of Albert Camus (1913–1960) about Kafka:

> A doctor with ideas as to psychiatric treatments asked him "if they were biting" to which he received the harsh reply: "of course not, you fool, since this is a bathtub."

And the explanation of Camus:

> Kafka's world is in truth an indescribable universe in which man allows himself the tormenting luxury of fishing in a bathtub, knowing that nothing will come of it.[56]

Kafka's work is torn between the conviction that the tragic fate of human existence is determined, on the one hand, and the frustrated desire to change it, on the other. Moreover, sometimes, like in "Kleine Fabel," we must look at Kafka's world from two points of view: the human being that does not lose his or her hope till the last moment, as against the metaphysical outlook, which does not see any refuge for the human being in this world. Here between the lines, and in accordance with Kafka's other writing, we meet the nostalgia for a lost paradise, or the concept of God, even if this God is not the same God that ʿAbd al-Ṣabūr yearns for. Both Kafka and ʿAbd al-Ṣabūr share the feeling of hope, since "it is not contradictory for fundamentally existentialist writing to find cause for hope."[57] Albert Camus succeeded in

be interesting to study the works of the Iraqi-Jewish writer Samīr Naqqāsh (1938–2004) against the background of Kafka's works: Naqqāsh focuses in his fiction on a specific and local reality, namely, the reality of Iraqi Jews, but at the same time, like Kafka, addresses universal themes that characterize the human condition in the twentieth century. His works deal with the fate of man in a universe without boundaries or providence, and with man's illusory pursuit of reason and scientific achievement following the collapse of his spiritual and religious world. Kafka and Naqqāsh describe modern man as bereft of divine providence and abandoned to the helplessness of his human nature (see, e.g., the Kafkaesque metamorphosis as reflected of Naqqāsh in Elimelekh 2013, pp. 323–42).

56 Camus 1942, p. 179 (English translation: Camus 1955, p. 96).

57 Myers 1986, p. 83.

clarifying this point by saying that it is strange that works like those of Kafka should in the long run lead to that tremendous cry of hope; it is through humility that hope enters in. For the absurd in this existence assures them a little more of a supernatural reality. If the course of this life leads to God, there is an outcome after all:

> Kafka refuses his God moral nobility, evidence, virtue, coherence, but only the better to fall into his arms. As I see once more, existential thought in this regard, and contrary to current opinion, is steeped in a vast hope, the very hope which at the time of early Christianity and the spreading of the good news inflamed the ancient world ... (His work) is universal because its inspiration is religious. As in all religions, man is freed of the weight of his own life.[58]

There is no doubt that the human being is confronted with a desperate situation, but, as Camus says, "the word 'hope' used here is not ridiculous. On the contrary, the more tragic the condition described by Kafka, the firmer and more aggressive that hope becomes."[59]

5. CONCLUSION

In the two fables in question, there is a synthesis of strangeness; alienation; wondering about the meaning and purpose of life; deep depression after the tragic nature of human existence, from which there is no escape; hope; and religious quest. Both of the writers offer, in different ways, a salvation in which death could be the gate to the true life. 'Abd al-Ṣabūr offers the yearning for God, which is the only refuge from the hopelessness of the materialistic world—the true union with God, as the unitive state (i.e., the attainment of the absolute, according to the mystics)[60]—is impossible without the death of the despised bodily prison and the escaping of the soul that will merge with its divine source. In some sense, Kafka offers us a similar refuge with a spiritual dimension.[61] His work is imbued with the conviction that there is no hope for human existence in our hopeless world, and that there is no mercy to be expected from it. The acknowledgment of man's hopeless condition is not, however, a sign of weakness, but it is instead a courageous, if futile, protest against this condition and a craving for refuge. If there is a refuge and if there is an agent of mercy in our desperate situation, it can only be the unknowable and ineffable God or any absolute essence. Here, despite the differences between the two writers, we find the common yearning. The

[58] Camus 1942, pp. 185–7 (English translation: Camus 1955, pp. 100–1).
[59] Camus 1942, p. 184 (English translation: Camus 1955, p. 99).
[60] Underhill 1961, pp. 413–43.
[61] Cf. Myers 1986, pp. 94–5.

human being is called to believe and be patient, as was written in the inscription on the gravestone of the old commandant of the penal colony in Kafka's well-known story:

> Here rests the Old Commandant. His supporters, who now have no name, dug him this grave, and set this stone for him. It is prophesied that after a certain number of years, the Commandant will rise again, and from these premises here, lead his followers on to the reconquest of the colony. Believe and be patient![62]

[62] Kafka 2007, p. 180.

Chapter 7

Reception: Stream of Consciousness[1]

And she felt that she had been given a present, wrapped up,
and told just to keep it, not to look at it.
– Virginia Woolf

1. INTRODUCTION

There is a good deal of research on the formative stage of modern Arabic literature, mostly the second half of the nineteenth century, when the Arab world set about creating responses to the growing impact and domination, political as well as cultural, of the West. Most of the studies are in both Arabic and English, but one can find as well comprehensive studies in other languages, such as German, French, and Spanish.[2] It was during the late nineteenth century that Western literary forms, such as the novel and the short story, were "borrowed" by Arabic literature, though I have shown in several studies that this "import" was by no means a pure import because Arab culture had had approximately the same genres or similar ones in their own local versions. Unlike poetry, which parted ways only gradually with traditional "sacred" norms, the development of fiction has faced no major obstacles. Within less than one century, traditional canonical prose genres, such as the *maqāma* and *risāla*, totally disappeared from the Arabic literary system,[3] and ever since the short story and the novel have become the leading

[1] This chapter uses material that first appeared in Snir 1999, pp. 6–7.

[2] See references in Snir 2017.

[3] Among the few writers of *maqāmāt* in the twentieth century, mention should be made of the Egyptian *zajal* poet Bayram al-Tūnisī (1893–1961) (al-Tūnisī 1976, vols. 8 and 9 of his *Complete Works*). On his *maqāmāt*, see Armbrust 1996, pp. 55–8) and his compatriot Fu'ād Qā'ūd (1936–2006) ('Abd al-Fattāḥ 1993b, pp. 165–96). For references on the *maqāma* and *risāla* in general, see Snir 2017, p. 206, n. 129.

prose genres. Together with other classical genres,[4] both the *maqāma* and *risāla* played a role in the development of the new prose genres, but the exact nature of that role is still a matter of dispute. What is clear is that the new genres developed quickly thanks to the popularity of non-canonical narrative literature, with *Alf Layla wa-Layla*, *Siyar al-Anbiyā'*, and the various epics of 'Antara, Baybars, and Banū Hilāl all paving the way for the modern narrative genres.[5] The spread of novels translated into Arabic and original Arabic works of popular fiction during the second half of the nineteenth century and the first quarter of the twentieth century was a necessary stage in the development of the novel as a canonical genre. Much has already been written about the development of Arabic narrative discourse, and the short story and the novel in particular, and there are a number of studies on the changing norms in dialogue and narration.[6] There is, however, surprisingly little research on the contemporary Arab literary scene as to Western borrowings or interference. The concept of "stream of consciousness" is a salient example—it is clearly present in Arabic literature by the 1960s, but no one has so far followed its trajectory from the West to the Arab East, not least regarding particular prominent authors involved in such a move. The following, therefore, is only a preliminary survey of the presence of one of these major authors, Virginia Woolf (1882–1941), whose impact on Arabic literary writing has been beyond any doubt.

Woolf made an original contribution in general to the form of the novel and was one of the most distinguished critics of her time. After her novels *The Voyage Out* (1915) and *Night and Day* (1919) appeared, she began to experiment in her creative writing, stressing the continuous flow of experience, the indefinability of character, and external circumstances as they impinge on consciousness. She was also interested in the way time is experienced both as a sequence of disparate moments and as the flow of years and of centuries. From *Jacob's Room* (1922) onward, she tried to convey the impression of time present and of time passing in individual experience and also of the characters' awareness of historic time. In *Mrs. Dalloway* (1925) and more so in *To the Lighthouse* (1927), which was written after Woolf had read *Ulysses* (1922) by James Joyce (1882–1941), she extended her technical mastery; above all, she gave to each of these novels a tightly organized form, partly by using poetic devices, such as recurrent images, and partly by restricting the time of the action. In her long essay, "A Room of One's

4 Such as *ayyām al-'Arab*, *qiṣaṣ al-anbiyā'*, *al-faraj ba'da al-shidda*, as well as various parts of the *adab* literature.
5 See Selim 2019.
6 See, for example, Snir 2017, pp. 206–18, and the references there.

Own" (1929), she described the difficulties encountered by women writers in a man's world. Returning to the art of the novel, in *The Waves* (1931) she confined herself to recording the stream of consciousness. The reader lives within the minds of one or the other of six characters from their childhood to their old age. Human experience of the "seven ages of man," rather than character or event, is paramount. In the present chapter, I will refer to the presence of Virginia Woolf in Arab culture as a metaphor for the place of Western culture in the Arab world and the significant role of the West and its cultural agents in changing Arab culture. The translations of her works into Arabic and their impact on Arabic literary writing may be considered against the background of the massive translation movement that has taken place in the Arab world since the nineteenth century, which is a fundamental factor in the changes that Arab culture has been undergoing. I will try to present several issues that the translators grappled with and the difficulties of Woolf's reception by Arab authors and readers.

2. "UNRESTRAINED, UNORGANISED MOVEMENTS OF THE MIND"

The translation of Virginia Woolf's works into Arabic, many years after their original publication, only started to receive attention in the Arab world with the rising critical interest in modernist writing techniques and the benefits Arab authors started to gain from psychology in terms of successfully presenting characters, expressing their moods, and bringing the reader into the psychological dimension of human reality. One of the first times in which we find a reference to Virginia Woolf in Arabic scholarship is in an English essay that was published by the Iraqi-Jewish writer Nissīm Rajwān (Rejwan) (1924–2017) on July 4, 1948 in the English newspaper *Iraq Times* in Baghdad. In a review of *Guide to Modern Thought* (1948) by Cyril Edwin Mitchinson Joad (1891–1953),[7] Rejwan refers to the chapter "The Invasion of Literature by Psychology," where the author pointed out the inadequacy and obscure nature of most of modern English writers, such as James Joyce (1882–1941), D. H. Lawrence (1885–1930), Aldous Leonard Huxley (1894–1963), and Elizabeth Bowen (1899–1973), in addition to Virginia Woolf. Rejwan refers to Joad's central argument that these writers, especially the novelists, are trying to come closer to life by recording, in the words of Virginia Woolf, "the atoms as they fall upon the mind in the order in which they fall, by tracing the pattern, however disconnected and incoherent in appearance, which each sight or incident scores upon the consciousness"; that they have therefore given their readers, without selection or emphasis, the complete

[7] Joad 1948.

contents of a mind at a given moment; and that this method, besides presenting many difficulties, has obvious defects. Further, "the unrestrained, unorganised movements of the mind are like dreams. People who tell their dreams are a public nuisance, and the psychical lives of these characters in a novel, interesting, perhaps, to the persons who experience them, interesting even to the novelists who record them, are to the reader simply boring." Rejwan reacts to the aforementioned with the following:

> Now this, to say the least, sounds simply unconvincing, since it is difficult to see how anyone save a truly original artist can possibly impart "the unrestrained, unorganised movements of the mind." Moreover, has Dr. Joad ever come across one of those who tell their dreams, who can also tell them with even a hundredth of the power and the charm of Mrs. Blooms's internal monologue at the end of Joyce's *Ulysses*?[8]

In his review, Rejwan seems to be one of the first of the Arab intellectuals and critics that noted the great power of the stream of consciousness trend in literature.[9] Fifty-six years later, describing in his autobiography the intellectual life in Baghdad during the 1940s, Rejwan says:

> As far as my views and attitudes on these matters were concerned, I was fiercely avant garde and rather rash with my judgments. It was in those days that Elie [Kedourie][10] and I stumbled on Virginia Woolf's essay, "Middlebrow," in which she coined that word to indicate all that she found obnoxious and objectionable in culture. She herself, she wrote, was a "highbrow" and rather proud of it. As such, she was able to appreciate, respect and even enjoy "lowbrow" culture and literary works. "Middlebrow," however, was something else again. Neither here nor there, neither fish nor fowl, she held it in contempt. And she was outspoken enough to name names, relegating the works of Arnold Bennett, H. G. Wells and Somerset Maugham to the middlebrow variety—and into the dustbin. He seemed to us in those days to be the nearest thing to a personal challenge—always dismissive and scornful of the new and the avant garde and letting no opportunity slip of savaging such of our idols as T. S. Eliot, James Joyce, and Virginia Woolf while openly admiring and praising everything that was traditional and "middlebrow" in literature and the theater.[11]

Another Jewish writer inspired by the writings of Virginia Woolf was Isḥāq (Isaac) Bār-Moshe (1927–2003), whose stories probe the complexity of the human soul in an attempt to understand the psychological motives behind

[8] *Iraq Times*, July 4, 1948.

[9] Cf. also his words in the Hebrew magazine *Kesher* 17 (May 1995), p. 111, regarding his admiration of Virginia Woolf.

[10] Elie Kedourie (1926–1992) was an Iraqi-Jewish scholar (on him, see Kedourie 1998; Rejwan 2004, pp. 122–3, 150–68).

[11] Rejwan 2004, p. 160.

people's actions. Detailed interior monologues inspired by Woolf appear frequently in Bār-Moshe's writings—most of his protagonists, or better antiheroes, are outsiders living in their own world of misery or on the margins of society, not willing to compromise their principles. Some of them suffer from schizophrenia and other psychological disorders, which sometimes lead them to find refuge in the worlds of the imagination and dreams, which sometimes prove to be nothing other than other nightmares. Generally stripped of any signifier of space or ethnicity, they are introvert personalities marked by alienation and strangeness with hardly any interest in matters outside their own feelings and thoughts.[12] In his fiction, Bār-Moshe also frequently refers to spiritual–metaphysical issues, such as the eternal and mysterious forces that direct people's actions and shape their future and their relationships, addressing existential questions through the prism of mysticism and fantasy. Many of his stories are spiritual journeys into the conscious or subconscious mind, in which the action takes place within the character's soul or imagination.[13]

It was expected that Woolf would inspire female writers in the Arab world, both with her ideas and literary techniques, as she had inspired various feminist female writers throughout the world. Unfortunately, the impact of Woolf's writing in the Arab world was delayed for some decades especially because of the delay in the emergence of Arabic literature written by women. Moreover, the emergence of original Arabic literature that was not only written by women but that also touched on feminist issues was delayed even more and grew into an important research topic only in the 1970s, when the study of women in the Middle East was firmly established as a separate field[14] as a result of what the Syrian writer and scholar Kamāl Abū Dīb (Abu-Deeb) (b. 1942) calls "the collapse of totalizing discourses and the rise of marginalized/minority discourses."[15] Only during recent decades has the literary scene, as Roger Allen points out, been changing and women have been contributing in significant ways to experimental modes of literary creativity.[16] The first translations of Woolf's works into Arabic were in the 1960s,[17] mainly following the critical attention to her fiction in various Arabic books

[12] See Snir 2005a, pp. 102–35.
[13] Elimelekh 2014, pp. 426–41.
[14] Cf. Baron 1996, pp. 172–86. On the start of the interest in feminist studies in the Middle East, see Nikki Keddie's observations in Gallagher 1994, pp. 143–4. Leila Ahmed stresses the significance of women as writers in shaping cultural production and altering conventional mainstream discourses (Ahmed 1992, p. 214. Cf. al-Ali 1993, p. 119). On the discourse of "Islamic feminism," see Hatina 2011, p. 9.
[15] Abu-Deeb 2000, p. 348.
[16] Allen 2007, p. 257. On feminist Arabic literature, see Snir 2017, pp. 101–2.
[17] See, for example, Woolf 1968; Woolf 1968b.

and periodicals.[18] In her important scholarly contribution about Woolf's representation through the translation of her works into Arabic, Hala Kamal (Hāla Kamāl) indicates that the history of Woolf in Arabic can be defined in terms of two historical periods, the 1960s and the 1990s; each marks a different specific aspect of Woolf's writings:

> In the 1960s, critics and scholars were interested in introducing Woolf to an Arab audience as a modernist writer, which ultimately affected the selection of the texts to be translated and available. This came at a moment when Arabic literature was developing beyond the first generation of the Arabic novel which had emerged at the beginning of the twentieth century and was marked by its realism, depiction of Egyptian society and imitation of the nineteenth-century Western and Victorian form of the novel. The 1960s witnessed the rise of a new phase in Arabic fiction that was characterised by postcolonial and postmodern concerns and techniques. In the 1990s, with the emergence of the third wave of feminism in Egypt, Woolf came to life again in Egypt and the Arab world through the translation of *A Room of One's Own*, as well as the re-translation of some of her novels.[19]

Nevertheless, we can sense the start of the impact of Woolf and other stream-of-consciousness writers on female Arabic writers already during the 1960s—one of the first female writers to be inspired by her was the Lebanese writer Laylā Baʿlabakkī (b. 1936). From the personal, social, and cultural respects, Baʿlabakkī was completely different from Woolf, but her writing was inspired not only by Woolf's literary insights but also by her life story and her traumatic sexual abuse as a child, which apparently caused her ongoing mental health issues. We may see that inspiration in her novel *Anā Aḥyā* (*I Am Alive*) (1958), where she tried to employ the same techniques used in Woolf's novel *Mrs. Dalloway*.[20] However, it seems that Baʿlabakkī expressed her inspiration from Woolf most prominently in her collection of short stories *Safīnat Ḥanān ilā al-Qamar* (*A Space Ship of Tenderness to the Moon*), which was first published in 1963.[21] The collection includes twelve stories with a short introduction in which the author refers to the circumstances of the writing of the stories between 1960 and 1963. The introduction also illustrates her stream of consciousness as a result of which the stories were born. The first story was written in Paris:

18 See, for example, al-Amīr 1964, pp. 61–4; Ṭāhā 1965, pp. 23–42; Shalash 1966, pp. 50–9; Ṭāhā 1966. Cf. Kamal 2021, p. 166.

19 Kamal 2021, p. 167.

20 Cf. Shaʿbān 1999, pp. 99–100. On Baʿlabakkī, see Cohen-Mor 2005, pp. 92–6, 199–204 (translation of two of her stories); Abudi 2011, pp. 274–5. On feminism throughout her fiction, see Igbaria 2013; Igbaria 2015, pp. 152–64.

21 Baʿlabakkī 2010 [1963].

لم أقرّر، الآن سأكتب قصّة قصيرة. فكتبت قصّة قصيرة. لا. لم أضع مخطّطا لها ولا تفاصيل. جلست أمام آلتي الكاتبة، فانهمرت الحروف السّوداء على أوراقي كالرّذاذ الّذي لا ينقطع في مدينة عجيبة. كنت مرتاحة وأنا أكتبها، كنت ملتذّة، كنت أتنفّس فيها، كنت ألحق اكتشافات صغيرة.

> I did not decide, I will write now a short story, and then I wrote it. Not at all! I did not plan the scheme and details. I sat down before my typewriter and suddenly the black letters flowed into my papers like a light rain that does not stop in a mysterious city. I was relaxed when I was writing, I was enjoying, I was breathing into it, I was achieving little discoveries.

Then she returned to Beirut and traveled between countries, and throughout the next year she did not write anything; suddenly, the second story came, "When the Snow Falls," in which, according to her, "I reached an important thing related to my creative work—I found the solution to my literary characters: in dreams." And then came the other stories:

كان أشخاصها ينغلون كالجنّ في يديّ وعلى حروف آلتي الكاتبة. كنت أراهم يصرخون معا ويقفزون ويضطجعون ويبكون بصمت. وكانت صعوبتي الوحيدة فيها، هي أن أكمش واحدة بيد أكتبها، وبيدي الأخرى أضمّ القصص الباقية أداعبها، ألهيها، أمنعها من الهرب.

> Their characters were going wild like demons in my hands and on the letters of my typewriter. I was watching them shouting together, jumping and making noise, and crying in silence. My only problem was to grasp one of them in one hand to write it, and in my other one to gather the rest of the stories, caressing and entertaining them, preventing them from escaping.

Each story, according to the author, was like a chapter in a novel, and when the author reached the last story, the title story of the collection, "A Space Ship of Tenderness to the Moon,"[22] "the seeds of the novel were still alive inside me." Finishing all the stories, she reached a sense of satisfaction like one feels following sexual intercourse:

نعمت بالرّاحة والفرح. كنت أعرف أنّني اكتشفت فيها أشياء جديدة وطرقا وبشرا، وأكثر من تذكرة سفر. اكتشفت سفن حنان إلى القمر.

> I felt delight and happiness. I knew that I discovered in them new things and paths and human beings, more than a travel card. I discovered space ships of tenderness to the moon.[23]

[22] Ba'labakkī 2010 [1963], pp. 179–90. For English translations of the story, see Johnson-Davies 1967, pp. 130–6; Fernea and Bezirgan 1977, pp. 274–9; Jones and Williams 1996, pp. 182–7; Khalaf 2006, pp. 25–32. On the reception of the entire collection and the tendency to judge it as "a social document," thus compromising its value as a work of art, see Abū al-Najā 2017, pp. 74–95.

[23] The quotation is from the introduction to the book (Ba'labakkī 2010 [1963], pp. 5–7).

The sexual atmosphere of the collection is highly expressed in the last lines of the story:

> وعندما أصبح قربي، واقفا كبرج هائل في محطّة إطلاق صواريخ، خفق قلبي وتمتمت له أنّني أعشق جسده عاريًا. عندما يرتدي ثيابه، خصوصًا عندما يعقد ربطة عنقه، أحسّه شخصًا غريبًا جاء إلى البيت في زيارة لسيّد البيت. فتح ذراعيه، وانحنى. فهجمت إلى حضنه أهذي: أحبّك. أحبّك. أحبّك. أحبّك. أحبّك. أحبّك. وهو يهمس في شعري (أنت لؤلؤتي). ثم نشر راحة يده على شفتيّ، وشدّني إليه بيده الأخرى، وأمرني (هيّا لنصعد أنا وأنت إلى القمر).

> And when he was near me, standing like a massive tower at a rocket-firing station, my heart throbbed and I muttered to him that I desired his body when he was naked. When he put on his clothes, especially when he tied his tie, I felt he was a stranger coming to pay a visit to the head of the house. He opened his arms and leaned [them] over me. I rushed into his embrace, mumbling crazily: "I love you, I love you, I love you, I love you, I love you," while he whispered into my hair: "You're my pearl." Then he spread the palm of his hand over my lips, drawing me to him with the other hand, and ordering me: "Let us take off, you and me, to the moon."[24]

One can sense in these lines the feminist insights of Virginia Woolf but, at the same time, the sexual energy embedded in the writings of D. H. Lawrence (1885–1930) that Ba'labakkī no doubt read and was aware of. In the aforementioned concluding lines of "A Space Ship of Tenderness to the Moon," I hear the echoing of several dialogues from Lawrence's *Women in Love* (1920). For example, in chapter 4 of the novel on a rainy Saturday morning, Ursula and Gudrun walk to Willey Water, the lake at Shortlands, the Criches' estate. All of a sudden Gerald springs out of the boathouse and dives into the water. Gudrun is envious of the freedom and happiness Gerald has to be alone in the water. This freedom, where he has a whole other world to himself, is his because he is a man. Gudrun exclaims with envy:

> You're a man. You want to do a thing, you do it. You haven't the *thousand* obstacles a woman has in front of her.[25]

Ursula, who does not share Gudrun's desire to enter the cold water, is confused by her sister's intense reaction, but Ba'labakkī's female protagonist adopts Gudrun's wishful desire: "You want to do a thing, you do it." The daring writing of Ba'labakkī was so exceptional at the time that she was involved in one of the most famous examples of the morality-based censorship of Arabic literature. The public prosecutor of the Lebanese Court of Appeal, Sa'īd al-Barjawī, summoned the writer in accordance with section

[24] Ba'labakkī 2010 [1963], p. 190 (the translation is according to Johnson-Davies 1967, pp. 135–6, with some modifications).

[25] Lawrence 2005 [1920], ch. 4.

532 of the Lebanese Criminal Code, and he accused her of harming public morality and demanded that the court hand down a sentence of between one to six months in prison and that she pay a fine of 10 to 100 liras. At the same time, members of the Beirut Vice Squad confiscated the remaining copies of the book from bookstores. On August 23, 1964, however, after discussing the case, the court's unanimous verdict was to stop proceedings against Ba'labakkī, to waive the payment of any fine, to overturn the original decision to confiscate the copies of the book, and to return the confiscated books to their rightful owners.[26] It should be noted that copies of the Hebrew translation of Ba'labakkī's novel *Anā Aḥyā* (*I Am Alive*) (1958), published in 1961, were also confiscated from bookstores in Israel for harming public morality and for the alleged anti-Jewish sentiment expressed in the novel.[27] Although Ba'labakkī was eventually acquitted in Beirut, it seems that the cultural persecution she experienced was apparently behind her decision to stop publishing works of fiction since then. In his essay "Laylā Ba'labakkī Established the Feminist [Arabic] Novel and Retired,"[28] the Lebanese literary critic 'Abduh Wāzin (b. 1957) tries to speculate why Ba'labakkī stopped writing, but at last left the question open.

Apart from Ba'labakkī's creative inspiration from Woolf's personal experiences and literary works and critical essays, other female Arabic authors started to turn their attention to ideas and insights introduced by Woolf. At the same time, Arab scholars of English and Arabic literature started to investigate the comparative aspects of both literatures from the point of view of the stream-of-consciousness method. Some scholars discussed the role of Woolf in reviving Arabic writing. For example, in his book on fiction writers in modern English literature, the Egyptian Ṭāhā Maḥmūd Ṭāhā (1929–2002) devotes a chapter to Joseph Conrad (1857–1924), Edward Morgan Forster (1879–1970), David Herbert Lawrence (1885–1930), Aldous Leonard Huxley (1894–1963), and Virginia Woolf.[29] The author discusses Woolf's life and literary work, especially *Jacob's Room* (1922), *Mrs. Dalloway* (1925), *To the Lighthouse* (1927), and *The Waves* (1931). Ṭāhā is an example of the tendency of Arab scholars who have studied the works of Woolf and published their research (in English and Arabic) to totally ignore her impact on Arab

[26] For an account of the trial and the court decision, see Fernea and Bezirgan 1977, pp. 280–90; Allen 1987, pp. 72–3.

[27] Cf. Amit-Kochavi 1999, pp. 269–72. On the uproar that the novel created in Beirut due to Ba'labakkī's outspokenness and her critical approach to most aspects of Lebanese society, see Salem 2003, p. 59.

[28] See *Dīwān al-'Arab*, March 6, 2008, available at: https://www.diwanalarab.com/%D9%84%D9%8A%D9%84%D9%89-%D8%A8%D8%B9%D9%84%D8%A8%D9%83%D9%8A-%D8%A3%D8%B3%D8%B3%D8%AA, last accessed April 25, 2020.

[29] Ṭāhā 1966, pp. 92–129.

authors and the reception of her works in Arabic literature.[30] The reason for this trend seems to be the narrow scholarly interests of those scholars, who felt that their expertise in English literature did not necessitate the widening of the scope of their research to include Arabic literature. The same may be said of Makram Shākir Iskandar, who in 1992 published a study on writers who had committed suicide. Chapter 4 of the same book gives an outline of the biography of Woolf,[31] concentrating on psychological aspects of her life (i.e., her childhood, her father's death, her marriage to Leonard Woolf, her several attempts at suicide because of depression and mental disturbances, and her final successful suicide attempt by drowning). Writing on *To the Lighthouse* (1927) and inspired by Western critical studies, the author argues that the arrival to the lighthouse denotes the unconscious wish to return to the womb and to be born again as a man.[32] Here, too, no connections are made between the study of Woolf's literary work and her impact on Arabic literature or her reception by Arab readership. The same tendency is found in shorter sections on Woolf geared toward Arab audiences, such as Mūrīs Ḥannā Sharbal's *Mawsūʿat al-Shuʿarāʾ wa-l-Udabāʾ al-Ajānib* (*Encyclopedia of Foreign Poets and Writers*), which was published in Tripoli in Lebanon by Jarrūs Press.[33] An exceptional attitude can be found in a critical study by Diana Royer discussing the works of the Egyptian feminist writer Nawāl al-Saʿdāwī (1931–2021) and the connections between al-Saʿdāwī and Woolf.[34]

To sum up, until the late twentieth century, only a few Arab writers read English classics in the original, and most of them have become familiar with English literature through translations. Thus, when tracing the impact of English authors on Arabic literature, Woolf's works included, it is important to pay attention to the availability of the translations, and in this regard it is important to indicate that almost all of Woolf's literary and critical works have been translated into Arabic.

3. "IN ME TOO THE WAVE RISES"

Very few studies have been conducted on Woolf in translation into Arabic; the earliest among them is a short article by the present writer dealing with Woolf's modernist impact on Arabic literature but not on her feminist

30 For other studies by him, see Ṭāhā 1975, pp. 249–72; Ṭāhā 1979, pp. 225–56.

31 Iskandar 1992, pp. 58–70.

32 Iskandar 1992, pp. 71–97. The novel *To the Lighthouse* was translated by Isabel Kamāl as *Ilā al-Fanār* (Woolf 2015).

33 Sharbal 1996, pp. 456–7.

34 Royer 2001, pp. 139–61.

conceptions.[35] Another study is by Paola Viviani focusing on Fāṭima Nāʿūt's (b. 1964) translation of Woolf's "An Unwritten Novel' (1920) – apart from her concern with the technical rendering of Woolf's style and literary technique, Viviani suggests that Nāʿūt employs a conscious intervention in the text such as establishing a female voice as narrator and allowing the protagonist to appropriate the narrator's neutral voice in the original text.[36] In the following, some comments will be introduced regarding some of Woolf's famous novels.

Virginia Woolf's most experimental work, *The Waves*,[37] which consists of soliloquies spoken by the novel's six characters, explores concepts of individuality, self, and community. Each character is distinct, yet together they compose an organized whole that is perceived as more than the sum of its parts, a sort of *Gestalt* about a silent central consciousness. The novel was translated by Murād al-Zumar, revised by Aḥmad Khākī (1907–1993), and published in Cairo in 1968. The translator seriously tried to stay as close as possible to the original, which results in a text that only few would consider reasonable literary prose. For example, the beginning of the original novel runs as follows:

> The sun had not yet risen. The sea was indistinguishable from the sky, except that the sea was slightly creased as if a cloth had wrinkles in it. Gradually as the sky whitened a dark line lay on the horizon dividing the sea from the sky and the grey cloth became barred with thick strokes moving, one after another, beneath the surface, following each other, pursuing each other, perpetually.[38]

In Murād al-Zumar's translation, we find the following (the Arabic text is printed here and below exactly as it appears in the original):

> لم تكن الشّمس قد أشرقت بعد. البحر والسّماء لا يكادان يتميّز بعضهما عن بعض إلّا من حيث أنّ البحر يتجعّد قليلا وكأنّه قطعة من القماش المتكسّر. وبينما كان لون السّماء يتحوّل إلى البياض تدريجيا، كان هناك خطّ قاتم مضطجع في الأفق يفصل بين السّماء والبحر، وأصبح القماش المعتّم مستورا بخطوط كثيفة تتحرّك تحت السّطح واحدا إثر آخر، متتابعة متعاقبة في غير انقطاع[39]

The end of the original novel is as follows:

> And in me too the wave rises. It swells; it arches its back. I am aware once more of a new desire, something rising beneath me like the proud horse whose rider first spurs and then pulls him back. What enemy do we now perceive advancing against us, you whom I ride now, as we stand pawing this stretch of pavement?

35 Snir 1999, pp. 6–7.
36 Viviani 2012, pp. 145–55.
37 Woolf 1963.
38 Woolf 1963, p. 5.
39 Woolf 1968, p. 3 (the title of the novel appears, separately, on p. 2).

It is death. Death is the enemy. It is death against whom I ride with my spear couched and my hair flying back like a young man's, like Percival's, when he galloped in India. I strike spurs into my horse. Against you I will fling myself, unvanquished and unyielding, O Death!

The waves broke on the shore.

THE END[40]

In Murād al-Zumar's translation, we find the following:

وأنا أيضا ترتفع الموجة بين *جوانحى* . . انها تتلاطم *وتحنى* ظهرها هأنذا مرة أخرى *أرانى* واعيا مدركا، شاعرا برغبة جديدة، بشيء ما من *تحتى* وكأنه جواد مختال يكزه راكبه بادئ الأمر بالمهماز ثم يعود فيرده الى الوراء .
خبرنى يامن أمتطيك الآن: أى عدو ذلك *الذى* نراه مقبلا نحونا ونحن نذرع هذا الطوار؟ انه الموت . . الموت هو العدو . . انه العدو الذى أنقض عليه رافعا رمحى *وشعرى* يتطاير الى الوراء كشعر رجل فى ربيع شبابه . . كشعر بيرسيڤال عندما كان يركض بجواده فى الهند . هأنذا أكثر *جوادى* بالمهانة وأنقض عليك أيها الموت دون أن أتقاعس أو ألين».

تحطمت الأمواج على الشاطئ

انتهت والحمد لله[41]

Here are several observations regarding the translation:

1. The translation does not pay attention to the poetic language of the original and provides the reader with a literal translation without the "spirit" of the Woolf text. For example, the sentence "except that the sea was slightly creased as if a cloth had wrinkles in it" was translated into

إلّا من حيث أنّ البحر يتجعّد قليلا وكأنّه قطعة من القماش المتكسّر.

Which reflects the following English meaning:

except with respect to the fact that the sea is slightly wrinkled as if it is a piece of broken cloth.

Leaving aside the poetic characteristics of the text, this specific translation as well is not literally correct—if we want to be close to the original, we can expect the following Arabic translation:

سوى أنّ البحر كان يتجعّد قليلا وكأنّ قطعة من القماش احتوت على تجاعيد.

The connection between the sea and the cloth in the original is not in any doubt, and therefore the addition of *wa-ka'annahu* (as if it is) in the translation is not necessary at all.

40 Woolf 1963, p. 211.
41 Woolf 1968, p. 220 (only the words in *italics* are my emphasis).

2. The translator ignored the original division into passages and added titles, such as "Introduction for Chapter 1"; "Chapter 1"; "Introduction for Chapter 2"; "Chapter 2"; etc. Sections in the original that appeared in small print became "introductions" to the "chapters" that follow them.

3. From a technical point of view, instead of ي in the end of words (in *italics*) we find ى, and the use of the *hamza* is not systematic. Also, two points (. .) are used as a punctuation mark in the translated text, but this is not acceptable in English. At the end of the novel, we find the addition of والحمد لله (praise to God).

4. Throughout the translation, we can find footnotes in the margin explaining Western terms or even rare Arabic words used in the translation. For example, on p. 15 of the translation (original, p. 16) the translator mentions that the word *ahilla* in Arabic is the plural of *hilāl* (crescent); on p. 51 (original, p. 51), the translator adds that Sophocles is "the greatest ancient Greek writer"; on p. 65 (original, p. 64), the translator explains that a sonnet is "a poem of fourteen lines"; and on the street name Shaftesbury Avenue (translation, p. 146; original, p. 140) the translator says in the margins: "street of literature in London; full of book stores."

To sum up, the Arabic translation of Virginia Woolf's *The Waves* published in 1968 reflects the state of the art in the field of Arabic translation from English at the time, and one can hardly refer to any particular attitude to Woolf's works and the status she had gained in English literature. It goes without saying that the inspiration that Arabic authors received from Woolf's writings was at the time very limited. The case of later translations of her works into Arabic would be different, as I will discuss below with regard to her aforementioned novel *Mrs. Dalloway*.

4. "WHAT A SHAME TO SIT INDOORS!"

Detailing a day in the life of Clarissa Dalloway, a fictional high-society woman in post-First World War England, *Mrs. Dalloway*, published in 1925, is one of Woolf's best-known novels. It was translated and published in Arabic in two versions: the first, by ʿAbd al-Karīm Maḥfūḍ (1935–2007), was published in Homs, Syria, in 1994, and the second, by ʿAṭā ʿAbd al-Wahhāb (1924–2019), was published in Beirut in 1998. ʿAbd al-Karīm Maḥfūḍ has taken some liberties with the original. In order to compare the style of these translations and their conception, we will check two versions of two excerpts. The first one is as follows:

She stood by the fireplace talking, in that beautiful voice which made everything she said sound like a caress, to Papa, who had begun to be attracted rather against his will (he never got over lending her one of his books and finding it soaked on the terrace), when suddenly she said, "What a shame to sit indoors!" and they all went out on to the terrace and walked up and down. Peter Walsh and Joseph Breitkopf went on about Wagner. She and Sally fell a little behind. Then came the most exquisite moment of her whole life passing a stone urn with flowers in it. Sally stopped; picked a flower; kissed her on the lips. The whole world might have turned upside down! The others disappeared; there she was alone with Sally. And she felt that she had been given a present, wrapped up, and told just to keep it, not to look at it—a diamond, something infinitely precious, wrapped up, which, as they walked (up and down, up and down), she uncovered, or the radiance burnt through, the revelation, the religious feeling!—when old Joseph and Peter faced them:

"Star-gazing?" said Peter.

It was like running one's face against a granite wall in the darkness! It was shocking; it was horrible!

Not for herself. She felt only how Sally was being mauled already, maltreated; she felt his hostility; his jealousy; his determination to break into their companionship. All this she saw as one sees a landscape in a flash of lightning—and Sally (never had she admired her so much!) gallantly taking her way unvanquished. She laughed. She made old Joseph tell her the names of the stars, which he liked doing very seriously. She stood there: she listened. She heard the names of the stars.

"Oh this horror!" she said to herself, as if she had known all along that something would interrupt, would embitter her moment of happiness.[42]

The Arabic texts in the following translations of the aforementioned paragraphs are printed here exactly as they appear in the original translations. In ʿAbd al-Karīm Maḥfūḍ's translation, we find the following:

كانت واقفة قرب الموقد ومتحدثة بذلك الصوت الجميل الذي *كان يجعل* كل ما تقوله يبدو مداعبة لبابا الذي بدأ ينجذب إليها، ورغم إرادته على الأرجح (ولكنه ما غفر لها أبدا غلطتها حين أعارها أحد كتبه ووجده مبللا بالماء في الحاكورة)، حين قالت فجأة «يا للعار من الجلوس في البيت» وخرج الجميع إلى الحاكورة وبدأوا يسيرون جيئة وذهابا. بيتر ولش وجوزيف بريتكوف ثابرا على التحدث عن فاغنر. هي وسالي تلكأتا قليلا خلفهما. وعندئذ جاءت أروع لحظة في كل حياتها وهي تمر بقرب جرة حجرية فيها ورد. وهنا توقفت سالي، قطفت وردة، وقبلتها على شفتيها. بدت الدنيا كلها وكأنها تنقلب عاليها سافلها. اختفى الآخرون، و*كانت هناك* وحيدة مع سالي. وشعرت بأنها أعطيت هدية، هدية مغلفة، وطلب منها صيانتها وحسب، لا النظر إليها—جوهرة، شيئا ثمينا جدا لا يقدر بثمن، شيئا مغلفا، بيد أنهما، و*هما* تسيران (جيئة وذهابا، جيئة وذهابا)، كشفت عنه، أو أن الإشراق نفذ إلى الداخل بعد حرق الغلاف، أو الوحي، أو الشعور الديني — حينما جاءا، جوزيف العجوز وبيتر، وجها لوجه معهما:

«اتحدقان بالنجوم؟» قال بيتر.

[42] Woolf 1925, pp. 52–3.

كان وقع ذلك السؤال كوقع اصطدام وجه المرء بجدار غرانيتي في الظلمة، كان مثيرا للصدمة، كان مثيرا للرعب.

لا لها هي. كل ما شعرت به كان الفظاظة التي عوملت بها سالي، إساءة المعاملة، كما شعرت بنزعته العدوانية، بحسده، بتصميمه على اختراق عشرتهما. هذا كله رأته كما يرى المرء مشهدا طبيعيا، ابان ومضة برق — وسالي (التي ما أعجبت بها من قبل قدر هذا الإعجاب) سارت في طريقها، غير هيابة، غير مهزومة. قهقهت عاليا جعلت جوزيف العجوز يقول لها أسماء النجوم الذي جاءا. أداه بمنتهى الجد. وقفت هناك: أصغت. سمعت أسماء النجوم.

«أواه من هذا الرعب» قالت فيما بينها وبين نفسها، وكأنها أدركت توًّا أن شيئا ما سوف يعترض لحظة سعادتها، ويصيبها بالمرارة.[43]

'Aṭā 'Abd al-Wahhāb's translation of the above passage is as follows:

لقد وقفت بجنب الموقد تتحدث، بذلك الصوت الجميل الذي يجعل من أي شيء تقوله يبدو كأنه غزل — وتتكلم مع بابا، الذي أخذ ينجذب إليها ضد إرادته نوعا ما (لم ينس لها إعارته إياها أحد كتبه ثم وجده مبللا في الشرفة)، فقالت فجأة: «عيب يا ناس ان نجلس هنا في الداخل!» فخرجوا جميعا الى الشرفة يسيرون ذهابا وإيابا. استمر بيتر ولش وجوزيف بريتكوف يتحدثان عن واغنر. تأخرت هي وسالي خلف الآخرين قليلا ثم جاءت ارهف لحظات حياتها كلها وهما تمران بقلة حجرية ذات عروة فيها أصص من زهور. سالي توقفت؛ قطفت زهرة، قبلت كلاريسا من الشفتين. لكأن العالم انقلب رأسا على عقب! الآخرون اختفوا: ها هي وحدها مع سالي. فشعرت انها قد منحت هدية، مغلفة، وقيل لها ان تحتفظ بها لا غير، والا تنظر اليها — فصًا من ماس، شيئا نفيسا كل النفاسة، يضم الالهام والشعور الديني! ففتحت غطاءه وهما تسيران (ذهابا وايابا، ذهابا وايابا)، او ان التالق اتقد اتقادا من باطنه—حين واجهها جوزيف نفسه وبيتر: سألهما هذا الأخير: «تنظران في النجوم»؟

كان ذلك كمن يرتطم وجهه بجدار من صوان في الظلام. *كان أمرا مروعا؛ كان فظيعا*، ليس بالنسبة اليها. انها شعرت فقط كيف ان سالي تُخاشَن اساسا، تُساء معاملتها، شعرت بمعاداة بيتر؛ بغيرته؛ بتصميمه على التدخل في شؤون صحبتها. كل هذا رأته كما يرى المرء الطبيعة في وهجة برق—وسالي (*وقد بلغ اعجابها بها أقصاه!*) لا تنهزم وتمضي في طريقتها ببسالة. لقد ضحكت وجعلت جوزيف العجوز يخبرها بأسماء النجوم، الأمر الذي يحب القيام به بكل جدية. لقد وقفت هناك: واصغت. سمعت اسماء النجوم.

قالت كلاريسا في نفسها «يا لهذه الفظاعة!» كما لو انها قد عرفت طوال الوقت ان شيئا ما سيقطع عليها سعادتها. سيشيع فيها المرارة.[44]

In order to characterize the traits of both Arabic translations, it would be useful to bring a translation into another language, Hebrew:

היא עמדה ליד האח, משוחחת, באותו קול מקסים שהפך כל שאמרה ללטיפה, עם אבא, שהחל נמשך בעל-כורחו (לעולם לא נרגע מן העובדה שהשאיל לה אחד מספריו ומצאו ספוג מים על המרפסת), כאשר לפתע אמרה, ״איזה פשע לשבת בפנים!״ וכולם יצאו למרפסת והחלו פוסעים עליה הלוך ושוב. פיטר וולש וג׳וזף ברייטקופף המשיכו לשוחח על ואגנר. היא וסאלי פיגרו מעט מאחור. ואז בא הרגע הנפלא ביותר בחייה, בעברן על פני כד-פרחים עשוי אבן. סאלי עצרה; קטפה פרח; נשקה לה על שפתיה. העולם כולו נהפך על פיו! כל האחרים נעלמו! היא נותרה לבדה עם סאלי. וחשה כמי שהוענק לו שי, ארוז היטב, ונאמר לו לשמרו בלבד, לא לפתוח אריזתו—כעין יהלום, דבר-מה יקר מפז, ארוז היטב, אשר, תוך כדי טיולן (הלוך

43 Woolf 1994, pp. 42–3 (the words in *italics* are my emphasis. The errors in grammar, syntax, and spelling are in the original).

44 Woolf 1998, pp. 41–2 (the words in *italics* are my emphasis).

ושוב, הלוך ושוב), גילתה אותו, או הברק הוא שהבקיע דרך לעצמו, ההארה, החוויה הדתית!
— כאשר לפתע ג'וזף הזקן ופיטר התיצבו עמן פנים אל פנים:
"חוזות בכוכבים?" אמר פיטר.
היה זה כאילו הוטחו פניה בקיר של שחם באפלה! היה זה מזעזע! היה זה מחריד!
ולא לדידה. רק חשה כיצד סאלי נפצעת כבר, מתקפחת; חשה בעוינותו; קנאתו; בדעתו הנחושה להתפרץ אל תוך ריעותן. כל זאת ראתה כראות נוף בהבזק הברק—ואת סאלי (מעולם לא העריצה אותה כבאותה שעה!) הממשיכה באבירות בדרכה, לא-מובסת. היא צחקה. אילצה את ג'וזף הזקן לקרוא לה בשמות הכוכבים, דבר שנהנה לעשות מתוך רצינות יתירה. עמדה לה: האזינה. שמעה את שמות הכוכבים.
'הו, איזו זוועה!' אמרה בלבה, כמו ידעה כל העת כי דבר-מה עתיד להפריע, למרר את רגע האושר שלה.[45]

Here are some comments about the translations of the above excerpt that could help us reflect on their nature:

1.'Abd al-Karīm Maḥfūḍ preferred to use for the first two words of the first sentence—"she stood"—a copulative verb, namely, *kānat wāqifa,* while 'Aṭā 'Abd al-Wahhāb uses a simple verb with an assertive particle: *laqad waqafat.* Astonishingly, both of them preferred not to use the simple necessary translation—*waqafat.* The Hebrew translation, *hi amda,* is the closest to the original. Both Arabic translators tended to limit the ability of each Arabic reader to construct his or her own personal meaning of the original text, which is peculiar to each author, certainly to Woolf. Both of them tended to be more interpretative, but Maḥfūḍ was much more so in this regard as might be seen as well in the words between brackets in the opening of the paragraph "(he never got over lending her one of his books and finding it soaked on the terrace)"—the word "lending" was interpreted as if she made a mistake for which he never forgave her. Also the word "terrace" was translated as *ḥākūra* (vegetable garden). Unlike him, the other Arabic translation and the Hebrew one kept much closer to the original.

2. The translations of the last sentence in the excerpt reflect the same tendencies of the translators. Here is the original sentence:

> "Oh this horror!" she said to herself, as if she had known all along that something would interrupt, would embitter her moment of happiness.

'Abd al-Karīm Maḥfūḍ's translation is the following:

«أواه من هذا الرعب» قالت فيما بينها وبين نفسها، وكأنها أدركت توًا أن شيئا ما سوف يعترض لحظة سعادتها، ويصيبها بالمرارة.

[45] Woolf 1974, pp. 32–3.

ʿAṭā ʿAbd al-Wahhāb's translation is the following:

> قالت كلاريسا في نفسها «يا لهذه الفظاعة»! كما لو انها قد عرفت طوال الوقت ان شيئا ما سيقطع عليها سعادتها. سيشيع فيها المرارة.

Both of them unjustifiably added meanings that do not exist in the original: Maḥfūḍ translated "she said to herself" to what could be translated back into English as "she said between her and herself," while ʿAbd al-Wahhāb translated what could be translated back into English as "Clarissa said in herself." The end of the sentence, in both translations, is much more interpretative than the original. Conversely, the Hebrew translation is very faithful to the original:

> ”הו, איזו זוועה!“ אמרה בלבה, כמו ידעה כל העת כי דבר-מה עתיד להפריע, למרר את רגע האושר שלה.

The second excerpt from *Mrs. Dalloway* that I selected here to be compared with its translations is as follows:

> She stood quite still and looked at her mother; but the door was ajar, and outside the door was Miss Kilman, as Clarissa knew; Miss Kilman in her mackintosh, listening to whatever they said.
>
> Yes, Miss Kilman stood on the landing, and wore a mackintosh; but had her reasons. First it was cheap; second, she was over forty; and did not, after all, dress to please. She was poor, moreover; degradingly poor. Otherwise she would not be taking jobs from people like the Dalloways; from rich people, who liked to be kind. Mr. Dalloway, to do him justice, had been kind. But Mrs. Dalloway had not. She had been merely condescending. She came from the most worthless of all classes—the rich, with a smattering of culture. They had expensive things everywhere; pictures, carpets, lots of servants. She considered that she had a perfect right to anything that the Dalloways did for her.[46]

In ʿAbd al-Karīm Maḥfūḍ's translation, we find the following:

> وقفت ساكنة تمامًا تنظر إلى أمها، بيد *أن* الباب *كان* منفرجًا، وخارج الباب *كانت الآنسة* كيلمان، كما كانت تعرف كلاريسا، الآنسة كيلمان بمعطفها الواقي من المطر، كلها آذان صاغية لكل ما قد تقولانه. فأولًا *كان المعطف رخيصًا*، وثانيًا *كانت فوق الأربعين*، وأخيرًا *ما كانت تختار ملابسها لتكون متعة للناظرين*. *كانت فقيرة*، لا بل فقيرة فقرًا مدقعًا. ولولا ذلك لما كانت تؤدي بعض الخدمات للناس كآل دلووي، لأناس أغنياء ممن *كانوا يتظاهرون* باللطافة. السيد دلووي، إنصافًا له، *كان لطيفًا*. ولكن السيدة دلووي ما كانت على غراره. كانت تتصنع الكياسة وحسب. لقد انحدرت من أتفه الطبقات قاطبة ـــ طبقة الأغنياء، بنتفة من الثقافة. *كانوا* يمتلكون أشياء نفيسة في كل مكان، صورًا، سجاجيد، عددًا كبيرًا من الخدم. *كانت تعتبر أن* لها ملء الحق بأي شيء يفعله لها آل دلووي.[47]

46 Woolf 1925, pp. 186–7.

47 Woolf 1994, p. 141 (the words in *italics* are my emphasis).

'Aṭā 'Abd al-Wahhāb's translation of the above passage is as follows:

> وقفت ساكنة تمامًا ونظرت إلى أُمّها، *لكن* الباب منفرج قليلًا، وخارج الباب تقف الآنسة كيلمان، كما تعرف كلاريسا؛ الآنسة كيلمان بمعطفها المطري، وهي تسترق السمع لما تقولان.
> أجل الآنسة كيلمان تقف في صحن السلم بمعطفها المطري؛ *لكن* لديها أسباب. اولا، *إنه* رخيص الثمن؛ ثانيًا؛ *إنها* تجاوزت الأربعين؛ *وهي* على أية حال لا تلبس لكي تسر الناظرين. *وهي* فضلًا عن ذلك فقيرة؛ فقيرة بشكل مهين. وإلا لما *كانت تتقبل* اعمالًا من أناس من أمثال آل دالاواي؛ من أناس أغنياء يريدون أن يكونوا لطفاء. وإنصافًا *كان* السيد دالاواي لطيفًا. أما السيدة دالاواي فلا. *إنها* محض متلطفة بترفع. إنها تنحدر من أحط الطبقات طرًا—طبقة الأغنياء مع ثقافة سطحية. *إن* لديهم أشياء غالية الثمن في كل مكان: تصاوير، سجادًا، مع كثير من الخدم. وهي تعدّ *أن* لديها حقًّا كاملًا في أي شيء قام به آل دالاواي من أجلها.[48]

And here is the Hebrew translation of the aforementioned excerpt:

> עמדה בלי נוע ובחנה את אמה; ואולם הדלת *היתה* פתוחה כסדק, ומעבר לדלת עומדת העלמה קילמן, זאת ידעה קלריסה; העלמה קילמן במעיל-הגשם שלה, מאזינה לכל דבריהן.
> כן, העלמה קילמן עמדה אמנם על הסף, לבושה מעיל-גשם; אך *היו* לה סיבות טובות לכך. ראשית, *היה* זה מעיל; שנית, היא עברה את שנתה הארבעים; ואחרי ככלות הכל, לא התלבשה כדי לשאת חן. יתר על כן, *היתה* עניה; עניה באופן משפיל. שאלמלא כן לא *היתה* נענית למשרות המוצעות על-ידי אנשים דוגמת הדאלוויים; אנשים עשירים, האוהבים לגלות גילויי נדיבות. מר דאלווי, יש לומר לזכותו, אמנם גילה נדיבות. אך לא כן מרת דאלווי. אינה אלא נוטה חסד. ומוצאה מן המעמד חסר-הערך שבכולם—מעמד העשירים, שלהם תרבות של קצה-המזלג. חפצים יקרי-ערך להם בכל פינה ;תמונות, שטיחים, המון משרתים. סבורה *היתה* שזכאית היא לחלוטין לכל מה שהדאלוויים עשו למענה.[49]

Here are some comments about the aforementioned translated paragraphs:

1. In 'Abd al-Karīm Maḥfūḍ's translation, as we can find as well in his translation of the previous paragraph, there is ample use of *kāna wa-akhawātuha* (fourteen occurrences), while in 'Aṭā 'Abd al-Wahhāb's translation there is plenty of employment of *inn wa-akhawātuha* (eight occurrences), together with using four times the personal pronoun *wa-hiya* (and she), which is parallel to إنها. In this sense, Maḥfūḍ was much more interpretative than 'Abd al-Wahhāb, who preferred not to provide the reader in each sentence with the past tense of the events.

2. Maḥfūḍ combined the two passages of the original into one, omitting the sentence "Yes, Miss Kilman stood on the landing, and wore a mackintosh; but had her reasons." He translated the sentence incorrectly: "And did not, after all, dress to please." Still, the Arab reader gets a vivid sense of Woolf's writing.

48 Woolf 1998, pp. 132–3 (the words in *italics* are my emphasis).
49 Woolf 1974, pp. 100–1 (the words in *italics* are my emphasis).

3. In the whole of Maḥfūḍ's translation, there are only three explanatory notes in the margins, all referring to Arabicized words: on p. 57 (original, p. 72), the Arabicized word *frāk* (*frac* in French) for "tail-coat" with the marginal notes: "this is the traditional English long dress." "Sirens" (translation, p. 67; original, p. 86) was Arabicized into *sīrānāt* with the explanation in the margins: "a kind of marine animals" (sic!). "Muff" (translation, p. 142; original, p. 188) was Arabicized into *mūfa* with the explanation in the margins: "a woolen cylinder open at both ends used to keep the hands warm."

4. The translations differ in handling the last sentence of the paragraph:

> They had expensive things everywhere; pictures, carpets, lots of servants. She considered that she had a perfect right to anything that the Dalloways did for her.

'Abd al-Karīm Maḥfūḍ's translation is the following (the *italics* below are mine):

> *كانوا يمتلكون* أشياء نفيسة في كل مكان، صورًا، سجاجيد، عددًا كبيرًا من الخدم. كانت تعتبر *أن* لها ملء الحق بأي شيء يفعله لها آل دلووي.

'Aṭā 'Abd al-Wahhāb's translation is the following:

> *إن* لديهم أشياء غالية الثمن في كل مكان: تصاوير، سجادًا، مع كثير من الخدم. وهي تعدّ *أن* لديها حقًّا كاملًا في أي شيء قام به آل دالاواي من أجلها.

And here is the Hebrew translation:

> חפצים יקרי-ערך להם בכל פינה ;תמונות, שטיחים, המון משרתים. סבורה היתה שזכאית היא לחלוטין לכל מה שהדאלוויים עשו למענה.

In line with the aforementioned discussed styles, Maḥfūḍ's translation begins with *kānū yamtalikūna* and afterwards *kānat ta'tabiru*, while 'Abd al-Wahhāb translates *inna ladayhim* and *wa-hiya ta'uddu*. Unlike the Arabic translations, the Hebrew one keeps close to the original, providing the reader as much as possible with the feeling the English reader would have regarding the various nuances of the text. To sum up, the Arabic translations of Woolf are still lacking the subtle and sophisticated nuances that characterize the stream-of-consciousness trend.

5. CONCLUSION

A unique feature of modern Arabic literature is that it, in virtually all its aspects, has remained closely connected to its ancient roots. This means, among other things, that no Arab poet, writer, or playwright is able to win recognition if his or her work does not show a deep knowledge of a heritage that goes back 1,300 years. There have been changes and innovations, but these too were always based upon or introduced against the achievements of the past, at least in the eyes of readers born in the twentieth century, simply because the Arabic language has not undergone yet any essential changes during the last centuries. The nature of this relationship between modern and classical literature is fundamental to any understanding of the contemporary Arabic literary scene.[50] Perhaps this partially explains why the impact that Woolf's oeuvre has so clearly had on contemporary Arab writers has as yet to cause ripples among critics and scholars.

Significantly, almost every reader of Arabic who is familiar with Virginia Woolf's works senses her spirit in the many short stories and novels that use stream-of-consciousness techniques. As there is almost comprehensive consensus in this respect among scholars of Arabic literature, it is all the more astonishing that one can hardly find even one in-depth study dealing with the impact Woolf has had on contemporary Arab writers. Scholars who do mention Woolf often reveal a lack of interest in conducting such research into her works besides briefly mentioning her name as someone who has had a great impact on Arabic literature without any constructive or helpful comments. For example, the Palestinian scholar Maḥmūd Ghanāyim (1949–2021), from Tel Aviv University, mentions Woolf's novels as an important source of inspiration for the stream of consciousness in the modern Arabic novel, which he traces back to the early 1960s,[51] but refrains from providing and exploring any detailed evidence. In a study on foreign "influences" on modern Arabic literature, Ḥilmī Badīr, from Manṣūra University, Egypt, mentions Western influence on the rise of stream of consciousness in Arabic literature, especially the use of interior monologues, but mentions no writers in particular.[52]

Woolf has significantly inspired Arabic literary production and it clearly derives also from the translations of her critical works, but here also no one, to my knowledge, has investigated the impact of her literary conceptions, which undoubtedly existed in many Arabic literary works. Moreover, the significant scholarly contributions on Woolf in the Arab world have not been published by scholars of Arabic literature, but by female feminist scholars of English literature. One of them was published by the Syrian feminist academic and literary critic Buthayna Sha'bān (b. 1953)—her article offers a comparative study between Woolf and the Syrian writer

[50] On this relationship, see Snir 2017, pp. 176–93.
[51] Ghanāyim 1992, pp. 56, 117.
[52] Badīr 1982, p. 67.

Ghāda al-Sammān (b. 1942).[53] Sha'bān argues that instead of asserting their feminism, both al-Sammān and Woolf seem to embrace androgyny through their emphasis on human beings having elements of both masculinity and femininity—an idea introduced by Woolf and adopted by al-Sammān as a way of asserting their presence in the male-dominated literary mainstream.[54] In a critical note, the aforementioned Hala Kamal indicates that Sha'bān's article reveals, at times, "her inaccurate knowledge of Woolf's life and writing as she accuses Woolf of failing to establish relationships with women even though she had many strong connections with women." Also, Sha'bān wrongly suggests that "Woolf's writings were almost totally dominated by her concern with the experience of war, which is a very limited understanding of Woolf, whose writings express her pacifist, anti-fascist views in addition to her feminist ideology and modernist technique."[55]

Another significant scholarly contribution on Woolf was published by the aforementioned Hala Kamal herself, a professor of English and Gender Studies at Cairo University, who has been engaged in Egyptian civil society feminist activism and gender-education programs.[56] Her research interests and publications in both Arabic and English are in the areas of feminist literary criticism, autobiography studies, women and gender studies, and the history of the Egyptian feminist movement but not in Arabic literature as illustrated in her studies. Kamal's contribution is a chapter published in *The Edinburgh Companion to Virginia Woolf and Contemporary Global Literature* (2021)—it is not concerned with the critical reception of Woolf's work in the Arab world; instead, the chapter focuses on Woolf's representation through the translation of her writings into Arabic, and, thus, offers a feminist critique of the strategies used in translating Woolf's work into Arabic. One of the conclusions of Kamal in her study is that the Arabic translation of Woolf's fictional work has been performed by men, mostly professional literary translators, while, on the other hand, Woolf's critical writings were translated by academic women. This gender division in publication corresponds with the marked separation in the reception of her work between those who read and wrote about Woolf the modernist author or Woolf the feminist critic.

Only two of Woolf's non-fiction books were translated into Arabic and published: the first was *The Common Reader*, translated as *al-Qāri' al-'Ādī:*

[53] Sha'bān 1986, pp. 64–89.
[54] Sha'bān 1986, pp. 66–7.
[55] Kamal 2021, p. 167.
[56] See Kamal 2021, pp. 166–82. The following discussion is partly based on Kamal's study.

Maqālāt fī al-Naqd al-Adabī by ʻAqīla Ramaḍān and edited by Suhayr al-Qalamāwī (1911–1997).[57] This collection of essays was published in two series, the first in 1925, the second in 1932. Woolf originally published most of her essays in such publications as the *Times Literary Supplement, The Nation, Athenæum, New Statesman, Life and Letters, Dial, Vogue*, and *The Yale Review*. The title of the collection indicates Woolf's intention that her essays be read by the "common reader" who reads books for personal enjoyment. Using the sympathetic persona of "the common reader," Woolf treats literary and cultural topics. In her introduction, Ramaḍān mentions the difficulties she encountered because Woolf's text is "full of figurative expressions and metaphors." Now and then, she decided not to follow the original literally "in order to clearly convey the meaning the author intended."[58]

The second of Woolf's non-fiction books translated into Arabic was the polemic *A Room of One's Own* (1929)—it was introduced in Arabic in Cairo in 1999, in the context of women's and feminist writing within a national translation initiative, translated by Sumayya Ramaḍān under the title *Ghurfa Takhuṣṣu al-Mar' Waḥdahu*.[59] Another Arabic version of the book under the same title appeared in Damascus in 2017, translated by ʻAhd Ṣabīḥa; and seems to offer an edited version of Sumayya Ramaḍān's translation.[60] The Arabic title sounds odd, and faced criticism because the word *al-mar'* as an equivalent to the impersonal pronoun "one" in Woolf's original title is inaccurate since in Arabic this impersonal pronoun is grammatically masculine.[61] The word *al-mar'—imra'* and *imru'* with the definite article *al*—appears in dictionaries as a man; person, human being; also frequently for the English "one" as يظنّ المرء (one would think).[62] Sumayya Ramaḍān was aware of the untranslatability of the book's title and in her introduction to the translation, she explains her phrasing of the title as a desire to maintain Woolf's intentional ambiguity and generalization in the English title conveyed through the use of the impersonal pronoun "one."[63] Nevertheless, and although both of Woolf's non-fiction books were translated into Arabic and published, we have not yet found any significant traces of the impact of these books on the scholarship of Arabic literature in any

57 Woolf 1971.
58 Woolf 1971, p. 4.
59 Woolf 2009a.
60 Woolf 2017.
61 Kamal 2021, p. 174.
62 Wehr 1976, pp. 901–2.
63 On the issue of the the untranslatability of the title of the book, see Kamal 2021, pp. 174–5.

language. One may hope that the impact of Virginia Woolf's oeuvre, both her literary and critical works, on Arabic literature will be widely investigated in the near future—it will probably cause many more ripples among the vast community of critics and scholars. Such a task promises to be both a fascinating and thankful one.

Chapter 8

Import: Science Fiction[1]

The human race must know:
The phones of the world have just rung.
– Arthur C. Clarke

1. INTRODUCTION

Out of all the various cases introduced in the present part of the book related to interactions and interplay between Arabic literature and Western culture, the case of the emergence of science fiction (SF) in Arabic is the most evident illustration of an imported genre. At least from the point of view of the beginnings of the genre, it grew by borrowing the Western pattern of the genre, though at a later stage, as I will show, the genre would pass through a process of Arabization and even Islamization. Science fiction[2] in Arabic has been around only since the 1970s, a relatively very late time if we take into account that the genre first emerged in the West already in the nineteenth century. As with most genres of popular non-canonical Arabic prose, the scholarly academic research about Arabic literature in the Arab world and outside it has paid little or no attention to it. The present chapter attempts to partly fill that gap, approaching the topic within the theoretical framework for the study of Arabic literature discussed in the Introduction.

SF originated in the United States, and, as many things American, quickly proved to be a valuable export item; it did not take long for SF to be written, published, read, and studied throughout the world. *The Penguin World Omnibus of Science Fiction* (1986), edited by Brian Aldiss and Sam J. Lundwall,

[1] This chapter uses material that first appeared in Snir 2000b, pp. 263–85; Snir 2002a, pp. 209–29.
[2] In Arabic: *adab ʿilmī* or *khayāl ʿilmī* or *al-qaṣaṣ al-ʿilmī al-taṣawwurī* or *al-riwāya al-mustaqbaliyya.*

"a collection of science fiction stories from all over the world,"[3] includes twenty-six SF stories from, in order of presentation, Czechoslovakia, Chile, Brazil, Japan, Great Britain, Israel, the United States, Romania, Poland, Norway, India, Sweden, West Germany, the Soviet Union, Yugoslavia, Uruguay, Italy, Bulgaria, China, Colombia, Singapore, Hungary, Holland, France, Australia, and Ghana. This is a truly impressive array of countries, except for the absence of countries representing the vast population of hundreds of millions of Arabs. The editors have only one legitimate answer: they could find not one single work of SF in Arabic while they were putting the collection together. They may even have found justification also in the Western scholarly work written about Arabic literature up until the mid-1980s: there was, and in fact still is, almost no mention there of SF as existing in Arabic literature.[4] Only in *The Encyclopedia of Science Fiction* (1995), edited by John Clute and Peter Nicholls, did I manage to find anything: four short passages on Arabic SF written by Jaroslav Olša, Jr.[5] To illustrate this dearth, I offer a brief look here at *An Overview of Modern Arabic Literature* by Pierre Cachia (1921–2017), which was published in 1990. Based upon a survey of the *New York Times Book Review* between November 1988 and May 1989 and an inventory available to Arab readers, Cachia deals with "unwritten Arabic fiction and drama."[6] Pointing out that a dizzying range of fictional literature is available in English, including SF, he compares the situation of the American reader with that of his Arab counterpart: "Needless to say, this literary wealth belongs to a populous country with a very high level of literacy, where more than 50,000 books and hundreds of journals are published every year. With this, the resources of Arab writers are in no way comparable. It is instructive nevertheless to search for gaps in Arab fiction and drama, especially since these genres reached maturity."[7] Cachia then finds that modern Arabic literature is virtually all about Arabs, alluding to the paucity of a literature of mere entertainment, "unless love stories and

[3] Aldiss and Lundwall 1986, p. 15.

[4] Cf. Snir 1998, pp. 111–12.

[5] Olša 1995, p. 49. Only in 2000 did the first English-language examination of Arabic SF appear (Snir 2000b, pp. 263–85). On Arabic SF, see also ʻAsāqla 2003; ʻAsāqla 2006; ʻAsāqla 2011; Dick 2016; Barbaro 2017, pp. 31–49; Blasim 2017; Barbaro 2021, pp. 351–71; Labanieh 2021, pp. 8–12. Significant among the scholalry contributions in the field is Campbell 2018, which includes chapters on definitions and origins, criticism and theory, postcolonial literature, and Arabic SF, as well as chapters on several prominent Arabic SF authors. See also *Journal of Science Fiction* 4.2 (February 2021), dedicated to science fiction in the Middle East. On SF and dystopia, see Bakker 2021, pp. 79–94. On literary masculinities in contemporary Egyptian SF and dystopian fiction, see Viteri Marquez 2020.

[6] Cachia 1990, pp. 171–8.

[7] Cachia 1990, p. 172.

historical novels be reckoned as such." Noting that no Arab has made a name as a writer of detective, spy, Gothic, SF, sport, or adventure stories, or even humor, Cachia indicates that "the comparative disinterest of Arab writers in genres that might have been expected to attract a wide readership and financial reward is particularly impressive." He concludes:

> The programme which Arab intellectuals have been proclaiming for about a hundred years is modernity, broadly understood as the realization of the values of Western civilization, and these values are most powerfully cemented together by nationalism. More recently, socialism has become an almost integral part of it. By some unspoken consensus, writers eschew those aspects of reality that may cast doubt not only on the validity of their idealizations, but even on the extent to which they have been actualized. It is between these self-set limits that they allow themselves to probe the depths.[8]

The way Cachia presents Arabic literary production illustrates the traditional, narrow concept to which critics and scholars, especially Western critics and scholars, engaged in the study of contemporary Arabic literature generally adhere. They continue to pay attention almost exclusively to those literary types and genres that have been recognized by the literary establishment[9] as belonging to highbrow culture. In the way it ignores how prolific and diverse contemporary Arabic literary production is, Cambridge's *Modern Arabic Literature* (1992), edited by Muhammad Mustafa Badawi (1925–2012), is a typical exponent of this limited concept: not only is Arabic SF not mentioned even once in this 571-page volume, but out of its fourteen chapters only one is devoted to non-formal literature.[10] A survey that was carried out on doctoral dissertations in Arabic literature submitted to North American universities from 1938 to 1984 furthermore reveals that only three out of about fifty deal with poetry in the vernacular, and none of them deal

[8] Cachia 1990, pp. 177–8.

[9] I use the term "establishment" here and below advisedly. As much as a political establishment is based not only on merit but on power as well, so too a cultural and/or literary establishment refers not just to cultural and literary elements within the community, but to the power relations that structure it as well. It is that hegemonic group in a society's culture that has succeeded in establishing its interpretative authority over all other cultural groups, that is, a minority group of individuals within society, such as major critics and scholars, editors of literary periodicals, publishers, and major educators who, from the sociocultural point of view, are acknowledged as superior in some sense and who influence or control most segments of culture. Although the people-in-the-culture share in the process of defining sociocultural distinctions, it is the above cultural and literary elite that have the decisive role in that process (Snir 1998, p. 93). In Israel, the cultural and literary establishment closely parallels the hegemonic Zionist structure of the state itself and is predominantly Ashkenazi and Western-oriented. On cultural and literary establishments, see Snir 2017 (index).

[10] Booth 1992, pp. 463–82. For a review article of the book, see Snir 1994, pp. 61–85.

with other popular lowbrow types and genres.[11] As the whole *habitus* of the intellectuals' field tends implicitly to dismiss the importance and seriousness of what falls under the rubric of popular literature, no serious aesthetic attention is being given to non-canonical works. Even when they have significant aesthetic qualities, such works tend to go unnoticed or their importance is minimized, which only reinforces the basic dismissive attitude toward popular literature and its writers. It is interesting that even Arab writers ignore the production of Arab SF. Trying to explain that, the Iraqi writer Khālid al-Qashṭīnī (b. 1929), for example, says that the literature of advanced and flowering nations is full of SF works, because they reflect their scientific and technological expectations from the future, while in backward nations, such as "our Arab nations," you cannot find such literary works, and "that is clear because we do not have scientists from whom we can expect great achievements."[12]

Yet, a short visit to any book fair held anywhere in the Arab world reveals a totally different picture: we find overwhelming quantities of original and translated books in various popular fields, such as spy literature, journalistic literature, and semiliterary types, large amounts of original and translated children's literature, and vast quantities of SF.[13] Moreover, even if one accepts his narrow limits of Arabic literature, several of the gaps mentioned by Cachia are not gaps at all.[14] Detective stories and novels, spy thrillers, monster and SF stories, pornographic and erotic literature, and comic books, all of them enjoy a huge circulation.[15] The inventory of non-canonized original

[11] *The Arab World: A Catalogue of Doctoral Dissertations, 1938–1984* (University Microfilms International 1985), pp. 33–4.

[12] Al-Qashṭīnī 2004, p. 3.

[13] See already in the 1990s the details about the sales in the 1994 Beirut International Book Fair published in *al-Quds* (*Jerusalem*), January 19, 1994, p. 15.

[14] See Snir 1998, pp. 88–9.

[15] Many outstanding Arab writers were, when young, ardent readers of detective novels. Najīb Maḥfūẓ, for example, even attempted to imitate Ḥāfiẓ Najīb's (1883–1948) detective stories, which were popular while he was young (Somekh 1973a, p. 37. Cf. El-Enany 1993, pp. 11, 198; Mahfouz 2001, pp. 3–21, 30; Dhinī 2002, p. 92; al-Ghīṭānī 2006, pp. 140–1; Ayalon 2016, pp. 321–2). According to Saad Elkhadem, the detective novel (in his words, the "mystery novel") experienced in Egypt two golden periods of translations from English and French: the first, from the dawn of the twentieth century to the First World War; and the second, from 1936, with the establishment of the series *Riwāyāt al-Jayb* (*Pocket Novels*), to the end of the Second World War (Elkhadem 2001, p. 23). On the popularity of the detective novels in the Arab world, see also al-Faytūrī 1979, p. 11; Schami 1996, pp. 206–7; and the interview with ʻAbd al-Wahhāb al-Bayyātī in *al-Ḥayāt*, August 7, 1999, p. 18. The Egyptian Bahā' Ṭāhir (1935–2022) writes that "all readers, no matter what their intellectual and cultural level are likely from time to time to spend time reading detective novels or any other amusing work" (Ṭāhir 2006, p. 8). The Jewish writer of Iraqi origin Shimon Ballas (Shamʻūn Ballāṣ) (1930–2019) wrote in his youth a detective novel in Arabic titled *al-Jarīma al-Ghāmiḍa* (*The Mysterious Crime*); however, he burned it before immigrating to Israel in

texts for children includes police stories, adventure thrillers, SF, and comics books. However, despite the abundance of non-canonized literary texts, most genres of popular culture still suffer from total neglect on the part of scholarly research.[16] The canonical center of the Arabic literary system still refers to most of these popular genres as messengers of "aggressor cultures" (*thaqāfāt ghāziya*).[17] At the same time, in a study of the Arabic comics for children, one of the few genres of Arab mass culture that has been investigated in depth, Allen Douglas and Fedwa Malti-Douglas (b. 1946) state that:

> the individuals who create Arab comics are among the best that their societies have produced in literature and the arts. Often they have already made a name for themselves as serious writers, painters or political cartoonists. They are motivated by the need for self-expression ... by political ambition ... but they are also concerned about the future of contemporary culture and particularly that of the children of their society.[18]

1951 (personal communication in Haifa, April 4, 2001; and S. Ballas, "Ṣuwar Mutaḥarrika," *Mashārif* [Haifa] 21 [Summer 2003], p. 22). Fedwa Malti-Douglas tried to find a similar genre in the classical Arabic heritage (Malti-Douglas 1988, pp. 108–27 [= Malti-Douglas 2001, ch. 9]; Malti-Douglas 1988a, pp. 59–91 [= Malti-Douglas 2001, ch. 7]). See also Cooperson 2004, pp. 20–39. On the detective Arabic novel, see also Rāghib 1981, pp. 95–102; Smolin 2013, pp. 695–714; Smolin 2013a (Smolin translated into English two detective novels by the Moroccan writer ʿAbd al-Ilāh al-Ḥamdūshī [b. 1958]: *al-Rihān al-Akhīr* [al-Ḥamdūshī 2001; Hamdouchi 2008] and *al-Dhubāba al-Bayḍā'* [al-Ḥamdūshī 2000; Hamdouchi 2016]. For an interview with al-Ḥamdūshī, see Guyer 2014, pp. 1–4); Farānish (Faranesh 2015; Bawardi and Faranesh 2018, pp. 23–49; Selim 2019, pp. 11, 19, 29, 131, 136; Ghosn and Tadié 2021, pp. 195–206; and the studies included in Ghosn and Tadié 2021. On detective stories and their contribution to the process of Arab nation-building at the turn of the twentieth century, see Selim 2004a, 75–89; Zachs and Bawardi 2019, pp. 1–23. Also, a symposium on the Arab detective narrative was held on March 28–29, 2019 at the Institut National des Langues et Civilisations Orientales (INALCO), Paris. Attention should be turned as well to the emergence of Arabic noir fiction, a subgenre of crime fiction, in which right and wrong are not clearly defined, while the protagonists are seriously and often tragically flawed. See, for example, *Baghdad Noir* (Shimon 2018), which was published within the *Akashic Noir* series, available at: http://www.akashicbooks.com/subject/noir-series, last accessed June 13, 2021.

16 The non-canonical narrative genre that has gained the most attention from scholars is the folktale, although this has generally been for historical, social, and anthropological considerations, and not always for literary considerations; see, for example, Pacha 1968; El-Shamy 1980; Watson 1992; Early 1993; Shaʿlān 1993; Hejaiej 1996. On Arabic popular literature and legitimation, see Snir 2017, pp. 14–19. On approaches to Arabic popular culture in general, see Konerding et al. 2021.

17 Abū al-Saʿd 1994, pp. 26–8. The term *ghazw thaqāfī* (cultural aggression) frequently appears in Islamist writings. One of the attempts to define this term is found in Muḥammad 1994, p. 16. On cultural aggression or cultural imperialism, see also Kishk 1966; al-Ḥājj 1983; al-ʿAẓm 1992, pp. 153–62. A critical approach to the above, particularly with regard to the Gulf crisis in the 1990s, can be found in Makiya 1993, pp. 278–83.

18 Douglas and Malti-Douglas 1994, pp. 5–6. The religious establishment, however, has been very suspicious toward such artistic expressions as seen in the attitude even to the

Twenty-five years later, Emanuela De Blasio writes:

> Nowadays comics are not only a means of mass communication, but also a narrative form able to express formal values and offer compositions of undoubted aesthetic level. Many authors publish their works online, not only for the immediacy, speed and ease that the network implies, but also to potentially reach a worldwide diffusion, an audience as wide as possible and to escape possible state controls, which, in a more or less intense way depending on the countries, limit the freedom of expression. Starting in the 2000s and even more following the revolutions, the Arab world offers a rich scene in the production of local comics. The current culture of comics in the Arab world is represented by young artists who publish comics aimed at a wider audience and, contrary to what happened in the past, suitable for a mature audience, since they deal with [such] issues as religion, politics and sex in formats such as graphic novels, magazines and anthologies. The linguistic register used has changed over time in relation to the historical-political context: during the years of pan-Arabism the artists, subsidized by the State, used standard Arabic, the language spoken by the whole Arab nation; from the 2000s and then even more during the Arab revolutions, the authors used the local dialectal variety, since it represents an instrument closest to the readers and which best expresses the everyday reality.[19]

As to SF, Magdi Wahba's (1925–1991) English–French–Arabic *A Dictionary of Literary Terms*, unlike the other terms it contains, defines SF without alluding at all to any Arabic examples.[20] The same goes for Nabīl Rāghib's

religiously inspired comic book series *al-Tisʿa wa-l-Tisʿūn* or *al-99* (*The Ninety-Nine* or *The 99*), which was created by Nāyif al-Muṭawwaʿ (b. 1971) and published by Tashkīl Comics (Teshkeel Comics). The series was published in forty-eight issues between 2007 and 2014, and it featured a team of superheroes with special abilities based on the ninety-nine attributes of Allāh in their pursuit of social justice and peace against the forces of chaos and evil. The Grand Mufti of Saudi Arabia, ʿAbd al-ʿAzīz Āl al-Shaykh (b. 1943), said that "the 99 is a work of the devil that should be condemned and forbidden in respect to Allah's names and attributes." See details in Wikipedia and other websites on the Internet as well; unfortunately, only a few scholarly studies have been published on the series, among them Enderwitz 2009, pp. 42–3; Enderwitz 2011, pp. 83–96; Enderwitz 2015, pp. 127–34. See also Akbar 2015, who explains how "ironically, he has hardline detractors in both America and the Arab world, though they hate him for opposing reasons. To US conservatives, he is a terrorist and a pawn of hardline Islam; to Islamist Arabs, he is a heretic and a pawn of the liberal West."

19 De Blasio 2020, pp. 125–6. On comics in contemporary Arab culture, see also Bellino 2017, pp. 183–206; Høigilt 2019. Over the past two decades, an increasing number of young Arab writers have adopted comics as their main means of artistic expression; see, for example, the report on five notable graphic novels and comics published in 2021, which deal with issues as diverse as beach gentrification in Lebanon and the ghouls of Tunisia in *Middle East Eye*, December 20, 2021; as well as the special issue of *Mizna* 21.2 (2021), and the report on the Beirut Comic Art Festival, which took place between October 6 and 10, 2021, in *The Comics Journal*, October 28, 2021.

20 Wahba 1974, p. 503.

(1940–2017) *A Guide for the Literary Critic* published in 1981.[21] Research into the development of SF in Arabic literature is limited to a few studies by Arab scholars who generally do not belong to the canonical center of the literary system. Even when writing on SF, some Arab critics do not mention at all the emergence of this genre; an Arabic reader might think that this genre is completely absent from the Arabic literary system.[22]

The first serious article written about the topic came not from an academic scholar but from an Egyptian short-story writer, Yūsuf al-Shārūnī (1924–2017). Titled "Science Fiction in Arabic Literature," the article was published in 1980 in *'Ālam al-Fikr*, a somewhat marginal non-professional magazine published in Kuwait, remote from the centers of Arab culture.[23] Al-Shārūnī, who already in 1971 noticed the emergence of SF in Arabic literature,[24] seems to have been one of the most dedicated Arab researchers of the genre. Since the 1980s, he has frequently written and lectured on the topic, as, for example, when he visited China in October 1996.[25] However, most references to the topic that we come across, including al-Shārūnī's, are descriptive and leave out the study of the narrative conceptions as well as the background of how this genre developed through the stimuli it got from Western literature, movies, and television programs.[26] Finally, as in the West,[27] the definition of SF in the Arabic literary system is not always clear, and problems of definition have been raised by a majority of SF writers and critics. Some critics confuse it with fantasy;[28] furthermore, there

21 Rāghib 1981, pp. 103–12.

22 Darrāj 2004, p. 17.

23 Al-Shārūnī 1980, pp. 243–76.

24 Alluding to several novels of the Egyptian Muṣṭafā Maḥmūd (1921–2009), al-Shārūnī wrote that they could be considered as "the first attempts in our literature dealing with science dreams (*aḥlām 'ilmiyya*), as dealt before by Western writers, such as Jules Verne and [H. G.] Wells" (al-Shārūnī 1971, p. 11). It seems that al-Shārūnī paid attention to SF as part of his interest in Surrealism and non-canonical literature as well as part of his tendency toward scientific topics, such as the structure of the atom and quantum theory (Faraj 1971, pp. 50–2).

25 *Akhbār al-Adab*, October 13, 1996, p. 3. However, it is not coincidental that a 468-page book devoted to al-Shārūnī on his 70th birthday, with dozens of articles on his contributions both in creative writing and in research (see Faraj 1995) does not mention his preoccupation with SF.

26 One exception is a PhD thesis written by Mahā Maẓlūm Khaḍr at Cairo University and approved in April 1999 (according to *Majallat Kulliyyat al-Ādāb, Jāmi'at al-Qāhira* 59.2 [July 1999] pp. 375–6). The thesis was published in book form two years later (Khaḍr 2001).

27 For example, see Knight 1977, pp. 62–9; Cuddon 1986, p. 608. Paul Kincaid writes: "The more comprehensively a definition seeks to encompass science fiction, the more unsatisfactory it seems to those of us who know the genre" (Kincaid 2005, p. 43).

28 See Qāsim 1993, esp. pp. 199–255; Rāghib 1981, pp. 103–12; 'Azzām 1994, pp. 9–11; Bahī 1994 (arguing that Tawfīq al-Ḥakīm [1898–1987] in fact wrote SF. On al-Ḥakīm as an SF

is no definition of SF that excludes fantasy.[29] Others consider time-travel literature as SF,[30] and some consider certain stories in *Alf Layla wa-Layla* (*A Thousand and One Nights*) as "proto-science fiction."[31] Even the philosophical tale *Ḥayy ibn Yaqẓān* by Abū Bakr Ibn Ṭufayl (1100–1185)[32] has been considered as some sort of early example of Arabic-Islamic SF.[33]

2. TRANSLATION AND ADAPTATION

Original Arabic SF emerged following the growing public interest in and fascination with various aspects of outer space, especially as of the second half of the twentieth century. Four years before the first manned spaceflight (Yuri Gagarin [1934–1968] in Vostok 1; April 12, 1961), the Iraqi poet Mīr Baṣrī (1911–2006) published a poem titled "Riḥlat al-Qamar" ("The Trip to the Moon"), in which the imagination of the persona is possessed by the possible forthcoming explorations of outer space ("We shall raid stars, much bigger than Earth"), together with thought about human existence ("We are only a grain in an endless ocean / In our science, we have striven to an aim beyond the strength of human beings").[34] There appeared great demand for stories about outer space created by the many recent technological advances, and it was partly fulfilled by translations, especially from English,[35] or by original scientific works.[36] Trips by astronauts to outer space and the moon led to a

writer, see also ʿAzzām 2000, pp. 20–4; Giacconi 2018, pp. 112–25; Tabur 2019, pp. 63–90); Olša 1995, p. 49 (that considers Imīl Ḥabībī's *al-Waqāʾiʿ al-Gharība fī Ikhtifāʾ Saʿīd Abī al-Naḥs al-Mutashāʾil* [Ḥabībī 1974; English translation: Habiby 1982; Habiby 1985] as SF). On Arabic literature of fantasy and the difference between it and science fiction, see Kassem and Hashem 1985 (2nd edn, Kassem and Hashem 1996); Barbaro 2018, pp. 181–202; De Blasio 2019, pp. 29–39.

29 See Clute and Nicholls 1995, pp. 407–11.

30 On Arabic time-travel literature, see Cooperson 1998, pp. 171–89.

31 For example, see Olša. 1995, p. 49. See also Khaḍr 2001, pp. 18–19. On proto-SF in general, see Clute and Nicholls 1995, pp. 965–7 (p. 967: "The attempt to identify a coherent tradition of proto SF is vain, in more than one sense of that word").

32 Ibn Ṭufayl 1940. For an English translation of this tale, see Goodman 1972, pp. 95–166. On an earlier translation by the Elder Edward Pococke (1604–1691), see Nahas 1985, pp. 88–90.

33 See also Khaḍr 2001, pp. 16–18.

34 *Al-Adīb*, June 1958, p. 41.

35 For example, see Leonard 1957 (translation of Leonard 1953); Haggerty and Woodburn 1964 (translation of Haggerty and Woodburn 1961); Grey and Grey 1966 (translation of Grey and Grey 1962); Hirsch 1972 (translation of Hirsch 1966).

36 For example, see Shaʿbān 1993. One of the chapters of the book (pp. 467–87) deals with the contribution of Islam to the understanding of the universe and outer space. On November 8, 1989, the Kalinga Prize, the UNESCO Science Prize, for the popularization of science was awarded to the author. For the first time in the history of this prize, a representative of the Arab region was selected as the winner. In his speech at the award ceremony, Federico

stream of books and articles in the late 1960s and 1970s, among them Michael Collins' *Carrying the Fire: An Astronaut's Journeys* (1974), which was published in Arabic in 1978.[37] One of the main issues was the position of Islam vis-à-vis the trips to outer space.[38] In December 1972, the Egyptian popular magazine *al-Hilāl* dedicated a complete issue to the moon in an attempt to prove, as the editor Ṣāliḥ Jawdat (1912–1976) states in the preface to the issue, that the technological advances were not contradictory to belief in God.[39] Among the items in the issue were poems about the moon,[40] articles on the moon and outer space in Arab culture,[41] and scientific essays on the trips to outer space.[42] It was not surprising to find in the same issue an advertisement for the SF Arabic novel *Qāhir al-Zaman* (*The Conqueror of Time*) by Nihād Sharīf (1930–2011).[43]

After several months, *al-Hilāl* dedicated another issue to the topic, the title of which was *al-Madīna al-Fāḍila* (*The Perfect State*). It contained pieces on utopian literature, including some pieces on outer space.[44] Classical utopias, such as *Risāla fī Mabādi' Ārā' Ahl al-Madīna al-Fāḍila* (*An Epistle on the Principles of Opinions of the People of the Virtuous City*) by Abū Naṣr al-Fārābī (872–950),[45] have been considered as some kind of SF.[46] Moreover, it can be argued that all utopias are SF, "in that they are exercises in hypothetical sociology and political science."[47]

The growing public interest in the Arab world in strange phenomena,[48] such as flying saucers, created a market for popular books, such as the series *Aghrab min al-Khayāl* (*Stranger than Fiction*) by Rājī 'Ināyat (1929–2020),

Mayor, Director General of UNESCO, said that Sha'bān "has been engaged for over 35 years in propagating scientific and technological culture on the broadest possible basis in Egypt and the Arab world ranging out from his fields of special competence—electrical engineering aviation and space—into the large number of adjacent fields of science (according to Sha'bān 1993, p. 511).

37 See Collins 1978. Collins was a member of the three-man crew of the Apollo 11 lunar-landing mission (July 16–24, 1969).

38 For example, see Ismā'īl Ḥaqqī's essay in *al-Majalla* (Cairo), October 1969, pp. 89–92.

39 See *al-Hilāl*, December 1972, p. 4.

40 See *al-Hilāl*, December 1972, pp. 29, 42–3, 73, 106, 147, 156–7.

41 See *al-Hilāl*, December 1972, pp. 5–11, 12–21, 22–8.

42 See *al-Hilāl*, December 1972, pp. 30–41, 66–72.

43 See *al-Hilāl* December 1972, p. 63.

44 For example, one of the poems in the issue is "Markabat al-Faḍā'" ("The Space Vessel") by Zuhayr Far'ūn (*al-Hilāl*, February 1973, p. 29).

45 Translated by R. Walzer as *Al-Farabi on the Perfect State* (Oxford, 1985).

46 For example, see Olša 1995, p. 49; Khaḍr 2001, p. 15. Cf. 'Asāqla 2003, pp. 61–2.

47 Clute and Nicholls 1995, p. 1260. On utopias in general, see also al-Khaṭīb 1995.

48 For example, see Ayyūb 1971, which is a review of Erich von Däniken's book *Erinnerungen an die Zukunft* (*Chariots of the Gods*) (Däniken 1968; Däniken 1970). See also Sarḥān 1990, pp. 20–3.

published by Dār al-Shurūq (Cairo and Beirut), which by 1995 included sixteen books, among them *Sirr al-Aṭbāq al-Ṭā'ira* (*The Secret of the Flying Saucers*) (1980); *La'nat al-Farā'ina Wahm am Ḥaqīqa* (*The Curse of the Pharaohs: Illusion or Truth*) (1983); *Aḥlām al-Yawm Ḥaqā'iq al-Ghad* (*The Dreams of Today Are the Realities of Tomorrow*) (1984); and *al-Ashbāḥ al-Mushāghiba* (*The Subverter Ghosts*) (1995).[49] Most of the books in the series went through more than one printing: *La'nat al-Farā'ina Wahm am Ḥaqīqa*, for example, saw at least five printings.

The aforementioned publications, together with the growing frequency of televised Western SF programs, paved the way for the infiltration of SF into the Arabic literary system. Arab readers initially became familiar with the genre through translations and adaptations of Western SF short stories published in journals or in special anthologies.[50] To this, we may add articles in various magazines about SF since it first appeared in the West,[51] as well as about major figures of Western SF, such as Herbert George (H. G.) Wells (1866–1946)[52] and Ray Bradbury (1920–2012).[53]

One of the SF stories translated into Arabic was "al-Walīd al-Mur'ib" ("The Dreadful New-Born Baby") by the aforementioned Rājī 'Ināyat, and it was published in 1976 by the Kuwaiti popular magazine

[49] See 'Ināyāt 1980; 'Ināyāt 1984; 'Ināyāt 1993 [1983]; 'Ināyāt 1995.

[50] For example, see Silverberg 1986 (a translation of Silverberg 1983).

[51] For example, see 'Īsā 1979, pp. 199–232; Qāsim 1990, pp. 285–301.

[52] For example, see *al-'Arabī*, December 1966, pp. 72–5 (to commemorate the centenary of the birth of H. G. Wells [1866–1946]); *al-Jadīd* (Cairo), April 15, 1976, pp. 43–7 (written by Nihād Sharīf, who would later become one of the central figures of Arabic SF). Several SF novels by Wells were published by Dār al-Hilāl in Cairo in the 1950s and 1960s (Badrān 1972, pp. 341–2). It is assumed that the first of his novels in Arabic translation was *The Food of the Gods* (1904), which was translated into *Ṭa'ām al-Āliha* by Muḥammad Badrān and published in 1947 (according to details on the cover of the new edition of the translated novel published by Dār al-Madā in Damascus, 2001). The first SF literary work translated into Arabic was H. G. Wells' short story "The Valley of Spiders," which was published as "Wādī al-'Anākib" in *al-Hilāl*, December 1959, pp. 55–61 (no mention of the translator). It is interesting that the impact of Wells' SF works may be found on political Arab thinkers such as the Palestinian historian 'Ārif al-'Ārif (1892–1973)—in his essay *Ru'yāy* (*My Vision*) (al-'Ārif 1943), he describes in SF style the Arab world in the very distant future, in fact in the year 2160, more than 200 years after the publication of the essay. Eli Osheroff points to the connections between al-'Ārif's essay and Wells' works in the general context of Palestinian cultural life and political thought of the Mandate period with regard to sovereignty, minority rights, and religious difference ("Indigenous Literature as Global Literature: Palestinian Science Fiction Between 'Arif al-'Arif and H.G. Wells," Departmental Colloquium, Ben-Gurion University of the Negev, January 4, 2022).

[53] For example, see *al-Jadīd* (Cairo), November 15, 1977, pp. 46–7. For more on the stage of translation and adaptation of SF in Arabic literature, see 'Asāqla 2003, esp. pp. 30–53, 63–75.

al-'Arabī.[54] That Rājī 'Ināyat, together with his *Stranger than Fiction* series, also engaged in translating Western SF into Arabic shows how Arabic SF emerged against the background of a growing public interest in strange phenomena from outer space. The original Western text in this regard was "Dial F for Frankenstein," written in June 1963 by Arthur C. Clarke (1917–1997), and was incorporated into his collection *The Wind from the Sun* (1972).[55] 'Ināyat's translation reflects the path that the new genre took in order to be considered acceptable by the reading public, a situation that is reminiscent of the nineteenth century, when Arabic translations of Western literature opened the way for new generic conceptions.[56] As the different title shows, the translation was prepared with the awareness of the horizons of the relevant readers. The original title was chosen by Clarke apparently for his confidence that it would evoke in the minds of his Western readers the meaning of a person who creates a monster or a destructive agency that he cannot control that eventually brings about his own ruin.[57] Being aware that most Arab readers did not know the significance of the name Frankenstein, the translator preferred to give the story another title, one that would evoke the same meaning, "The Dreadful New-Born Baby," that is, a new-born baby is always a hoped-for creature but to describe him at the same time as dreadful means that a destructive agency is unacceptably revealed in him, as in the person of Frankenstein. In his efforts to provide the story with the same effect the original had when it had been published, the translator changed its beginning. The original story starts as follows:

> At 0150 GMT on December 1, 1975, every telephone in the world started to ring (p. 67).

The following is the beginning of 'Ināyat's translation:

> في السّاعة الواحدة والدّقيقة الخمسين بعد منتصف اللّيل، بتوقيت جرينيتش، من صباح الأوّل من ديسمبر 1977، أطلقت جميع تليفونات العالم أجراسها.

[54] See *al-'Arabī*, August 1976, pp. 138–40. It should be noted that in the 1970s and the 1980s *al-'Arabī* became one of the major Arab magazines that encouraged the SF genre, with more than twenty translated stories and articles relating to the topic.

[55] Clarke 1972, pp. 67–73. *Al-'Arabī* published other stories by Clarke in translation, such as "The Secret" ("al-Sirr," published in September 1976, pp. 42–6, trans. by Rājī Ināyat); and "Love That Universe" ("Miḥnat al-Najm al-Aswad" ["The Black Star's Ordeal"] (sic!), November 1977, pp. 135–7, trans. Rājī 'Ināyat).

[56] For example, see Tājir 1945 (= Tājir 2014); al-Shayyāl 1950; al-Shayyāl 1951; 'Anānī 1976, pp. 8–25; Peled 1979, pp. 128–50; Somekh 1982, pp. 45–59; Cachia 1990, pp. 29–42; Ostle 1991, pp. 33–44; Somekh 1991, pp. 75–82; Hill 2015, pp. 177–201; Hill 2019, pp. 95–211.

[57] After the novel *Frankenstein* (1818) by Mary Shelley (1797–1851).

> At 0150 GMT on December 1, 1977 in the morning, all the telephones in the world started to ring (p. 138).

As we can see, the translation is very close to the original with the exception of the year: the original was written in 1963, and the event in the story happens twelve years later. The translation was published in 1976, and, in order to give the readers the feeling that the story was about a future event, the year was changed to 1977. The original names were generally retained in the translation. However, instead of the BBC (original, p. 73) the translator used the term "the broadcasting station/s" (translation, p. 142). He presumably thought that not every reader would understand that BBC stands for British Broadcasting Corporation. As for the omission of passages, for example, when Smith asks Williams: "Are you suggesting that the world telephone system is now a giant brain?" (original, p. 69; translation, p. 140), Williams gives a scientific explanation:

> "That's putting it crudely—anthropomorphically. I prefer to think of it in terms of critical size." Williams held his hand out in from of him, fingers partly closed.
>
> "Here are two lumps of U-235. Nothing happens as long as you keep them apart. But bring them together"—he suited the action to the words—"and you have something *very* different from one bigger lump of uranium. You have a whole half a mile across."
>
> "It's the same with our telephone networks. Until today, they've been largely independent, autonomous. But we've suddenly multiplied the connecting links, the networks have all merged together, and we've reached criticality." (Original, p. 69)

In the translation, we find the following:

> أجاب الدّكتور وليامز «ليس بالضّبط، ما أريد أن أشرحه، هو أنّ التّليفونات حتّى أمس كانت مجموعة من الشّبكات الآليّة. لكنّها الآن وبعد أن حقّقت فيما بينها هذا الاتّصال الوثيق، تضاعفت طاقتها إلى حدّ وصلت بنا إلى اللّحظة الحرجة».

> Dr. Williams replied: "Not exactly, what I want to explain is that the telephones until yesterday were a group of automatic networks. But now after they made between them that strong communication, their strength has been multiplied till it brought us to this critical moment." (Translation, p. 69)

The heart of the story is that the telephone networks that the human being invented for his daily use became a destructive agency that he cannot control and eventually would bring about his own ruin. The original story ends with the following:

> But he knew already that it was far, far too late. For *Homo sapiens*—the species to which all modern human beings belong—the telephone bell had tolled.

The translation ends with:

فعلى الجنس البشريّ أن يدرك: لقد دقّت تليفونات العالم أجراسها.

The human race must know: the phones of the world have just rung.

The end result, however, was more than sufficient for Arab readers to realize what SF was all about, and it was the growing demand for more translations that paved the way for the emergence of original SF in Arabic.

3. ORIGINAL SF

Original Arabic works of SF were limited in the beginning to the short-story genre, and only later included novels. As of the late 1980s, Arabic SF can be divided into two trends: the first offers mere entertainment value and is published to attract a wide readership and to provide quick financial reward, while the second represents a form of literature that consciously attempts to acquire canonization in the literary system.

The first trend might be illustrated by the series *Milaff al-Mustaqbal* (*The Future File*), which was written by Nabīl Fārūq (1956–2020) and published by al-Mu'assasa al-ʿArabiyya al-Ḥadītha in Cairo with illustrations by Ismāʿil Diyāb (1936–2005). The series began appearing in the mid-1980s, would include more than one hundred books, and is defined as offering "detective novels of SF for the young." The circumstances of its inception are instructive: Fārūq, till then a physician unknown as a writer, saw in *ʿĀlam al-Kutub* a notice by al-Mu'assasa al-ʿArabiyya al-Ḥadītha inviting SF writers to submit novels for a competition. He sent in the novel *Ashiʿʿat al-Mawt* (*The Death Rays*), which won first prize among 160 participants. The same novel was published a year later as the first part of the series *Milaff al-Mustaqbal*.[58]

On the opening page of each volume of the series, we find the following statement: "This is an entirely Egyptian work containing absolutely no translation, quotation or adaptation of any European stories." The narrative of all novels clearly sets out on the series' Egyptian local patriotic nature through the "High Command of Egyptian Scientific Intelligence," which works for the "protection of the scientific secrets that are the guarantee for the progress of nations." The special crew selected to accomplish that mission consists of commander Nūr al-Dīn; Salwā, who is an expert in communications; Ramzī the expert in psychology; and Maḥmūd, a physicist, who is an expert in X-rays. Not only does the same crew appear in all novels of the series, but all of them also follow the same structure and formula,

[58] According to http://www.rewayat.com/S_Malaff_al_Mustaqbal.htm, last accessed August 5, 2019.

much like any popular Western television series. In addition, titles of chapters are geared to whet the readers' appetite. For example, number 79 in the series, *al-Taḥaddī* (*The Challenge*),[59] includes ten chapters beginning with "The Vanquishing" and ending with "The Fall." It forms Part 4 of a serial novel (within the general series of *The Future File*) whose other titles consist of 76: *al-Iḥtilāl* (*The Occupation*); 77: *al-Muqāwama* (*The Resistance*); 78: *al-Ṣirā'* (*The Struggle*); 79: *al-Taḥaddī* (*The Challenge*); and 80: *al-Naṣr* (*The Victory*). Number 97, titled *Lahīb al-Kawākib* (*The Flame of the Future*),[60] also includes ten chapters beginning with "The Promise" and ending with "The Confrontation." This is the first part of a serial novel, to be followed, as announced on the final page, by a second part titled *Nīrān al-Kawn* (*The Fire of the Universe*).[61] The aforementioned Nabīl Fārūq, the writer of this best-selling series, sees a didactic aim in his writing: to attract teenagers to books because they are more likely to benefit from the information woven into an adventure story or SF novel than an article or any scientific matter because the former appeals to their imagination more directly and can better sustain their attention than the latter.[62]

The same publisher, al-Mu'assasa al-'Arabiyya al-Ḥadītha, put out another series similar to *Milaff al-Mustaqbal* titled *Idārat al-'Amaliyyāt al-Khāṣṣa al-Maktab Raqam 19* (*The Special Missions Section No. 19*), which already includes dozens of novels. The fact that the same publisher put out two series of much the same nature and with dozens of novels in each series only testifies to the wide readership and the huge financial rewards involved. The series is written by Sharīf Shawqī with illustrations by the aforementioned Ismā'il Diyāb. Volumes in the series are based on much the same formula as *Milaff al-Mustaqbal* with commander Murād Ḥamdī and his associate Mamdūḥ 'Abd al-Wahhāb making up the constant crew of *The Special Missions Section No. 19*.

SF stories are included also in the series *Zūm* written by Nabīl Fārūq with illustrations by 'Abd al-Ḥalīm al-Miṣrī, which is also published by al-Mu'assasa al-'Arabiyya al-Ḥadītha. Each book consists of a miscellany of riddles, jokes, stories, crosswords, etc. in addition to SF stories. For example, number 3, titled *Lughz al-Kura al-Arḍiyya* (*The Riddle of the Globe*) includes a translation of an American SF story titled "al-Su'āl" ("The

59 See Fārūq n.d.1.

60 See Fārūq n.d.2.

61 Since this is the last in the series that I was able to obtain, I cannot say how many parts have made up this particular serial novel. Neither is there an indication in the list at the end of the novel (Fārūq n.d.2, p. 139), which gives one hundred titles.

62 *Al-Ahram Weekly*, January 29–February 4, 2004.

Question") without mentioning the original author.[63] In number 6 in the series, *Lughz al-Qiṭṭ al-Fiḍḍī* (*The Riddle of the Silvery Cat*), we can find a translation, but no mention of the original author, of an American SF story titled "al-Mustawā al-Thālith 'Ashar" ("The Thirteenth Level").[64] Another series put out by the same publisher and written again by Nabīl Fārūq and illustrated by Ismā'il Diyāb is *Kūktīl 2000* (*Cocktail 2000*), which occasionally includes material on SF. For example, number 20, titled *al-Ba'th wa-Qiṣaṣ Ukhrā* (*The Resurrection and Other Stories*), contains an article on creatures from outer space.[65]

Other similar SF series have been published in recent years throughout the Arab world. For example, *Mughāmarāt al-Jīl al-'Ilmiyya* (*SF Adventures by al-Jīl Publishing House*) is a series published by Dār al-Jīl in Beirut offering SF comics for children written by Rajā' 'Abd Allāh with drawings by 'Iffat Ḥusnī (b. 1942). Number 6 in the series, *al-Ukhṭubūṭ Raqam 11* (*Octopus Number 11*), tells the story of a huge octopus threatening mankind. Another SF series for children is *al-Sanābil—al-Mughāmarāt al-Muthīra* (*al-Sanābi—Exciting Adventures*) written by Samīra Abū Sayf and published in Cairo by al-Sharika al-Miṣriyya al-'Ālamiyya li-l-Nashr—Longman. Number 2 in the series is called *Mughāmara fī al-Faḍā'* (*Adventure in the Outer Space*) and is an adaptation of an American SF story.[66]

Arabic SF series are published not only in the Arab world but also in the West, as for example the series *Discovery*, which is written by Majdī Ṣābir (b. 1960) with illustrations by Amjad Ṣalāḥ al-Dīn and is published by Mid-Light in London. In number 6, titled *al-Qamar al-Mal'ūn* (*The Cursed Moon*), there is a picture of the author receiving a special award from Egypt's First Lady, Mrs. Susan Mubārak (b. 1941), in appreciation of his efforts in promoting children's literature, even though the series is not defined as children's literature. Since the 1980s, Mrs. Mubārak has been sponsoring international fairs for children's literature as well as annual competitions in the field and for illustrators of children's books. She has also founded a special prize for authors of SF for children. In 1990, the prize was granted to Maḥmūd Muḥammad Aḥmad Rifā'ī for his SF story "Safīnat al-Faḍā' al-Ghāmiḍa" ("The Obscure Space Vessel").[67] In fact, this story already belongs to the second trend of original Arabic SF, which does not in the first place seek a wide readership and financial reward but rather seeks to be accepted as part of the canonical literary

[63] Fārūq n.d.4, pp. 146–57.
[64] Fārūq n.d.5, pp. 134–45.
[65] Fārūq n.d.3, pp. 103–16.
[66] Abū Sayf 1987. On Arabic SF for children, see the collection of articles *Adab al-Ṭifl al-'Arabī* (Amman: Manshūrāt al-Ittiḥād al-'Āmm li-l-Udabā' al-'Arab, 1995).
[67] Rifā'ī 1990.

system. Thus, the book was published by al-Hay'a al-Miṣriyya al-ʿĀmma li-l-Kitāb, that is, the General Egyptian Book Organization, the most prominent representative of the canonical literary center in Egypt, whose head, Samīr Sarḥān (1941–2006), wrote the introduction for the book.

Within this second trend, we can even find SF written by Islamist authors to propagate Islamic concepts. This no doubt is due to the great impact the genre has had on the masses as well as to its "utopian" nature.[68] In his study on utopian writing in the prisons of Jamāl ʿAbd al-Nāṣir, Christian Szyska analyzes the play *al-Buʿd al-Khāmis* (*The Fifth Dimension*) of the Egyptian writer and historian Aḥmad Rā'if (1940–2011), which was written in 1967 but published for the first time only in 1972.[69] The play tells the story of its three main characters' flight from Earth to Mars, where they find a utopian society. Their encounter with leading members of the Martian society asserts their hypothesis about the existence of a metaphysical "Fifth Dimension," which more adequately explains the world than purely materialist ideas.[70] However, the marginal status that children's literature and the Islamist writers occupy in the literary system makes it unlikely that they will soon become part of the canon. This can be achieved only by secular writers, SF specialists, whose works do not contradict the principles of the canonical center of the literary system.

The prolific Egyptian writer Muṣṭafā Maḥmūd (1921–2009) has been considered by critics as the "father of Arabic SF."[71] Among his SF works are three SF novels he published in the 1960s: *al-ʿAnkabūt* (*The Spider*) (1965);[72] *al-Khurūj min al-Tābūt* (*Coming Out of the Coffin*) (1965); and the best known of the three, *Rajul Taḥta al-Ṣifr* (*A Man Under Zero*) (1966).[73] However, Maḥmūd is by no means an SF specialist; he wrote on many other issues, love, politics, and religion among them. And even some of his SF works cannot be referred to as SF in the Western sense. Additionally, in an autobiographical note he considered his SF writing as only one passing

68 The genre of SF for the propagation of Islamic ideas is also employed by non-Arabic Muslim writers (e.g., the Turkish novel *Uzay Çiftçileri* [*Space Farmers*] by Ali Nar [b. 1941]). See Szyska 1995, pp. 96–125. On Islam and science fiction, see Determann 2021, pp. 5–26.

69 Rā'if 1972. For another edition, see Rā'if 1987.

70 See Szyska 1997–1998, pp. 115–42.

71 See Olša 1995, p. 49. On Muṣṭafā Maḥmūd, see Campbell 1996, II, pp. 1194–98; ʿAzzām 2000, p. 24; Malti-Douglas 2001, p. 8; Campbell 2018, pp. 153–84.

72 On the novel, see Khaḍr 2001, pp. 51–6, 66–7, 83–6.

73 The novel, which in 1970 was awarded the Egyptian State Prize in Literature, was published at least in three editions by Dār al-Maʿārif in Cairo and another edition by Dār al-ʿAwda in Beirut. On the novel, see Khaḍr 2001, pp. 148–57.

stage in his development as a writer.[74] Maḥmūd started his literary career as a Marxist, and his book *Allāh wa-l-Insān* (*God and Human Being*) (1956) was banned by an Egyptian court. The book—a collection of articles first serialized in the magazine *Rūz al-Yūsuf* in October–November 1955—deals with social and religious topics "in a philosophical secular way and with an existentialist outlook on life."[75] The book was confiscated at the request of al-Azhar University, which considered the book to be against Islam.[76] After moving from Marxism to scientific issues in his scholarly works, and SF in his literary writing, he gradually adapted a clear Islamic worldview. Moreover, toward the end of the third edition of the aforementioned SF novel *A Man Under Zero* (1985 [1966]) he added two additional sentences: "She was bowing in worship, praying, and weeping. She was the only one in the world of blasphemy that believed in the existence of Allāh."[77] Also, in an interview published in 1984 he did not pay much attention to his own SF works, concentrating instead on his intellectual contributions to Islam.[78]

Among other SF writers, we can mention the Syrian Ṭālib 'Umrān (b. 1948), who is described as an SF specialist and who has published five SF novels, fifteen short-story collections, and eight studies in book form;[79] the Egyptian Maḥmūd Qāsim (b. 1949), who has published at least five SF novels;[80] and the Libyan Yūsuf al-Quwayrī (1938–2018).[81] Jaroslav Olša, Jr., mentions also the Syrian Walīd Ikhlāṣī (b. 1935), the Egyptians Yūsuf Idrīs (1927–1991) and 'Alī Sālim (1936–2015), and the Tunisian 'Izz al-Dīn al-Madanī (b. 1938).[82] However, those writers cannot be considered as SF specialists, since the bulk of their literary work is by no means SF. Even their SF works, or what is described to be SF, can be somehow regarded as contributing to their general worldviews that are expressed in their other

[74] Campbell 1996, II, p. 1195. In that stage, he also published several books on scientific issues and on the meaning of life and death (e.g., Maḥmūd 1959; Maḥmūd 1960; Maḥmūd 1961; Maḥmūd 1961a).

[75] Stagh 1993, p. 146.

[76] On the banning of the book, see Stagh 1993, pp. 145–56.

[77] Maḥmūd 1985, p. 98.

[78] See Ghurayyib 1984, pp. 156–74. In the introduction to his *Ziyāra li-l-Janna wa-l-Nār* (1996), which can be considered as an attempt to present some kind of Islamic SF, he justifies his resort to *khayāl* (imagination) by alluding to the *Divine Comedy* by Dante (1265–1321) and *Risālat al-Ghufrān* (*The Epistle of Forgiveness*) by Abū al-'Alā' al-Ma'arrī (973–1058) (Maḥmūd 1996, pp. 7–8). On the relationship of al-Ma'arrī's epistle and modern SF, see Khaḍr 2001, pp. 15–16.

[79] According to Olša 1995, p. 4, and 'Azzām 2000, which brings on pp. 203–4 a detailed list of 'Umrān's writings. On 'Umrān, see Campbell 2018, pp. 253–75.

[80] Qasim 1991; Qasim 1993; Qasim 1995; Qasim 2001; Qasim 2004.

[81] See al-Quwayrī 1997.

[82] Olša 1995, p. 49.

works. A good example of this is Idrīs' play *al-Jins al-Thālith.*[83] In addition, it should be noted that in the entries dedicated to them in his *Contemporary Arab Writers: Biographies and Autobiographies* (1996), Robert B. Campbell does not mention them as having any SF expertise. At the same time, the fact that ʻUmrān, Qāsim, and al-Quwayrī are not mentioned by Campbell at all could serve as an indication of the status of SF in the Arabic literary system in the mid-1990s.

In the following section, I will present one of the few SF specialists in Arabic literature, the Egyptian writer Nihād Sharīf (1930–2011), who is probably the most dedicated writer of original Arabic SF.

4. CANONIZATION

For Nihād Sharīf, who did his best to improve the status of SF in the literary system,[84] the roots of the genre are Arabic: "The origin from which the first Western SF was transmitted was an Arabic one ... but due to neglect and amnesia, the Arabs never spoke about this and let others claim that SF originated by Western writers."[85] Sharīf sees a direct relationship between the popular stories from Arabic folklore, especially the *Arabian Nights*, which his grandmother used to tell him when he was a child, and modern "Western" SF.[86]

That none of the dictionaries of Arab writers and encyclopedias of modern Arabic literature[87] include Sharīf's name only goes to show how marginal the status of SF is in the Arabic literary system. Still, the scope of Sharīf's activities has been very wide indeed; he has published several collections of short stories, among them *Raqam Arbaʻa Ya'murukum* (*Number 4 Commands You*), *Alladhī Taḥaddā al-Iʻṣār* (*The Man Who Stands up against the Hurricane*), and *Anā wa-Kā'ināt Ukhrā* (*I and Other Creatures*). He also wrote four novels: *Qāhir al-Zaman* (*The Conqueror of Time*),[88] *Sukkān al-ʻĀlam al-Thānī* (*The Inhabitants of the Second World*), *al-Shay'* (*The Thing*), and *Ibn al-Nujūm* (*The Son of Stars*).[89] Also, Sharīf is considered to be

83 Idrīs 1988 [1971].
84 On Nihād Sharīf's views concerning the reservations of the canonical center of Arabic literature regarding SF, see the interview with him in *al-Qāhira*, July 15, 1988, pp. 40–3. On Sharīf as an SF writer, see ʻAzzām 2000, pp. 25–31; Barbaro 2013, pp. 39–49.
85 See *al-Qāhira*, July 15, 1988, p. 41.
86 Sharīf 1981, p. 7.
87 For example, see Campbell 1996; Meisami and Starkey 1998.
88 On the novel, see also Khaḍr 2001, pp. 57–61, 67–75, 86–90; Campbell 2018, pp. 119–52. A film based on the novel was produced in Egypt (*al-Qāhira*, July 15, 1988, p. 40).
89 On Sharīf's SF, see Bahī 1982, pp. 57–65; ʻAzzām 1994, pp. 124–6; Khaḍr 2001.

part of the canonical sector of Arabic literature, as was shown by the literary prizes he was awarded in appreciation of his literary output.[90]

Sharīf's short story "Imra'a fī Ṭabaq Ṭā'ir" ("A Woman in a Flying Saucer"), from his collection *Alladhī Taḥaddā al-I'ṣār* (1981), is a good example of the stage original SF has reached in Arabic after the period of translation and adaptation.[91] It is about an Egyptian city-dweller who decides to escape for a few hours from the noisy bustle of big city life in a way that is reminiscent of the retreat and seclusion medieval Muslim ascetics (*zuhhād*) and mystics (*Ṣūfīs*) strove after (as I have already pointed out, the Muslim heritage would soon become an integral part of Arabic SF). He drives his car up into the mountains around Cairo like a mystic searching for peace and calm in the wilderness and the deserted forests and the peaks of the mountains:

> هناك، حيث ينتهي صعودي، حيث دوامات الهواء المصفّى والبعد عن ضجيج العاصمة القاتل، يوجد عالمي دنياي المتّسعة باتّساع الكون وترامي أنحائه المجهولة.

> There, where my ascent will end, where whirlpools of clean air are blowing about, far away from the deadly noise of the capital, there I'll find my world. My world is as wide as wide the world itself and like it has far unknown limits. (p. 121)

This is the spatial and temporal context in which usually in classical Ṣūfī Arabic literature the mystical vision arises.[92] But instead, or perhaps as its modern equivalent, the narrator suddenly sees a beautiful woman:

> لمحتها تستند بكتفها العاري إلى نتوء صخريّ وقد راحت تلوّح بأصابع رخصة موسيقيّة الأطراف لكن هل لفظتها سحابة ضباب فأين أطراف السّحابة وما حجمها؟ أم انبثقت من قلب نافورة دخان تبخّر تكوينها على الفور؟

> I saw her leaning with her naked shoulder on a jutting rock signaling to me with her soft musical-edged fingers. Yet, had she been thrown by a cloud of fog, where was that cloud and where were its edges and what was its size? Or had she been born from the heart of a fountain of smoke whose structure vanished at once? (p. 122)

The sight of a beautiful woman does not necessarily contradict a mystical vision; Arabic literature frequently sees the mystical and sexual experiences as somehow connected.[93] The narrator then recounts how struck he was by

[90] See *al-Qāhira*, July 15, 1988, p. 40.

[91] Sharīf 1981, pp. 121–33.

[92] Cf. the ascetic and mystical experiences of Ibrāhīm ibn Adham (d. 776), one of the first Muslim mystics (al-Qushayrī 1940, p. 8).

[93] Cf. Snir 2005a, pp. 108–9. On the erotic symbolism in Sufism, see Snir 2006, p. 86; Snir 2013a, p. 212.

the woman who "was swimming toward the car" and came and sat beside him. Without a word, she signaled him to drive his car onto a side road while in her eyes there was "a desperate anxious glance." The description that the narrator gives of the woman leaves no doubt about who she is: he was giving a lift to a woman-saint who was encircled by a "vague halo of breaking of light and darkness, though the time was noon" (p. 122).[94] Still, the narrator continues to describe her in clearly sexual terms: "her red-wine skin"; "rosy lips"; "waves of coal-black hair"; "narrow clothes that reveal in detail her symmetrical body which is crowned by full and round breasts" (p. 123).

After the narrator changed direction, the car went down the mountain, while the woman's face remained unchanged. The narrator tried to speak to her in Arabic, but she answered only by moving her head to indicate whether or not she understood the questions. Anxious to know the nature of the strange woman, he suddenly became fascinated by a view whose description may throw some light on how the genre emerged from Western translated and televised SF serials:

> فيما وراء التّبّة، فوق منبسط من الرّمال السّوداء، أو المحترقة لدرجة السّواد، قبع ساكنا جسم لامع يبلغ حدّ الإعجاز في انسيابيّته واستدارة حوافّه، **ومن كثرة وألفة ما تقرأ وتشاهد يوميّا** عرفت في الحال أنّني بإزاء طبق طائر يجثم حقيقة أمامي وليس في حلم أو خيال عابر. فهل أنا أيضا بإزاء كائنة يحتمل قدومها من كوكب بعيد؟

> Behind the hill, above a black plateau of sand, or burned sand, a fantastically stream-lined, round shining body was lying quietly. *Based on what we frequently read and view everyday*, I immediately knew that I had come face to face with a flying saucer, and that this was not a dream or a passing imagination. Am I before a female probably coming from a distant star? (p. 124; my emphasis)

Near the flying saucer, the narrator saw lying three ostensibly dead persons who needed help; he wanted to help them, but the woman asked him to come with her into the flying saucer; inside he saw a hall "similar to those at computer centers in Cairo" (p. 125); lying on a bed, he saw a second woman who seemed to be the twin of the other, who now asked him to inject some liquid into the forehead of her twin, whereupon the two women become one, as though through mystical union. At this moment, the narrator, for the first time, hears the woman speak. Robot-like with a pause after each word, she uttered in *fuṣḥā* (standard Arabic) the following sentence:

> أشكر. لك. صنيعك. لقد. أنقذت. حياتي.

> I. Thank. You. For. Your. Act. You. Have. Saved. My. Life.

[94] Cf. the final description of women in the SF novel *Lamsat al-Ḍaw'* (*The Touch of Light*) by the Lebanese Qāsim (Qasim 1993, p. 87).

And when the narrator seems not to understand, she continues:

بل. أنقذت. حياة. طاقم. السّفينة. بأكمله.

Indeed. You. Have. Saved. The. Life. Of. The. Vehicle's. Entire. Crew. (p. 127)[95]

Then both of them hurriedly leave the vehicle, where the woman with some magical instrument saves the men lying on the ground. She then tells the narrator, always in the same robotic intonation, that their vehicle has come from Deimos, and, for the first time in the story, we learn that the narrator's name is Ṭal'at al-Shirbīnī, and that he is not a mystic but an astronomer from the observatory center of al-Quṭṭāmiyya near Cairo. Admittedly, the plot is a bit weak: although the narrator is an astronomer by profession, he refers to Deimos as a moon of Jupiter, while the woman does not correct him that it is actually a moon of Mars.

A love story now develops between them, but the central idea of the story is not in any doubt: the crew of the vehicle came to Earth in order to save it from destruction, given the belligerent nature of human beings. They came with the pacifist message that war should and could be abolished. It was, moreover, the constant threat of nuclear war that encouraged the people from outer space to do their utmost to prevent this danger, as it would also destroy the people of Deimos, who desperately need some special gas found only on Earth. The woman from outer space even elaborates on how they planned to prevent such a catastrophe: they would destroy any violent nation as they had done, so she claims, with the people of Atlantis, that mythical island first mentioned by Plato as having existed in the Atlantic Ocean west of Gibraltar that sank to the bottom of the sea. As she tells him, they fired upon Atlantis "two hundred Neutron missiles and so destroyed all its inhabitants" (p. 132). The love story between the narrator and the woman from outer space reaches both its climax and its conclusion in a hot sensual kiss, after which, with the woman having presented her people's pacifist message, he sees the vehicle take off and disappear in an ash-colored cloud.

While the way the story is built is a clear attempt at having SF canonized, it incorporates some aspects of popular Arabic literature, making it at times read as a detective or romantic story. Sharīf uses these popular aspects to make it attractive to Arab readers familiar with Western SF on television.

Sharīf's *Imra'a fī Ṭabaq Ṭā'ir* became the nucleus for his SF novel *al-Shay'* (*The Thing*)[96]—one of the pre-eminent examples of Arabic SF intended to

[95] The English translation follows the Arabic text with robot-like speaking using a pause after each word, although for obvious reasons there is no correspondence in the English translation between the two texts.

[96] Sharīf 1989.

have the genre considered part of the canon. The novel was also inspired by the American film *The Thing from Another World* (1951), the most influential of the films that sparked the SF and monster-movie boom of the 1950s.[97] In his introduction to the novel, whose pacifist message is evident, the author says:

> لغة إنسان اليوم حقًا وصدقا هي لغة العنف، لكن رغم سيادة هذه اللّغة، ورغم غلظة إيقاعها ومدى تغلغلها وسطوتها وكونها ممقوتة ملعونة، فإنّ دولاً شعوباً بشرا لا يزالون وسط المدّ المكتسح على نقائهم الرّبّانيّ وصفائهم الفكريّ وهم حكماء شجعان يتكلّمون لغة مغايرة لم تباد للآن قوامها كلمات الهدوء والمنطق والعقلانيّة والسّلام، أمّا الأزرار والأزناد فإنّها آخر ما يلجأون إليه فقط للدّفاع عن النّفس. وهذه اللّغة وحدها في يقيني هي الّتي تعرفها كذلك كائنات متشابهة أو مختلفة مقارّها عبر السّماوات والأكوان النّائية وإلى الأقاصي المتوارية في ملكوت كلّ الأشياء. فإلى متكلّمي اللّغة الأخيرة أهدي سطوري.

> The language of contemporary human beings is truly the language of violence. Nevertheless, despite the hegemony of this language, and despite the rudeness of its rhythm, the range of its penetration and strength, and the fact that it is disgusting and cursed, there are states, nations, and peoples, who, against the sweeping rise of the flood, preserve their divine purity and intellectual clarity. They are brave heroes who speak a different language which has not appeared openly yet. This is a language whose basic vocabulary consists of words of tranquility, logic, rationality and peace. Buttons and hammers are only their final resort, used only in self-defense. This is the only language, in my opinion, that is spoken by those creatures, different or similar, that live beyond the skies, in faraway universes, in the hidden distances of the kingdom of all things. To those who speak this very language, I dedicate the following pages. (p. 6)

Sharīf belongs to those representatives of the SF genre, like Jules Verne (1828–1905), whose heroes are apprehensive about the fate of mankind. As in the aforementioned story, this theme is central in this novel. Suffice it to mention that the Thing in the story, which comes from outer space, is actually a divine alert. The novel presents in detail the daily reactions of the Egyptian people and authorities to the Thing after it has turned Egypt into the center of the world by choosing its territory as its landing place. The plot branches out into subplots intended to make the central figures and the narrated events look plausible. Significant too is that events of the plot stretch

97 Clute and Nicholls 1995, p. 1218. The film was actually directed by Howard Hawks (1896–1977) (though Christian Nyby [1913–1993] received the directing credit). It starred Kenneth Tobey, Margaret Sheridan, Robert Cornthwaite, Douglas Spencer, and James Arness. The screenplay, by Charls Lederer, is based on "Who Goes There?" (1938) by Don A. Stuart. About thirty years later, John Carpenter directed *The Thing* (1982)—another version of Stuart's story—with screenplay by Bill Lancaster, starring Kurt Russell, A. Wilford Brimley, T. K. Carter, Richard Dysart, Charles Hallahan, and Richard Masur (Clute and Nicholls 1995, pp. 1218–19).

out over seven days, as in the creation of the world, while there is an unspecified period of time before and after these seven days. Interesting also is the content of the message that the robots inside the Thing after leaving Egypt sent to the High Command of their outer star, which is phrased in terms usually reserved for Allāh. The robots' impression from what they found in Egypt is that they are "happy, glad, good and pacifist," which makes them call Earth "the star of happiness" (p. 115).

Sharīf's SF novel *al-Shay'* may be seen as one of the first steps in the process of the canonization of Arabic SF, especially as it was published by the prominent representative of the canonical literary center in Egypt, the General Egyptian Book Organization. Five years after the publication of this novel, another step would be taken in the aforementioned process when the latter published a collection of more SF novels by Sharīf.[98]

5. CONCLUSION

Though the bulk of Arabic SF literature is still generally referred to in the Arab world as "stories for children and adventures of young men,"[99] Arabic SF has already taken its first steps on the road toward canonization. Its emergence is mostly due to the impact of Western popular culture and the advent of modern technology, but the contribution SF can make to Arab society goes far beyond literature, such as getting readers accustomed, in the words of Isaac Asimov (1920–1992), to the thought of "the inevitability of continuing change and the necessity of directing and shaping that change rather than opposing it blindly or blindly permitting it to overwhelm us."[100] At the same time, as in the efforts toward the decolonization of African literature, Arab authors and critics in this field might also stop being mesmerized by the West and improve the quality of their writing: "The half-baked ideas, unexamined assertions, wild speculations, mystification, careless thinking, muddled logic, vague generalities, slippery argumentation and other intellectual misdemeanors to which they are prone are a gross disservice to their own intelligence and to [their] literature and its readership."[101]

We may meanwhile have seen "the collapse of universally applicable standards of aesthetic judgment,"[102] but as long as we tend to think of

98 Sharīf 1994.
99 See the introduction by the translator Fidā' Dakrūb to the translation (Asimov 1994) of Isaac Asimov's *The Complete Robot* (Asimov 1982) (according to *al-Bilād*, March 1994, p. 43).
100 Quoted in Knight 1977, p. 61.
101 Chinweizu and Madubuike 1983, pp. 302–3.
102 Cartmell et al. 1997, p. 1.

canonical literature only in terms of its more celebrated works of genius, SF will remain typically identified with literature's most mediocre and standardized products. Yet, just as high literature is not an unblemished collection of masterpieces, so too SF should not be discarded as an undifferentiated abyss of tastelessness or a genre that cannot be judged by aesthetic criteria. In each genre or literary type, "there is room and need for aesthetic discriminations of success and failure."[103] Also, history clearly shows that the popular entertainment of one culture can become the high classics of a subsequent age. Even within the very same cultural period, a given work can function either as popular or as high literature, depending on how it is interpreted and appropriated by its public.[104] In addition, we can often notice Arab canonical writers drawing on elements of SF in their works, as in the writing of the Iraqi author Muḥammad Khuḍayyir (b. 1942).[105]

The common denominator of SF written by Arab authors who strive to make their work part of the canonical literature is the aspiration for a utopian society; the means they employ separates them into different ideologically motivated camps.[106] At any rate, as in other languages, all the works of SF of this sort contain indications of their national and cultural origins. As Aldiss and Lundwall have it, "the manner of telling throws light on something of the conditions of the country from which they have emerged."[107] Unlike in the SF of the West,[108] Arabic SF in general has as yet not generated any serious inquiry into the nature of contemporary social reality, and most of the writers, instead of using this genre as a "medium for social comment,"[109] are still too prone to serve entertainment or didactic purposes. Exceptions among Islamist SF authors attempt to build a utopian Muslim society on Earth, whereby, as in social Western SF, "background is foreground."[110]

103 Shusterman 1993, p. 217.

104 For example, see the case of *Alf Layla wa-Layla* (see Snir 1998, pp. 114–15). In nineteenth-century America, Shakespeare was both Vaudeville and high theater (Levine 1988, pp. 13–81).

105 Rossetti 2017, pp. 1, 13, 257–8, 269.

106 In this regard, I should mention an interesting exceptional short story written by the late Libyan leader Muʿammar Qadhdhāfī (1942–2011) titled "The Suicide of the Astronaut." The story is by no means an SF story, but by expressing the view that the exploration of outer space is of no avail to life on Earth, we can understand as well the total rejection of SF literature (Qaddafi 1998, pp. 59–62). On Qadhdhāfī and other rulers and political figures engaging in literary writing, see Snir 2017, p. 104, n. 22. In December 2017, the Centre for the Study of Manuscript Cultures (CSMC) at the University of Hamburg organized a workshop titled "Rulers as Authors in the Islamic World: Knowledge, Authority and Legitimacy" with nineteen contributions covering a period of 1,200 years.

107 Aldiss and Lundwall 1986, pp. 15–16.

108 For example, see Milstead et al. 1974.

109 Beckson and Ganz 1990, p. 251.

110 McNelly 1974, p. 21.

Also, we can find in Arabic SF the rebellion against the spiritual emptiness in contemporary human society, such as in the novel *al-Sayyid min Ḥaql al-Sabānik* (*The Mister from the Spinach Field*) by the Egyptian writer Ṣabrī Mūsā (1932–2018).[111] The novel deals with the conflict between the programmed mechanical system in contemporary societies and the frustrated human being who refuses the slavery imposed by such a system. The novel describes a society divided into classes, committees, centers, and bodies run by a general supreme robotic system establishing a fixed daily program for each person from the moment he rises until he goes to bed. Such a mechanical system becomes the master of the universe, while the real human being turns into a mechanical slave that obeys and performs its instructions without any thinking. The protagonist, Homo[112]—the name used here as a kind of characterization[113]—tries to break this programmed track, since it nullifies the humans' creativity, negates their personal freedom within the concept of "discipline," and prevents them from following their whims.[114]

As for the issue of language, although SF is referred to as non-canonical literature, nearly all the original (and translated) SF in Arabic uses *fuṣḥā* (standard Arabic) and not *ʿāmmiyya* (the spoken Arabic), which is the main characteristic of non-canonicity in Arabic literature. Throughout its history, Arabic culture has regarded works written in *fuṣḥā* as canonical and those written in *ʿāmmiyya* or in a mixture of *ʿāmmiyya* and *fuṣḥā* as subliterary. At the same time, not every text written in *ʿāmmiyya* is considered non-canonical and not every text written in *fuṣḥā* is canonical—canonicity and non-canonicity are also dependent on other aesthetic and non-aesthetic considerations and constraints. Prose is generally referred to as non-canonical if it deals with popular and so-called "non-suitable" themes, even if written in *fuṣḥā*.

Egypt is the center of both types of Arabic SF—the popular one whose aim is quick financial reward as well as the more serious one that seeks canonization. As far as I know, we cannot find even one Arab female author devoted only to the writing of SF,[115] while, in the West, over the past few years, some

111 Mūsā 1987. The book was serialized in the Egyptian *Ṣabāḥ al-Khayr* magazine between August 1983 and January 1984 and was published in book form only in 1987.

112 A reference to *Homo sapiens*, the species to which all modern human beings belong.

113 Cf. Gordon 1917; Rudnyckyj 1959, pp. 378–82; Auden 1970, p. 267. See also above.

114 On the novel, see ʿAsāqla and Masalha 2018, pp. 129–45; Alkhayat 2021, pp. 230–48.

115 On April 25, 2006, a conference on Arabic SF was held in Casablanca; among the questions discussed were the peculiarities of Arabic SF, and why there is not enough awareness of this genre in Arabic literature in addition to studies of the writings of the pioneers in Arabic SF, such as the Egyptians Nihād Sharīf (1930–2011) and Ra'ūf Waṣfī (1939–2006), the Moroccan Aḥmad ʿAbd al-Salām al-Baqqālī (1932–2010) (on him, see Campbell 2018, pp. 219–52) and ʿAbd al-Raḥīm Bahīr (b. 1953), the Tunisians Muṣṭafā al-Kaylānī and

new and progressive blood has been injected by women into the English-language SF genre.[116] As for the field of criticism and scholarly work, one of the encouraging phenomena is that the topic has become the subject of discussion of groups on the Internet. For example, the science fiction novel *Dune* (1965) by Frank Herbert (1920–1986) evoked discussions among Arab and Muslim scholars and critics not only because it symbolically refers to the dependence of the West on Arab oil and the power struggles to control this valuable resource. In the novel's fictional universe, the author draws attention to the landscape and the inhabitants of a desert planet while borrowing many terms from Arabic and Islamic culture, or using Arabic-sounding names.[117] Also, in June 1996 a long discussion about SF and fantasy in the Middle East developed on the *Adabiyat* list, which deals with the literatures of the Middle East. It is assumed that scholarly efforts will be also dedicated to the emergence in recent years of French SF by Arab writers,[118] especially as French literature by Arab writers occupies a unique position in both the Arabic and the French literary systems. Finally, as there now is a marked awareness among Western SF writers to stay away from stereotypes and to

al-Hādī Thābit (b. 1942), the Mauritanian Moussa Ould Ebnou (Mūsā Wuld Ibnū) (b. 1956), and the Syrian Ṭālib ʿUmrān (b. 1948); there was also a mention of two female writers, the Kuwaiti Ṭayyiba Aḥmad al-Ibrāhīm (1945–2011) and the Egyptian Umayma Khaffājī (according to www.elaph.com/Culture, April 28, 2006).

116 For example, see Cartmell et al. 1997, pp. 48–65.

117 On the novel and the discussions related to Arabic and Islamic issues, accompanied by links and references, see Bahayeldin 2004; Ryding 2021, pp. 106–23. Based on the novel, the French Canadian filmmaker Denis Villeneuve (b. 1967) directed the film *Dune* (2021), the first of a planned two-part adaptation of the book. Zaina Ujayli, a scholar of Arab American history and Arab and Muslim representation, tweeted that *Dune* is a racist, white savior narrative that relies on people's ignorance of Arab Islamic history to make itself creative (see at: https://twitter.com/zainaujayli/status/1091519388166041600, last accessed October 30, 2021). The film was also accused of erasing Middle Eastern actors—German-Palestinian filmmaker Lexi Alexander (b. 1974) tweeted: "A film about Middle East culture, shot in the Middle East, without a single Middle Eastern actor in sight" (see at: https://www.colorlines.com, September 10, 2020). Other examples of Islam in SF literature have been collected by Muhammad Aurangzeb Ahmad; see his website "Islam and Science Fiction: On Science Fiction, Islam and Muslims," available at: http://www.islamscifi.com, last accessed April 26, 2021. See also "100 Years of Science Fiction in the Islamicate World"—a webinar held by Aurangzeb on July 16, 2020 with the American Pakistani Foundation and hosted by APF President Shamila Chaudhary, availabe at: https://sinaiandsynapses.org/multimedia-archive/100-years-of-science-fiction-in-the-isl amicate-world, last accessed April 26, 2021.

118 For example, see the novels by the aforementioned Mauritanian author Moussa Ould Ebnou, such as Ebnou 1990; Ebnou 1994. On him, see Isabella 1997, pp. 331–40. Another writer in the field is the Algerian Hacène Farouk Zéhar (b. 1939); see Olša 1995, p. 49. On the Algerian poet and novelist Muḥammad Dīb (1920–2003) and science fiction, see Yanat 1985, pp. 197–203.

introduce authentic Arab and Muslim characters into their works,[119] it may not be long before scholarly communities, in both the West and East, will start taking up the challenge to systematically explore Arabic SF, synchronically and diachronically, in various parts of the Arab world.[120]

Among the recent scholarly developments in the field of Arabic SF, we can mention the attempt to widen the boundaries of the genre to include works whose authors and Arabic readers never identified as SF. One example is Aḥmad Saʿdāwī's (b. 1973) novel *Frankenstein fī Baghdād* (*Frankenstein in Baghdad*) (2013), winner of the International Prize for Arabic Fiction (2014), and one of the six shortlisted novels for the 2018 Man Booker International Prize. Throughout its nineteen chapters, the novel tells the story of the scavenger Hādī al-ʿAttāk, who collects human body parts in the rubble-strewn streets of US-occupied Baghdad and stitches them together to create a corpse. His goal, he claims, is for the government to recognize the parts as people and give them a proper burial. But when one corpse goes

119 I found the following message by SF writer Jack McDevitt (b. 1953) on the Arabic-L Internet list (January 16, 1998): "I am currently working on a novel with several Arabic characters. There will be a very few lines for which I require translation from English into Arabic. And I know there will be occasional questions about Arabic culture and manners. If you can recommend someone who would be willing to help, to advise me, I'd be grateful." See also the Call for Papers for the conference in Buffalo, NY (April 7–8, 2000) titled "Orientalism in Science Fiction: Persistence or Resistance?" The call, published on the "Adabiyat: Middle Eastern Literary Traditions" Internet list (July 9, 1999), ended with the question: "Has science fiction learned anything from the emergence of postcolonial studies?"

120 On July 12, 2019 at the SOAS, scholars hosted a discussion on the topic of Arabic SF, attempting to shift the discussion from lamenting the supposed lack of Arabic texts in the genre to exploring nuanced ideas of dystopia and alternate temporalities in future-oriented Arabic fiction. In the words of organizer Tasnim Qutiat, the conference, whose title was "Science Fiction Beyond the West: Futurity in African and Asian Contexts," centered on "the contested space of the future, how it is envisioned and theorized, and what this reveals about our present moment." The program's speakers extended the critical and theoretical discussion about futurity in the early twenty-first century to regions that have tended to fall under a framework of exceptionalism and developmental rhetoric (see at: https://arablit.org/2019/08/29/science-fiction-in-conversation-with-al-atlal, last accessed September 13, 2019). The Saudi city of Jeddah has submitted a bid to host the 2022 Worldcon—the annual convention of the World Science Fiction Society (WSFS). It was first held in 1939 and, after a hiatus during the Second World War, has been held continuously since 1946. For the website of the Saudi bid, see at: https://jeddicon.com, last accessed August 29, 2020. However, a group of writers, led by the British author Anna Smith Spark, have protested against Saudi Arabia's bid to host the 2022 World Science Fiction Convention, citing the Kingdom's human rights abuses and discriminatory laws. In a letter to the WSFS, eighty science fiction authors said that the "Saudi regime is antithetical to everything SFF [science fiction and fantasy] stands for" (see at: https://www.middleeasteye.net/news/saudi-arabia-worldcon-science-fiction-jeddah, last accessed August 29, 2020). Winning 517 of the 587 ballots, Chicago won the site vote and will host the 80th Worldcon, Chicon 8, to be held on September 1–5, 2022, available at: https://locusmag.com/2020/07/chicago-wins-worldcon-site-bid, last accessed August 30, 2020.

missing, a wave of eerie murders sweeps the city, and reports stream in of a horrendous-looking criminal who, though shot, cannot be killed. Hādī soon realizes he has created a monster, one that needs human flesh to survive—first from the guilty, and then from anyone who crosses its path. The reader has no doubt that Hādī al-ʿAttāk's activities are only a metaphor for the hopes of Baghdad's people to regain Baghdad's glory, and each episode in the novel encapsulates something of the history of Baghdad during the last decades before its publication. For example, this novel illustrates the demise of the Iraqi-Jewish community as *all* the mentions of the Jewish traces in Baghdad[121] are of a remote past that is hardly recognized and will probably never return. Chapter 13, called "al-Kharāba al-Yahūdiyya" ("The Jewish Ruin"), may be considered as representing a Jewish ruined past in Iraq. Nothing substantial about the glorious Iraqi-Jewish cultural and social past is mentioned in the novel. Nevertheless, in a study of the novel, Ian Campbell argues that it uses the historically most common trope of Arabic SF, double estrangement, to critique not only the acute crisis of sectarian violence but also "the long-term stagnation and decline of scientific and technological development in Iraq since its Golden Age a thousand years ago." While any reader can by no means ignore the social and political messages of the novel, one can hardly see how the novel concentrates on the stagnation and decline of scientific and technological development in Iraq. At any rate, Campbell refers to the novel as demonstrating "the full maturity of Arabic SF."[122] With such a method of widening the boundaries of SF, one may refer to numerous other Arabic novels written during the current and the previous centuries as SF although they have been never considered as such. Nevertheless, to quote Rawad Alhashmi in her review of Campbell's book, against the background of the dearth of scholarship on the subject and the growing interest in this genre, especially after the Arab Spring, Arabic SF has become "a self-conscious genre and hence constitutes serious literature."[123]

121 For example, Saʿdawī 2013, pp. 20, 30–1, 105, 187, 226–7, 240–1, 298, 303–4. On the demise of Arab-Jewish identity and culture, see Snir 2015.

122 Campbell 2018, pp. 1–26. The quotations are from pp. 1 and 26, respectively. On the novel, see also Teggart 2019, pp. 1–30, which does not mention any connection between Saʿdawī's novel and the SF genre.

123 *Mashriq & Mahjar* 8.2 (2021), pp. 111–14. For an understanding of the experience of trauma lived by people in Egypt since the cataclysmic violence of the Arab Spring as it is expressed in the speculative fiction that has flooded the Egyptian literary scene in the aftermath of the 2011 uprisings, see de Wringer 2020. Speculative fiction—an umbrella term for fiction in which the author speculates about what could happen when stepping outside the realm of reality—includes science fiction, fantasy, utopian and dystopian fiction, (post) apocalyptic fiction, and horror and is usually set in the future (on the classification of speculative fiction, see Gill 2013, pp. 71–85).

Epilogue

Arabic Literature and World Literature[1]

I wanted to live outside the history that Empire
imposes on its subjects, even its lost subjects.
– John Maxwell Coetze

As an epilogue to the present project, which summarizes my studies in the field of Arabic literature during the last fifty years, I will discuss below the conceptions and insights provided by Muhsin Jassim al-Musawi (Muḥsin Jāsim al-Mūsawī) (b. 1944) in his study *The Medieval Islamic Republic of Letters: Arabic Knowledge Construction* (2015).[2] The discussion of the book's conceptions and insights will refer as well to other contributions that deal with the same topics or other relevant issues,[3] in addition to review essays in English and Arabic on al-Musawi's scholalry contributions.[4] Because of the theoretical gist and drive of al-Musawi's book and articles, and due to his declared ambition to contribute to a better understanding of Arabic literature in its historical development, his contributions are important

[1] The Epilogue is based on Snir 2017, pp. 137–92.

[2] See al-Musawi 2015b. For a translation of the book, see al-Mūsawī 2020.

[3] Such as al-Musawi 2013, pp. 43–71; al-Musawi 2014, pp. 265–80; Ganguly 2015, pp. 272–81; Helgesson 2015, pp. 253–60; al-Musawi 2015, pp. 115–30; al-Musawi 2015b, pp. 281–6; El-Ariss 2015, pp. 260–6; Orsini 2015, pp. 266–72.

[4] For review essays of the book, see Mohammad Salama, "Bridging the Gap: A Review Essay of Muhsin al-Musawi's *The Medieval Islamic Republic of Letters*," *SCTIW Review* (November 19, 2015), pp. 1–6; Kristina Richardson's review essay in *Journal of Arabic Literature* 47.1/2 (2016), pp. 209–13 (the general editor of the journal is al-Musawi himself); Dana Sajdi's review in *Journal of Early Modern History* 20.2 (2016), pp. 589–92; Marilyn Booth's review essay in *Journal of Islamic Studies* 28.3 (2017), pp. 382–6; and Elizabeth Lhost's review essay in *Reading Religion*, website published by the American Academy of Religion (AAR) (May 19, 2017). See also, in Arabic, Shīrīn Abū al-Najā's review essay in *al-Ḥayāt*, February 28, 2016. Since the publication of the book in Arabic translation (al-Mūsawī 2020), it is expected that additional reviews will be published in Arabic; in fact, the first of them has already been published by Aḥmad Ma'mūn (*al-'Arabī al-Jadīd*, June 9, 2020).

not only for the study of premodern Arabic literature, but for the study of modern Arabic literature as well. In several studies, I explained the significance of the continuity and uninterruptedness of the Arabic literature from ancient times until the present day—in fact, since the emergence of the Arabic language long before the Arabic poetry known to us emerged in the fifth century.[5]

In *Modern Arabic Literature* (2017), I argue that Arabic literature can be more adequately analyzed as a historical phenomenon when conceived of as a system that replaces the search for data about material aspects of literary phenomena with the uncovering of the functions that these aspects have. Arabic literature has been postulated to constitute a system or polysystem—a heterogeneous, multistratified, and functionally structured system-of-systems—kept in motion by a permanent struggle between canonical and non-canonical texts and models. The evaluation of the systems of successive periods springs from the oscillating movement between the periphery of the system and its center (here I could employ, instead of "system," the term "republic" as this term will be explained below). Such a system is inclusive and consists of all *literary* texts regardless of any hierarchies of value, namely, all texts that in a given culture or community have been imbued with cultural value—something that allows for higher levels of complexity and significance in the way they are constructed. Each text forms a system and at the same time is an element of a larger system, which is itself, in turn, a part of the greater system of the Arabic literary environment. That is to say, in each given period a given text is placed at a particular point in the Arabic literary system according to its synchronic relative value. Diachronic value is assigned to the text by its paradigmatic position in the succession of synchronic systems, which acquire retrospective significance. Here, as previously indicated, my analysis avoids as much as possible any personal subjective evaluative assessments, and at the same time it reflects the values and judgments of the relevant communities toward their literary texts in different stages and periods. Sociocultural distinctions of text production in the proposed system are conceptualized in terms of literary stratification: canonized versus non-canonized texts. By canonized texts, I mean literary works that have been accepted by dominant circles within Arab culture, that have become part of a community's historical heritage, and that have entered into its collective memory. Conversely, non-canonized texts are those literary works that have been rejected by the same circles as illegitimate or worthless

[5] For example, Snir 2017, pp. 182–93. As for the linguistic situation among the Arabs before the rise of Islam, see the contributions by Jan Retsö 2003, pp. 591–599; and Retsö 2013, pp. 433–450.

and that are often in the long run forgotten by the community. This means that canonicity is not seen as an *inherent feature* of textual activities on any level, although canonicity in Arabic literature depends in general—but not always—on the language of production: *fuṣḥa* (the pan-Arab standard language) is the basic medium of canonized texts, whereas *'āmmiyya* (local dialect) is that of non-canonized texts. In addition, it means that, if not from the synchronic point of view, certainly from the diachronic respect we obviously lack the ability to explore most of the non-canonized texts that were created, certainly not all of them.

In my book, I propose three categories of investigation for modern Arabic literature. The first is the investigation of the literary dynamics in synchronic cross-section—potential inventories of canonized and non-canonized literary texts in three sections: texts for adults, texts for children, and translated texts for adults and children. The resulting six subsystems—three canonized and three non-canonized—are seen as autonomous networks of relationships and as interacting literary networks on various levels. The internal and external interrelations and interactions between the various subsystems need to be studied if we wish to arrive at a comprehensive understanding of the modern Arabic literary system. The second category consists of the study of the historical outlines of the modern Arabic literary system's diachronic intersystemic development, namely, the need to refer to the changes and interactions with various extra-literary systems that have determined the historical course of Arabic literature since the nineteenth century. The space between the text, its author, and the reader is understood as constituting both an economic environment (e.g., literary markets, publishing, distribution) and a sociocommunicative system that passes the meaning potential of the text through various filters (e.g., criticism, literary circles, groups, salons, public opinion) in order to concretize and realize it. All spaces related to literary production and consumption should be considered. For example, in order to determine the general characteristics of the historical development of Arabic literature from the start of the nineteenth century, we should look at the interaction of literature with extra-literary systems, such as religion, territory, nation-state, language, politics, economy, philosophy, gender, electronic media, Internet technologies, and social networks, as well as with other foreign literary and cultural systems. Finally, the third category is intended to concentrate on the historical diachronic development that each genre underwent and on the relationships between the various genres. Since literary genres do not emerge in a vacuum, the issue of generic development cannot be confined to certain time spans; emphasis must be put on the relationship between modern literature, on the one hand, and classical and medieval literature, on the other. Crucial in this regard is the concept of periodization, that is, how one is to delimit and define "literary periods." The complete study of literary dynamics in historical, diachronic development requires an analysis of every genre and subgenre separately, of the interrelationships and interactions between the genres, and of the interrelationships and interactions between the genres and the subgenres.

In the following, I will look more closely at al-Musawi's scholarly project in the context of relevant theoretical contributions and within the framework of the study of Arabic literature in general. Al-Musawi opens the introduction (*Khuṭbat al-Kitāb*, lit. "Preliminary Discourse") to his book as follows:

> This book argues that the large-scale and diverse cultural production in Arabic in the post-classical era (approximately the twelfth through the eighteenth centuries) was the outcome of an active sphere of discussion and disputation spanning the entire medieval Muslim world. I explore this production over a long temporal stretch and across a vast swathe of Islamic territories. My focus is on the thematic and genealogical constructions that were of greatest significance to the accumulation of cultural capital, which, I argue, constitutes a medieval Islamic "republic of letters."[6]

In his conclusion, al-Musawi explains that his medieval Islamic republic of letters "implies an umbrella—literary world-systems that existed across Asia and Africa."[7] In what follows, I will further develop and expand upon some of the points that I made in my book in addition to new relevant ones.

1. GENERAL THEORETICAL CONTEXTS

Al-Musawi's use of the term "republic of letters" (*république des lettres*) relies on the meaning of the term established in two books, one by Dena Goodman (b. 1952) (*The Republic of Letters: A Cultural History of the French Enlightenment*)[8] and the other by Pascale Casanova (1959–2018) (*The World Republic of Letters*).[9] Coined by Pierre Bayle (1647–1706) to indicate a network of intellectuals who create and sustain cultural exchange,[10] this

[6] Al-Musawi 2015b, p. 1.
[7] Al-Musawi 2015b, p. 305.
[8] Goodman 1994.
[9] Casanova 2004.
[10] See also the project "Mapping the Republic of Letters" at the Stanford Humanities Center (Stanford University); the following is from its website (http://republicofletters.stanford.edu/index.html, last accessed July 23, 2020): "Before email, faculty meetings, international colloquia, and professional associations, the world of scholarship relied on its own networks: networks of correspondence that stretched across countries and continents; the social networks created by scientific academies; and the physical networks brought about by travel. These networks ... facilitated the dissemination and the criticism of ideas, the spread of political news, as well as the circulation of people and objects ... [The project] aims

term is used by al-Musawi to refer to "a conceptual framework, an edifice, to account for a literary world-system in which Arabic functions as the dominating language." However, al-Musawi is careful to state that "its appropriation in this book entails no equation between Latin and Arabic in relation to national languages."[11] Casanova's conceptions are mentioned throughout al-Musawi's book in a mixture of hidden gratitude (probably for inventing the attractive title for her book and, then, for enabling him to use it in his project) and visible disagreement (emphasizing his own postcolonial non-Eurocentric theoretical conceptions). That is why we frequently encounter in al-Musawi's study utterances indicating that Casanova's model of world literature cannot be applied to "Arabic knowledge construction" but, at the same time, we see him refer to her model's parameters to delineate the Islamic world—although in the latter case, some of these references are inapposite—for example, Cairo is compared with Paris as the Greenwich Meridian of literature, and Arabic is compared with Latin in relation to national languages. However, anyone who has read Casanova's study would see that al-Musawi deals only superficially with her conceptions without delving deeply into her arguments, or even, sometimes, without fully comprehending their meanings and implications. He or she would also see that al-Musawi overlooks the many insightful studies and critical reviews written about Casanova's book following its original publication in French (1999), its translation into Arabic (2002), and especially after its release in English by a distinguished publisher (2004). Without referring to these studies and reviews and the in-depth contributions in this regard to various literary and cultural systems, any attempt to use her conceptions is inadequate and unsatisfactory.

Casanova's study and the notion of a "republic of letters" captured the attention and interest of a range of scholars with regard to their approaches to the study of literature and the production of literary value, all of them treating culture as a field, a structure, or an economy. Drawing on the language of politics, it reminds us that this is a field constituted by power and competition, a hierarchical structure. The study was praised by Bill Marx as "a marvelously stimulating look at the realpolitik of world literature and the authorities who run the marketplace of ideas."[12] Perry Anderson refers to it as "path-breaking":

to create a repository for metadata on early-modern scholarship, and guidelines for future data capture."

11 Al-Musawi 2015b, p. 9.

12 Bill Marx, "Review of *The World Republic of Letters*," *Words without Borders* (n.d.), available at: http://www.wordswithoutborders.org/book-review/the-world-republic-of-letters, last accessed October 30, 2017.

> Here the national bounds of Bourdieu's work have been decisively broken, in a project that uses his concepts of symbolic capital and the cultural field to construct a model of the global inequalities of power between different national literatures, and the gamut of strategies that writers in languages at the periphery of the system of legitimation have used to try to win a place at the centre. Nothing like this has been attempted before.[13]

Others approached Casanova's study from various critical angles, some even arguing that her theory was erratic and implausible.[14] In brief, Casanova's point of departure is that, historically, the study of literature in the *modern* era has been dominated by nationalism. She believes that while we have been encouraged to think of literature exclusively in terms of *national* literatures, this approach is increasingly at odds with the realities of a *globalizing* world. As might be expected, she more or less ignores the question of official nationalism, which is one way of accounting for her avoidance, as Nergis Ertürk correctly observes, for example, of Turkey and Turkish literature.[15] Thence, her book is dedicated to moving beyond nationalism in literary study and looking instead at how all books and authors participate in what she thinks of as a *world literary system*.[16]

Casanova (and even Franco Moretti before her)[17] tried to theorize the literary field as one global phenomenon and to propose new structures of interaction between literature and history.[18] Casanova's central hypothesis, as she argues at the very beginning of her book, "is that there exists a 'literature-world,' a literary universe relatively independent of the everyday world and its political divisions, whose boundaries and operational laws are not reducible to those of ordinary political space." The world literary space is autonomous and "endowed with its own laws,"[19] and the aesthetic map of the world does not overlap with the political one. Casanova describes a Darwinian literary market, where, in the battle for survival, outsiders crash

[13] Anderson 2004, p. 18.

[14] For important critiques of Casanova's model, see Prendergast 2001, pp. 100–21; Prendergast 2004; and the special issue of *New Literary History* titled "Literary History in the Global Age" (39.3/4 [2008]). Following her death, the *Journal of World Literature* published a special volume (5.2 [2020]) with the title "Pascale Casanova's World of Letters and Its Legacies," edited by Gisèle Sapiro and Delia Ungureanu. In one of the articles, David Damrosch examines Casanova's responses to the varied responses to her book, and suggests that her subsequent books should be understood as embodying a resulting mixture of resistance and rethinking of her earlier positions (Damrosch 2020, pp. 174–88).

[15] See Ertürk 2010, p. 634. Cf. Snir 2017, pp. 160–74.

[16] The last emphasized terms demonstrate the irrelevance of Casanova's conceptions to the literary texts and the activities al-Musawi deals with in his book.

[17] Moretti 1996.

[18] López 2011, pp. 69–88.

[19] Casanova 2004, pp. xii and 350, respectively.

in while insiders fend off challenges to their authority: "It is the competition among its members that defines and unites the system while at the same time marking its limits," and "not every writer proceeds in the same way, but all writers attempt to enter the same race, and all of them struggle, albeit with unequal advantages, to attain the same goal: literary legitimacy."[20] She deals with the transnational literary market and with the critical discourse on world literature as an autonomous, transnational, unipolar system ruled by the literary Greenwich Meridian.[21] Casanova discusses the concept of "symbolic and literary capital" on an international scale, asking what the components of literary capital might be: literacy rates and prizes, numbers of books published and sold, numbers of publishers and bookstores, judgments, and reputations. Language would be a major component of literary capital: "Certain languages, by virtue of the prestige of the texts written in them, are reputed to be more literary than others, to embody literature."[22]

Scholars have attempted to explore the implications of Casanova's book with regard to specific local literatures, exactly as al-Musawi has tried to do with Arabic literature, but most of them did it with much more attentiveness to its conceptions. Peter Kirkpatrick and Robert Dixon, for example, grapple with the notion of "world literature" and its meaning for Australian literary studies. While they frequently allude to Casanova's views, their book presents a far more pluralistic vision of *literary community*. They attempt to juxtapose "world literature" with the very different forms of "community" created by writers' circles, little magazines, and the like. They acknowledge the "slippage" between these two concepts: while the term "community" suggests *shared values and interests*, the "republic of letters" draws on the language of politics, reminding us that this is a field constituted by *power*

[20] Casanova 2004, p. 40. Cf. Damrosch 2009, p. 335.

[21] On the concept of world literature and the various positions, see the following selected publications: Elster 1901, pp. 33–47; Elster 1986, pp. 7–13; Moretti 2000, pp. 54–68; Damrosch 2003; Schildgen et al. 2007; Damrosch 2009; Damrosch 2009a; Apter 2013; D'haen et al. 2013; Ganguly 2015, pp. 272–81. One of the definitions of world literature excludes any evaluative judgments or hierarchies of value, namely, "all of the world's literature, without pronouncing on questions of quality and influence" (D'haen et al. 2013, p. xi). On Arabic fiction and world literature, see Rooke 2011, pp. 201–13; Parr 2021, pp. 167–83. On Arabic poetry and world literature, see Fakhreddine 2017, pp. 147–54. On how Arabic literature has been introduced into world literature anthologies, see Khalifah 2017, pp. 512–26. On extending the paradigm of world literature beyond hegemonic global centers and attending to the trajectories that shape "literature in the world," see Helgesson 2015, pp. 253–60. On world literature and the demise of national literatures, see Clüver 1986, pp. 14–24; Clüver 1988, pp. 134–9; Clüver 1988a, pp. 143–4; Konstantinovic 1988, pp. 141–2; Steinmetz 1988, pp. 131–3.

[22] Casanova 2004, p. 17.

and competition.[23] Hayden White refers to Casanova's attempt to ground her history of literature in an idea of "literary temporality" and the way in which modern literature, originally identified with politics and nationalism, managed, "through a gradual accumulation of autonomy, to escape the ordinary laws of history." This allows her to define literature "both as an object that is irreducible to history and as a historical object, albeit one that enjoys a strictly literary historicity,"[24] but White points to the ambiguity in her use of the word "literary" and raises questions about the difference between the phrases "*literary* history of literature" and "*historical* history of literature."[25] Most criticism of Casanova, however, has referred to the book's claims for creating a method of canonicity for world literature, and thus has predictably focused on her neglect of certain authors and genres. The most thorough engagement with her work can be found in the collection edited by Christopher Prendergast.[26]

There is almost nothing of the above discussion in al-Musawi's study or articles. Although he acknowledges Casanova's work as an inspiration, al-Musawi does not take the book's theory as a point of departure either as a conceptual focus or even as a thesis to be rejected. It seems that what greatly captured al-Musawi's interest was Casanova's attractive title; otherwise, it is difficult to understand how he ignores even what could have served his arguments quite well.[27] Good examples for dealing with theoretical conceptions of world literature with regard to Arabic literature can be found in four studies, one appearing before the publication of al-Musawi's book and the three others appearing after its publication. The first is an article by Nadia al-Bagdadi (b. 1963) in which she discerns three distinct phases and types of globalization: (1) *Oikumenical globalization* of late antiquity to the end of the Abbasid period; (2) *Expanding globalization* of the Imperialist age of the late eighteenth to the twentieth century; and (3) *Dispersal globalization* of the current age. Confining literary movements to these three forms of globalization is a simplified scheme of more complex historical developments, al-Bagdadi says, but "the heuristic advantage, however, opens up historical and theoretical perspectives on literacy, literature, and interpretation at the

23 Kirkpatrick and Dixon 2012, p. v.

24 Casanova 2004, p. 350.

25 White 2008, pp. 738–9. In addition, White offers Ami Elias' insights in her book *Sublime Desire: History and Post-1960s Fiction* (Elias 2001).

26 Prendergast 2004.

27 Such as the hope Casanova expresses at the very end of her book that her study will be a "critical weapon in the service of all deprived and dominated writers on the periphery of the literary world" in their struggle "against the presumptions, the arrogance, and the fiats of critics in the center, who ignore the basic fact of the inequality of access to literary existence" (Casanova 2004, pp. 354–5).

interface of crossing cultures and civilizations. It will suffice here to sketch out the three phases with regard to the question under consideration."[28] Unlike al-Bagdadi, who does not refer at all to Casanova's conceptions, although she deals with issues mentioned in her book, the other three studies discuss directly these theoretical conceptions as they relate to Arabic literature, with full awareness of their complexities. Rebecca Carol Johnson uses Aḥmad Fāris al-Shidyāq's (1804–1887) semi-autobiographical fictional travel narrative *al-Sāq 'alā al-Sāq fī mā Huwa al-Fāryāq* (*Leg upon Leg Concerning That Which Is al-Fāryāq*) (1855) in order to examine critically world literature paradigms that see literary modernity as the entrance into world literary space's zones of equivalence. Providing many examples from the book, she argues that literary modernity is a world that Arab authors accumulated in their texts by re-aggregating literary history as a collection of translations of texts and by reading them:

> The worldedness of literary reference in al-Shidyāq's sense is not one that supplants or is in conflict with national or local identifications. Nor is it universal style, form, or reason in disguise. He gathers styles, forms, and reasons—"connects the disconnected"—into an unstable archive of modernity that cannot be positioned within a single or uniform genealogy. Through a series of productive misreadings—by incorporating European modes and genres into his work as European, by creating fractured and heterogeneous audiences within his text, and by bringing Arabic literary standards to pass judgment on European texts—al-Shidyāq creates an aggregated global literary sphere and reminds us that the "world" in world literature is not a given; it must be manufactured, and from a particular and historically contingent location. In doing so, al-Shidyāq shows us how to take modern Arabic literature out of filiative or vertical narratives of development, and instead situate it within a larger network of transnational or horizontal associations that are embedded in, but not bound by, the material interactions that accompany them.[29]

Madeleine Dobie examines Casanova's theory, as well as those of Fredric Jameson and Franco Moretti. Focusing on the case of Algerian literature, she argues that narratives of world literature have tended to overemphasize the center–periphery divide, neglecting other geographies of production and circulation. Guided by a logic of mimesis, theories of world literature have often "derived their definition of literature from the western canon and then sought equivalents and tributaries in the rest of the world." They "approach non-western literature as an offshoot or extension of European culture and make little effort to explore other cultural forms or alternative

[28] Al-Bagdadi 2008, pp. 437–61. The quotation is from pp. 448–9.
[29] Johnson 2017, pp. 44–5. Cf. Johnson 2021, pp. 113–22.

sites of production and reception."[30] It is interesting that both Rebecca Carol Johnson and Madeleine Dobie do not refer to al-Musawi's book. Although it is unreasonable to assume that they were not aware of its appearance and its direct relevance to their studies—one can by no means rule out that the reason is not disconnected from what will be argued below concerning al-Musawi's influential and prestigious status in the scholarship of Arabic literature. Another study, by Marie Thérèse Abdel-Messih, does not mention explicitly Casanova's conceptions but refers to theories of world literature as well as to al-Musawi's arguments about the epistemological shifts effected by vocational cultural practices, such as those in rituals, recitations, slogans, odes, songs, banners, and colors, while elaborating upon them as they existed throughout the epochs of the Islamic republic of letters. However, when dealing specifically with world literature, she avoids referring to the gaps in al-Musawi's understanding of the principles of the relevant theories, maintaining that "the formation of a universal canon should be founded on a cross-cultural reading of mainstream and peripheral literary models from world literature, while engaging critics and scholars from the North and the South in the process of theorization." She concludes that

> restricting epistemology within a classical heritage or narrowed vocational practices related to an exclusive geographical location impedes access to a global dialogue. Rethinking critical approaches to Arabic initially requires rereading Arabic from a comparative perspective of distinct practices, within their continual intra-regional exchanges. Decolonizing the vocational from centralization, as well as hegemonic epistemic limitations, would enable scholars of Arabic to participate in the debate and address problems of global canon formation.[31]

In the following, I will refer to al-Musawi's study in the context of available scholarship on Arabic literature, and from time to time, when relevant, I will refer to world literature's theories and conceptions. According to the definition of David Damrosch, "I take world literature to encompass all literary works that circulate beyond their culture of origin, either in translation or in their original language ... a work only has an effective life as world literature whenever, and wherever, it is actively present within a literary system beyond that of its original culture."[32]

[30] Dobie 2017, pp. 78–90. The quotation is from p. 87.
[31] Abdel-Messih 2018, pp. 192–209. The quotations are from pp. 205 and 206–7, respectively.
[32] Damrosch 2003, p. 4.

2. TERMINOLOGY

For a study considered to be, as Suzanne P. Stetkevych writes in her endorsement of al-Musawi's book, "the starting point for a new generation of scholarship" on premodern Arabic literature, the intelligible use of terms and the appropriate justifications for the use of each term are crucial. That is why it is important to clarify in detail what makes the term "republic of letters" suitable, besides its decorative attractiveness, as an "umbrella term"[33] in a study on *Arabic* literature. Moreover, if the term's appropriation, according to al-Musawi himself, "entails no equation between Latin and Arabic in relation to national languages," one has to ask what justifies the borrowing of this very term from a specifically "literary world-system," where the relationship between the major language (Latin) and the national languages is fundamental.[34] Casanova's conceptions, which are indebted to world-systems theory as developed by the French historian and a leader of the Annales School Fernand Braudel (1902–1985), with his concept of an "economy-world" and especially to Pierre Bourdieu's concept of literature as an autonomous social field in which competitions for symbolic capital in the cultural field supersede yet as well mirror the wider competition for power,[35] make a case for an international theory space, which has developed its own standards, canons, and values operating separately from national literary systems. According to Dena Goodman, the "French Republic of Letters rose with the modern political state out of the religious wars of the sixteenth century, out of the articulation of public and private spheres, citizen and state, agent and critic." The basics of this "Republic" were established in the "Parisian salons, from which networks of social and intellectual exchange were being developed to connect the capital with the four corners of France and the cosmopolitan republic." Its aim was "to serve humanity and [its] project was Enlightenment."[36]

33 Al-Musawi 2015b, p. 305.

34 Some of al-Musawi's statements regarding the comparison between Arabic and Latin are obscure and ambiguous. Take, for example, the following: "Although Arabic remained a language of conversation and discussion among writers and scholars, *it was so only in the shadow of other empires and city-states*; hence, it cannot be compared to Latin. Its relation to other competing and challenging vernaculars is a dialectical one, *a record of give and take*, but also as the most recognized by scholars from non-Arab regions" (al-Musawi 2015a, p. 283 [my emphasis]). For the interaction between Latin and Arabic as linguistic systems throughout the centuries and the equation between Latin and Arabic in relation to national languages, see König 2016, pp. 419–93.

35 Bourdieu 1992; Bourdieu 1996.

36 Goodman 1994, pp. 2 and 52, respectively. On literary and cultural salons as "the spirit and soul of a public sphere" within the *Nahḍa* project as well, see Khaldi 2009, pp. 1–36 (quotation from p. 5).

However, apart from brief references to both studies in his *Preliminary Discourse* and some quotations from Casanova's book in subsequent pages, nowhere does al-Musawi provide any coherent explanation for the shared views and conceptions between either Goodman's or Casanova's concepts of the term "republic of letters" and his own. At the same time, in justifying his focus on rhetoric, in a visible attempt to imitate the authors of the post-classical and premodern periods,[37] al-Musawi refers to the Arabic translation of the term "republic":

> The recourse in rhetoric to indirection, or *laḥn al-qawl* (i.e. implicitness), and to *taʿrīḍ* (dissimulation, connotation, concealment) signifies the other side of written and verbal transactions in this *jumhūr* (majority) of littérateurs, which is the basis for Arab and Muslim modernists' application of the term *jumhūriyyah* (i.e. republic). In this verbal domain, the root and conjugation of the verb *jamhara* also connote dissimulation. Hence, both verb and noun are loaded in Arabic in a binary structure, negation, or *taḍadd* (based on opposites or contrasts—*aḍdād*), implying both revelation and concealment.[38]

Al-Musawi implies here that the etymology of the Arabic term for "republic" is relevant to his conception of the "republic of letters" and that, since "both verb and noun are loaded in Arabic in a binary structure, negation, or *taḍadd*," negation is also relevant to it. Al-Musawi, however, does not further elaborate on his claim. The original meaning of the verb *jamhara*, from which the term *jumhūriyya* (republic) is derived, is "[to collect] together a thing or earth, or dust." The same verb also denotes dissimulation: thus, "*jamhara ʿalayhi* (or *lahu* or *ilayhi*) *al-khabara*" means "he acquainted him with a part of the news, or story, and concealed what he desired or meant," or "he acquainted him with a part of the news, or story, incorrectly, or not in the proper manner, and omitted what he desired or meant."[39] In *one* source only, there is a view that the verb *jamhara* is of the category *aḍdād*, which is to say that it is a *ḍidd* (plural: *aḍdād*), the Arabic term for a word with two basic meanings but with one meaning being the opposite of the other (i.e., a contronym): thus, "*jamhar lak al-khabara jamharatan*" means "he acquainted you with a minor part of the news and concealed its main part."[40] However, this is *not* an obvious case of the category of *aḍdād*, since *jamhar* in its main meaning, from which the word *jumhūriyya* is derived, as

[37] Hereafter, the terms "postclassical" and "premodern" are in general used interchangeably. On what makes that period both postclassical and premodern, see Allen 2006, pp. 8–17. For a critical approach to the use of the term "postclassical" applied to the literary production of the Mamluk period, see Bauer 2007, p. 71. See also Bellino 2020, pp. 123–4.

[38] Al-Musawi 2015b, pp. 2–3.

[39] Lane 1968 [1863–1893], I.2, pp. 461–2 (*jamhar*).

[40] al-Lughawī 1963, p. 182.

well as in its marginal meaning, does not connote a meaning and its total opposite, such as, for example, the word *jawn*, which means both "black" and "white," or *jalal*, which means both "great" and "small," or *ḍidd* itself, which ironically has the contrary meanings "opposite" and "equal."[41] On the other hand, it is not clear at all what the benefit is to al-Musawi's argument for the "republic of letters" if "both verb and noun are loaded in Arabic in a binary structure, negation, or *taḍadd*."[42]

In any case, al-Musawi writes about a period when the term "*jumhūriyya*" did not exist and the terms concerning literary and cultural activities were different from those that have been used since the late nineteenth century (see my discussion of the term "*adab*" below). Thus, there is a need to clarify the terms al-Musawi uses throughout his study, such as "cultural production" and "cultural activity," as well "literary production," "literary life," and "literary value." The aforementioned term "literary world-system" is also used without clear definition, sometimes by an indirect allusion to Casanova's arguments or to an interpretation of one of her book's reviews.[43] In my recent book, I explain what I mean by terms, such as "literary system,"

41 Lane 1968 [1863–1893], p. 1775 (*ḍidd*).

42 In an interview with the Arabic press before the publication of his book, al-Musawi referred to its title as *Jumhūriyyat al-Adab fī al-ʿAṣr al-Islāmī al-Wasīṭ* (*al-Sharq al-Awsaṭ*, January 22, 2013), but after its publication he preferred to translate it as *Jamharat al-Ādāb fī al-ʿAṣr al-Islāmī al-Wasīṭ* (*al-Khalīj*, June 30, 2015). He justifies the use of *Jamharat al-Ādāb* for "republic of letters" by arguing wrongly(!) that the term alludes to the contrary meanings of *jamʿ wa-tafrīq* ("joining and separating") (*al-Bayān*, June 30, 2015):

> لأن جمهر تعني الجمع والتفريق، وهي أصل للجمهوريّة كمفردة توازي ما درج عليه الفرنسيّون، فدلالتها ديمقراطية لاسيّما أنها تشتمل على الضدّين، وتتيح عبر الجمع والتفريق، الاحتجاج واختلاف الرأي والجدل والمناقشة. وبالتالي، إحياء الفضاء العام اللازم لتنامي الظواهر المختلفة مؤسساتيًّا ومعرفيًّا.

In another interview after the publication of the Arabic version of the book, al-Musawi reiterates the same wrong argument, available at: https://www.youtube.com/watch?v=161bCQvJzV4, September 21, 2021, last accessed December 19, 2021. In a review of the book, Shīrīn Abū al-Najā translates its first part as *al-Jumhūriyya al-Islāmiyya li-l-Ādāb* (*al-Ḥayāt*, February 28, 2016). Casanova's book was translated into Arabic as *al-Jumhūriyya al-ʿĀlāmiyya li-l-Ādāb* (trans. Amal al-Ṣabbān) (Casanova 2002).

43 Al-Musawi 2015b, p. 89, where al-Musawi bases his argument on a partial and inaccurate quotation from Cleary 2006, p. 202. In an article published two years before he published his book, al-Musawi refers to Casanova's arguments but only mentions Cleary's review in a footnote. The article opens with two sentences about the "major restructuration and hence proliferation of the literary world-system" that are "motivated and driven by the corporate effort of grammarians and writers, an effort that in the case of English drew impetus from a sustained privileging of literature in a self-assertive nationalism" (al-Musawi 2013, p. 43). Cleary mentions "the efforts of men of letters, grammarians and lexicographers" (Cleary 2006, p. 202), but in a different context. It is debatable as to how al-Musawi actually "applies" this, in the next sentence, to the medieval and premodern Islamic cultural world-system, when he argues "that grammar, lexicography, and literary production assume *even more significance* as evidenced in the massive production and demand" (my emphasis).

"literary text," and "culture,"[44] among others, and my definitions evidently differ from those of al-Musawi, since his are—and they are, as I have been arguing—rather vague.

3. TEMPORAL SPACES AND BORDERS

Al-Musawi's book refers to the "postclassical era (approximately the twelfth through the eighteenth centuries),"[45] but one has to wonder about the uniformity of this long time span and the assumed difference between it—or a section of it—and between other periods, such as the eleventh and the nineteenth centuries. For example, the essential characteristics of *literary* production in Arabic did not dramatically change between the tenth and twelfth centuries. Furthermore, in chapter 2, al-Musawi deals with the tenth-century encyclopedic work *Ikhwān al-Ṣafāʾ* (*The Brethren of Purity*), considering it as the "prototype for an Islamic republic of letters"[46] and thus complicating the issue of the temporal spaces and borders of his imagined "republic." In any event, before the late nineteenth century, modern literary conceptions had not as yet penetrated Arabic literature, and therefore it is important that the particular characteristics of the "twelfth through the eighteenth centuries" and how they can be distinguished from those of other periods, both previous and subsequent, be fleshed out. Here, theoretical studies dealing with periodization, as mentioned above, may help as well as contributions by other scholars of Arabic literature who have dealt with this issue. For example, in the introduction to *Arabic Literature in the Post-Classical Period* (2006), Roger Allen, the most prominent experienced contemporary scholar in the field of Arabic literature, eloquently explains in detail why the volume he edited together with D. S. Richards treats "the vast period between approximately 1150 and 1850 as a separate entity."[47] In addition, in my recent book I deal with the topic of periodization from a *literary* point of view, and the parameters I use to distinguish between periods may also be relevant to al-Musawi's research project.[48]

[44] See Snir 2017, pp. 2–3, 4, 11 (n. 11), and 2–3, respectively.
[45] Al-Musawi 2015b, p. 1.
[46] Al-Musawi 2015b, p. 15.
[47] Allen and Richards 2006, p. 20. For a review article of the book, see Bauer 2007, pp. 137–67. And see as well the response of Salma Khadra Jayyusi, whose article in the book (Jayyusi 2008, pp. 193–207) was described by Bauer (p. 159) as falling "far short of scholarly standards."
[48] See Snir 2017, pp. 176–81.

4. TERRITORIAL, PHYSICAL, AND METAPHORICAL SPACES

Casanova's book, on which al-Musawi relies, is concerned with what one might call the "geopolitics of literature." In his review of the book, Terry Eagleton writes the following:

> Literary works, so it claims, are never fully intelligible in themselves; instead, you have to see them as belonging to a global literary space, which has a basis in the world's political landscape, but which also cuts across its regions and borders to form a distinctive republic of its own. Like geopolitical space, this literary republic has its frontiers, provinces, exiles, legislators, migrations, subordinate territories and an unequal distribution of resources. It is a form of intellectual commerce in which literary value is banked and circulated, or transferred from one national currency to another in the act of translation ... like the political sphere, too, the republic of letters is wracked by struggle, rivalry and inequality between the literary haves and the have-nots. There are "peripheral" or "impoverished" literary spheres ... Such underdeveloped pockets are poor in literary capital, lacking publishers, libraries, journals and professional writers. Dominating their cultural resources is Old Europe, with its literary capital located firmly in Paris.[49]

Al-Musawi refers to Cairo of the postclassical era as the literary capital of the medieval Islamic republic of letters—a "cosmopolitan" city by virtue of its place and by virtue of its being a "nexus that witnesses a dialogue among schools of thought, scholastic controversies, scientific achievements, poetic innovations and shifts in expression, the massive use of prose for statecraft, and soaring heights of Ṣūfī poetry that simultaneously derive and refract worldliness from common tropes."[50] In addition, "the influx of scholars, poets, travelers, and entrepreneurs continued markedly into the nineteenth century and played a significant role in giving the city its

[49] *New Statesman*, April 11, 2005, available at: http://www.newstatesman.com/node/198469, last accessed October 30, 2017.

[50] In his review of al-Musawi's book, Mohammad Salama argues that "one of the book's persuasive arguments is that we give Egypt, especially Cairo, its long overdue literary recognition that Casanova assigns exclusively to Paris" ("Bridging the Gap," p. 2). However, it seems that al-Musawi does not see Paris and Cairo as competing on the same track; he argues that Cairo "stood to the postclassical Islamic world *as* Paris stood to Europe" (al-Musawi 2015b, p. 7 [my emphasis]). In his over-praising of al-Musawi's book and wholesale adoption of his arguments, Salama attributes to al-Musawi several achievements and accomplishments that the latter had never wished or intended to realize. For example, Salama writes that al-Musawi criticizes Casanova for resorting to "Eurocentric statements" and then quotes a sentence by al-Musawi regarding Paris (p. 2), which can by no means be understood as critical of Casanova. Salama's review of the book, which lacks critical perspective, is typical of most if not all the reviews of al-Musawi's studies during the last two decades (see below).

cosmopolitan features." Scholars from all over the Islamic world "settled in Cairo or at least stopped there for a while. Others were satisfied with an imaginary stopover, which was sustained and given shape through Ṣūfī networks and an innovative reliance on the antecedent tradition of poetry and writing." Additionally, Cairo escaped destruction and as "a safe enclave, it functioned in a way similar to its multiplying compendiums and lexicons."

However, can we *truly* consider Cairo to be a "cosmopolitan space," as al-Musawi argues, against the backdrop of his own argument that following the fall of Baghdad the "Arab center could not hold for long"? Al-Musawi does admit that the emergence of "an alternative center in Cairo was accepted, but not as wholeheartedly as had been the case with Baghdad."[51] Here, the status of Paris in Casanova's model, from which al-Musawi drew his inspiration to refer to Cairo as cosmopolitan, is very important. In Casanova's view, because of its long accumulation of literary prestige and its relative freedom from political concerns, Paris serves as the Greenwich Meridian of literature, which "makes it possible to estimate the relative distance from the center of the world of letters of all those who belong to it."[52] Casanova and Moretti have tried to establish new paradigms that recreate a globalist literary discourse and a systematic apparatus that can render a literary world comprehensible while distancing itself from the discourse of postcolonial studies. The aim, as Silvia L. López correctly mentions, is to "reinstate models of a global understanding of literary production that have in the long run a depoliticizing effect, be this achieved through the adoption of an empirical Darwinian model of the evolution of literary forms or through the redeployment of the concept of literary autonomy, this time with all the clocks set to the Greenwich Meridian."[53] Cairo, however, can by no means be considered as the Greenwich Meridian of Arabic literature during the postclassical or premodern periods.

For Casanova's republic, the central hypothesis is that "there exists a 'literature-world,' a literary universe relatively independent of the everyday world and its political divisions, whose boundaries and operational laws are not reducible to those of ordinary political space."[54] In short, it has its own specific politics. That being said, the "literature-world" is not, as Joe Cleary explains in his review of Casanova's book, "some free-floating cosmopolitan cultural zone that transcends or is independent of political space either." It has "its own capitals, its own core and peripheral cultural regions, and its

[51] Al-Musawi 2015b, pp. 6–7, 45–6, 51, 71, 25, and 132, respectively.
[52] Casanova 2004, p. 88.
[53] López 2011, p. 70.
[54] Casanova 2004, p. xii.

own laws of canonization and capital accumulation."[55] We can measure the power, prestige, and volume of linguistic and literary capital of a language not in terms of "the number of writers and readers it has, but in terms of the number of cosmopolitan intermediaries—publishers, editors, critics, and especially translators—who assure the circulation of texts into language or out of it." In addition, "the great, often polyglot, cosmopolitan figures of the world of letters act in effect as foreign exchange brokers, as they are responsible for exporting from one territory to another texts whose literary value they determine by virtue of this very activity."[56]

Theoretical research on the topic of cosmopolitanism has seen significant developments during recent decades, including its use in relation to the Middle East; this has been shown concerning Alexandria as a cosmopolitan city at the turn of the twentieth century and concerning subsequent periods, such as the developments and changes following the "cosmopolitan turn" and the intensified globalization during the last few decades.[57] It is assumed that there is a need for certain urban, social, and cultural dimensions for a city to be considered as cosmopolitan or for a global society to have cosmopolitan features. Also, as it has been proven in various societies, cosmopolitanism in general, certainly in the pre-globalization world, is the product of very limited periods, certainly not of long periods of six or seven centuries.[58] Such was the case, for example, with Baghdad after its establishment in 762, when the city enjoyed, for a limited time span, a pluralistic and multiconfessional atmosphere with multicultural ethnic and religious gatherings of Muslims, Christians, Jews, Zoroastrians, Pagans, Arabs, Persians, and various other Asian populations. That cosmopolitan atmosphere was inspired by the leadership of the Caliph al-Mansur (754–775), who from Baghdad propagated an open and multicultural policy toward religious minorities.[59] The political, religious, and cultural supremacy of Baghdad as the center of the flowering of Mansur's Islamic empire encouraged and inspired the multicultural environment not only in the city itself, but also throughout other cities, close and remote alike. A contemporary text describing typical gatherings that would take place in the southern city of Basra in the year 156H (772/773) may serve to illustrate such a pluralistic environment (the fact that those gatherings were held in Basra, the site of the production of the aforementioned encyclopedic work *Ikhwān al-Ṣafā'* [*The Brethren of Purity*], which was depicted

[55] Cleary 2006, p. 199.
[56] Casanova 2004, p. 21.
[57] Snir 2017, pp. 267–9. And see now also Tal 2017, pp. 237–54, where the author connects cosmopolitanism with the term "Levantinism."
[58] Cf. Snir 2017, p. 267.
[59] Micheau 2008, pp. 219–45.

by al-Musawi as a "prototype for an Islamic republic of letters," is not a coincidence):

> Khalaf ibn al-Muthannā related: Ten persons used to meet in Basra regularly. There was no equivalent to this gathering for the diversity of the religions and sects of its members: al-Khalīl ibn Aḥmad—a *sunnī* (Sunni), and al-Sayyid ibn Muḥammad al-Ḥimyarī—*rāfiḍī* (Shiite), and Ṣāliḥ ibn 'Abd al-Qaddūs—*thanawī* (dualist), and Sufyān ibn Mujāshi'—*ṣufrī* (Khārijī), and Bashshār ibn Burd—morally depraved and impudent, and Ḥammād 'Ajrad—*zindīq* (heretic), and the exilarch's son—a Jew, and Ibn Naẓīra—*mutakallim al-naṣārā* (a Christian theologian), and 'Amrū the nephew of al-Mu'ayyad—*majūsī* (Zoroastrian), and Rawḥ ibn Sinān al-Ḥarrānī—*ṣābi'ī* (Gnostic). At these gatherings, they used to recite poems, and Bashshār used to say: your verses, Oh man, are better than *sūra* this or that [of the Qur'ān], and from that kind of joking and similar things, they declared Bashshār to be a disbeliever.[60]

Not in its literary heritage, and nowhere in the historical chronicles of Cairo, could we find any text related to similar pluralistic "cosmopolitan" gatherings.[61] Notwithstanding the fact that the glorious and multicultural cosmopolitan image of Baghdad concealed a day-to-day reality of a city that suffered from all kinds of difficulties and troubles, just like any other medieval city, its cosmopolitan nature remained in the Arab cultural imagination for many centuries to come, but was not for a long period a reality on the ground. For example, European travelers visiting Baghdad during the sixteenth and seventeenth centuries reported that several of its quarters were neglected, although the city was still at the time a center of commerce with an international atmosphere, where three main languages (Arabic, Persian, and Turkish) were spoken. Even during the 1920s and 1930s, as well as

60 Al-Dhahabī 1988, p. 383. For another version of this episode, see Ibn Taghribirdī 1930, II, p. 29 (= edition 1992, II, pp. 36–7); on that liberal cultural atmosphere, see also Yāqūt 1991, III, pp. 242–4. For another translation and some remarks, see Tobi 2004, pp. 33, 62. On the atmosphere of freethinking in Basra and on the participants in such gatherings, see also Ibn Warraq 2003, pp. 254–6, who uses the historical materials for his own purposes. Ibn Warraq (b. 1946) is the pen name of a secularist author of Pakistani origin and founder of the Institute for the Secularization of Islamic Society; he believes that the great Islamic civilizations of the past were established in spite of the Qur'ān, not because of it, and that only a secularized Islam can deliver Muslim states from "fundamentalist madness." On the open debate in the classical Muslim world, which included the Jews, see also Fischel 1938, pp. 181–7; Baron 1957, V, pp. 83–5; MacDonald 1960 [1903], p. 194; al-Ḥumaydī 1989, I, pp. 175–6; Wasserstrom 1995, p. 113 and the references in n. 71.

61 The closest text we can find is about the Fatimid vizier of Jewish origin Ya'qūb ibn Killis (930–991), a gifted administrator and a lover of Arabic *belles lettres* who wrote books on Islamic law and the Qur'ān; he used to hold weekly Tuesday gatherings, *majlis* sessions, at home and provided stipends for scholars, writers, poets, jurists, theologians, and master artisans participating in them. Fridays he would convene sessions at which he would read his own works (Cohen and Somekh 1990, pp. 283–314).

during the 1960s, Baghdad was known for its remarkable religious tolerance, multicultural atmosphere, and ability to bear witness to the peaceful coexistence of all of its inhabitants,[62] but this was for very short periods.

Also, al-Musawi argues that the pervasive Islamic consciousness that takes the Arabic language as its pivotal point seems more important here than a metropolitan–peripheral demarcation:

> Under precarious and ever-shifting politics, centers at any given time may be replaced by other centers, and scholars are compelled to develop their own counterstrategies in a vast Islamic domain where theological studies hold sway. Thus, the issue of centers and peripheries is secondary in relation to cultural activity.[63]

Apart from the premise that the very use of the term "republic of letters" demands the adoption of the center–periphery binary, it seems unlikely that the issue of centers and peripheries could be "secondary in relation to cultural activity" in any "republic of letters." Studies of the hierarchy of cultural activities indicate that the idea of any literary or cultural system is based on the hypothesis that, although the activities within a periphery, any periphery, essentially differ from those at the center, all cultural activities should be taken into account—those of the center as well as those of the periphery.[64] According to Casanova's study, Paris established itself as the center, namely, as the city with the most literary prestige on the face of the earth: "The exceptional concentration of *literary* sources that occurred in Paris over the course of several centuries gradually led to its recognition as the center of the *literary* world."[65] Quoting this very sentence, al-Musawi writes that "such description is no less applicable to Cairo; it stood to the postclassical Islamic world as Paris stood to Europe,"[66] but no scholar of Arab-Islamic civilization can testify to that. Moreover, al-Musawi does not refer only to *literary* texts and activities, for he states that his "interdisciplinary critique conforms to a contemporaneous definition of the term *adab*, one through which aesthetics, the sciences, and crafts of professions transform the cultural landscape at the same time as they undergo ruptures and shifts."[67] The term *adab* resists precise definition despite many attempts by scholars—in fact, as Bilal Orfali indicates, each attempt at a definition has resulted in excluding some work that a medieval scholar would have considered *adab*.

62 Duclos 2012, pp. 391–401. See also Snir 2013, pp. 5–8.
63 Al-Musawi 2015b, p. 2.
64 As proposed in Snir 2017, pp. 35–99.
65 Casanova 2004, p. 54 (my emphasis).
66 Al-Musawi 2015b, p. 7.
67 Al-Musawi 2015b, p. 14.

But, "nearly all proposed definitions agree, however, that moral and social upbringing, intellectual education, and entertainment are key ingredients of *adab*."[68] In chapter 6, al-Musawi refers to an ancient definition for the same term that was offered by Muḥammad ibn Ibrāhīm ibn al-Akfānī (d. 1348) in the translation of George Makdisi (1920–2002):

> *Adab* is a field of knowledge by virtue of which mutual understanding of what is in the minds is acquired through word-signs and writing. The word and writing are its subject-matter with respect to their communication of ideas. Its benefit is that it discloses intentions in the mind of one person, communicating them to another person, present or absent. *Adab* is the ornament of the tongue, and of the finger tips. By virtue of *adab,* man is distinguished from the rest of the animals. I have begun with *adab* because it is the first element of perfection; he who is devoid of it will not achieve perfection through any of the other human perfections.[69]

Al-Musawi adds the following:

> The term *adab* refers to both a field and a practice, meaning that there is a littérateur, *adīb*, who is distinctly different from the "scientist" or *'ālim*, especially when both terms can be inclusive of all learned people ... Throughout the course of Islamic history and before the advent of a European modernity, the term *adab* as literature was inclusive of poetry and prose but not restricted to them. Its semantic field included refinement and good manners, in the tradition of the notion of *belles lettres,* while at the same time partaking of an all-inclusive network of knowledge with no specific boundaries. It was only with the arrival of European modernity through colonization or incorporation that *adab* became institutionalized as a term referring specifically to literary writing, a process mediated through colleges fashioned after French and British models, all the way to the Higher Teachers' Colleges in Egypt and later Baghdad. Those colleges also happened to include among their graduates the most influential literary figures associated with literary modernity.[70]

Unlike Casanova, and because there is no equation between *belles lettres* and *adab* in its premodern sense, al-Musawi argues that the premodern Islamic

68 Orfali 2012, pp. 29–30, and see the references in n. 1.

69 Makdisi 1990, p. 93. It is quoted from Ibn al-Akfānī's *Kitāb Irshād al-Qāṣid ilā Asnā al-Maqāṣid* (Ibn al-Akfānī 1998, p. 18. Cf. al-Musawi 2015b, pp. 180–1, where Makdisi's translation is quoted, according to al-Musawi, "with some editorial changes" (n. 7, on p. 369), which, in my view, are unnecessary.

70 Al-Musawi 2015b, pp. 181–2 (for other references and indications for the term *adab*, see also pp. 369–70, n. 7). See also Makdisi 1981, pp. 79, 214, 306–7, 309; and the numerous mentions in Makdisi 1990 (see index); Bray 2011, pp. 383–413. On *adab* and the tradition of Islamic encyclopedic writing, see Muhanna 2017, pp. 7–11, 38–42. See also Bauer 2013a, pp. 38–42; Orfali and Baalbaki 2015, pp. 1–26; Bellino 2020, p. 124, n. 3. On *adab* and history, see Toral-Niehoff 2015, pp. 61–85.

republic is not merely *literary*.[71] With respect to *adab* in its *modern* sense—the *literary* dimensions of cultural production—one can perhaps agree that Cairo in the modern period, at least during the first half of the twentieth century,[72] stood in relation to the Arab world as Paris did to Europe. However, there is no consensus among scholars regarding Cairo as the *literary* center throughout the time span of the postclassical Islamic era, particularly against the backdrop of the fragmentation of the Arab literary center after the fall of Baghdad.

Also, it is difficult to write about any "republic of letters" in the postclassical era without being aware of several significant studies in the field of world literature, including *Before European Hegemony* by the American sociologist Janet Abu-Lughod (1928–2013). In her book, Abu-Lughod deals with the formation of a "world system" in the thirteenth and fourteenth centuries, referring to the network of contacts from northwest Europe to China across the Middle East and India. This system consisted of eight subsystems; the Middle East was a geographic fulcrum with strategic world cities like Baghdad and Cairo. They stood out "as dual imperial centers, but their linkages through overland and sea routes tied them selectively to an 'archipelago' of hinterlands."[73] The studies of the German historian of science Sonja Brentjes (b. 1951) are also important: dealing with the interests of the (West European) republic of letters in the Middle East, one cannot ignore her insight about the flexible and permeable boundaries of any republic:

> The Republic of Letters—its territory with its centers and peripheries, its population and their hierarchies, its values, norms, and codes of behavior, and its cognitive projects—has been described in recent studies ... as universal, but West European; as non-denominational, but Western Christian; as liberal, socially mobile, and apolitical, but authority-worshipping, group-conscious, and involved in politico-religious intrigues and battles; and as favoring "right" behavior over "right" knowledge. In other words, it appears to have been a fairly close-knit community which by weaving various conflicting hopes, dreams, and beliefs into patterns of "correct" behavior and speech tried to gain independence

[71] It is important in this regard to mention the view that the Arabic concept of *adab* carries much the same sense as eighteenth-century French literature: "learning and good breeding" (D'haen et al. 2013, p. 321).

[72] See Snir 2005, p. 75, n. 192. See also the findings that came out of a special project initiated by the Egyptian magazine *al-Risāla* in 1936: writers from all over the Arab world were asked to report on the state of the "literary life" (*al-ḥayāt al-adabiyya*) in their region. This report was published in successive issues of *al-Risāla*; most of the reports mentioned the central status of Egypt in Arabic culture and the marginality of other regions (cf. Snir 2017, pp. 151n, 168n, 246n).

[73] Abu-Lughod 1989; the quotation is from p. 14. And see also Allan 2016, and the insightful review by Hoda El Sharky in *Journal of Arabic Literature* 48 (2017), pp. 327–49.

> and protect itself from the harsh West European social, religious, economic, and political realities. While there is no reason to doubt that the members of the Republic of Letters indeed tried to cope with life by drawing clear and at times even solid boundaries, the description of those boundaries as given by [number of studies] on early modern history of science is ... much too rigid. It tends to simplify the complexity of the relations between the values, norms, and codes of behaviors and the quests for knowledge that governed and motivated the Republic of Letters. The territorial, cognitive, and religious boundaries were much more flexible and permeable than their confinement to Western Europe implies.[74]

5. THE CORPUS

Unlike the body of texts investigated in Casanova's model, the "extensive corpus" of texts that al-Musawi examines "through various lenses"[75] and the potential texts that he considers as belonging to his "republic" do not include only *literary* texts, as we have just seen from the latter's definition of the term *adab*. Notwithstanding my view that, like Plato's ideal republic, a republic of letters is something that can exist only in literature,[76] when the texts al-Musawi deals with are *literary*—whatever definition of the term is adopted—they are in fact largely limited to what I describe in my book as non-canonical literature.[77] Indeed, because of the diglossia that exists in the Arabic language, there is no doubt that literary production in *ʿāmmīyya* should be an important part of the Arabic corpus in any "Islamic republic of letters." Such non-canonical production has unfortunately been largely ignored by most "canonical" scholarship, and from this point of view al-Musawi's study is very important against the backdrop of traditional scholarship, especially in its refusal to ignore literary texts in *ʿāmmīyya* within their relevant contexts. Arabic underwent, as al-Musawi correctly writes, "some of its most serious transformations ... in the form of nonclassical modes and practices," as well as the "upsurge of the so-called *ʿāmmī* (colloquial) poetry." And also: "There was an equally large production of works of *lesser merit* over these centuries, which were intended to nourish a broad populace in quest of knowledge." No less important is the awareness that these activities "are no less

74 Brentjes 1999, pp. 464–5. See also Brentjes 2001, pp. 121–48; Brentjes 2010.

75 Al-Musawi 2015b, p. 8.

76 Partly because, as Jacques Derrida argues, literature can be thought of as being "the institution which allows one to *say everything, in every way*" ("This Strange Institution Called Literature: An Interview with Jacques Derrida," trans. Geoffrey Bennington and Rachel Bowlby, in Attridge 1992, p. 36).

77 Snir 2017, pp. 65–89.

foundational for cultural capital than the belletristic cultural tradition" and that, along with bringing canonical works into communal use, poetry and rhetoric "are no longer the monopoly of the elite."[78] The cultural creativity of the "street" (quotation marks in the original) and popular responses to literature are mentioned as "part of this vibrant encounter and unfolding" within the "republic of letters" and are contrasted to the literary production of "scholars and other elites."[79] This "cultural creativity" refers to popular performances in public urban spaces, such as markets, mosques, hospices, and colleges, as well as Ṣūfī *dhikr*, mourning rituals, festivities, and epics (along with an increasing awareness in compendiums of such activities).[80] All these activities allude to the "democratization of space as a central characteristic of the republic of letters" and the "increasing power of the Arab-Islamic street."[81] Also, the "street," understood as the language of the common people, "made its way into the writing and compilations of highly recognized scholars and poets." The "street" is "the stage on which the body and its physiological expressions in terms of eating and drinking practices are given free rein, which takes them far beyond normative conservative restraints."[82] According to al-Musawi, the republic of letters transcends the boundaries of learned scholars and reaches into the very fringes of society:

> Nonclassical poetic subgenres, especially the ones with street registers, cover the lands of Islam from Andalusia and North Africa to Mosul in the North of Iraq and bring into circulation words, images, and rhythms that also raise serious questions regarding the efforts of current scholarship to assign specific geographical and territorial locations and identities to popular literature.[83]

Also, the republic of letters "was forced to expand its parameters so as to host the street, and it did so in the relative absence of the court, whose role as a literary and cultural center had diminished since the decline of the caliphate."[84]

Unfortunately, no chapter of al-Musawi's book focuses on the *zajal* or *muwashshaḥ* genres. Also, various popular cultural activities of the period, such as the semi-theatrical forms of entertainment, should have been mentioned.[85] One of the literary works included in the non-canonical corpus that

[78] Al-Musawi 2015b, pp. 7, 11 (my emphasis), 50, and 166–7, respectively.
[79] Al-Musawi 2015b, pp. 9, 43, and 62.
[80] Al-Musawi 2015b, pp. 17–18, 48–50, 79, 120, 270–2, 298–303.
[81] Al-Musawi 2015b, pp. 43 and 119–20, respectively. On "street poetry," see pp. 263–70.
[82] Al-Musawi 2015b, pp. 245 and 286, respectively.
[83] Al-Musawi 2015b, p. 134.
[84] Al-Musawi 2015b, p. 263.
[85] See, for example, Moreh 1992; Snir 1993, pp. 149–70. In his book, al-Musawi mentions incidentally and cursorily the assemblies and memorial processions and practices to

al-Musawi examined is *A Thousand and One Nights,* on which he had already published extensively.[86] But al-Musawi uses these stories only for thematic purposes, such as for "a testimony to the power of knowledge." When referring to their "successful entry into Europe," he should have noted that their entry into Europe would later be the cause of the gradual change of their status in the Arabic literary system.[87] The emergence of popular genres and the achievements of the "street" poets and writers in the postclassical era justify the rejection of the Orientalist discourse regarding the decadence and decline of Arab culture during this period.[88] That very Orientalist discourse reflects the paradigm that sees political changes as pivotal in their effects on cultural life. For example, the destruction of Baghdad in 1258 by Hulagu has been unjustifiably engraved on the Arabs' memory as the fundamental reason for what was seen as the destruction of their great medieval civilization and the cause of its cultural stagnation until the *Nahḍa* in the nineteenth century.[89] Prompted by European Orientalists, Arabs placed emphasis on the aforementioned descriptions of the killing of many of the local scholars and men of letters by the Mongol army, the demolition of cultural institutions, the burning of libraries, the throwing of books into the Tigris, and the using of these books as a bridge to cross the river. While I was writing the introduction for *Baghdad: The City in Verse* (2013), I encountered many such texts in historical narratives and literary histories, as well as in a variety of other sources in both poetry and prose. Furthermore, as mentioned above, modern Arab leaders and officials have used the devastation caused by Hulagu for their own "patriotic" aims, one prominent example of this being the late Egyptian president Jamāl 'Abd al-Nāṣir (1918–1970). In another example, a high-level Syrian government official was quoted as saying that "if the Mongols had not burnt the libraries of Baghdad in the thirteenth century, we Arabs would have had so much science, that we would

commemorate the tragedy at the Battle of Karbalā' in 680, which "possessed sufficient resilience to resist elite censorship or repression," and scholars tend to regard them as being separate from literary culture. Brief mentions are also made of several popular epics (pp. 48–50) and of *khayāl al-ẓill* (puppet shadow theater) (p. 26).

86 See, for example, al-Musawi 1981; al-Musawi 1986; al-Musawi 2000; al-Musawi 2009b; al-Musawi 2016. On the growth of modern Arabic fiction against the background of the increasing interest in *A Thousand and One Nights,* see also al-Musawi 2003.

87 Al-Musawi 2015b, pp. 12 and 311, respectively. On this, see also the references in Snir 2017, pp. 91n, 93n.

88 Al-Musawi mentions briefly, without any detailed elaboration, popular epics, such as *Sayf ibn Dhī Yazan, al-Amīra Dhāt al-Himma, al-Sīra al-Hilāliyya,* and *al-Ẓāhir Baybars* (p. 50); the colloquial *mawwāl* (p. 96); and the *zajal* (p. 126).

89 On this, see Allen 2006, p. 13: "[W]ithin a literary-historical context the year 1258 cannot serve as a useful divide ... the most significant processes of change in that context belong to an earlier period."

long since have invented the atomic bomb. The plundering of Baghdad put us back centuries."[90]

The emphasis laid by al-Musawi on non-canonical literature is a very fresh approach to the scholarship of Arabic literature—my book provides the rationale and reasoning for the inclusion of non-canonical production from the point of view of aesthetic legitimization as well as from the standpoint of the actual people who are constituent of Arab culture.[91] Nevertheless, the "layered structure," according to al-Musawi, which held together the "seemingly disparate modes of writing, rewriting, compilation, revision, commentary, and disputation in nearly every field of knowledge,"[92] seems to be incomplete and unbalanced, as there is paradoxically almost *no mention* of what was considered in the premodern period to be *canonical* poetry and prose. This absence in such a study that aspires to explore "the large-scale and *diverse* cultural production in Arabic in the postclassical era" (my emphasis) is unjustifiable, certainly when it is expected to inspire the new generation of scholars of premodern Arabic literature. A brief look at the contents of Allen and Richards' *Arabic Literature in the Post-Classical Period* (2006) reveals the wealth of "elite poetry" and "elite prose" that existed side by side with "popular poetry" and "popular prose."[93] Thomas Bauer's contributions in this regard are extremely important as well.[94]

6. THE "REVOLUTIONARY VERNACULARIZING THRUST"

Al-Musawi argues that the concentration of scholars, authors, and copyists in Cairo and other Islamic centers valorized Arabic but also prompted what he calls, borrowing Casanova's words, the "revolutionary vernacularizing thrust" noticeable throughout the Islamic world. Al-Musawi refers to that "thrust" as making

> heavy use of lexical transmission, appropriation, and transference of Arabic grammar, rhetoric, and poetics. National languages also brought into Arabic their own distinctive traits ... Arabic itself underwent some of its most serious transformations, in the form of nonclassical modes and practices that were

[90] On Hulagu's destruction of Baghdad and what has been engraved in the Arabs' collective memory, see Snir 2013, pp. 26–31. On the topos of Baghdad's destruction, see also above, Chapter 3, Section 4.

[91] See Snir 2017, pp. 14–19.

[92] Al-Musawi 2015b, p. 8.

[93] Allen and Richards 2006, pp. v–vi. See also Allen 2006, pp. 17–21.

[94] See, for example, Bauer 2005, pp. 105–32; Bauer 2007, pp. 137–67. See also a special issue of *Annales Islamologiques* (vol. 49 [2016]) under the title "Arabic Literature, 1200–1800: A New Orientation," edited by Monica Balda-Tillier and Adam Talib.

> theorized by several prominent scholars, and in the upsurge of the so-called *'āmmī* (colloquial) poetry. Hence, in spite of linguistic divergence, a common Islamic literary, theological, and symbolic field emerged that warrants the present discussion of an Islamic republic of letters. The massive production that *has unsettled Arab modernists* attests to this cultural space.[95]

I will refer below to al-Musawi's campaign against the "modernists," which "necessitates" his argument that "the massive production [has] unsettled Arab modernists," and only concentrate here on his approach to the "vernacularizing thrust." Casanova, while engaging the prior work of Benedict Anderson on nationalism,[96] speaks of the "revolutionary vernacularizing thrust of capitalism" as the first stage in the genesis of a *world literary space* that "saw the exclusive use of Latin among educated men give way first to a demand for intellectual recognition of vulgar tongues, then to the creation of modern literatures claiming to compete with the grandeur of ancient literatures."[97] The second major stage in the enlargement of the literary world, according to Casanova, corresponds to the "philological-lexicographic revolution" that saw the appearance in Europe of new nationalist movements associated with the invention or reinvention of national languages and the creation of popular literatures. The third and final stage was the process of decolonization, which marked "the entry into international competition of contestants who until then had been prevented from taking part."[98] Almost nothing of these three stages exists in al-Musawi's analysis of the genesis of world *Islamic* literary space. Here, it is instructive to refer to an observation by the Moroccan scholar Abdelfattah Kilito (b. 1945) regarding the importance of understanding the literary output of the postclassical period on its own terms, because it is relevant in the present context:

> To us it seems more appropriate to regard Arabic poetics on its own terms and so to avoid treating the subject as some kind of deviation from a model realized in other times and under other skies. The governing principle should be derived from characteristics that are intrinsic to it, not those of works from some other poetics.[99]

95 Al-Musawi 2015b, p. 7 (my emphasis).
96 Anderson 1991, p. 39.
97 Casanova 2004, pp. 47–8.
98 Casanova 2004, p. 48.
99 Kilito 1983, p. 136. Translation according to Allen 2006, p. 20. For the Arabic translation, see Kilito 1993, p. 114. Cf. Phillips 2008, p. 297, regarding the attempt to apply Gérard Genette's model of hypertextuality to Najīb Maḥfūẓ's *Malḥamat al-Ḥarāfish* (1977). For the need for "homegrown modernity" and the issue of extroversion and introversion, see Helgesson 2015, pp. 253–60. See also Ricci 2011. Unlike al-Musawi, who posits his analysis as a counter-narrative to the European impact on Arabic literary modernity, Ricci deals with the inter-Asian travels of Arabic and brings into focus an Arabic cosmopolis in south

In this regard, the experience of Henry Louis Gates, Jr., concerning Black discourse of criticism is illuminating:

> The Western critical tradition has a canon, as the Western literary tradition does. I once thought it our most important gesture to *master* the canon of criticism, to *imitate* and *apply* it, but I now believe that we must turn to the black tradition itself to develop theories of criticism indigenous to our literatures.[100]

7. THE ROLE OF SUFISM

Al-Musawi frequently mentions the challenge posed to dominant ways of thought through the agency of Sufism because it "involved a liberated sensibility in a loving God's universe" and because it was "a challenge to official schools of thought since it disturbs and unsettles their paradigms of self-righteousness and dogma."[101] Also, "Ṣūfi terminology strips language of its denotative role and sets it free. Words and nature leave their signifiers behind and assume new life in the soaring of the liberated Ṣūfi experience, which may be seen as a partial anticipation of *postmodern musings on madness and poetry.*" Ṣūfi orders as well "turned Sufism into *a poetic enterprise and practice in a God-loving universe* ... its significance for the republic of letters extends even beyond its deconstruction of the prosaic and the mundane; for its striking freedom and newness in vision and illumination also necessarily downplay structures of authority and power."[102] Because I have extensively written on the intersection of Arabic literature and Sufism from the latter's rise until the second half of the twentieth century,[103] I can say here that one

and southeast Asia, underscoring as well "the power of literature to create, enable, and sustain far-reaching transformation" (Ricci 2014, p. 504. Cf. Ganguly 2015, pp. 278–9). See also Thomas Bauer's suggestion concerning the need to "listen patiently to Mamluk authors and carefully analyze their texts, to elucidate their own aesthetic standards, and judge their texts by this rather than apply a yardstick of heroism that does not match the participational aesthetics of the Mamluk middle class" (Bauer 2013, pp. 21–2. Cf. Bauer 2007, p. 144). In her review article of the aforementioned Allen and Richards 2006 and Khaled al-Rouayheb's *Before Homosexuality in the Arabic-Islamic World 1500–1800* (al-Rouayheb 2005), Hilary Kilpatrick emphasizes "the need to abandon modern concepts that stand in the way of understanding the texts and contexts of the period under discussion, and to analyse perceptively the terms used by the people of the time" ("Beyond Decadence: Dos and Don'ts in Studying Mamluk and Ottoman Literature," *Middle Eastern Literatures* 12.1 [2009], p. 78).

100 Gates 1985, p. 13.

101 Al-Musawi 2015b, pp. 78–9.

102 Al-Musawi 2015b, pp. 142–3 (my emphasis), 309 (my emphasis), respectively.

103 See, for example, the following studies: Snir 1986; Snir 2002; Snir 2006. On the Sufi experience and on "musings on madness and poetry," which are not necessarily postmodern, see Snir 1993, pp. 74–88.

must distinguish between the role of early Sufism in reviving Arab society and culture, the various literary genres included in this revival, and the negative phenomena later attributed to Ṣūfī orders, especially in the premodern period.

8. IDENTITARIAN MARKERS IN THE MAKEUP OF "MODERNITY" AND THE *NAHḌA* PROJECT

In a follow-up article to his book, al-Musawi refers to three sociocommunal markers of formative presence in the makeup of "Arab modernity" and its concretization in the nation-state: first, "the use of a poem from the medieval period to provide the structure and syntax of the Arab national flag in the fight for independence from the Ottomans"; second, "the reclamation of the Mamluk terms of parity between state administration and the role of the intelligentsia"; and, third, "the generation of lexical conversation and lexicographic production with deep roots in both genealogical tradition and rhetorical ancestry." According to al-Musawi, these three instances "are strongly linked to identitarian politics and hence also raise questions regarding the complexity of the so-called 'Awakening' (*nahḍah*) project, with its many preoccupations, concerns, methodologies, and conspicuous appropriations from colonial culture." Al-Musawi shows how these three markers were deployed in the Arab world at the end of the nineteenth century against a landscape most often "grounded in negativity, shrouding the period in concepts of decadence and loss, blotting it out as [an] unfortunate anticlimax to an otherwise golden age."[104]

The fact that these three "identitarian markers" from the premodern period are reproduced in the nineteenth century by intellectuals that contributed to the Arab "Awakening" by no means implies *any* overall attitude toward the premodern period. On the contrary, these intellectuals found themselves drawn to leading conceptualizations and tropes that "differ in a significant way from the dominant disparagement of the [premodern] period" *only because they were glancing unbiasedly toward their past heritage*, choosing and picking what they considered suitable for their contemporary needs. That is why I utterly disagree with al-Musawi's abstruse or simply superfluous argument:

> Unless we are willing to conceive the consolidated and intense conversation at the turn of the nineteenth and early twentieth century between religious thinkers, secularists like Faraḥ Anṭūn [1874–1922] and Yaʿqūb Ṣarrūf [1852–1927], and journalists and writers as being a site of vigorous national awareness, we

[104] Al-Musawi 2014, p. 272. More details about these markers appear on pp. 272–80.

> are bound to overlook not only the permeation of the culture of the middle period into the "modernity" project, but also the relevance of the politics of the medieval Islamic republic of letters. Even when seemingly subdued, that earlier cultural tradition, with its many paradigmatic and axial categories, continued to inform the modernity project and at times unsettle its excessive internalization of Western orientations.[105]

This is a one-sided and unbalanced reflection on the culture and politics of "the medieval Islamic republic of letters" and their relevance to the "modernity project" at the turn of the nineteenth and early twentieth centuries, which unnecessarily overemphasizes the "unsettling" of the "excessive internalization of Western orientations." The most current research on the period has by no means challenged the conception that the "modernity project" used *all means at its disposal* without distinguishing between various orientations and periods.

9. LEXICONS AND TRANSLATION

Referring to the just-mentioned "lexicographic production with deep roots in both genealogical tradition and rhetorical ancestry," in chapter 3 of his book, al-Musawi writes about the "lexicographic turn in cultural capital." The diligence shown by scholars during the nineteenth century in their pursuit of lexicography and the deep roots of their production in both genealogical tradition and rhetorical ancestry are presented against the backdrop of massive lexicons and encyclopedic dictionaries composed across the Islamic lands during the premodern period. The scholarly and academic neglect of this "lexicographic turn," according to al-Musawi, speaks to an "educational failure":

> The textual archeological archive, visible at its clearest in its lexical component, is usually bypassed in modern academic discussions, not only inside the Arab world but also in Western academies that instead are exclusively focused on periodicals, narratives, and text-based disciplines. People tend to forget that the lexicographical presence presupposes not only grammatical and linguistic knowledge, but also a full-scale corpus of aural and literate culture.[106]

Al-Musawi's attitude toward lexicographic production, however, is by no means consistent. Referring, for example, to Edward William Lane's (1801–1876) efforts in producing his lexicon, al-Musawi writes that the

[105] Al-Musawi 2014, p. 275.
[106] Al-Musawi 2015, p. 116.

"purpose and expediency" behind these efforts could not have been lost on Arab intellectuals and scholars:

> What could be more conducive to *imperial expansion* than the training of its personnel in Arabic and to have *empire philologists* on demand to explain and justify means and notions of *command, control, and ultimate takeover*? ... The *empire* generates its interests through a lexical mapping that preserves *verbal utility* in the colonized lands through a pragmatic use of native languages under the positivist drive. In the colonial production of lexicons and their implementation in teaching colonial personnel, *the defining criteria involve utility and interest.*[107]

Against the background of this negative attitude toward the author of one of the best Arabic–English dictionaries in scholarly research, the lexicographic efforts of "early advocates of Arab modernity" to bring Arabic into "the domain of the struggle for independence" are described by al-Musawi in the most favorable terms:

> The link between these initiatives and the earlier lexicographical movement that was so noticeably strong in the middle period is the new emphasis on social groups, their use of language, and their actual practices ... From Buṭrus al-Bustānī and al-Shartūnī to Fāris al-Shidyāq and Father Anāstās Mārī al-Kirmilī (sic!) and beyond, *the lexicon now became more or less a verbal reconstruction of the nation. In a deft and highly conscious systematization, verbal roots with meanings relevant to nation building increase in number in keeping with needs and priorities.*[108]

This Manichean distinction between the wicked "colonial production of lexicons" and the blessed "verbal reconstruction of the nation" is so biased and one-sided from the academic scholarly point of view, that al-Musawi's far-out conceptualizing could not possibly induce any change in the current certitude of serious scholars that Lane's dictionary is irreplaceable, certainly as compared with other relevant dictionaries, among them those mentioned by al-Musawi himself (although Lane died before completing it and the sections completed by his nephew, after the root QD, are not on par with the rest of the book).[109] In line with the postcolonial, or better postscholarly character of the way al-Musawi discusses this issue, one can be sure that if instead of Edward William Lane the name here had been Anwar Walīd Labadī, he would have never dared utter any critical remark against this dictionary or its author. Exposing another important scholar to the danger

[107] Al-Musawi 2014, p. 278 (my emphasis).
[108] Al-Musawi 2014, p. 279 (my emphasis).
[109] Arab scholars as well referred to the great merits of Lane's dictionary; see, for example, Nūr 1973, pp. 237–54.

of being labeled as an "empire philologist" who should be considered part of "the colonial production of lexicons and their implementation in teaching colonial personnel," I will quote what A. J. Arberry (1905–1969) wrote about Lane's dictionary:

> Lane's *Lexicon* is a work of such fundamental importance and of such matchless excellence that praise for it is quite superfluous ... It is certainly true to say, that every work produced in this century relating in any way to Arabic studies has drawn heavily upon the *Lexicon*. It is a sufficient tribute to its unique greatness, that to this day it remains supreme in the field of Arabic lexicography: *no scholar or group of scholars has produced anything to supplant it.*[110]

Al-Musawi develops the evil–good dichotomy into what he describes obscurely as "an ironic twist of fortune" whereby paronomasia and antithesis establish a presence in imperial rhetoric, the word *empire* (i.e., lexicons) being put into the service of a world empire, and the word *qāmūs* (dictionary) itself grew genealogically over time and became "no longer only a container of lexis, but rather a *generator of identity and nationhood*."[111] However, there is another dimension to this false Manichean distinction, and it concerns al-Musawi's xenophobic attitude toward non-Arab philologists, since this is the only reason for which Lane is described as an "imperial" opportunist, whose scholarly criteria involve nothing but "utility and interest." Had al-Musawi troubled himself to read Lane's scholarship without such prejudices, he would have discovered the great difference between Lane, for example, and Richard Burton (1821–1890), the translator of the first unexpurgated English version of *Alf Layla wa-Layla* (1885–1888). Burton projected, according to the British Syrian cultural historian Rana Kabbani (Ranā Qabbānī) (b. 1958), every imaginable kind of sexual perversion onto the Orient using the *Arabian Nights* "to express himself, to articulate his sexual preoccupations" as well as to "serve as an occasion for documenting all manner of sexual deviation." Moreover, his fascination with the *Arabian Nights* "was greatly enhanced by the fact that they upheld his own views on women, race and class."[112] On the other hand, Lane was by no means what

[110] Arberry 1960, p. 116 (my emphasis).

[111] Al-Musawi 2014, pp. 279 (my emphasis) and 280 (my emphasis), respectively.

[112] Kabbani 1986, pp. 7, 60–1, and 48, respectively. On the association of the Orient with sexual fantasies, see Said 1985 [1978], p. 190; Hopwood 1999, pp. 180–2. Cf. Snir 2017, p. 94. Anna Ziajka Stanton argues that Burton's translation is neither a faithful nor an original translation of *Alf Layla wa-Layla*, but rather an English text whose "aesthetic enjoyment is proffered as an affective engagement with the literary aesthetics of the source text, translated through Burton's own pleasurable experiences of Arabic literary language." Framing the reception of Burton's translation, through the Arabic concept of *ṭarab*, as a process of iterative cycles of pleasure that move between the translator and his readers, she contends that "what makes Burton's Nights enjoyable to read also makes it scandalous

al-Musawi calls an "empire philologist," as he never offered his services "to explain and justify means and notions of command, control, and ultimate takeover," and his lexicon did not serve to teach "colonial personnel" with the defining criteria involving "utility and interest." Lane explained his decision to translate the *Arabian Nights* as follows:

> I consider myself possessed of the chief qualifications for the proper accomplishment of my present undertaking, from my having lived several years in Cairo, associating almost exclusively with Arabs, speaking their language, conforming to their general habits with the most scrupulous exactitude, and received into their society on terms of perfect equality.[113]

Accordingly, he even saw it fit to "domesticate" and "sanitize" the texts of the stories, removing or changing "objectionable" tales and anecdotes—thus rendering them "so as to be perfectly agreeable with Arab manners and customs."[114] Against the negative attitude of al-Musawi toward Lane, certainly inspired by Edward Said's campaign against the "Orientalists," Lane included,[115] here is how Leila Ahmed concludes her study of Lane's life and works and of the British ideas of the Middle East in the nineteenth century:

> To disclose a living culture to the members of another, to disclose it so as to show its ways and beliefs as entirely intelligible, to respect, in the presentation of these, their intrinsic validity—to the extent that a native of that culture can assent to the general accuracy of the presentation—is a formidable achievement. It is the more formidable, and the more urgent, in relation to a people and a culture respecting which the author's native culture, as is the case with the Europeans and the peoples of the Near East, possesses a rich and assorted heritage of myths, legends, and emotively highly charged and often hostile traditions. And although the dissipation on [the] literary level of many of the myths and legends relating to the Arab world by no means automatically entailed the eradication of emotional and imaginative attitudes and habits pertaining to it—habits, some of them, ingrained over centuries and so remarkably pertinacious—Lane's work created for his compatriots a clearing within which such

to the world literary system within which it has circulated" (Stanton 2021, pp. 45–64. The quotation is from p. 45).

113 Lane 1914 [1859], I, p. xii.

114 Lane 1914 [1859], I, pp. xvii. Cf. Naddaff 2014, pp. 489–90.

115 Although Said credits Lane as a scholar who used his residence in Egypt "for the specific task of providing professional Orientalism with scientific material," he does not hesitate to write that "[Lane's] identity as counterfeit believer and privileged European is the very essence of bad faith, for the latter undercuts the former in no uncertain way" (Said 1985 [1978]), pp. 157–8 and 161, respectively). For a more balanced attitude toward Lane, see Dhabab 2005, pp. 56–9.

attitudes could not easily and openly flourish, and equipped them with the means to thrust further back the darkness.[116]

The issue of translation presents another example of al-Musawi's biased methodology. In his campaign against the "modernists" (to which I will refer in detail below), al-Musawi dedicates long sections to the 1920 preface by Ṭāhā Ḥusayn (1889–1973) to the Arabic version of Johann Wolfgang von Goethe's (1749–1832) *Die Leiden des jungen Werthers,* translated from the French by Aḥmad Ḥasan al-Zayyāt (1885–1968),[117] as well as to the issue of translation in general.[118] Referring to Ṭāhā Ḥusayn's preface, al-Musawi writes about the implications of negativism, "as they lead to a *deliberate negligence* on the part of some *nahḍah* scholars to overlook significant and in fact groundbreaking contributions to the theories of translation as laid down by al-Jāḥiẓ, for example." Furthermore, Ṭāhā Ḥusayn, to whom al-Musawi refers in the aforementioned quotation, "may be excused for his indiscriminate critique of some nineteenth-century verbosity that sounds jarring enough to those acquainted with Abbasid and European-informed prose writing, [but] there is little reason to justify his *repression* of the Abbasid source on translation."[119] And how al-Musawi reached this "insight" is very instructive and may give us an illuminative hint about the prejudiced motives of his campaign against the "modernists." The great "sin" of Ṭāhā Ḥusayn, according to al-Musawi, is that in his aforementioned preface he did not mention al-Jāḥiẓ's contributions to the theories of translation. Reading the preface, one cannot understand how several sentences therein, whose general aim is to praise al-Zayyāt for the translation of the book, could have led al-Musawi to build such a house of cards. The preface *was not written for the scholarly community,* but rather for a wider readership, and it was not meant to be a scientific introduction to the book. As it was a popular preface addressed to the common reader, any discussion about theories of translation would have undoubtedly been a troublesome distraction.

10. EXTROVERSION–INTROVERSION AND THE IMPACT OF "COLONIAL MODERNITY"

In his response to al-Musawi's contribution in the "Forum on Literary World Systems" of the *Cambridge Journal of Postcolonial Literary Inquiry*, the South

[116] Ahmed 1978, p. 199.
[117] Goethe 1968.
[118] Al-Musawi 2015, pp. 121–30.
[119] Al-Musawi 2015, pp. 115 (my emphasis) and 121 (my emphasis), respectively.

African scholar Stefan Helgesson (b. 1966) argues that the crucial theoretical question raised by al-Musawi's study concerns tensions between extroversion and introversion. He summarizes al-Musawi's argument as follows: the *Nahḍa* scholars should have been more introverted—instead of adopting the values and ideals of the European Enlightenment, the deep time of the Arab Republic of Letters when "monographs, massive lexicons, and encyclopedic dictionaries" were produced across the lands of Islam, the writers in question could have supplied the *Nahḍa* with the basis for a homegrown modernity.[120] According to Helgesson, an *attentiveness* to the dynamic relationship between extroversion and introversion affords the most promising theoretical point of departure for a world-literary study that remains alert to the diversity of literatures in the world and yet evades the risk of reifying national or linguistic provenance. Enlisting two examples to illustrate his argument—the Sudanese writer al-Ṭayyib Ṣāliḥ (Tayeb Salih) (1929–2009) and the South African author Sol Plaatje (1876–1932)—Helgesson concludes his essay with the following:

> What we are learning as we extend the paradigm of world literature beyond hegemonic languages and global centers of (cultural) capital is the inherent potential of reconfiguring the problem not just from within any given geohistorical location, or, for that matter, through a recognition of the diachrony of reception as a "thick" history in its own right, but ultimately by *attending to the combined, contradictory, and proliferating trajectories that shape literature in the world.*[121]

Al-Musawi's response to this engagement implies a misunderstanding of Helgesson's argument:

> For a cultured society, Arabic was "cosmopolitan" and universal, even when rulers were not necessarily bound to this practice. Hence, Stefan Helgesson's point is valid in trying to navigate between "extroversion and introversion" *as a third space between one model and another.* No culture can have its world systems or universal and cosmopolitan spread without this reach-out in regions other than its hinterland; the Arabic model with its Afro-Asian multiple centers had its knowledge construction and cultural capital beyond ethnicity and boundaries. Hence, it was wider than any of its components and more complex than regional or city-state formations.[122]

Helgesson talks about attentiveness to the "combined, contradictory, and proliferating" trajectories of the extroversion–introversion dynamics as a theoretical point of departure for a world-literary study, presenting al-Ṭayyib

[120] Helgesson 2015, p. 254.
[121] Helgesson 2015, p. 260 (my emphasis).
[122] Al-Musawi 2015a, p. 285 (my emphasis).

Ṣāliḥ and Sol Plaatje as good examples. Al-Musawi refers to "a third space between one model and another." Helgesson speaks neither about spaces between models, nor about "reach-out in regions other than its hinterland" but simply about the means of scholarly approaches to the literatures of the world at large.

In her own response to al-Musawi's contribution, the Italian scholar of South Asian literature Francesca Orsini (b. 1966) writes that the echoes of al-Musawi's arguments can also be found in South Asian scholarship and public debates, many of which are over the impact of "colonial modernity" and the issue of the "amnesia" that afflicted intellectuals and scholars. The summation of her comments is as follows:

> [M]ore productive than a *critique of modern intellectuals and their "amnesia,"* or a historical narrative about the inevitable rise of the juggernaut English (or French) and the obliteration of everything else in their wake, is to be wary of *single-strand and monolingual historical narratives* (Arabic existed in a multilingual world, too), and conceive of space, whether local or further flung/wider, as the "multiplicity of stories so far," and attend to those stories and the different configurations they produce.[123]

Referring to premodern periods described as "dark middle ages" of "religious and cultural oppression," Orsini argues that the consolidation of colonial power in India, for example, ended the age-old power of Sanskrit learning to shape Indian intellectual history. Instead of responding to Orsini's main argument, or paying attention to the difference between the colonial role in India and that in the Muslim world, where it failed to erode the status of *fuṣḥa*, al-Musawi's response implies, to say the least, a misunderstanding of Orsini's meticulous arguments:

> While, as Francesca Orsini argues, Sanskrit flourished on the eve of colonialism, and continued to do so for some time, *Arabic had struggled to sustain its circulation among rhetors, grammarians, poets, jurists, and philosophers.* From the twelfth to the end of the eighteenth centuries, Arabic was the language of lettered societies. But what Sheldon Pollock argues *can be applicable when we try to*

[123] Orsini 2015, p. 272 (my emphasis). Orsini attributes "the *multiplicity* of stories so far" to Doreen Massey's definition in *For Space* (London: Sage, 2005, p. 9 [my emphasis]). From the three propositions Massey offers in order to make the case for an alternative approach to space, the first refers to space as "the product of interrelations," the second understands space as "the sphere of the possibility of the existence of multiplicity," while the third asserts that "perhaps we could imagine space as a *simultaneity of stories-so-far*" (p. 9 [my emphasis]. On p. 89, Massey writes that "any 'simultaneity' of stories-so-far will be a distinct simultaneity from a particular vantage point").

> *account for dissemination and limit.* For a cultured society, *Arabic was "cosmopolitan" and universal, even when rulers were not necessarily bound to this practice.*[124]

One can hardly follow the rationale of al-Musawi's response, in which everything becomes mixed and confused. Orsini argues that, due to the multilingual and multicultural nature of the world and due to the fact that no single language was completely hegemonic, the early modern Indian story could also be told as a story of the *persistence* of the high languages of Sanskrit and Persian in particular, and in fact the story of the wider dissemination of Persian well into the colonial period. Al-Musawi refers to Sheldon Pollock's "argument," which is irrelevant to Orsini's engagement—she mentions Pollock's scholarship in regards to "Sanskrit knowledge systems on the eve of colonialism" as a "cosmopolis" that was eroded in the historical process of "vernacularization" only to offer an example of a premodern system similar to al-Musawi's premodern republic. When al-Musawi insists on presenting Arabic as always being "cosmopolitan and universal"—something with which no serious scholar can agree—he misunderstands Pollock's conception as well. Much more importantly, following Shu-Mei Shih[125] Orsini refers to the "technologies of recognition" that "selectively and often arbitrarily confer world membership on literatures." Those technologies are "mechanisms in the discursive (un)conscious—with bearings on social and cultural (mis)understandings—that produce 'the West' as the agent of recognition and 'the rest' as the object of recognition, in representation."[126] Here, al-Musawi could have used these technologies as analytical modes to support his argument "with respect to the need to explore other formations of world systems beyond the specific models that scholars of European literature have presented,"[127] but he failed to do so. All in all, Orsini's response implies a strong reservation about al-Musawi's campaign against the "modernists" (see below): in her words, it is a "critique of modern intellectuals" and their "amnesia," which regretfully causes al-Musawi to sink, in her words, into "single-strand and monolingual historical narratives."

Both Helgesson and Orsini mention issues in world literature that need considerably more reflection and exploration, whereas al-Musawi avoids delving into the same significant issues and does not refer to the new turn

124 Al-Musawi 2015a, pp. 284–5 (my emphasis).

125 Shih 2004, pp. 16–30; reprinted in D'haen et al. 2013, pp. 259–74.

126 Shih 2004, pp. 16–17. Orsini identifies those technologies as "ignorance, distaste, and indifference," but in fact, these may be the result of the five modes of recognition that Shih refers to as belonging to the academic discourse and the literary market: the return of the systematic, the time lag of allegory, global multiculturalism, the exceptional particular, and post-difference ethics.

127 Al-Musawi 2015a, p. 282.

toward world literature in the last decade, which in some measure was a result of a disciplinary crisis in American comparative literature in the second half of the 1990s and the beginning of the 2000s. In the same regard, one can find an excellent survey in Dennis Sobolev's recent study, where he analyzes the problems of the textual volume of the corpus under investigation and the cross-cultural translation, the conceptual reflection and the principles of taxonomization, the sociologically oriented reshaping of literary studies and research methods, the problem of "cultural regions," and the homogenization and reification of the objects of study. According to Sobolev, the resultant theoretical complications and unsolved problems seem to outweigh the contribution of the school of world literature to the understanding of literary texts, processes, and structures. He underscores the necessity of returning to the disciplinary self-reflection of comparative literature, the reappraisal of its basic questions and tasks, as one of the major goals of the study of culture at the present moment.[128]

11. CULTURE, SCHOLARSHIP, AND ACCOUNTABILITY

Al-Musawi's book was nominated for the 2016 Sheikh Zayed Book Award for "Arabic Culture in Other Languages" because "it presents a compelling argument against the commonly held opinion that Arabic literature, since the glorious peak of the Abbasids, has somehow failed to be modern, and instead became locked in conventions that were stultifying and rarefied, created only for a small circle of initiates who were themselves censored and censuring."[129] In his endorsement of the book, Roger Allen writes that al-Musawi's study refutes "the orientalist-inspired notion of a 'period of decadence' in the Arabo-Islamic cultural heritage ... With al-Musawi's work, the medieval Arabo-Islamic 'slough of despond'—to cite Bunyan's well-known English phrase—can, one hopes, be forever laid to rest."[130] And al-Musawi is generally right in his rejection of the paradigm that sees political changes as pivotal in their effects on cultural life (although one may reject his decisive relevant statements).[131]

128 Sobolev 2017, pp. 20–53.

129 According to http://www.middle-east-online.com/english/?id=75978, last accessed July 17, 2016.

130 Roger Allen elaborates on what he terms the "decadence paradigm" in Allen 2018, pp. 15–26.

131 Al-Musawi argues that there was no cultural decline but only "political disintegration": the six centuries of political upheaval and loss of a specific or unitary Islamic discourse, according to al-Musawi, "pose a number of challenges to any positivist claims. *Undaunted by this upheaval,* cultural production and its multiplicity across large swathes and times require systematic reading to uncover significant epistemic shifts that should take us beyond a

Scholarship aside, however, one cannot ignore al-Musawi's sharp critical attitude throughout many sections of his book toward those he calls "Arab and Muslim modernists" or "architects of [Arab] modernity," who, in his words, failed to dissociate the "political disintegration" from "the ongoing cultural dissemination and exchange across the Islamic world."[132] He accuses them of misreading their past, of falling back "on a series of negations and denials of [its] merit," and of internalizing the "European Enlightenment disparagement of the Middle Ages ... in their zealous duplication of a seductive Europe."[133] The failure to connect effectively with the rich culture of the past and to establish emotive and cultural links with the Muslim populace, according to al-Musawi, can "easily induce *architects of regression* to involve regions and peoples in schisms and disorder."[134] Al-Musawi also holds the "modernists" *accountable for the failed education system* in the newly emerging *Islamic* nation-states because of the "depreciation of pre-modern Arabic cultural production," which "amounts to a substantial disengagement from a tradition that was much needed for the promotion of education and culture in the newly emerging *Islamic* nation-states."[135] In short, the experienced reader, certainly any scholar of Arab culture, has the feeling that al-Musawi functions here not only as an unbiased scholar and literary critic, but as an active participant in Arab cultural life and, moreover, as an integral part of the Arab-Islamic community in what is presented as the struggle against Western powers and their "internal collaborators."[136]

Unlike most Western scholars of Arabic literature, even those of Arab origin, al-Musawi could be seen as somewhat "justified" in the effacement of the borders between research and participation in a culture. Al-Musawi is now an integral part of the international Western community of scholars and critics of Arabic literature that warmly adopted him and, moreover, made him one of its doyens, perhaps the first one. Born in al-Nāṣiriyya in

blanket disparagement of an age of decadence and stagnation" (al-Musawi 2015a, p. 282 [my emphasis]).

132 Al-Musawi 2015b, p. 11 (see also p. 144).

133 Al-Musawi 2015b, pp. 5, 308–9, and 15, respectively.

134 Al-Musawi 2015b, p. 11 (my emphasis).

135 Al-Musawi 2015b, p. 45 (my emphasis).

136 More than forty years earlier, al-Musawi published a book on Iraqi oil, the struggle with the oil companies, and "the great robbery of the Iraqi people's treasures" (al-Mūsawī 1973; the quotation is from p. 7). One can sense the parallel lines, according to al-Musawi, between the material and spiritual robbery of Arab-Islamic treasures (cf. al-Mūsawī 1973, pp. 5–10; al-Mūsawī 1993; al-Mūsawī 2001; al-Mūsawī 2005, pp. 63–9). Several years ago, al-Musawi had mentioned his plan to publish a monograph titled *Arab Modernists' Struggle with the Past* (according to al-Musawi 2015a, p. 282). However, apart from a lecture he delivered on the topic at Columbia University on October 15, 2015, I have not found any additional publications or presentations by him related to that issue.

Iraq in 1944, and having obtained his PhD from Dalhousie University in Nova Scotia, Canada, in 1978, al-Musawi now holds the prestigious Chair for Arabic Literature at Columbia University. Since 1999, he has been a member of the editorial board of the *Journal of Arabic Literature* (*JAL*), the only professional journal dedicated to the study of Arabic literature, and in recent years he has been serving as its general editor. On January 2022, he was awarded the prestigious King Faisal Prize for Arabic language and literature. Before moving to the West, physically, metaphorically, and spiritually, al-Musawi had, for more than two decades, been an integral part of the literary, cultural, and academic Arab life and its *jumhūr* of littérateurs, sensing its vibrant rhythm and vivacious beating heart, feeling its pains, and looking for ways to push it forward. As an active writer, he published five Arabic novels, and as a scholar he published numerous scholarly books and articles in Arabic. He taught at major Arab universities, such as Baghdad University, Amman National University, San'a University, Tunis University, and the American University of Sharjah. Also, he played a dominant role in government cultural institutions in Baghdad during the regime of Ṣaddām Ḥusayn (1937–2006),[137] serving as the director of the publishing house Dār al-Shu'ūn al-Thaqāfiyya al-'Āmma, the president of the board of directors of another publishing house, al-Adīb al-'Arabī, and the editor-in-chief of the journal *Istishrāq*. He also served as the editor-in-chief of *Āfāq 'Ārabiyya* in Tunis.

But who are those "modernists" whom al-Musawi holds accountable for the failed education system in the newly emerging Islamic nation-states? And with whom does al-Musawi debate, sometimes less as an unbiased critic and literary historian and more as an active proponent with a very clear agenda for the present and particularly for the future? In his *Preliminary Discourse*, al-Musawi mentions Ṭāhā Ḥusayn (1889–1973), Aḥmad Ḥasan al-Zayyāt (1885–1968), and Salāma Mūsā (1887–1958) who, in his words, "have long internalized a European Enlightenment discourse and looked with suspicion and distrust in the past and its massive accumulation in cultural capital."[138] At the end of chapter 1, al-Musawi refers to the "hasty conclusions of the kind often encountered in the writings of many Arab and Afro-Asian

[137] Al-Musawi's brother 'Azīz al-Sayyid Jāsim (1941–1991) was executed in prison upon the orders of Ṣaddām Ḥusayn (for his profile, see al-Musawi 2006, pp. 144–6. On his views, see the same book, which is dedicated to his memory). Al-Musawi himself, who served in his various positions in Iraq under Ṣaddām Ḥusayn, was accused, for no fault of his own, of collaborating with the regime, even after the murder of his brother (see the reactions of readers to a report on al-Musawi, especially comments 2 and 7, at: http://www.alarabiya.net/articles/2011/07/14/157569.html, July 14, 2011, last accessed February 16, 2017).

[138] Al-Musawi 2015b, p. 5. For al-Musawi's first thoughts on the modernists, see the interview with the Saudi diplomat and journalist Turkī al-Dakhīl (b. 1973) at: https://www.youtube.com/watch?v=OHbmF3vS45o, July 25, 2011; last accessed September 16, 2020.

modernists," but, apart from the three names mentioned above, all of them Egyptian, he did not mention other names of those "many."[139] In one place in the book, he mentions the Christian-Lebanese Jurī Zaydān (1861–1914),[140] who was active mainly in Egypt, but he does not mention, for example, great Lebanese "modernists," such as Buṭrus al-Bustānī (1819–1883) and Aḥmad Fāris al-Shidyāq (1805–1887). In what follows, I will respectfully disagree with al-Musawi's position. I will do so not as a proponent of any agenda, of course, but as a student of Arabic literature who has read most, if not all, of his writings and those of the "modernists" he named in his recent work.

I mentioned above the unjustifiable attitude of some Orientalists to pre-modern Arabic literature at large as a "period of decadence," but nowhere could I find in the writings of al-Zayyāt, Mūsā, or Ḥusayn the sweeping statements that al-Musawi attributes to them, as, for example, that the *whole* "literary output of the medieval Arab and Islamic nation-states is *ineffectual*."[141] Feeling that literary sensibility should be altered in order to enable an overhaul of Arabic literature, they indeed rejected some literary values of the postclassical period, but they did so following previous writers who had in various ways already expressed their criticism of the state of the culture in their own eras. One of these writers was Yūsuf al-Shirbīnī (1591?–1688), whose *Kitāb Hazz al-Quḥūf bi-Sharḥ Qaṣīd Abī Shādūf* (*Brains Confounded*

[139] Al-Musawi 2015b, p. 58. In an article al-Musawi published before the release of his book, he referred to the Iraqi poet Badr Shākir al-Sayyāb (1926–1964) as a "modernist" as well (al-Musawi 2014, p. 268). In an interview before the publication of his book, al-Musawi argues that the project of the Arab *Nahḍa* had failed because of "the rupture between the rural areas (*rīf*) and the city, namely, the intellectual started to deem himself above his roots and despise them, like what Ṭāhā Ḥusayn has done in *al-Ayyām* (*The Days*)" (see at: https://www.alaraby.co.uk/portal, October 21, 2014). For an earlier version of al-Musawi's accusations against the "modernists," see al-Musawi 2013, pp. 51–2.

[140] Al-Musawi 2015b, p. 111.

[141] Al-Musawi 2015b, p. 5 (my emphasis). In a detailed note, al-Musawi quotes publications by the "modernists" in an attempt to prove that they "looked with suspicion and distrust at the [medieval Arab, and Islamic] past and its massive accumulation in cultural capital" (p. 324, n. 10). Sahar Ishtiaque Ullah duplicates al-Musawi's arguments, accusing the "modernists" of the "misreading of a massive corpus of evidence and at worst a deliberate neglect of an incredibly vast undertaking of postclassical literary production" (Ishtiaque Ullah 2016, pp. 203–25). Checking closely the references in the aforementioned note by al-Musawi, it is difficult to find how the relevant writings could support these sweeping arguments; suffice it here to mention Mūsā 1947, pp. 75–80; Mūsā 1962, pp. 137–41; al-Jābirī 1982, pp. 34–8; as well as what is cited in Allen 2006, pp. 14–15. One can find citations of Arab intellectuals who found themselves confronting the dilemmas of the cultural transformation that followed the interaction of the Arab world with the West (see, e.g., Amīn 1965, p. 7. Cf. Allen 2006, p. 2). However, even these citations should not be taken literally, but as another indication of the decline of the Arabs' cultural self-image and the huge gap between the august status enjoyed by Arab culture in the Middle Ages and its feeble modern counterpart (see Snir 2017, pp. 232–7).

by the Ode of Abū Shādūf Expounded)[142] is a humorous account of the lifestyles and habits of speech of peasants during the period of Ottoman rule in Egypt in a mixture of genres, styles, and dictions. Writing that this work "plays havoc with a solid canon that staunchly adhered to verisimilitude and truth, while at the same time enrolling in its ranks jurists of disputable and unreliable knowledge," al-Musawi himself refers to its "dashing satire on elitism, pedantry in scholarship, and the compendious and commentarial surplus, and its biting irony directed toward certain religious circles and sham Sufism."[143]

Referring to the "modernists" as the "reluctant heirs" of the medieval body of knowledge, al-Musawi argues that their "disillusion with [that] cultural production was primarily informed by a European discourse but was also driven by a misreading of the compendious and commentarial effort of the period." He explains that they

> could not discern the significant redirection of cultural capital to escape imitation, while simultaneously assimilating ancient and classical knowledge. In fact, by appropriating and classifying these sources rather than duplicating them, postclassical scholars and littérateurs embarked on what Pascale Casanova terms a "diversion of assets."[144]

Some observations are necessary here regarding the way al-Musawi understands the meaning of the term "diversion of assets": first, his argument that a "seductive Europe" was the root of all evil and the driving force behind the "modernists" in their role as "architects of regression" who internalized the "European Enlightenment disparagement of the Middle Ages" does not, to say the least, do Arab culture any justice. Kilito's aforementioned call "to regard Arabic poetics on its own terms" and "to avoid treating the subject as some kind of deviation from a model realized in other times and under other skies" should guide us here as well. In a short, brilliant essay, Tarek El-Ariss refers directly to al-Musawi's thesis, including the latter's argument about the *Nahḍa* as "the other appellation for Arab modernity,"[145] while suggesting that the *Nahḍa* texts be freed from the *Nahḍa* as a "'modernity' project" and from "the dominant narrative of rise and decline, and from their intertextual and ideological dependency on European modernity as a model to be borrowed or resisted." El-Ariss argues that the *Nahḍa*'s "civilizational practices could not be reduced to notions of civilization associated with Orientalism

142 See al-Shirbīnī 2005; al-Shirbīnī 2007. On al-Shirbīnī's work, see al-Musawi 2015b, pp. 147–74. See also Peled 1986, pp. 57–75; Abū Fāshā 1987; Omri 2000, pp. 169–96.

143 Al-Musawi 2015b, pp. 83 and 96, respectively.

144 Al-Musawi 2015b, p. 5.

145 Al-Musawi 2014, p. 265.

as [a] system of othering and cultural superiority." Instead, he refers to it as "this potential, this vague thing that everyone is practicing without knowing what it looks like or whether it will be achieved or not or to what end." Moreover, it is a speech-act: let there be *Nahḍa*! Therefore, there is a need to decolonize the *Nahḍa* and "allow it to make its own meaning, however contradictory and inconsistent with historical narratives and ideological critique."[146] Here we should also consider Michael Cooperson's observation:

> Today no serious historian speaks of "Islamic decadence" any more. But if one narrows the field a bit, the situation seems less clear-cut. In the study of Arabic literature ... it was long considered axiomatic that the Mongol, Mamluk, and Ottoman periods constituted one long age of decline. Today one finds vigorous arguments against this position, but no generally accepted counter-narrative, and some pushback from colleagues, who sense that some modern scholars, in their eagerness to disavow the old paradigm, "overcompensate by denying any reality" to nineteenth-century Arab accounts of the preceding two hundred years, "as a period of decline in Arabic letters and the institutions that sustained them" [Ahmed El Shamsy's personal communication]. There is also the awkward fact that the Orientalist paradigm, though the "Orientalists" themselves have largely abandoned it, remains the default position in Arabic-language literary histories and mass-culture references to the Arab and Islamic past, even if it has had, and continues to have, its critics.[147]

Second, the term "diversion of [literary] assets"[148] is used by Casanova, following the poet and critic Joachim du Bellay (1522–1560), to refer to the redirection of "the gains of Latinist humanism—a vast collection of knowledge

146 El-Ariss 2015, pp. 261, 264, 265, and 266, respectively. In his response to El-Ariss' intervention, al-Musawi does not refer directly to El-Ariss' major arguments regarding the *Nahḍa*, but mainly reiterates his accusations against the "modernists"—those "prominent intellectuals [who] thought of themselves as leaders of thought like the European Enlightenment figures, locating themselves in that European moment of a century earlier, cutting themselves doubly from their immediate history and the challenge to the age of reason brought about by the rising imperial culture of nineteenth-century Europe" (al-Musawi 2015a, p. 281). On the *Nahḍa* and modernity, see also El-Ariss 2013. On the "glocal" approach to the *Nahḍa* as a world literature, see Mahmoud 2019, pp. 557–72. See also the special issue of *Oriente Moderno* 99.1/2 (2019) titled "Nahḍah Narratives: Arab Literary Modernity and the Dialogue between Genres." On the transformation of the Arab region within the context of world history, looking beyond the well-worn categories of "traditional" versus "modern," see Hill 2020. Hill places the visions of the crucial intellectuals of the *Nahḍa* within the context of their local class- and state-building projects in Ottoman Syria and Egypt, which themselves formed part of a global age of capital. See also Patel 2013; Hanssen and Weiss 2016.

147 Cooperson 2017, p. 42.

148 Casanova 2004, p. 54. Casanova uses as well the terms "diversion of literary wealth" (p. 46), "diversion of [literary/symbolic] capital" (pp. 53, 99, 157, 235, 284), and "diversion of resources" (p. 233).

derived from translation and commentaries on ancient texts" to the profit of French, a language that was less "rich." As a result, by the time of Louis XIV France reigned as the "dominant literary power in Europe."[149] Nothing similar to that happened in what al-Musawi considers as the medieval Islamic republic of letters if only for the simple reason that, to use Casanova's words, the gains of Arab classical humanism, though they helped other Muslim nations consolidate their cultures, were by no means used to the benefit of another single specific language in a way that would result in the establishment of a new dominant literary power to replace Arabic. Furthermore, even if we adopt al-Musawi's use of Casanova's conception, as far as I know no "modernist," certainly not al-Zayyāt, Mūsā, or Ḥusayn, decried those works that successfully assimilated ancient and classical knowledge while redirecting cultural capital to escape imitation. They rightly decried texts that, in al-Musawi's words, failed in the act of "redirection of cultural capital to escape imitation." If there is any blame to be leveled against the "modernists," it is their elitist attitude toward the popular cultural production consumed by the masses, which in turn caused them to decry and even to ignore popular texts and activities.[150] According to the conceptions adopted in my studies, and in this respect I completely agree with al-Musawi, texts and activities of this nature should be considered as an integral part of any cultural system.

In a passionate apologetic section titled "The Fight for Culture: Compendiums and Commentaries,"[151] al-Musawi denounces the "modernists" for their tendency to negate rhetoric as superfluity and denigrate the tradition of commentaries and compendia in the premodern Arab-Islamic period.[152] Emphasizing the importance of the tradition of *shurūḥ* (commentaries), *dhuyūl* (supplements), and *ḥawāshin* (marginal notes)—"a paper empire, of words on words, and *kalām 'alā kalām* (metadiscourse)"[153]—which flourished during the postclassical period, al-Musawi takes refuge in Michel Foucault's (1926–1984) *The Order of Things: An Archaeology of the Human Sciences* (French: *Les mots et les choses: Une archéologie des sciences humaines*) (1966).[154] After Foucault, al-Musawi quotes Michel de Montaigne

149 Casanova 2004, pp. 53–4.

150 Ṭāhā Ḥusayn, who opposed the dialects in literature (see Snir 2017, pp. 28–31), pointed in a lecture delivered in front of the "Commission for the Arabic Language in Cairo" (Majma' al-Lugha al-'Arabiyya bi-l-Qāhira) in 1957, to the dangers inherent in exposing Arabic to the same evolution as Latin. The establishment of written Arabic dialects would disable communication between different Arabic societies and create rivalling national cultures (König 2016, pp. 464–5).

151 Al-Musawi 2015b, pp. 97–103.

152 Al-Musawi 2015b, pp. 98–9, 118.

153 Cf. Yaḥyāwī 2015.

154 Al-Musawi relies on Foucault 1966, pp. 38–46 ("The Writing of Things").

(1533–1592): "There is more work in interpreting interpretations than in interpreting things; and more books about books than on any other subject; we do nothing but write glosses about each other." Foucault comments on de Montaigne's words: "These words are not a statement of the bankruptcy of culture buried beneath its own monuments; they are a definition of the inevitable relation that language maintained with itself in the sixteenth century." Al-Musawi argues that Foucault's analysis is an attempt to define commentary and gloss as the infinite proliferation of the interpretation that justifies what Foucault describes as the "sovereignty of an original text." It is the text "that offers its ultimate revelation as the promised reward of the commentary." Thus, it is the "interstice occurring between the primal Text and the infinity of Interpretation" that accounts for the proliferation in interpretation, commentary, and gloss, which take writing to be a substantial part of the "fabric of the world."[155] Al-Musawi relies as well on Jorge Luis Borges's (1899–1986) idea of "a minutely drawn map that negates the original" and Christine Brooke-Rose's (1923–2012) argument that "disclaiming rhetoric is itself a figure of rhetoric."[156] He suggests that the "strikingly widespread recourse to compendiums, the rise of the polymath, and the vogue of *shurūḥ*, of explications of an original text, all suggest a process in which designated classification and centers of institutionalized knowledge were being undermined."[157] In short, arguing that the "lengthy pre-modern era remains relatively understudied, especially in terms of what Brinkley Messick associates with a 'calligraphic state',"[158] al-Musawi makes use of texts by Foucault, Borges, and Brooke-Rose in defense of the tradition of commentaries and compendia of the premodern Arab-Islamic period.

These texts, however, by no means support al-Musawi's arguments. First, it seems that Messick's "calligraphic state" is irrelevant to al-Musawi' arguments. Messick traces "connections between the literary processes behind the constitution of authority *in* texts and the social and political processes involved in articulating the authority of texts." The types of text involved in Messick's research activity, intended to contribute to the specific history of Yemen, are basic manuals of *sharī'a* jurisprudence and their commentaries.[159] Second, there is a substantial difference between sixteenth-century European commentaries according to Michel de Montaigne and the *shurūḥ*

155 Al-Musawi 2015b, pp. 98–9. The quotations are from Foucault 1966, p. 45. For an earlier version of these arguments, see al-Musawi 2013, pp. 51–2.
156 Al-Musawi 2015b, p. 118.
157 Al-Musawi 2015b, p. 132.
158 Al-Musawi 2015b, p. 98.
159 Messick 1993, pp. 1–12.

tradition.[160] Moreover, the "modernists" voiced their criticism in real time when they were endeavoring to change the face of Arab culture and save it from what they considered to be the negative phenomena of the premodern tradition; al-Musawi's criticism of them is possible *thanks* to their efforts. Third, Yūsuf al-Shirbīnī's aforementioned *Kitāb Hazz al-Quḥūf bi-Sharḥ Qaṣīd Abī Shādūf* would not have parodied, in the words of al-Musawi, "an ongoing and firmly established *shurūḥ* tradition"[161] unless that tradition had seemed *at the time* to be superfluous in essence. That is why, even according to al-Musawi, al-Shirbīnī "dislodges the entire practice of these commentaries, not only by creating a distance between a hilarious ode and the commentator, but also by giving himself the freedom to poke fun at many practices that are normally buttressed by serious material or apocryphal detail."[162] And fourth, examining the few critical surveys of Arab scholars in the nineteenth century of contemporary literature, such as that by Syrian Jurjī Murquṣ (1846–1912), we find that their opinion of the poetry of the time, which is an extension of the previous century, was not high.[163] And this was many years before the emergence of the "modernists"!

All in all, al-Musawi speaks assertively against the "modernists" and about their "wholesale" and "sweeping" "resistance," "rejection," and "denigration" of their past and its "cultural values" and "intimidating cultural capital."[164] Additionally, in one section, referring to Casanova's book and one of the in-depth reviews of it, he finds fault with the "modernists" for the following reason:

> What is lost on modernists is a simple premise expressed by Casanova in her *The World Republic of Letters*: "It is necessary to be old to have any chance of being modern or of decreeing what is modern." In a review of her book, Joe Cleary puts this point as follows: "Only countries that can claim a venerable and distinguished historical stock of literary capital get to decree what is and is not 'fashionable' in literary terms."[165]

160 For a discussion of the trends of "compilation and elaboration" in the postclassical period against the backdrop of what had preceded them, see Allen 2006, pp. 8–13.

161 Al-Musawi 2015b, p. 158.

162 Al-Musawi 2015b, p. 153.

163 See Kilpatrick 2015, pp. 91–2. Cf. the instructive anecdote told by Ṭāhā Ḥusayn about his interview with Shukrī Bāshā, the Sulṭān's *chef de bureau* (*Ra'īs al-Dīwān al-Sulṭānī*), regarding the change in Arabic poetic sensibilities (Snir 2017, p. 159).

164 Al-Musawi 2015b, pp. 9, 11, 14, 24, 97–8.

165 Al-Musawi 2015b, pp. 11–12. See also al-Musawi 2015b, pp. 111–14: "A number of things that are lost on most modernists ... The enhanced devotion to rhetoric that has engendered so much negative criticism against the so-called age of superfluity" (p. 114. See also pp. 135, 142–3, and 159–62).

The context of Casanova's aforementioned "premise" is her argument that "the ability to decree without fear of challenge what is or is not 'fashionable,' in the domain of haute couture and elsewhere, permitted Paris to control one of the main routes of access to modernity ... Paris managed to sustain its position—at least until the 1960s—as the center of the system of literary time." Only then, Casanova adds the following:

> The temporal law of the world of letters may be stated thus: *It is necessary to be old to have any chance of being modern or of decreeing what is modern.* In other words, having a long national past is the condition of being able to claim a literary existence that is fully recognized in the present.[166]

In his review of her book, Joe Cleary refers to Casanova's argument, but unfortunately al-Musawi in the quote above does not cite Cleary's full text, which runs as follows:

> In other words, only countries that can claim a venerable and distinguished historical stock of literary capital get to decree what is and is not "fashionable" in literary terms. But, since what constitutes up-to-dateness or the literary present is constantly changing—"the only way in the literary world to be truly modern is to contest the present as outmoded—to appeal to a more present, as yet unknown, which thus becomes the newest certified present."[167]

In his attack against the "modernists," al-Musawi argues that they did not understand what Casanova describes as the "temporal law of the world of letters," namely, the condition of being able to claim a literary existence that is fully recognized in the present as having a long national past. But Cleary adds that this is because "what constitutes up-to-dateness or the literary present is constantly changing," and here he quotes, with some inaccuracies, Casanova's saying, in a section titled "What Is Modernity?," that "the only way in the literary *space* to be truly modern is to contest the present as outmoded—to appeal to a *still* more present, as yet unknown, which thus becomes the newest certified present."[168] In other words, contrary to what al-Musawi attributes to the "modernists," *they did exactly what Casanova recommends*—they tried to contest the outmoded present by appealing to another present in order to make it "the newest certified present." Moreover, when Casanova speaks about the "fashionable" in literary terms, she is only referring to *belles lettres*.[169]

166 Casanova 2004, pp. 89–90 (emphasis in the original).

167 Cleary 2006, pp. 199–200. The quotation is from Casanova 2004, p. 91.

168 Casanova 2004, p. 91. The words in *italics* are those in which Cleary does not quote Casanova accurately.

169 See the aforementioned anecdote told by Ṭāhā Ḥusayn about his interview with Shukrī Bāshā, the Sulṭān's *chef de bureau* (*Ra'īs al-Dīwān al-Sulṭānī*) (Snir 2017, p. 159).

Another charge al-Musawi levels against the "modernists" is that they adopted a basic equation between secularism, on the one hand, and humanism and modernism, on the other.[170] And here, al-Musawi expresses his opposition to the argument presented by the Iranian scholar Hamid Dabashi (b. 1951) that Arab humanism "remained canonical in its commitment to the imperially imposed language of the Arab conquerors and their tribal racism."[171] Al-Musawi has reservations about defining Arab humanism as necessarily being tied to conquest and gain:

> The republic as the dialogic space for poetics and politics claims its freedom from power as the condition for its humanist conversations. Hence, the use of Arabic and the spread of a culturally oriented Islamic identification in no way negate the racial manipulation of genealogical divides to ensure privilege in times of conquest.[172]

Reading carefully the relevant texts and scholarship, Hamid Dabashi's included, and closely examining and analyzing al-Musawi's aforementioned argument leave no doubt that this charge is totally unjustified. Due to a lack of space, this is all I will say on this topic.

12. COGNITIVE DISSONANCE AND COMMON FALLACIES

Having been a student of Arabic literature for the last forty-five years, and having read almost everything written by the major Arab thinkers and writers in the formative period of modern Arabic literature, I am greatly disturbed by al-Musawi's unjustifiable and biased campaign against the "modernists." But, much more than that, I am very dismayed by the *almost complete and utter silence of the entire academic community involved in the study of Arabic literature*, whose major scholars, as revealed in their published works and in private, first-hand knowledge, very much appreciate these "modernists" that al-Musawi labels "architects of regression." Communicating with various scholars, both distinguished and young, I could not find even one who does not have serious reservations regarding al-Musawi's campaign, about which, unfortunately, no scholar has so far dared to write with the exception of Marilyn Booth, who writes as follows:

> Such wholesale dismissal of these individuals' bodies of thought, which are not monochromatic, along with dismissal of a presumably larger group labelled simply as "modernists," does not do justice to the nuanced—if at times

170 Al-Musawi 2015b, pp. 310–11.

171 Dabashi 2012, pp. 79–80 (quoted in al-Musawi 2015b, p. 54. See also pp. 40, 46–7, and 54–7).

172 Al-Musawi 2015b, p. 56.

> ambivalent—relationship that many Arab intellectuals of the past two centuries have had to the past that al-Musawi excavates. *Even those modernists (as a group they are memorably called "architects of regression" [p. 11]) who embraced intellectual heritages of western Europe and saw this as the road to their own societies' modern future did study and honour their own past*—its "middle" period as well as that of the earlier "golden age."[173]

Also, some reviewers of *The Medieval Islamic Republic of Letters: Arabic Knowledge Construction* could not avoid making critical comments even if extremely cautious: as already shown in brief above, under the polite cover of praise, Tarek El-Ariss presented significant counterarguments, mostly between the lines. Tipping her hat to the author "for his erudition and Herculean capacity for tackling multitudes—perhaps hundreds—of authors and voluminous texts," Dana Sajdi writes that "one cannot be but in awe" of al-Musawi's project, but she indicates that he "bites off more than he can chew, or perhaps more than he is able to share with his readers." Among the gaps in the book, for example, the reviewer mentions that "the book's employment of the 'republic of letters' seems to be a ploy to reconcile two frameworks that do not necessarily fit: on the one hand, an open premodern world-system ... and Mamluk imperial consolidation and centralization," on the other. Also al-Musawi ignores significant contributions by scholars, such as Janet Abu-Lughod, and he cites others without engaging with their work: "Had the various contributions of Khaled al-Rouayheb and Nelly Hanna been integrated, as opposed to merely cited, into the book, some of the observations about the later period would have been different."[174] Elizabeth Lhost writes that "the author's tendency to re-articulate his position, relative to Casanova, in seemingly every chapter hinders his ability to replace the tired narrative of European ascendance—which tends to discredit Arabic literature from the medieval period altogether—with an engaging account of his alternative vision, or to provide the reader with a sense of the rich textures, delightful details, and fascinating tidbits that populate the literature he praises."[175] Charles Burnett writes that al-Musawi takes terms and concepts from Pascale Casanova and Michel Foucault but one is left to draw his own "conclusions as to how the Islamic 'Republic of Letters' differs from the early modern European phenomenon with the same name. Al-Musawi provides plenty of material on which to make these comparisons. Yet, in the last analysis, the value of his book is not so much that it argues for a European-style

[173] *Journal of Islamic Studies* 28.3 (2017), p. 385 (my emphasis).

[174] *Journal of Early Modern History* 20.2 (2016), p. 591.

[175] *Reading Religion*, website published by the American Academy of Religion (AAR) (May 19, 2017), available at: http://readingreligion.org/books/medieval-islamic-republic-letters, last accessed October 16, 2017.

'Republic of Letters' in the Islamic area, as that it draws attention to the richness of Islamic literature in a neglected period, and describes its themes, its continuities and ruptures, and its distinctive characteristics."[176] The other scholars mentioned above that expressed reservations toward al-Musawi's arguments (i.e., Helgesson, Orsini, and Ganguly) do not belong to the scholarly community of Arabic literature, and they did so in spite of being unfamiliar with the relevant scholarship.

This unfamiliar academic "silence" in the scholarship on Arabic literature could not conceivably occur in the scholarship on any other literature whatsoever, wherein its founding fathers were defamed in such an aggressive manner and with such unbalanced and biased scholarly theses being generated. But, and I can testify to this from my own personal experience of several decades, the scholarship on Arabic literature is a "special case," more especially against the backdrop of the waves of pressure generated in Middle Eastern scholarship by Edward Said, the Indian literary theorist Gayatri Spivak (b. 1942), and the Indian English theorist Homi Bhabha (b. 1949), who have come to be seen as what the South African scholar Dennis Walder (b. 1943) calls "the three police officers of the postcolonial."[177] Said's *Orientalism* (1978), together with his academic reputation and total immunity from criticism whatsoever by *all* scholars of Arabic literature—a blind worship of a god-like scholar not to be found among any other similar international scholarly communities of *critics* of any other literature—as well as Said's nationalist Palestinian agenda, have left a deep imprint on the scholarship in the field.[178] One of the consequences of the inspiration Said's book, which is an indictment of Western scholars for purveying a false image of the Arab world as static, backward, and uncivilized, is the "generous" attitude toward Arab scholars and academics by the Western scholarly community—a generosity colored by a compulsion to apply less rigorous critical judgment to them. Unlike, for example, Israeli-Jewish scholars in the field of Arabic literature, who have collectively suffered from the effects of the Boycott, Divest, Sanction (BDS) movement, even if they fiercely oppose Israeli governmental policy, Arab scholars are immune to any criticism save for very

[176] *Erudition and the Republic of Letters* 2.3 (2017), pp. 351–4. The quotation is from p. 353.

[177] Walder 1998, p. 4.

[178] "There are signs that his impact may eventually rank on a par with, if not surpass, the *nahda* spearheaded in the late nineteenth century by Jamaleddeen Afghani, and continued by Muhammad Abduh" (Rice and Hamdy 2008, p. 22). On Said's impact on the scholarship of Arabic literature, see also Tresilian 2008, pp. 21–2. According to Robert Spencer, "the backlash against Said's work has the aim of discrediting the radical pedagogical and, ultimately, political potential of [his] ideas. It would discourage the practice of questioning and self-questioning, which after all is what scholarship is all about" (Spencer 2013, p. 170).

rare cases.[179] It is only in this light that I can at all understand how some of al-Musawi's slander and defamatory statements against great Arab intellectuals were published three years ago, so far without almost any significant response, even though al-Musawi presents arguments that are quite unacceptable in academic scholarly discourse. For example, more than once al-Musawi refers insultingly to the "modernists" as using straw man arguments:

> Although *nahḍah* intellectuals needed a *straw man to justify their call for transformation and discontinuity with the [premodern] past*, they could not bypass some of its landmarks—that being the case with lexicons, for example. Entrenched in between, they either come up with *illogical proposals and selective categorizations* or end up by indulging in a sweeping denial of any cultural significance in the cultural production of the past five centuries ... If the study of the Abbasid past produced significant readings and discussions, they were primarily intended to problematize other questions, such as the ninth-tenth century translation movement from the Hellenistic tradition. In other words, the seeming *nahḍah* espousal of an Abbasid Golden Age (750–978), with its widely proclaimed indebtedness to Greek philosophy and science, partially duplicates a comparable proclaimed European filiation with a Greco-Latin tradition.[180]

And, again, in the same article:

> [Ṭāhā Ḥusayn] needs to prove his thesis that the West leads the Enlightenment and hence the cultural dependency of Egypt. Another is *a latent desire to repress sources of power in an Arab/Islamic cultural tradition in order to use the recent past, the Mamluk and premodern periods, as his straw man, to be beaten and dismissed as unwanted past*, an awkward memory to be dumped forever in order to align consciousness with an enlightened Europe that has put its medieval past behind [it]. As a leading figure in the *nahḍah* movement, Ṭāhā Ḥusayn is the sum-up of anxieties, contradictions, and achievements that happen to be a translational interstice.[181]

And in another article:

> Arab modernists show an enormous anxiety that is common in periods of transition, especially under the impact of British and French cultural achievement. The desire to be their Other, the European, and the need to retain native magnanimity drove them to the classical past of an Abbasid empire, a Golden Age, a lighthouse that justifies importation of a colonial culture in times of regression and decadence that the recent past signifies for them in terms similar to what the Middle Ages signify to the Enlightenment.[182]

[179] Such as Thomas Bauer's critique of Salma Khadra Jayyusi's article in *Mamlūk Studies Review* 11.2 (2007), pp. 137–67.

[180] Al-Musawi 2015, pp. 117–18 (my emphasis).

[181] Al-Musawi 2015, p. 127 (my emphasis).

[182] Al-Musawi 2015a, p. 283.

Reading closely al-Musawi's recent studies and exploring his arguments against the background of his scholarly and other activities before and after his moving to the West, several points seem to be in order. First, notwithstanding his proven academic and scholarly excellence, during the last two decades al-Musawi has enjoyed exclusive privileges no one else has had in the scholarship of Arabic literature. The only explanation for that *immunity* is that he is an Arab scholar publishing in English in a scholarly community characterized by a culture of confrontation and suffering from a specific "cognitive dissonance"[183] known from other similar communities.[184] Those who comprise the international Western scholarly establishment of Arabic literature, which prides itself on being pluralistic and leftist-liberal-oriented, are, most if not all of them, with postcolonial allegiances and, in general, eager to be generous toward the literary and scholarly production of the "other"—the subject of their investigation, in this case Arab writers and scholars—avoiding as much a possible voicing of any disparaging or critical attitude toward them. Among the dozens of reviews written on al-Musawi's many books, one cannot find even one with any real significant reservations, without enveloping them in a lot of praise and flattery. At the same time, just for comparison, as an Israeli-Jewish student of Arabic literature, together with my colleagues, we frequently suffer from the results of BDS activities,[185] but also from other exclusionary actions and operations not related to the boycott against Israel. For example, we are not on the list of scholars who deserve to be invited to conferences, to participate in scholarly projects, to be members of editorial boards, to write reviews, or simply worthy to be mentioned in their publications. The latter exclusion is backfiring on them because a scholar who is writing on a specific topic and does his or her best to avoid mentioning a book or an article published on the same very topic only damages his or her own reputation as a true scholar. Surprisingly, or perhaps not, scholars in the Arab world, Palestinian included, are eager to cooperate with us in all scholarly fields, while Western scholars, or Arab scholars adopted by the Western establishment with only a few exceptions (Roger Allen is a towering example!), are hesitant, to say the least, in their connections with Israeli-Jewish scholars.

Second, al-Musawi presents contradictory arguments without being exposed to any criticism. For example, he writes about the "paradoxical intersection" that leaves the *Nahḍa* intellectual in a liminal space, in perpetual trial, even when "voicing triumph and targeting others with sardonic

[183] According to Festinger 1957, esp. pp. 1–31.
[184] See, for example, Snir 1995, pp. 163–83; Snir 2001, pp. 197–224.
[185] See Snir 2017, p. 274.

sarcasm as Ḥusayn did in his seminal autobiography, *The Days*." According to al-Musawi, "autobiography signals unease, not contentment. Otherwise, how can we understand the massive growth of autobiographical writing?" But immediately afterwards, al-Musawi mentions that "this autobiographical stream speaks of an unverified belief in one's role, a mastery of one's fate, worth communicating and circulating widely to help justifying one's role for posterity." The following is also unintelligible:

> Ṭāhā Ḥusayn's struggle against his blindness and the limits it imposed on his life generated a search for a larger vision, more comprehensive and encompassing, to involve the liberation of a nation ... *Biographical, autobiographical, or narrative accounts signify a self writ large to account for communal or national issues*. As a significant threshold to nation, the act of narration provides us also with conditions of possibility and estrangement. *The Days* of Ṭāhā Ḥusayn, for example, could not become so seminal for subsequent writing without its power to incite, invite, and demarcate venues for self-dependency, sovereignty, and acclamation of Orientalists' knowledge and methods in approaching and even reading Arabic.[186]

Third, on the whole, al-Musawi's arguments against the "modernists" suffer from certain common fallacies. For example, they use *ad hominem* attacks and resort to offensive remarks that should scarcely be found in respectable scholarly and academic discourses: the "modernists" are the "architects of regression," the "reluctant heirs" of the medieval body of knowledge, and their arguments are nothing but "wholesale" and "sweeping" "resistance," "rejection," and "denigration" of their past and its "cultural values" and "intimidating cultural capital"; and they misread their past, and falling back "on a series of negations and denials of [its] merit," they internalize the "European Enlightenment disparagement of the Middle Ages ... in their zealous duplication of a seductive Europe." Moreover, al-Musawi, who accuses the "modernists" of using straw-man arguments, as seen above, himself uses such arguments. He frequently attributes to them distorted weaker arguments, misrepresenting their positions, only to "successfully" defeat them. It seems that al-Musawi is so aware of his undisputedly strong position among scholars of Arabic literature in the West, and is so certain that no one will dare to make any critical comments about his arguments (and he is right if we go by the reviews written during the last twenty years on his publications, his last book discussed in the present article inclusive), that he has allowed himself what no scholar would dare. This is undoubtedly a kind of the "argument from authority" fallacy.

[186] Al-Musawi 2015a, p. 283 (my emphasis).

13. CONCLUSION

Muhsin Jassim al-Musawi's *The Medieval Islamic Republic of Letters: Arabic Knowledge Construction* is a thought-provoking book and an eye-opener study for scholars of Arabic literature. His campaign against the "modernists," however, acts as an incentive to ponder his motivation as being more than just scholarly in nature. He refers to the "Islamic constellation of knowledge as a movement with its own identifiable features and regenerative processes that *could have nourished the present and led it safely out of wars, disasters, and colonial incursions*." And he alludes to the "complexity, diversity, and magnitude of medieval cultural production, which has daunted modernists and their counterparts in the West and caused them to fall back on a series of negations and denials of merit." Among the accusations he levels against the "modernists" is that they depreciated certain "Islamic practices," considering them to be "regressive and hence not conducive to progress and modernity."[187] In alluding to Jean Le Rond d'Alembert's (1717–1783) *Preliminary Discourse* that accompanied the first volume of Diderot's *Encyclopedia of Arts and Sciences* (1751), al-Musawi's *Preliminary Discourse* is instructive; it shows that he is not satisfied with academic investigations of the past alone, as seen from the fact that his sequential articles on the topic have the phrase "Arab modernity" in their subtitles. In this regard, the final lines of his *Conclusion* (*Al-Khātima*)[188] are illuminating because they speak not only on the past but on the present and the future as well:

> Hence, the long-established Western equation between secularism and humanism needs to be challenged whenever it is applied outside the specific domain of a European Renaissance. *Only through better engagement with this past, with rigorous interrogation of its successes and failures, can modernists build up a sustainable view of the present and thus be at peace with themselves.* Diversity and dissent constitute a marked feature of Islamic culture, one that valorizes and invigorates a republic of letters with its many conspicuous or discrete worlds in what amounts to no less than seismic *Islamica*.[189]

[187] Al-Musawi 2015b, pp. 306 (my emphasis), 308–9, and 310, respectively.

[188] In his *Khuṭbat al-Kitāb* (*Preliminary Discourse*) (pp. 1–20) and *Al-Khātima* (*Conclusion*) (pp. 305–11), al-Musawi imitates, mainly through the wording of the titles he selects, the style of the postclassical Arabic writers as well that of Jean Le Rond d'Alembert, who was until 1759 co-editor with Denis Diderot (1713–1784) of the *Encyclopédie* (*Encyclopedia of Arts and Sciences*) (1751–1772), one of the largest collaborative ventures of the republic of letters (see al-Musawi 2015b, p. 323, n. 2, as well as pp. 103 and 144).

[189] Al-Musawi 2015b, p. 311 (my emphasis, except for the last word).

I disagree with al-Musawi when he accuses the "modernists" of "a substantial disengagement from a tradition that was much needed for the promotion of education and culture," and of failing to engage with their past and build up "a sustainable view of the present." It is a simplification of the challenges that the "modernists" faced at the time. A brief look at the articles that Ṭāhā Ḥusayn published in the Egyptian press over a period of almost sixty years gives a completely different picture.[190] And, last, but not least, one should notice that al-Musawi has defamed *only* Egyptian and *only* dead "modernists," those that cannot respond to his arguments; he ignores others—including many Christian "modernists"—based on the parameters he set up, as well as those who are still active. That is why, in concluding the *Khātima* (*Conclusion*) of the present Epilogue, I will now quote some lines by the Syrian poet ʿAlī Aḥmad Saʿīd, better known as Adūnīs (b. 1930), perhaps the greatest of all contemporary Arab "modernists" (which does not mean that I agree with everything that Adūnīs writes!),[191] and unlike the false accusations leveled by al-Musawi against al-Zayyāt, Ḥusayn, and Mūsā regarding their attitude toward the premodern period,[192] the following lines are undoubtedly sweeping:

منذ سقوط بغداد وقيام السّلطنة العثمانيّة،
تحوّل الدّين إلى مجرّد أداة عنفيّة لخدمة السّلطة.
لا نجد، على سبيل المثل، في تاريخ السلطنة العثمانيّة كلّها، على مدى أكثر من
أربعة قرون، مفكّرًا عربيًّا واحدًا، أو فنّانًا واحدًا، أو موسيقيًا واحدًا، أو شاعراً واحداً، أو عالمًا
واحدًا.
هكذا كان لا بدّ من مجيء أتاتورك للأتراك،
ومن أن تبدأ حركة النّهوض العربيّ.

Since the fall of Baghdad and the establishment of the Ottoman Sultanate,
Religion has become only a harsh tool in the service of authority.
We do not find, for example, throughout the history of the Ottoman Sultanate, during more than

190 See *Turāth Ṭāhā Ḥusayn: al-Maqālāt al-Ṣuḥufiyya min 1908–1967* (Cairo: Maṭbaʿat Dār al-Kutub wa-l-Wathāʾiq al-Qawmiyya, 2002). From the numerous articles that refute al-Musawi's accusations, I will mention only two: an article published in *Majallatī* (June 1, 1936) titled "Tanẓīm al-Nahḍa" ("Organizing the Renaissance") (pp. 419–23); and another article published in *Musāmarāt al-Jayb* (January 18, 1948) titled "Mushkilat al-Lughāt al-Ajnabiyya" ("The Issue of Foreign Languages") (pp. 610–11).

191 In fact, I agree with most of the arguments put forth in Thomas Bauer's aforementioned review of Salma Khadra Jayyusi's theses (Bauer 2007, pp. 137–67).

192 In a recent article, al-Musawi discusses Salāma Mūsā's conceptions in an appropriate and balanced manner, and, more importantly, with more thorough scholarship with regard to the "modernists" than he does in his book reviewed here (al-Musawi 2018, pp. 174–91).

Four centuries, even one Arab intellectual, or one artist, or one musician, or one poet, or one scientist.
That is why it was necessary that Atatürk would come to the Turks,
And that the Arabic renaissance would start.[193]

[193] Adūnīs, "Madārāt: Lafẓ Yuwaḥḥid wa-'Amal Yubaddid," al-Ḥayāt, May 29, 2015. Cf. Adūnīs' sharp rhetorical question:

> ما الجديد الذي قدّمته وأسهمت به [الثقافة العربية] في بناء عالم المعرفة، على المستوى الكَونيّ، بدءاً من سقوط الخلافة في صورتها العثمانيّة، والتي سجَنَت عالم اللغة العربية في ظلماتٍ مُتَنَوّعة، على مدى أربعة قرون؟ (Adūnīs 2022).

References

The definite *al-* only at the beginning of a surname is not taken into consideration in the alphabetical order. It appears in this form throughout the book before solar and lunar letters. Titles of Arabic books and articles are transliterated into English. Titles of Hebrew books and articles are translated into English and identified as such at the end of the translated title.

Abāẓa, Tharwat. 1983 [1967]. *Shay' min al-Khawf.* Cairo: Dār al-Ma'ārif.

'Abbās, Ḥasan Maḥmūd. 1983. *Ḥayy ibn Yaqẓān wa-Robinson Crusoe: Dirāsa Muqārina.* Beirut: al-Mu'assasa al-'Arabiyya li-l-Dirāsāt wa-l-Nashr.

'Abbās, Iḥsān. n.d. [1956]. *Fann al-Sīra.* Beirut: Dār al-Thaqāfa.

——. 1969. *Ta'rīkh al-Adab al-Andalusī: 'Aṣr Siyādat Qurṭuba.* Beirut: Dār al-Thaqāfa.

——. 1977. *Malāmiḥ Yūnāniyya fī al-Adab al-'Arabī.* Beirut: al-Mu'assasa al-Jāmi'iyya li-l-Dirāsāt wa-l-Nashr.

——. 1985. *Ta'rīkh al-Adab al-Andalusī: 'Aṣr al-Ṭawā'if wa-l-Murābiṭīn.* Beirut: Dār al-Thaqāfa.

——. 1996. *Ghurbat al-Rā'ī.* Beirut: Dār al-Shurūq

al-'Abbāsī, 'Abd al-Raḥīm ibn Aḥmad. 1947. *Ma'āhid al-Tanṣīṣ 'alā Shawāhid al-Talkhīṣ,* ed. Muḥammad Muḥyī al-Dīn 'Abd al-Ḥamīd. Beirut: 'Ālam al-Kutub.

'Abbūd, 'Abduh. 1995. *Hijrat al-Nuṣūṣ: Dirāsāt fī al-Tarjama al-Adabiyya wa-l-Tabādul al-Thaqāfī.* Damascus: Manshūrāt Ittiḥād al-Kuttāb al-'Arab.

'Abd al-'Azīz, Aḥmad. 1983. "Athar Federico Gracia Lorca fī al-Adab al-'Arabī al-Mu'āṣir." *Fuṣūl* 3.4 (July–September), pp. 271–99.

'Abd al-Dā'im, Yaḥyā Ibrāhīm. 1975. *al-Tarjama al-Dhātiyya fī al-Adab al-'Arabī al-Ḥadīth.* Beirut: Dār Iḥyā' al-Turāth al-'Arabī.

'Abd al-Fattāḥ, Sayyid Ṣiddīq. 1993a. *Tarājim wa-Āthār Udabā' al-Adab al-Sākhir.* Cairo: al-Dār al-Miṣriyya al-Lubnāniyya.

——. 1993b. *Ḥayāt wa-A'māl Shu'arā' al-Adab al-Sākhir.* Cairo: al-Dār al-Miṣriyya al-Lubnāniyya.

'Abd al-Ḥalīm, Muḥammad. 2014. "Fī Ifādat Najīb Maḥfūẓ al-Fanniya min Lughat al-Qur'ān." *Journal of Qur'anic Studies* 16.3, pp. 104–26.

'Abd al-Ḥayy, Muḥammad. 1977. *al-Usṭūra al-Ighrīqiyya fī al-Shi'r al-'Arabī al-Mu'āṣir.* Cairo: Dār al-Nahḍa al-'Arabiyya.

'Abd al-Nāṣir, Jamāl. n.d. [1955]. *Falsafat al-Thawra.* Cairo: Dār al-Ma'ārif.

'Abd al-Ṣabūr, Ṣalāḥ. n.d. *Madīnat al-'Ishq wa-l-Ḥikma.* Beirut: Dār Iqra'.

——. 1957. *al-Nās fī Bilādī.* Beirut: Dār al-Ādāb.

——. 1964. *Aḥlām al-Fāris al-Qadīm.* Beirut: Dār al-Ādāb.

——. 1965 [1964]. *Ma'sāt al-Ḥallāj.* Beirut: Dār al-Ādāb.

——. 1969. *Ḥayātī fī al-Shi'r*. Beirut: Dār al-'Awda.
——. 1971. *Riḥla 'alā al-Waraq*. Cairo: Maktabat al-Anglo al-Miṣriyya.
——. 1972. *Dīwān*. Beirut: Dār al-'Awda.
——. 1972a. *Murder in Baghdad*, trans. Khalil Semaan. Leiden: Brill.
——. 1981. *al-Ibḥār fī al-Dhākira*. Beirut: Dār al-Shurūq.
——. 1981a. "Tajribatī fī al-Shi'r." *Fuṣūl* 2.1, pp. 13–18.
——. 1981 [1969]. *Ḥayātī fī al-Shi'r*. Beirut: Dār Iqra'.
——. 1981 [1969]a. *Musāfir Layl*. Beirut: Dār al-Shurūq.
——. 1982 [1968]. *Qirā'a Jadīda li-Shi'rinā al-Qadīm*. Beirut: Dār Iqra'.
——. 1982a. *Nabḍ al-Fikr*. Riyadh: Dār al-Mirrīkh.
——. 1983. *'Alā Mashārif al-Khamsīn*. Beirut: Dār al-Shurūq.
——. 1983 [1973]. *Ba'da an Yamūta al-Malik*. Beirut: Dār al-Shurūq.
——. 1986. *Shajar al-Layl*. Beirut and Cairo: Dār al-Shurūq.
'Abd al-Wahhāb, Zuhayr. 1995. "Ḥājatunā ilā al-Tarjama." *al-Qāfila* (al-Ẓahrān), July/August, pp. 10–12.
Abdel-Messih, Marie-Thérèse. 2009. "Hyper Texts: Avant-Gardism in Contemporary Egyptian Narratives." *Neohelicon* 36.2, pp. 515–23.
——. 2018. "Rethinking Critical Approaches to Arabic Comparatively, in a 'Post' Colonial Context." *Interventions: International Journal of Postcolonial Studies* 20.2, pp. 192–209.
Abdel Nasser, Tahia. 2017. *Literary Autobiography and Arab National Struggles*. Edinburgh: Edinburgh University Press.
Abdel Sabour, Salah. 1970. *A Journey at Night*, trans. Samar Attar. Cairo: al-Hay'a al-Miṣriyya al-'Āmma li-l-Ta'līf wa-l-Nashr.
Abdul Saboor, Salah. 1986. *Now the King Is Dead*, trans. Nehad Selaiha. Cairo: General Egyptian Book Organization Press.
Abdullah, Thabit. 1997. "Arab Views of Northern Europeans in Medieval History and Geography." In David R. Blanks (ed.). *Images of the Other: Europe and the Muslim World: Before 1700*, Cairo Papers in Social Science, vol. 19, Monograph 2, Summer 1996. Cairo: American University in Cairo Press, pp. 73–80.
Abdul-Razak, H. M. 1989. "Keats, Shelley and Byron in Nazik al-Mala'ikah's Poetry." PhD thesis, University of Glasgow.
Abel, A. 1965. "Dadjdjāl." *The Encyclopaedia of Islam*, 2nd edn. II, pp. 76–7.
Abi-Rached, Joelle M. 2020. *'Aṣfūriyyeh: A History of Madness, Modernity, and War in the Middle*. Cambridge, MA: MIT Press.
Abou-Bakr, Omaima. 1997. "The Religious Other: Christian Images in Sufi Poetry." In David R. Blanks (ed.). *Images of the Other: Europe and the Muslim World: Before 1700*, Cairo Papers in Social Science, vol. 19, Monograph 2, Summer 1996. Cairo: American University in Cairo Press, pp. 96–108.
Aboul-Ela, Hosam. 2001. "Challenging the Embargo: Arabic Literature in the US Market." *Middle East Report* 219 (Summer), pp. 42–4.
——. 2011. "Our Theory Split." *International Journal of Middle East Studies* 43.4 (2011), pp. 725–7.
Abrams, M. H. 1981. *A Glossary of Literary Terms*. New York: CBS Publishing Japan.
Abu-Deeb, Kamal. 2000. "The Collapse of Totalizing Discourse and the Rise of Marginalized/Minority Discourses." In Kamal Abdel-Malek and Wael Hallaq (eds.). *Tradition, Modernity, and Postmodernity in Arabic Literature: Essays in Honor of Professor Issa J. Boullata*. Leiden: Brill, pp. 335–66.
Abudi, Dalya. 2011. *Mothers and Daughters in Arab Women's Literature: The Family Frontier*. Boston, MA: Brill.
Abū Fāshā, Ṭāhir. n.d. *Alf Yawm wa-Yawm*. Cairo: Madbūlī.
——. 1987. *Hazz al-Quḥūf bi-Sharḥ Qaṣīdat Abī Shādūf*. Cairo: al-Hay'a al-Miṣriyya al-'Āmma li-l-Kitāb.

Abū Ḥadīd, Muḥammad Farīd. 1935. "Majālis al-Adab fī al-Qarn al-Thāmin 'Ashar." *al-Risāla*, February 11, pp. 205–7.

Abu-Haidar, Jareer. 1985. "*Awlād Ḥāratinā* by Najīb Maḥfūẓ: An Event in the Arab World." *Journal of Arabic Literature* 16, pp. 119–31.

——. 1991. "The *Muwaššaḥāt* in the Light of the Literary Life that Produced Them." In Alan Jones and Richard Hitchcock (eds.). *Studies on the Muwaššaḥ and the Kharja*. Reading: Ithaca Press, pp. 115–22.

——. 1992. "The *Muwashshaḥāt*: Are They a Mystery?" *Al-Qanṭara* 13, pp. 63–81.

——. 1993. "The Arabic Origins of the *Muwashshaḥāt*." *Bulletin of the School of Oriental and African Studies* 56.3, pp. 439–58.

——. 2001. *Hispano-Arabic Literature and the Early Provençal Lyrics*. Richmond: Curzon.

Abū Ḥannā, Ḥannā. 1988. *Qaṣā'id min Ḥadīqat al-Ṣabr*. Acre: n.p.

Abu-Lughod, Ibrahim. 1963. *Arab Rediscovery of Europe: A Study in Cultural Encounters*. Princeton, NJ: Princeton University Press.

Abu-Lughod, Janet L. 1987. "The Islamic City: Historic Myth, Islamic Essence, and Contemporary Relevance." *International Journal of Middle East Studies* 19, pp. 155–76.

——. 1989. *Before European Hegemony: The World System, A.D. 1250–1350*. New York: Oxford University Press.

Abū al-Najā, Shīrīn. 2017. "al-Istiqbāl al-Ṣuḥufī l-Khiṭāb Laylā Ba'labakkī al-Adabī." *Alif: Journal of Comparative Poetics* 37, pp. 74–95.

Abu-Remaileh, Refqa. 2021. "Country of Words: Palestinian Literature in the Digital Age of the Refugee." *Journal of Arabic Literature* 52, pp. 68–96.

Abū al-Sa'd, 'Abd al-Ra'ūf. 1994. *al-Ṭifl wa-'Ālamuhu al-Adabī*. Cairo: Dār al-Ma'ārif.

Abū Sa'ūd, Fakhrī. 1934. "al-Athar al-Yūnānī fī al-Adab al-'Arabī." *al-Risāla*, June 11, pp. 968–9.

Abū Sayf, Samīra. 1987. *al-Sanābil: al-Mughāmarāt al-Muthīra (2): Mughāmara fī al-Faḍā'*. Cairo: al-Sharika al-Miṣriyya al-'Ālamiyya li-l-Nashr—Longman.

Abū Shabaka, Ilyās. 1985. *al-Majmū'a al-Kāmila fī al-Shi'r*, ed. Walīd Nadīm 'Abbūd. Jounieh, Lebanon: Dār Ruwwād al-Nahḍa.

Abū Ṭālib, Ibrāhīm. 2016. "The Autobiographical Poem of the Yemenite Poet Ḥasan 'Abd Allāh al-Sharfī." *Muṭāraḥāt* 5, pp. 131–45.

Abū Tammām. n.d. *al-Ḥamāsa*. Cairo: Muḥammad 'Alī Ṣubayḥ.

Accad, Evelyne. 1990. *Sexuality and War: Literary Masks of the Middle East*. New York: New York University Press.

Achour, Christiane. 1991. *Dictionnaire des oeuvres algériennes en langue française: Essais, romans, nouvelles, contes, récits autobiographiques*. Paris: Éditions L'Harmattan.

Adab al-Ṭifl al-'Arabī. 1995. Amman: Manshūrāt al-Ittiḥād al-'Āmm li-l-Udabā' al-'Arab.

Adams, Hazard. 1971. *Critical Theory since Plato*. New York: Harcourt Brace Jovanovich.

Adūnīs (Adonis). 1965. *Kitāb al-Taḥawwulāt wa-l-Hijra fī Aqālīm al-Nahār wa-l-Layl*. Beirut: al-Maktaba al-'Aṣriyya.

——. 1971. *al-Āthār al-Kāmila*. Beirut: Dār al-'Awda.

——. 1971a. *Muqaddima li-l-Shi'r al-'Arabī*. Beirut: Dār al-'Awda.

——. 1971 [1961]. *Aghānī Mihyār al-Dimashqī*. Beirut: Dār al-'Awda.

——. 1974. *al-Thābit wa-l-Mutaḥawwil: al-Uṣūl*. Beirut: Dār al-'Awda.

——. 1978. *al-Thābit wa-l-Mutaḥawwil: Ṣadmat al-Ḥadātha*. Beirut: Dār al-'Awda.

——. 1980. *Fātiḥa li-Nihāyāt al-Qarn—Bayānāt min Ajl Thaqāfa 'Arabiyya Jadīda*. Beirut: Dār al-'Awda.

——. 1988 [1983]. *al-A'māl al-Shi'riyya al-Kāmila*. Beirut: Dār al-'Awda.

——. 1992. *al-Ṣūfiyya wa-l-Sīryāliyya*. Beirut: Dār al-Sāqī.

——. 1993. *Hā Anta, Ayyuhā al-Waqt*. Beirut: Dār al-Ādāb.

——. 2005. *al-Muḥīṭ al-Aswad*. Beirut: Dār al-Sāqī.

——. 2005a. *Sufism and Surrealism*. London: Saqi.

——. 2008. *Mihyar of Damascus: His Songs*, trans. Adnan Haydar and Michael Beard. Rochester, NY: BOA Editions.
——. 2008a. *Warrāq Yabīʿ Kutub al-Nujūm*. Beirut: Dār al-Sāqī.
——. 2008b. *Ra's al-Lugha Jism al-Ṣaḥrā'*. Beirut: Dār al-Sāqī.
——. 2012–2015. *al-Aʿmāl al-Shiʿriyya al-Kāmila*. Beirut: Dār al-Sāqī.
——. 2020. *Dafātir Mihyār al-Dimashqī*. Beirut: Dār al-Sāqī.
——. 2022. "al-Thaqāfa al-ʿArabiyya al-Rāhina Bayna al-Dhātiyya wa-l-Ākhariyya." *al-Sharq al-Awsaṭ*, January 17.
Adūnīs and Saʿīd, Khālida (eds.). 1982. *Aḥmad Shawqī*. Beirut: Dār al-ʿIlm li-l-Malāyīn.
al-ʿAfif, Aḥmad Khulayf. 2008. *al-Taṭawwur al-Idārī li-l-Dawla al-ʿIrāqiyya fī al-Intidāb al-Bariṭānī (1922–1932)*. Amman: Dār Jarīr li-l-Nashr wa-l-Tawzīʿ.
Agius, Dionysius and Hitchcock, Richard (eds.). 1993. *The Arab Influence upon Medieval Europe*. Reading: Ithaca Press.
Aḥjayūj, Muḥammad Saʿīd. 2019. *Kafka fī Ṭanja (Kafka in Tanjier)*. Cairo: Dār Tabārak li-l-Nashr wa-l-Tawzīʿ.
Ahmed, Hussam R. 2021. *The Last Nahdawi: Taha Hussein and Institution Building in Egypt*. Stanford, CA: Stanford University Press.
Ahmed, Leila. 1978. *Edward W. Lane: A Study of His Life and Works and of British Ideas of the Middle East in the Nineteenth Century*. London: Longman.
——. 1992. *Women and Gender in Islam: Historical Roots of a Modern Debate*. New Haven, CT: Yale University Press.
Akash, Munir and Mattawa, Khaled. 2000. *Post Gibran: Anthology of New Arab American Writing*. West Bethesda, MD: Kitab (distributed by Syracuse University Press).
Akbar, Arifa. 2015. "The All-Islamic Super-Heroes: Muslim Children Love 'The 99' Comics, but Hardliners Loathe Their Creator: Whose Trial for Heresy Is Looming?" *The Independent*, March 11.
Akhbār al-Ḥallāj. n.d. (ed.) ʿAbd al-Ḥāfiẓ ibn Muḥammad Madanī Hāshim. Cairo: Maktabat al-Jundī.
al-Akhḍar, Rafīq. 1986. "Lorca fī al-Dhikrā al-Khamsīn li-Mawtihi." *al-Shaʿb*, May 15, p. 4.
Aldiss, Brian and Lundwall, Sam J. 1986. *The Penguin World Omnibus of Science Fiction*. Harmondsworth: Penguin.
Al-Ali, Nadje Sadig. 1993. *Gender Writing / Writing Gender: The Representation of Women in a Selection of Modern Egyptian Literature*. Cairo: American University in Cairo Press.
Ali, Samer M. 2010. *Arabic Literary Salons in the Islamic Middle Ages: Poetry, Public Performance and the Presentation of the Past*. Notre Dame, IN: University of Notre Dame Press.
Alkhayat, Marwa Essam Eldin Fahmy. 2021. "Sabry Musa's *Lord of the Spinach Field* (1987): A Critique of Post-Colonial Utopianism." *Arab Studies Quarterly* 43.3, pp. 230–48.
Allan, Michael. 2016. *In the Shadow of World Literature: Sites of Reading in Colonial Egypt*. Princeton, NJ: Princeton University Press.
Allen, Roger. 1987. *Modern Arabic Literature*. New York: Ungar Publishing.
——. 1993. "The Impact of the Translated Text: The Case of Najīb Maḥfūẓ's Novels, with Special Emphasis on *The Trilogy*." *Edebiyât* 4, pp. 87–117.
——. 1994. "PROTA: The Project for the Translation of Arabic." *Middle East Studies Association Bulletin* 28.2 (December), pp. 165–8.
——. 1998. *The Arabic Literary Heritage: The Development of Its Genres and Criticism*. Cambridge: Cambridge University Press.
——. 2006. "The Post-Classical Period: Parameters and Preliminaries." In Roger Allen and D. S. Richards (eds.). *Arabic Literature in the Post-Classical Period*. Cambridge: Cambridge University Press, pp. 1–21.
——. 2007. "Rewriting Literary History: The Case of the Arabic Novel." *Journal of Arabic Literature* 38.3, pp. 247–60.

——. (ed.). 2010. *Essays in Arabic Literary Biography 1850–1950*. Wiesbaden: Harrassowitz Verlag.
——. 2018. "Transforming the Arabic Literary Canon." In Roger Allen et al. (eds.). *New Geographies: Texts and Contexts in Modern Arabic Literature*. Madrid: Ediciones Universidad Autónoma de Madrid, pp. 15–26.
Allen, Roger and Hillmann, Michael. 1989. "Arabic Literature in English Translation." *Literature East and West* 25, pp. 104–16.
Allen, Roger and Richards, D. S. (eds.). 2006. *Arabic Literature in the Post-Classical Period*. Cambridge: Cambridge University Press.
Allen, Sture (ed.). 1993. *Nobel Lectures in Literature 1981–1990*. Singapore: World Scientific Publishing.
al-Amīr, Ayman. 1964. "Dirāsa fī Adab Virginia Woolf." *al-Ādāb* 12.1, pp. 61–4.
Alter, Robert. 1975. *Partial Magic: The Novel as a Self-Conscious Genre*. Berkeley: University of California Press.
Altoma, Salih J. 1993. "The Reception of Najib Mahfuz in American Publications." *Yearbook of Comparative and General Literature* 41, pp. 160–79.
——. 1993a. *Modern Arabic Poetry in English Translation: A Bibliography*. Tangiers: King Fahd School of Translation.
——. 1996. "Contemporary Arabic Fiction in English Translation: A Chronological Survey: 1947–1996." *Yearbook of Comparative and General Literature* 44, pp. 137–53.
——. 1997. "Iraq's Modern Arabic Literature in English Translation: A Preliminary Bibliography." *Arab Studies Quarterly* 19.4, pp. 131–72.
——. 2000. "Arabic–Western Literary Relation in American Publications: A Selected Bibliography." *Yearbook of Comparative and General Literature* 48, pp. 221–62.
——. 2005. *Modern Arabic Literature in Translation: A Companion*. London: Saqi.
——. 2009. "Translating Contemporary Iraq's Arabic Literature: Ten Years of *Banipal*'s Record 1998–2008." *International Journal of Contemporary Iraqi Studies* 3.3, pp. 307–19.
——. 2010. *Iraq's Modern Arabic Literature: A Guide to English Translations since 1950*. Lanham, MD: Scarecrow Press.
al-Ālūsī, Jamāl al-Dīn. 1987. *Baghdād fī al-Shi'r al-'Arabī: Min Ta'rīkhihā wa-Akhbārihā al-Ḥaḍāriyya*. Baghdad: Maṭba'at al-Majma' al-'Ilmī al-'Irāqī.
Alwan, Mohammed Bakir. 1972. "A Bibliography of Modern Arabic Fiction in English Translation." *Middle East Journal* 26, pp. 195–200.
——. 1973. "A Bibliography of Modern Arabic Poetry in English Translation." *Middle East Journal* 27, pp. 373–81.
Amanṣūr, Muḥammad. n.d. "al-Riwāya al-Maghribiyya al-Mu'āṣira: Ḥafriyyāt fī al-Takwwun." *Maknasat: Revue de la Faculté des Lettres et des Sciences Humaínes de Université Moulay Ismaïl* (Meknés), pp. 79–98.
Amīn, Aḥmad. 1965. *Zu'amā' al-Iṣlāḥ fī al-'Aṣr al-Ḥadīth*. Cairo: Maktabat al-Nahḍa al-Miṣriyya.
Amin, Magda. 2000. "Stories, Stories, Stories: Rafik Schami's *Erzähler der Nacht*." *Alif: Journal of Comparative Literature* 20, pp. 211–33.
'Āmir, Ibrāhīm. 1970. "Najīb Maḥfūẓ Siyāsiyyan min Thawrat 1919 ilā Yūnyū 1967." *al-Hilāl*, February, pp. 26–37.
Amit-Kochavi, Hannah. 1996. "Israeli Arabic Literature in Hebrew Translation: Initiation, Dissemination and Reception." *The Translator* 2.1, pp. 27–44.
——. 1999. "Translations of Arabic Literature into Hebrew: Their Historical and Cultural Background and Their Reception by the Target Culture" (in Hebrew). PhD thesis, Tel Aviv University.
——. 2000. "Hebrew Translations of Palestinian Literature—From Total Denial to Partial Recognition." *Études sur le texte et ses transformations* 13.1, pp. 53–80.

——. 2003. "Strangers and Enemies or Partners? Hebrew Translations of Palestinian Literature: Writers, Contents and Texts" (in Hebrew). *Jamaʻa: Interdisciplinary Journal of Middle East Studies* 10, pp. 39–68.

——. 2006. "Israeli-Jewish Nation Building and Hebrew Translations of Arabic Literature." In Yasir Suleiman and Ibrahim Muhawi (eds.). *Literature and Nation in the Middle East.* Edinburgh: Edinburgh University Press, pp. 100–9.

Amo, Mercedes del. 2010. "La traducción al español de la literatura marroquí escrita en árabe (1940–2009)." *Miscelánea de Estudios Árabes y Hebraicos (Sección Árabe-Islam)* 59, pp. 239–57.

ʻAnānī, Muḥammad Zakariyyā. 1976. "Rifāʻa al-Ṭahṭāwī wa-l-Adab: Tarjamat Télémaque." *al-Kātib* (Cairo) 189 (December), pp. 8–25.

And, Metin. 1963–1964. *A History of Theatre and Popular Entertainment in Turkey.* Ankara: Forum Yayinlari.

Anders, Gunther. 1965. *Franz Kafka*, trans. A. Steer and A. K. Thorby. London: Bowes.

Anderson, Benedict. 1991. *Imagined Communities: Reflections on the Origin and Spread of Nationalism.* London: Verso.

Anderson, Jon W. 2005. "Wiring Up: The Internet Difference for Muslim Networks." In Miriam Cooke and Bruce B. Lawrence (eds.). *Muslim Networks from Hajj to Hip Hop.* Chapel Hill: University of North Carolina Press, pp. 252–63.

——. 2011. "Electronic Media and New Muslim Publics." In Robert W. Hefner (ed.). *The New Cambridge History of Islam: Muslims and Modernity Culture and Society since 1800*, vol. 6. Cambridge: Cambridge University Press, pp. 648–60.

Anderson, Margaret (ed.). 1980. *Arabic Materials in English Translation.* Boston, MA: G. K. Hall.

Anderson, Perry. 2004. "Union Sucrée." *London Review of Books* 26.18, p. 18.

Anidjar, Gil. 2002. *"Our Place in al-Andalus": Kabbalah, Philosophy, Literature in Arab Jewish Letters.* Stanford, CA: Stanford University Press.

Anishchenkova, Valerie. 2014. *Autobiographical Identities in Contemporary Arab Culture.* Edinburgh: Edinburgh University Press.

Anṭūn, Sinān. 2010. *Layl Wāḥid fi Kull al-Mudun.* Cologne: Al-Kamel Verlag.

Apter, Emily. 2013. *Against World Literature: On the Politics of Untranslatability.* London: Verso.

ʻAql, Saʻīd. 1935. "Al-Shiʻr al-Lubnānī bi-l-Lughati al-Fransawiyya." *al-Mashriq* 33 (July/September), pp. 381–93.

Arberry, Arthur J. 1960. *Oriental Essays: Portraits of Seven Scholars.* London: George Allen & Unwin.

——. 1965. *Arabic Poetry: A Primer for Students.* Cambridge: Cambridge University Press.

——. (ed.). 1969. *Religion in the Middle East: Three Religions in Concord and Conflict.* Cambridge: Cambridge University Press.

——. 1979 [1950]. *Sufism.* London: Mandala Books.

——. 1979 [1964]. *The Koran Interpreted.* Oxford: Oxford University Press.

Arendt, Hannah. 1974. *Rahel Varnhagen: The Life of a Jewish Woman*, trans. Richard and Clara Winston. New York: Harcourt Brace Jovanovich.

al-ʻĀrif, ʻĀrif. 1943. *Ru'yāy.* Jerusalem: Maṭbaʻat al-Ābā' al-Fransīsiyīn.

Aristotle. 1967. *Poetics.* ed. and trans. G. F. Else. Ann Arbor: University of Michigan Press.

——. 1968. *Poetics*, ed. D. W. Lucas. Oxford: Clarendon Press.

Arjomand, Saïd. 2011. "Islamic Resurgence and Its Aftermath." In Robert W. Hefner (ed.). *The New Cambridge History of Islam: Muslims and Modernity Culture and Society since 1800*, vol. 6. Cambridge: Cambridge University Press, pp. 173–97.

Armbrust, William. 1996. *Mass Culture and Modernism in Egypt.* Cambridge: Cambridge University Press.

——. 2012. "A History of New Media in the Arab Middle East." *Journal for Cultural Research* 16.3, pp. 155–74.

Arslan, C. Ceyhun. 2016. "Translating Ottoman into Classical Arabic: *Nahḍa* and the Balkan Wars in Aḥmad Shawqī's 'The New al-Andalus.'" *Middle Eastern Literatures* 19.3, pp. 278–97.

'Asāqla (Asaqli) 'Iṣām (Eisam). 2003. "Wilādat Adab al-Khayāl al-'Ilmī fī al-Adab al-'Arabī." MA thesis, University of Haifa.

——. 2006. "Binā' al-Shakhṣiyyāt fī Riwāyāt al-Khayāl al-'Ilmī fī al-Adab al-'Arabī." PhD thesis, University of Haifa.

——. 2011. *Binā' al-Shakhṣiyyāt fī Riwāyāt al-Khayāl al-'Ilmī fī al-Adab al-'Arabī.* Amman: Azmina li-l-Nashr wa-l-Tawzī'.

'Asāqla (Asaqli) 'Iṣām and Masalha, Mariam. 2018. "*al-Sayyid min Ḥaql al-Sabānikh*: Personal Freedom versus Mechanical System." *International Journal of Advanced Research* 6.6, pp. 129–45.

Asfour, John Mikhail (ed.). 1988. *When the Words Burn: An Anthology of Modern Arabic Poetry 1945–1987*. Dunvegan, ON: Cormorant Books.

'Āshūr, Raḍwā. 1998. *Thulāthiyyat Ghranāṭa*. Beirut: al-Mu'assasa al-'Arabiyya li-l-Dirāsāt wa-l-Nashr.

Asimov, Isaac. 1982. *The Complete Robot*. Garden City, NY: Doubleday.

——. 1994. *Isti'rāḍ al-Rūbūṭ*, trans. Fidā' Dakrūb. Beirut: Dār al-Ḥadātha.

Athamneh, Waed. 2017. *Modern Arabic Poetry: Revolution and Conflict*. Notre Dame, IN: University of Notre Dame Press.

'Aṭiyya, Aḥmad Muḥammad. 1970. "Liqā' Ma'a Najīb Maḥfūẓ." *al-Ādāb*, January, pp. 27–9.

——. 1977. *Ma'a Najīb Maḥfūẓ*. Beirut: Dār al-Jīl.

Attridge, Derek. 1992. (ed.). *Acts of Literature*. London: Routledge.

Auden, W. H. 1970. *A Certain World*. London: Faber & Faber.

Avino, Maria. 2001. "La traduzione letteraria dall'italiano in arabo, fino alla vigilia della seconda guerra mondiale. (Abstract: Literary Translation from Italian into Arabic Up to World War II)." *Traduttore Nuovo* 56.1, pp. 53–66, 115.

al-'Awīṭ, 'Aql. 2021. *Āb Aqsā al-Shuhūr Yush'ilu al-Laylak fī al-Arḍ al-Kharāb*. Beirut: Dār Nelson.

'Awwād, Tawfīq Yūsuf. 1984 [1939]. *al-Raghīf*. Beirut: Maktabat Lubnān.

Ayachi, Khedija Kchouk. 2012. "L'héritage du soufisme dans la poétique arabe contemporaine." PhD thesis, Université de Strasbourg.

Ayalon, Ami. 1987. *Language and Change in the Arab Middle East*. Oxford: Oxford University Press.

——. 2011. "The Press and Publishing." In Robert W. Hefner (ed.). 2011. *The New Cambridge History of Islam: Muslims and Modernity Culture and Society since 1800*, vol. 6. Cambridge: Cambridge University Press, pp. 572–96.

——. 2016. *The Arabic Print Revolution: Cultural Production and Mass Readership*. Cambridge: Cambridge University Press.

——. 2021. "Children's Leisure Reading in the *Nahḍah*." *Journal of Arabic Literature* 52, pp. 372–93.

Ayyad, Shukry and Witherspoon, Nancy. 1999. *Reflections and Deflections: A Study of the Contemporary Arab Mind through Its Literary Creations*. Cairo: Prism.

Ayyūb, Dhū al-Nūn. 1971. "Kitāb al-Shahr: 'Arabāt al-Āliha." *al-Ādāb*, May, pp. 12–13.

al-A'ẓamī, Aḥmad 'Izzat. 1932. *al-Qaḍiyya al-'Arabiyya: Asbābuhā, Muqaddimātuhā, Taṭawwuruhā wa-Natā'ijuhā*. Baghdad: Maṭba'at al-Sha'b.

al-'Aẓm, Ṣādiq Jalāl. 1992. *Dhihniyyat al-Taḥrīm: Salmān Rushdī wa-Ḥaqīqat al-Adab*. London: Riyāḍ al-Rayyis.

al-Azmeh, Aziz. 1996. *Islams and Modernities*. London: Verso.

Azouqa, Aida. 2001. "Defamilarization in the Poetry of 'Abd al-Wahhāb al-Bayātī and T. S. Eliot: A Comparative Study." *Journal of Arabic Literature* 32.2, pp. 167–211.

'Azzām, Muḥammad. 1994. *al-Khayāl al-'Ilmī fī al-Adab*. Damascus: Dār Ṭalās.

——. 2000. *Khayāl bi-lā Ḥudūd: Ṭālib 'Umrān Rā'id Adab al-Khayāl al-'Ilmī*. Beirut: Dār al-Fikr al-Mu'āṣir.

al-'Azzāwī, 'Abbās. 1996. *Ta'rīkh al-Adab al-'Arabī fī al-'Irāq*. Baghdad: Āfāq 'Arabiyya.

al-'Azzāwī, Fāḍil. 1997. *al-Rūḥ al-Ḥayya: Jīl al-Sittīnāt fī al-'Irāq*. Damascus: Dar al-Madā.

Badawi, M. M. 1975. *A Critical Introduction to Modern Arabic Poetry*. Cambridge: Cambridge University Press.

——. 1975a. "Ten Modern Arabic Poems." *Journal of Arabic Literature* 6, pp. 130–9.

——. 1985. *Modern Arabic Literature and the West*. London: Ithaca Press.

——. 1985a. "The Father of the Modern Egyptian Theatre: Ya'qūb Ṣanū'." *Journal of Arabic Literature* 16, pp. 132–45.

——. 2000. "Perennial Themes in Modern Arabic Literature." In Derek Hopwood (ed.). *Arab Nation, Arab Nationalism*. Basingstoke: Macmillan, pp. 129–53.

al-Badawī al-Mulaththam. 1963. *al-Bustānī wa-Ilyādhat Hūmīrūs*. Cairo: Dār al-Ma'ārif.

Badīr, Ḥilmī. 1982. *al-Mu'aththirāt al-Ajnabiyya fī al-Adab al-'Arabī al-Ḥadīth*. Cairo: Dār al-Ma'ārif.

Badr, 'Abd al-Muḥsin Ṭāhā. 1983. *Taṭawwur al-Riwāya al-'Arabiyya al-Ḥadītha fī Miṣr (1870–1938)*. Cairo: Dār al-Ma'ārif.

Badrān, Ḥusayn.1972. *al-Thabt al-Biblūjrāfī li-l-A'māl al-Mutarjama 1956–1967*. Cairo: al-Hay'a al-Miṣriyya al-'Āmma li-l-Kitāb.

Badrān, Muḥammad Abū al-Faḍl. 2001. *Adabiyyāt al-Karāma al-Ṣūfiyya: Dirāsa fī al-Shikl wa-l-Maḍmūn*. al-'Ayn, UAE: Markaz Zāyid li-l-Turāth wa-l-Ta'rīkh.

al-Bagdadi, Nadia. 2008. "Registers of Arabic Literary History." *New Literary History* 39.3, pp. 437–61.

Bahayeldin, Khalid. 2004. "Arabic and Islamic Themes in Frank Herbert's 'Dune.'" Baheyeldin.com, January 22, 2004, available at: https://baheyeldin.com/literature/arabic-and-islamic-themes-in-frank-herberts-dune.html, last accessed April 26, 2021.

Bahī, 'Iṣām. 1982. "Riwāyat al-Khayāl al-'Ilmī wa-Ru'ā al-Mustaqbal." *Fuṣūl* 2.2 (January–March), pp. 57–65.

——. 1994. *al-Khayāl al-'Ilmī fī Masraḥ Tawfīq al-Ḥakīm*. Cairo: al-Hay'a al-Miṣriyya al-'Āmma li-l-Kitāb.

al-Bahnassī, 'Afīf. 1997. *al-'Umrān al-Thaqāfī Bayna al-Turāth wa-l-Qawmiyya*. Damascus: Dār al-Kitāb al-'Arabī.

Baḥr, Samīra. 1979. *al-Aqbāṭ fī al-Ḥayāt al-Siyāsiyya al-Miṣriyya*. Cairo: Maktabat al-Anglo al-Miṣriyya.

Bakker, Barbara. 2021. "Egyptian Dystopias of the 21st Century: A New Literary Trend?" *Journal of Arabic and Islamic Studies* 21, pp. 79–94.

Ba'labakkī, Laylā. 2010 [1963]. *Safīnat Ḥanān ilā al-Qamar*. Beirut: Dār al-Ādāb.

Ballas, Shimon. 1980. *La littérature arabe et le conflit au proche-orient (1948–1973)*. Paris: Éditions Anthropos.

Ballas, Shimon and Snir, Reuven (eds.). 1998. *Studies in Canonical and Popular Arabic Literature*. Toronto: York Press.

Balqāsim, Khālid. 2000. *Adūnīs wa-l-Khiṭāb al-Ṣūfī*. Casablanca: Dār Tūbaqāl.

Bamia, Aida. 1992. "The North African Novel: Achievements and Prospects." *Mundus Arabicus* 5, pp. 61–88.

Barakat, Halim. 2000. "Explorations in Exile and Creativity: The Case of Arab-American Writers." In Kamal Abdel-Malek and Wael Hallaq (eds.). *Tradition, Modernity, and Postmodernity in Arabic Literature: Essays in Honor of Professor Issa J. Boullata*. Leiden: Brill, pp. 304–20.

Barbaro, Ada. 2013. "Marginality as a Genre: Science Fiction in the Arab Literature and the Case of the Egyptian writer Nihad Sharif." In Lawrence Denooz and Xavier Luffin (eds.). *Aux marges de la littérature arabe contemporaine*. Helsinki: Academia Scientiarum Fennica, pp. 39–49.

——. 2017. "Where Science Fiction and *al-Khayāl al-ʿIlmī* Meet." In Esterino Adami et al. (eds.). *Other Worlds of Science Fiction and the Narrative Construction of Otherness*. Milan: Mimesis International, pp. 31–49.

——. 2018. "Between Fantasy and Science Fiction: Saudi Society through the Eyes of a Jinn." In Roger Allen et al. (eds.). *New Geographies: Texts and Contexts in Modern Arabic Literature*. Madrid: Ediciones Universidad Autónoma de Madrid, pp. 181–202.

——. 2021. "I Will Tell You My History: Rewriting to Revolt in the Process of *al-Tārīkh al-badīl* (Allohistory)." *Journal of Arabic Literature* 52.3/4, pp. 351–71.

al-Bāridī, Muḥammad. 1997. "al-Sīra al-Dhātiyya fī al-Adab al-ʿArabī al-Ḥadīth—Ḥudūd al-Jins wa-Ishkālātuhu." *Fuṣūl* 16.3 (Winter), pp. 68–80.

Baron, Beth Ann. 1996. "A Field Matures: Recent Literature on Women in the Middle East." *Middle Eastern Studies* 32.3, pp. 172–86.

Baron, Salo Wittmayer. 1957. *A Social and Religious History of the Jews*. Philadelphia: Jewish Publication Society of America.

Barrāda, Muḥammad. 1996. *As'ilat al-Riwāya As'ilat al-Naqd*. Casablanca: al-Rābiṭa.

Barthes, Roland. 1977 [1967]. "The Death of the Author." In Stephen Heath (ed. and trans.). *Image—Music—Text*. New York: Farrar, Straus & Giroux, pp. 142–8.

Bashkin, Orit. 2006. "'When Muʿawiya Entered the Curriculum'—Some Comments on the Iraqi Education System in the Interwar Period." *Comparative Education Review* 50.3, pp. 346–66.

Bāsīlī, Būluṣ. 1999. *al-Aqbāṭ: Waṭaniyya wa-Ta'rīkh*. Cairo: Dār Nūbār li-l-Ṭibāʿa.

Baṣrī, Mīr. 1991. *Aghānī al-Ḥubb wa-l-Khulūd*. Jerusalem: Rābiṭat al-Jāmiʿiyyīn al-Yahūd al-Nāziḥīn min al-ʿIrāq.

Bassiouney, Reem and Walters, Keith. 2021. *The Routledge Handbook of Arabic and Identity*. New York: Routledge.

Batatu, Hanna. 1978. *The Old Social Classes and the Revolutionary Movements of Iraq*. Princeton, NJ: Princeton University Press.

Bauer, Thomas. 2005. "Mamluk Literature: Misunderstandings and New Approaches." *Mamlūk Studies Review* 9.2, pp. 105–32.

——. 2007. "In Search of 'Post-Classical Literature': A Review Article." *Mamlūk Studies Review* 11.2, pp. 137–67.

——. 2013. "'Ayna Hādhā min al-Mutanabbī!': Toward an Aesthetics of Mamluk Literature." *Mamlūk Studies Review* 17, pp. 5–22.

——. 2013a. "Adab and Islamic Scholarship after the 'Sunni Revival'." In *Encyclopaedia of Islam*, 3rd edn. pp. 38–42.

Bawārdī (Bawardi), Bāsīlyūs Ḥannā. 1998. "Bayna al-Ṣaḥrā' wa-l-Baḥr: Baḥth fī Ta'thīr al-Qawmiyyatayn al-Lubnāniyya-al-Fīnīqiyya wa-l-Sūriyya ʿalā al-Adab al-ʿArabī al-Muʿāṣir." MA thesis, University of Haifa.

——. 2000–2001. "Adab al-Qawmiyya al-Lubnāniyya al-Fīnīqiyya: *al-Taṣwīnī*, Awwal Riwāya bi-l-Lugha al-Lubnāniyya ka-Namūdhaj Naṣṣī." *al-Karmil: Studies in Arabic Language and Literature* 21/22, pp. 7–79.

——. 2008. "First Steps in Writing Arabic Narrative Fiction: The Case of *Ḥadīqat al-Akhbār*." *Die Welt des Islams* 48, pp. 170–95.

——. 2016. *The Lebanese-Phoenician Nationalist Movement: Literature, Language and Identity*. London: I. B. Tauris.

Bawārdī (Bawardi), Bāsīlyūs Ḥannā and Faranesh, Alif. 2018. "Non-Canonical Arabic Detective Fiction: The Beginnings of the Genre." *Journal of Arabic and Islamic Studies* 18, pp. 23–49.

al-Bayyātī, ʿAbd al-Wahhāb. 1954. *Abārīq Muhashshama*. Baghdad: Manshūrāt al-Thaqāfa al-Jadīda.

——. 1968. *Tajribatī al-Shiʿriyya*. Beirut: Manshūrāt Nizār Qabbānī.

——. 1969 [1954]. *Abārīq Muhashshama*. Beirut: Dār al-Ādāb.

——. 1979. *Dīwān*. Beirut: Dār al-ʿAwda.

——. 1984 [1975]. *Qamar Shīrāz*. Cairo: al-Hay'a al-Miṣriyya al-'Āmma li-l-Kitāb.
——. 1984 [1979]. *Mamlakat al-Sunbula*. Cairo: al-Hay'a al-Miṣriyya.
——. 1995. *Kitāb al-Marāthī*. Beirut: al-Mu'assasa al-'Arabiyya li-l-Dirāsāt wa-l-Nashr.
Beard, Michael and Haydar, Adnan (eds.). 1993. *Naguib Mahfouz: From Regional Fame to Global Recognition*. Syracuse, NY: Syracuse University Press.
Beckson, Karl and Ganz, Arthur. 1990. *Literary Terms*. London: Andre Deutsch.
Beinin, Joel. 1998. *The Dispersion of Egyptian Jewry: Culture, Politics, and Formation of a Modern Diaspora*. Berkeley: University of California Press.
Bell, Daniel A. and de-Shalit, Avner. 2011. *The Spirit of Cities: Why the Identity of a City Matters in a Global Age*. Princeton, NJ: Princeton University Press.
Bellino, Francesca. 2017. "Ra's al- Ghūl, the Enemy of 'Alī and Batman: Upturned Narratives from Arabic Literature to American Comics." In Esterinp Adami et al. (eds.). *Other Worlds of Science Fiction and the Narrative Construction of Otherness*. Milan: Mimesis, pp. 183–206.
——. 2020. "Arabic Encyclopaedias and Encyclopaedism in the Ottoman Period: Forms, Functions and Intersections between Adab and Modernity." In Catherine Mayeur-Jaouen (ed.). *Adab and Modernity: A "Civilising Process"? (Sixteenth–Twenty-First Century)*. Leiden: Brill, pp. 123–67.
Benarab, Abdelkader. 1995. *Les Voix de l'Exil*. Paris: L'Harmattan.
Ben Driss, Hager. 2021. "Poetics of the Virtual: Technology and Revolution in the Poetry of Sghaier Ouled Ahmed." In Eid Mohamed et al. (eds.). *Cultural Production and Social Movements after the Arab Spring: Nationalism, Politics, and Transnational Identity*. London: I. B. Tauris, pp. 83–99.
Benedict, Ruth. 1934. *Patterns of Culture*. Boston, MA: Houghton Mifflin.
Benjamin, Walter. 1969. "Theses on the Philosophy of History." In Hannah Arendt (ed.). *Illuminations*, trans. Harry Zohn. New York: Schocken, pp. 253–64.
Benjamin II, Rabbi Israel-Joseph. 1856. *Cinq années de voyage en orient, 1846–1851*. Paris: Michel Levy Frères.
Ben Jelloun, Tahar. 1987. *La nuit sacrée*. Paris: Éditions du Seuil.
——. 2006. "Mahfouz, the Middle Man." *New York Times*, September 3.
Benn, Gottfried. 1997. *Qaṣā'id Mukhtāra*, trans. Khālid al-Ma'ālī. Cologne: Al-Kamel Verlag.
Bennett, Andrew and Royle, Nicholas. 2004. *An Introduction to Literature, Criticism and Theory*. Harlow: Pearson Longman.
Bergson, Henri. 1954. *Creative Evolution*, trans. Arthur Mitchell. London: Macmillan.
——. 1968. *The Creative Mind*, trans. Mabelle L. Andison. New York: Greenwood Press.
Berman, Nina. 1998. "German and Middle Eastern Literary Traditions in a Novel by Salim Alafenisch: Thoughts on a Germanophone Beduin Author from the Negev." *German Quarterly* 71, pp. 271–83.
Bhabha, Homi K. 1994. *The Location of Culture*. London: Routledge.
Bialik, Hayyim Nahman. 1966. *Poems* (in Hebrew). Tel Aviv: Dvir.
Binder, Hartmut. 1966. *Motiv und Gestaltung bei Franz Kafka*. Bonn: H. Bouvier.
——. 1977. *Kafka Kommentar zu Samtlichen Erzahlungen*. Munich: Winkler.
Biran, Michal. 2019. "Libraries, Books and Transmission of Knowledge in Ilkhanid Baghdad." *Journal of the Economic and Social History of the Orient* 62.2/3, pp. 464–502.
al-Bishrī, Ṭāriq. 1988. *al-Muslimūn wa-l-Aqbāṭ fī Iṭār al-Jamā'a al-Waṭaniyya*. Cairo: Dār al-Shurūq.
Blasim, Hassan (ed.). 2017. *Iraq + 100: The First Anthology of Science Fiction to Have Emerged from Iraq*. New York: Tor Books.
Booth, Marilyn. 1992. "Poetry in the Vernacular." In M. M. Badawi (ed.). *Modern Arabic Literature*. Cambridge: Cambridge University Press, pp. 463–82.
Bosworth, C. Edmund. 1967. *The Islamic Dynasties*. Edinburgh: Edinburgh University Press.

——. 1996. "Arabic Influences in the Literature of Nineteenth and Early Twentieth Century Britain." In J. R. Smart (ed.). *Tradition and Modernity in Arabic Language and Literature*. Richmond: Curzon, pp. 155–64.
Boudot-Lamotte, Antoine. 1977. *Aḥmad Šawqī l'homme et l'oeuvre*. Damascus: Institut Français de Damas.
Boulus, Sargon. 1997. *Zeugen am Ufer*, trans. Khālid al-Ma'ālī and Stefan Weidner. Berlin: Das Arabische Buch.
Bouraoui, H. A. 1980. "Creative Project and Literary Projection in Francophone North Africa." In Issa J. Boullata (ed.). *Critical Perspectives on Modern Arabic Literature*. Washington, DC: Three Continents Press, pp. 129–44.
Bourdieu, Pierre. 1992. *Les règles de l'art: genèse et structure du champ littéraire*. Paris: Éditions du Seuil.
——. 1996. *Rules of Art: Genesis and Structure of the Literary Field*, trans. Susan Emanuel. Cambridge: Polity.
Bousset, Wilhelm. 1895. *Der Antichrist in der Vberlieferung des Judentums, des Newen Testaments und der Alten Kirche*. Gottingen: Vandenhoeck und Ruprecht.
——. 1896. *The Antichrist Legend: A Chapter in Christian and Jewish Folklore*. London: Hutchinson.
Boyle, J. A. (ed.). 1968. *The Cambridge History of Iran*, vol. V. Cambridge: Cambridge University Press.
Brann, Ross. 1987. "The 'Dissembling Poet' in Medieval Hebrew Literature: The Dimensions of a Literary Topos." *Journal of the American Oriental Society* 107.1, pp. 39–54.
——. 2000. "The Arabized Jews." In Maria Rosa Menocal et al. (eds.). *The Cambridge History of Arabic Literature: The Literature of al-Andalus*. Cambridge: Cambridge University Press, pp. 435–54.
——. 2013. "Andalusi 'Exceptionalism.'" In Suzanne Conklin Akbari and Karla Mallette (eds.). *Sea of Languages: Rethinking the Arabic Role in Medieval Literary History*. Toronto: University of Toronto Press, pp. 119–34.
——. 2021. *Iberian Moorings: Al-Andalus, Sefarad, and the Tropes of Exceptionalism*. Philadelphia: University of Pennsylvania Press.
Bray, Julia. 2011. "Arabic literature." In Robert Irwin (ed.). *The New Cambridge History of Islam: Islamic Cultures and Societies to the End of the Eighteenth Century*, vol. 4. Cambridge: Cambridge University Press, pp. 383–413.
Brentjes, Sonja. 1999. "The Interests of the Republic of Letters in the Middle East, 1550–1700." *Science in Context* 12.3, pp. 435–68.
——. 2001. "On the Relationship between the Ottoman Empire and the West European Republic of Letters (17th–18th Centuries)." In Ali Çaksu (ed.). *International Congress on Learning and Education in the Ottoman World, Istanbul, 12–15 April 1999: Proceedings*. Istanbul: IRCICA, pp. 121–48.
——. 2010. *Travellers from Europe in the Ottoman and Safavid Empires, 16th–17th Centuries: Seeking, Transforming, Discarding Knowledge*. Aldershot: Ashgate.
Brenner, Rachel Feldhay. 1999. "'Hidden Transcripts' Made Public: Israeli Arab Fiction and Its Reception." *Critical Inquiry* 26 (Autumn), pp. 85–108.
——. 2003. *Inextricably Bonded: Israeli Arab and Jewish Writers Re-Visioning Culture*. Madison: University of Wisconsin Press.
Broek, R. van den. 1972. *The Myth of the Phoenix according to Classical and Early Christian Traditions*. Leiden: Brill.
Browne, Edward G. 1951. *A Literary History of Persia*. Cambridge: Cambridge University Press.
Brugman, J. 1984. *An Introduction to the History of Modern Arabic Literature in Egypt*. Leiden: Brill.
Bsīsū, Mu'īn. 1988. *al-A'māl al-Shi'riyya al-Kāmila*. Acre: Dār al-Aswār.
——. 1988a. *al-A'māl al-Masraḥiyya*. Acre: Dār al-Aswār.

Bukhārī, Muḥammad ibn Ismā'īl. 1927. *Ṣaḥīḥ*. Cairo: n.p.

Bulliet, Richard W. 2011. "Muslim Societies and the Natural World." In Robert Irwin (ed.). *The New Cambridge History of Islam: Islamic Cultures and Societies to the End of the Eighteenth Century*, vol. 4. Cambridge: Cambridge University Press, pp. 209–21.

Būluṣ (Boulus), Sargon (Sarkūn). 1985. *al-Wuṣūl ilā Madīnat Ayna*. Athens: Manshūrāt Sāriq al-Nār.

——. 1997. *Zeugen am Ufer: Gedichte*, trans. Khalid Al-Maaly and Stefan Weidner. Berlin: Verlag Das Arab Buch.

——. 2003. *al-Wuṣūl ilā Madīnat Ayna*. Cologne: Manshūrāt al-Jamal.

——. 2008. *'Aẓama Ukhrā l-Kalb al-Qabīla*. Cologne: Manshūrāt al-Jamal.

al-Buraykī, Fāṭima. 2008. *al-Kitāba wa-l-Tiknūlūjiya*. Casablanca: al-Markaz al-Thaqāfī al-'Arabī.

al-Bur'ī, Muḥammad. 1978. *'Awdat al-Ams*. Cairo: Dār al-Fikr al-'Arabī.

Burt, Clarissa. 1995. "Classical Motifs and Cultural Intertextuality in Contemporary Egyptian Poetry." *Critique* 4.7, pp. 91–9.

Bushrū'i, Suhayl Badī'. 1982. *James Joyce*. Beirut: Dār al-Āfāq al-Jadīda.

——. 1987. *Kahlil Gibran of Lebanon*. Gerrards Cross: Colin Smythe.

——. 2000. *al-Adab al-'Arabī bi-l-Inglīziyya*. Beirut: al-Mu'assasa al-'Arabiyya li-l-Dirāsāt wa-l-Nashr.

Busse, Herbert. 1998. *Islam, Judaism, and Christianity: Theological and Historical Affiliations*, trans. Allison Brown. Princeton, NJ: Markus Wiener.

al-Bustānī, Buṭrus. 1859. *Khuṭba fī Ādāb al-'Arab*. Beirut: al-Maṭba'a al-Amīrkāniyya.

——. 1990. *al-Jam'iyya al-Sūriyya li-l-'Ulūm wa-l-Funūn 1847–1852*. Beirut: Dār al-Ḥamrā'.

al-Bustānī, Sulaymān. 1904. *Ilyādhat Hūmīrūs*. Cairo: Dār al-Hilāl.

——. 1996. *Naẓariyyat al-Shi'r: Muqaddimat Tarjamat al-Ilyādha*, ed. Muḥammad Kāmil al-Khaṭī. Damascus: Manshūrāt Wizārat al-Thaqāfa.

Cachia, Peirre. 1990. *An Overview of Modern Arabic Literature*. Edinburgh: Edinburgh University Press.

Calderwood, Eric. 2014. "The Invention of Al-Andalus: Discovering the Past and Creating the Present in Granada's Islamic Tourism Sites." *Journal of North African Studies* 19.1, pp. 27–55.

——. 2018. *Colonial al-Andalus: Spain and the Making of Modern Moroccan Culture*. Cambridge, MA: Harvard University Press.

Calvino, Italo. 1999. *Why Read the Classics?* trans. Martin McLaughlin. New York: Pantheon.

Camera d'Afflitto, Isabella. 1997. "Fantascienza in Mauritania: La storia di un uomo nato nel 1034 e morto nel 2055. 'Madīnat al-riyāḥ' di Mūsà Wuld Ibnū." *Oriente Moderno* 17.2/3, pp. 331–40.

——. 2001. "Letteratura araba contemporanea in Italia: un percorso personale (Abstract: Contemporary Arab Literature in Italy: A Personal Itinerary)." *Traduttore Nuovo* 56.1, pp. 11–16, 109–10.

Campbell, Ian. 2018. *Arabic Science Fiction Studies in Global Science Fiction*. New York: Palgrave Macmillan.

——. 2020. "Double Estrangement and Developments in Arabic Science Fiction: Aḥmad Sa'dāwī's *Frankenstein in Baghdad*." *Mashriq and Mahjar* 7.2, pp. 1–26.

Campbell, Robert B. 1996. *A'lām al-Adab al-'Arabī al-Mu'āṣir: Siyar wa-Siyar Dhātiyya*. Beirut: al-Ma'had al-Almānī li-l-Abḥāth al-Sharqiyya.

Camus, Albert. 1942. *Le mythe de sisyphe*. Paris: Gallimard.

——. 1955. *The Myth of Sisyphus*, trans. Justin O'Brien. New York: Vintage.

Canter, H. V. 1930. "The Figure Adynaton in Greek and Latin Poetry." *American Journal of Philology* 51, pp. 32–41.

Caracciolo, Peter L. (ed.). 1988. *The Arabian Nights in English Literature: Studies in the Reception of the Thousand and One Nights into British Culture*. London: Macmillan.
Carpentieri, Nicola. 2018. "*Adab* as Social Currency: The Survival of the *Qaṣīda* in Medieval Sicily." *Mediterranea: International Journal for the Transfer of Knowledge* 3, pp. 1–18.
Cariou, Morgane. 2014. "Le topos de l'ineffable dans les catalogues poétiques." *Revue de philologie, de littérature et d'histoire anciennes* 88.2, pp. 27–58.
Carter, Barbara L. 1986. *The Copts in Egyptian Politics*. London: Croom Helm.
Cartmell, Deborah et al. 1997. *Trash Aesthetics: Popular Culture and Its Audience*. London: Pluto Press.
Casanova, Pascale. 2002. *al-Jumhūriyya al-ʿĀlāmiyya li-l-Ādāb*, trans. Amal al-Ṣabbān. Cairo: al-Majlis al-Aʿlā li-l-Thaqāfa.
——. 2004. *The World Republic of Letters*, trans. M. B. DeBevoise. Cambridge, MA: Harvard University Press.
Cavafy, Constantine P. 1998. *Collected Poems*, trans. Edmund Keely and Philip Sherrard. London: Chatto & Windus.
Cervantes, Míguel de. 1972. *The Selected Works*, ed. and trans. Samuel Putnam. London: Chatto & Windus.
——. 2003. *Don Quixote*, trans. Edith Grossman. New York: HarperCollins.
Chejne, Anwar G. 1969. *The Arabic Language: Its Role in History*. Minneapolis: University of Minnesota Press.
——. 1980. "The Role of al-Andalus in the Movement of Ideas between Islam and the West." In Khalil Semaan (ed.). *Islam and the Medieval West: Aspects of Intercultural Relations*. Albany: State University of New York Press, pp. 110–33.
Chekhov, Anton. 1929. *The Works of Anton Chekhov*. New York: Black.
Chinweizu, Onwuchekwa Jemie and Madubuike, Ihechukwu (eds.). 1983. *Toward the Decolonization of African Literature: African Fiction and Poetry and Their Critics*. Washington, DC: Howard University Press.
Civantos, Christina. 2020. "Writing on Al-Andalus in the Modern Islamic World." In Maribel Fierro (ed.). *The Routledge Handbook of Muslim Iberia*. New York: Routledge, pp. 598–619.
Clarke, Arthur C. 1972. *The Wind from the Sun: Stories from the Space Age*. New York: Harcourt Brace Jovanovich.
Classe, Olive (ed.). 2000. *Encyclopaedia of Literary Translation into English*. London: Fitzroy Dearborn.
Cleary, Joe. 2006. "The World Literary System: Atlas and Epitaph." *Field Day Review* 2, pp. 197–219.
Cleveland, William L. 1971. *The Making of an Arab Nationalist: Ottomanism and Arabism in the Life and Thought of Satiʿ al-Husri*. Princeton, NJ: Princeton University Press.
Clute, John and Nicholls, Peter (eds.). 1995. *The Encyclopedia of Science Fiction*. New York: St. Martin's Griffin.
Clüver, Claus. 1986. "The Difference of Eight Decades: World Literature and the Demise of National Literatures." *Yearbook of Comparative and General Literature* 35, pp. 14–24.
——. 1988. "World Literature—Period or Type? In Response to Horst Steinmetz." *Yearbook of Comparative and General Literature* 37, pp. 134–9.
——. 1988a. "On Using Literary Constructs: In Response to Zoran Konstantinovic." *Yearbook of Comparative and General Literature* 37, pp. 143–4.
Coetzee, M. 1983. *Waiting for the Barbarians*. Harmondsworth: Penguin.
Cohen, Hayyim. 1973. *The Jews of the Middle East 1860–1972*. Jerusalem: Israel Universities Press.
Cohen, Mark R. and Somekh, Sasson. 1990. "In the Court of Yaʿqūb ibn Killis: A Fragment from the Cairo Genizah." *Jewish Quarterly Review* 80.3/4, pp. 283–314.

Cohen-Mor, Dalya (ed.). 2005. *Arab Women Writers: An Anthology of Short Stories*. Albany: State University of New York Press.

Coke, Richard. 1935 [1927]. *Baghdad: The City of Peace*. London: T. Butterworth.

Colla, Elliott. 2009. "How *Zaynab* Became the First Arabic Novel." *History Compass* 7.1, pp. 214–25.

——. 2011. "Field Construction." *International Journal of Middle East Studies* 43.4, pp. 722–4.

Collins, Michael. 1978. *Ḥamalū al-Nār min al-Qamar: Riḥalāt Rā'id al-Faḍā'*, trans. Mīshīl Taklā. Cairo: Maktabat al-Anglo al-Miṣriyya.

Comendador, María Luz, Luis Miguel Canada, and Miguel Hernando de Larramendi. 2000. "The Translation of Contemporary Arabic Literature into Spanish." *Yearbook of Comparative and General Literature* 48, pp. 115–25.

Comendador, María Luz and Fernández-Parrilla, Gonzalo. 2006. "Traducciones de literatura árabe al español 2001–2005." *Al-Andalus Magreb* 13, pp. 69–77.

Conant, Martha Pike. 1966 [1908]. *The Oriental Tale in England in the Eighteenth Century*. London: Frank Cass.

Conrad, Joseph. 1996. *Heart of Darkness*. New York: Palgrave Macmillan.

Cook, David. 2002. *Studies in Muslim Apocalyptic*. Princeton, NJ: Darwin Press.

——. 2017. (ed. and trans.). *"The Book of Tribulations: The Syrian Muslim Apocalyptic Tradition": An Annotated. Translation by Nu'aym b. Hammad al-Marwazi*. Edinburgh: Edinburgh University Press.

Cooperson, Michael. 1998. "Remembering the Future: Arabic Time-Travel Literature." *Edebiyât* 8, pp. 171–89.

——. 2004. *Classical Arabic Biography: The Heirs of the Prophets in the Age of al-Ma'mūn*. Cambridge: Cambridge University Press.

——. 2017. "The Abbasid 'Golden Age': An Excavation." *Al-'Uṣūr al-Wusṭā* 25, pp. 41–65.

Cooperson, Michael and Hassan, Waïl S. 2011. "To Translate or Not to Translate Arabic: Michael Cooperson and Waïl S. Hassan on the Criticism of Abdelfattah Kilito." *Comparative Literature Studies* 48.4, pp. 566–75.

Corrao, Francesca Maria. 2001. "Tradurre poesia araba oggi (Abstract: Translating Arabic Poetry Today)." *Traduttore Nuovo* 56.1, pp. 17–21, 110–11.

——. 2020. "La Méditerranée dans la poétique de Muḥammad Bannīs: un regard italien." In Maria Avino et al. (eds.). *Qamariyyāt: oltre ogni frontiera tra letteratura e traduzione. Studi in onore di Isabella Camera d'Afflitto*. Rome: Istituto per l'Oriente C. A. Nallino, pp. 121–30.

Creswell, Robyn. 2019. *City of Beginnings: Poetic Modernism in Beirut*. Princeton, NJ: Princeton University Press.

Cruz, Anna C. 2018. "In Memory of al-Andalus: Using the Elegy to Reimagine the Literary and Literal Geography of Cordova." In Nizar F. Hermes and Getchen Head (eds.). *The City in Arabic Literature: Classical and Modern Perspectives*. Edinburgh: Edinburgh University Press, pp. 103–23.

Cuddon, J. A. 1986. *A Dictionary of Literary Terms*. Harmondsworth: Penguin.

Curtius, Ernst Robert. 1952. *European Literature and the Latin Middle Ages*, trans. W. R. Trask. New York: Pantheon.

Dabashi, Hamid. 2012. *The Arab Spring: The End of Postcolonialism*. London: Zed Books.

al-Dahshān, Ismā'īl Sarā. 1983. *Bayna al-Jidd wa-l-Jayyid*. Cairo: al-Hay'a al-Miṣriyya al-'Āmma li-l-Kitāb.

Damrosch, David. 2003. *What Is World Literature*? Princeton, NJ: Princeton University Press.

——. 2009. *How to Read World Literature*. Chichester: Wiley-Blackwell.

——. 2009a. *Teaching World Literature*. New York: Modern Language Association of America.

——. 2020. "*La république mondiale des lettres* in the World Republic of Scholarship." *Journal of World Literature* 5.2, pp. 174–88.
Dana, Joseph. 1982. *Poetics of Medieval Hebrew Literature According to Moshe ibn Ezra* (in Hebrew). Jerusalem and Tel Aviv: Dvir.
Däniken, Erich von. 1968. *Erinnerungen an die Zukunft*. Düsseldorf: Econ-Verlag.
——. 1970. *Chariots of the Gods? Unsolved Mysteries of the Past*. New York: Souvenir Press.
Darrāj, Fayṣal. 2004. "Riwāyat al-Khayāl al-'Ilmī fī al-Azmina al-Ḥadītha." *al-Ḥayāt*, November 3, p. 17.
——. 2005. *al-Ḥadātha al-Mutaqahqira: Ṭāhā Ḥusayn wa-Adūnīs*. Ramallah: al-Mu'assasa al-Filasṭīniyya li-Dirāsat al-Dīmuqrāṭiyya.
Darwaza, Muḥammad 'Izzat. 1993. *Mudhakkirāt Muḥammad 'Izzat Darwaza: Sijjil Ḥāfil bi-Masīrat al-Ḥaraka al-'Arabiyya wa-l-Qaḍiyya al-Filasṭīniyya Khilāla Qarn min al-Zaman; 1305–1404H/1887–1984*. Beirut: Dār al-Gharab al-Islāmī.
Darwisch, Mahmud. 1996. *Weniger Rosen*, trans. Khalid Al-Maaly and Heribert Becker. Berlin: Das Arabische Buch.
Darwīsh (Darwish), Maḥmūd (Mahmoud). 1980. *The Music of Human Flesh*, trans. Denys Johnson-Davies. London: Heinemann.
——. 1985. *Ḥiṣār li-Madā'iḥ al-Baḥr*. Beirut: Dār al-'Awda.
——. 1987. *Dhākira li-l-Nisyān*. Acre: Dār al-Aswār.
——. 1987a. *Ward Aqall*. Acre: Dār al-Aswār.
——. 1988. *Dīwān*. Acre: Dār al-Aswār.
——. 1992. *Aḥada 'Ashara Kawkaban*. Beirut: Dār al-Jadīd.
——. 2003. *Unfortunately, It Was Paradise: Selected Poems*, ed. and trans. Munir Akash and Carolyn Forché, with Sinan Antoon and Amira El-Zein. Berkeley: University of California Press.
——. 2008. *Athar al-Farāsha*. Beirut: Riyāḍ al-Rayyis.
Darwīsh, Maḥmūd and al-Qāsim, Samīḥ. 1990. *al-Rasā'il*. Haifa: Arabesque.
Daoudi, Anissa. 2011. "Globalization, Computer-Mediated Communications and the Rise of e-Arabic." *Middle East Journal of Culture and Communication* 4.2, pp. 146–63.
Davidson, Cathy N. 2011. *Now You See It: How the Brain Science of Attention Will Transform the Way We Live, Work, and Learn*. New York: Viking.
Davidson, Efraim. 1972. *Our Mouth's Laughter: Anthology of Humour and Satire in Ancient and Modern Hebrew Literature* (in Hebrew). Holon: Biblos.
De Blasio, Emanuela. 2019. "A Preliminary Study about the Fantasy Genre in Contemporary Arabic Literature." *Folia Orientalia* 56, pp. 29–39.
——. 2020. "Comics in the Arab World: Birth and Spread of a New Literary Genre." *Anaquel de Estudios Árabes* 31, pp. 117–26.
——. 2021. "Poetry in the Era of Social Networks: The Case of Faraḥ Šammā." *Annali di Ca' Foscari. Serie orientale* 57, pp. 91–118.
Defoe, Daniel. 1906 [1719]. *Robinson Crusoe*. London: Dent.
Déjeux, Jean. 1973. *Littérature maghrébine de langue française*. Ottawa: Éditions Naaman.
Deleuze, Gilles and Guattari, Felix. 1987. *A Thousand Plateaus: Capitalism and Schizophrenia*, trans. Brian Massumi. Minneapolis: University of Minnesota Press.
Derrida, Jacques. 1976. *Of Grammatology*, trans. Gayatri Chakravorty Spivak. Baltimore: Johns Hopkins University Press.
——. 1986. "Racism's Last Word." In Henry Louis Gates, Jr., Appiah Gates, and Kwame Anthony (eds.). *"Race," Writing and Difference*. Chicago: University of Chicago Press, pp. 329–38.
Determann, Jörg Matthias. 2021. *Islam, Science Fiction and Extraterrestrial Life: The Culture of Astrobiology in the Muslim World*. London: Routledge.
de Wringer, Anouck. 2020. "Trauma as a Life-World: Lived Experiences of Space, Time and the Body in *The Queue* and *Otared*." MA thesis, University of Amsterdam.

DeYoung, Terri. 1992. "Language in Looking-Glass Land: Samīḥ al-Qāsim and the Modernization of *Jinās*." *Journal of the American Oriental Society* 112.2, pp. 183–197.
——. 1998. *Placing the Poet: Badr Shakir al-Sayyab and Postcolonial Iraq*. Albany: State University of New York Press.
——. 2000. "T. S. Eliot and Modern Arabic Poetry." *Yearbook of Comparative and General Literature* 48, pp. 3–21.
——. 2016. "*Iterations of Loss: Mutilation and Aesthetic Form, Al-Shidyaq to Darwish*, Written by Jeffrey Sacks." *Journal of Arabic Literature* 47.1/2, pp. 222–6.
——. 2018. *Mahmud Sami al-Barudi: Reconfiguring Society and the Self*. Syracuse, NY: Syracuse University Press.
DeYoung, Terri and St. Germain, Mary (eds.). 2011. *Essays in Arabic Literary Biography 925–1350*. Wiesbaden: Harrassowitz Verlag.
Dhabab, Mansour M. A. 2005. "Representations of the Western Other in Early Arabic Novels (1900–1915)." PhD thesis, University of Leeds.
al-Dhahabī, Muḥammad ibn Aḥmad. 1988. *Ta'rīkh al-Islām wa-Wafayāt al-Mashāhīr wa-l-A'lām, Ḥawādith wa-Wafayāt 141–160H*. Beirut: Dār al-Kitāb al-'Arabī.
Dhinī, Sihām. 2002. *Tharthara ma'a Najīb Maḥfūẓ*. Cairo: Dār Akhbār al-Yawm.
Di-Capua, Yoav. 2012. "Arab Existentialism: An Invisible Chapter in the Intellectual History of Decolonization." *American Historical Review* 117.4, pp. 1061–91.
——. 2018. *No Exit: Arab Existentialism, Jean-Paul Sartre, and Decolonization*. Chicago: University of Chicago Press.
Dick, Barbara. 2016. "Modern Arabic Science Fiction: Science, Society and Religion in Selected Texts." PhD thesis, Durham University.
DiMeo, David. 2016. *Committed to Disillusion Activist Writers in Egypt from the 1950s to the 1980s*. Cairo: American University in Cairo Press.
Disraeli, Benjamin. 1844. *Coningsby, or The New Generation*. Philadelphia: Carey & Hart.
Diyāb, Ḥannā. 2021. *The Book of Travels: Volume One*, ed. Johannes Stephan, trans. Elias Muhanna. New York: New York University Press.
——. 2021a. *The Book of Travels: Volume Two*, ed. Johannes Stephan, trans. Elias Muhanna. New York: New York University Press.
Dobie, Madeleine. 2017. "Locating Algerian Literature in World Literature." *Middle Eastern Literatures* 20.1, pp. 78–90.
Dobrişan, Nicolae. 2004. "Extratextuality and the Translation of Fictional Work from Arabic into Romanian." *Romano-Arabica* 4, pp. 29–32.
D'Ohsson, C. 1834–1835. *Histoire des Mongols depuis Tchinguiz-Khan jusqu'a Timour Bey ou Tamerlan*. The Hague: Les Frères Van Cleef.
Dols, Michael W. 1992. *Majnūn: The Madman in Medieval Islamic Society*. Oxford: Clarendon Press.
Dougherty, James. 1980. *The Fivesquare City: The City in the Religious Imagination*. Notre Dame, IN: University of Notre Dame Press.
Douglas, Allen and Malti-Douglas, Fedwa. 1994. *Arab Comic Strips: Politics of an Emerging Mass Culture*. Bloomington: Indiana University Press.
Drory, Rina. 2000. "The Maqama." In Maria Rosa Menocal et al. (eds.). 2000. *The Cambridge History of Arabic Literature: The Literature of al-Andalus*. Cambridge: Cambridge University Press, pp. 190–210.
Duclos, Diane. "Cosmopolitanism and Iraqi Migration: Artists and Intellectuals from the 'Sixties and Seventies Generations' in Exile." In Jordi Tejel et al. (eds.). *Writing the Modern History of Iraq: Historiographical and Political Challenges*. Hackensack, NJ: World Scientific, pp. 391–401.
Duri, Abdel 'Aziz. 1980. "Governmental Institutions." In R. B. Serjeant (ed.). *The Islamic City*, selected papers from the Colloquium held at the Middle East Centre, Faculty

of Oriental Studies, Cambridge, United Kingdom, from 19 to 23 July 1976. Paris: UNESCO, pp. 52–65.
——. 2012. "Baghdad." In *Encyclopaedia of Islam*, 2nd edn. Leiden: Brill Online.
Dūs, Madīḥa and Davies, Humphrey (eds.). 2013. *al-ʿĀmmiyya al-Miṣriyya al-Maktūba*. Cairo: al-Hay'a al-Miṣriyya al-ʿĀmma li-l-Kitāb.
Duwāra, Fu'ād. 1963. "Maʿa Najīb Maḥfūẓ fī ʿĪdihi al-Dhahabī." *al-Kātib* 22, pp. 4–24.
——. 1965. *ʿAsharatu Udabā' Yataḥaddathūna*. Cairo: Dār al-Hilāl.
Early, Evelyn A. 1993. *Baladi Women of Cairo: Playing with Egg and a Stone*. Boulder, CO: Lynne Rienner.
Ebileeni, Maurice. 2019. "Breaking the Script: The Generational Conjuncture in the Anglophone Palestinian Novel." *Journal of Postcolonial Writing* 55.5, pp. 628–41.
Ebnou, Moussa Ould. 1990. *L'amour impossible*. Paris: Éditions L'Harmattan.
——. 1994. *Barzakh*. Paris: Éditions L'Harmattan.
Eco, Umberto. 1980. *Il Nome Della Rosa*. Milan: Gruppo Editoriale Fabbri.
——. 1984. *The Name of the Rose*, trans. W. Weaver. London: Picador.
Eickelman, F. Dale. 1974. "Is There an Islamic City?" *International Journal of Middle Eastern Studies* 5, pp. 274–94.
Eickelman, F. Dale and Anderson, Jon W. (eds.). 2003. *New Media in the Muslim World: The Emerging Public Sphere*. Bloomington: Indiana University Press.
Einbinder, Susan. 1995. "The *Muwashshaḥ*-Like *Zajal*: A New Source for a Hebrew Poem." *Medieval Encounters* 1.2, pp. 252–70.
Eksell, Kerstin. 2011. "The Legend of Al-Andalus: A Trajectory across Generic Borders." In Kerstin Eksell and Stephan Guth (eds.). *Borders and Beyond Crossings and Transitions in Modern Arabic Literature*. Wiesbaden: Harrassowitz Verlag, pp. 103–26.
El-Ali, Saleh Ahmad. 1970. "The Foundation of Baghdad." In Albert H. Hourani and S. M. Stern (eds.). *The Islamic City: A Colloquium*, held at all Souls College, June 28–July 2, 1965. Oxford: Bruno Cassirer, pp. 87–101.
El-Ariss, Tarek. 2010. "Hacking the Modern: Arabic Writing in the Virtual Age." *Comparative Literature Studies* 47.4, pp. 533–48.
——. 2012. "Fiction of Scandal." *Journal of Arabic Literature* 43.2/3, pp. 510–31.
——. 2013. *Trials of Arab Modernity: Literary Affects and the New Political*. New York: Fordham University Press.
——. 2015. "Let There Be *Nahdah*!" *Cambridge Journal of Postcolonial Literary Inquiry* 2.2, pp. 260–6.
——. 2019. *Leaks, Hacks, and Scandals: Arab Culture in the Digital Age*. Princeton, NJ: Princeton University Press.
El-Azma, Nazeer. 1968. "The Tammūzī Movement and the Influence of T. S. Eliot on Badr Shākir al-Sayyāb." *Journal of the American Oriental Society* 88, pp. 671–8.
——. 1980. "The Tammūzī Movement and the Influence of T. S. Eliot on Badr Shākir al-Sayyāb." In Issa J. Boullata (ed.). *Critical Perspectives on Modern Arabic Literature*. Washington, DC: Three Continents Press, pp. 215–31.
Elbaz, Robert. 1988. *The Changing Nature of the Self: A Critical Study of the Autobiographic Discourse*. London: Croom Helm.
——. 1996. *Thahar ben Jelloun ou l'inassouvissement du désir narratif*. Paris: Éditions L'Harmattan.
El Beheiry, Kawsar Abdel Salam. 1980. *L'Influence de la littérature française sur le roman arabe*. Sherbrooke, QC: Éditions Naaman.
El-Enany, Rasheed. 1993. *Naguib Mahfouz: The Pursuit of Meaning*. London: Routledge.
——. 2006. *Arab Representations of the Occident: East–West Encounters in Arabic Fiction*. London: Routledge.
Eliade, M. 1959. *The Sacred and the Profane*. New York: Harcourt Brace Jovanovich.
Elias, Ami. 2001. *Sublime Desire: History and Post-1960s Fiction*. Baltimore: Johns Hopkins University Press.

Elimelekh, Geula. 2013. "Kafkaesque Metamorphosis as Reflected in the Works of Samīr Naqqāsh." *Journal of Semitic Studies* 58.2, pp. 323–42.

——. 2014. "Fantasy as 'Recovery, Escape and Consolation' in the Short Stories of Isaac Bar Moshe." *Middle Eastern Studies* 50.3, pp. 426–41.

Elinson, Alexander E. 2009. *Looking Back at al-Andalus: The Poetics of Loss and Nostalgia in Medieval Arabic and Hebrew Literature*. Leiden: Brill.

Eliot, T. S. 1950. *Selected Essays*. New York: Harcourt.

——. 1960 [1932]. *Selected Essays*. New York: Harcourt, Brace.

——. 1969. *The Complete Poems and Plays*. London: Faber and Faber.

El Janabi, A. K. 1996. *Stance in the Desert: Surrealist Writings (1974–1986)*. Paris: Gilgamesh.

Elkhadem, Saad. 1985. *History of the Egyptian Novel: Its Rise and Early Beginnings*. Fredericton, NB: York Press.

——. 2001. *On Egyptian Fiction: Five Essays*. Toronto: York Press.

Elmarsafy, Ziad. 2012. *Sufism in the Contemporary Arabic Novel*. Edinburgh: Edinburgh University Press.

El Sadda, Hoda. 1996. "Women's Writing in Egypt: Reflections on Salwa Bakr." In Deniz Kandiyoti (ed.). *Gendering the Middle East*. London: I. B. Tauris, pp. 127–44.

——. 2010. "Arab Women Bloggers: The Emergence of Literary Counterpublics." *Middle East Journal of Culture and Communication* 3, pp. 312–32.

——. 2012. *Gender, Nation, and the Arabic Novel: Egypt, 1892–2008*. Edinburgh: Edinburgh University Press.

El Saffar, Ruth Snodgrass. 1968. "The Function of the Fictional Narrator in *Don Quijote*." *MLN* 83.2, pp. 164–77.

El-Shamy, Hasan M. (ed.). 1980. *Folktales of Egypt*. Chicago: University of Chicago Press.

Elster, Ernst. 1901. "Weltlitteratur und Litteraturvergleichung." *Archiv für das Studium der Neueren Sprachen und Literatur* 107, pp. 33–47.

——. 1986. "World Literature and Comparative Literature (1901)," trans. Eric Metzler. *Yearbook of Comparative and General Literature* 35, pp. 7–13.

Emmerson, Richard Kenneth. 1981. *Antichrist in the Middle Ages*. Seattle: University of Washington Press.

Enderwitz, Susanne. 1998. "From Curriculum Vitae to Self-Narration: Fiction in Arabic Autobiography." In Stefan Leder (ed.). *Story-Telling in the Framework of Non-Fictional Arabic Literature*. Wiesbaden: Harrassowitz Verlag, pp. 1–19.

——. 1999. "The Mission of the Palestinian Autobiographer." In Stephan Guth et al. (eds.). *Conscious Voices: Concepts of Writing in the Middle East*. Beirut: Orient-Institut der DMG, pp. 29–50.

——. 2000. "Gibt es eine arabische Autobiographie?" In Verena Klemm and Beatrice Gruendler (eds.). *Understanding Near Eastern Literatures*. Wiesbaden: Reichert Verlag, pp. 189–99.

——. 2002. "Palestinian Autobiographies: A Source for Women's History." In Manuela Marín and Randi Deguilhem (eds.). Writing the Feminine: Women in Arab Sources. London: Bloomsbury, pp. 49–72.

——. 2009. "Die Helden der Steine. Der islamische Comic 'Die 99'." *Welt-Sichten* 11, pp. 42–3.

——. 2011. "'The 99': Islamic Superheroes: A New Species?" In Christiane Brosius and Roland Wenzlhuemer (eds.). *Transcultural Turbulences: Interdisciplinary Explorations of Flows of Images and Media*. Vienna: Springer, pp. 83–96.

——. 2015. "The Forces of Good and Evil in 'Islamic' Comic." In Michael Welker and William Schweiker (eds.). *Images of the Divine and Cultural Orientations: Jewish, Christian and Islamic Voices*. Leipzig: Evangelische Verlagsanstalt, pp. 127–34.

Engels, Odilo and Schreiner, Peter (eds.). 1993. *Die Begegung des Westens mit dem Ostens*. Sigmaringen, Germany: Jan Thorbecke Verlag.

Enquist, Anna. 2006. *Gedichten voor het hart: troostende woorden uit de Nederlandse en Vlaamse poëzie*. Amsterdam: Maarten Muntinga.
Ertürk, Nergis. 2010. "Those Outside the Scene: Snow in the World Republic of Letters." *New Literary History* 41.3, pp. 634–40.
Esposito, J. L. (ed.). 1995. *The Oxford Encyclopedia of the Modern Islamic World*. New York: Oxford University Press.
Etman, Ahmed. 1993. "Round Table—Naguib Mahfouz and Arabic Literature: Problems of Translation." *Graeco-Arabica* 5, pp. 355–8.
Even-Zohar, Itamar. 1990. "Polysystem Studies." *Poetics Today* 11.1 (the whole volume is by I. Even-Zohar).
——. 1990a. "Laws of Literary Interference." *Poetics Today* 11.1, pp. 53–72.
——. 1990b. "The Emergence of a Native Hebrew Culture in Palestine, 1882–1948." *Poetics Today* 11.1, pp. 175–91.
Faddul, Atif Y. 1992. *The Poetics of T. S. Eliot and Adunis: A Comparative Study*. Beirut: Al-Hamra.
Fahd, Toufic. 1993. "La traduction arabe de l'*Iliade*." *Graeco-Arabica* 5, pp. 259–66.
Fähndrich, Hartmut. 2000. "Viewing 'The Orient" and Translating Its Literature in the Shadow of *The Arabian Nights*." *Yearbook of Comparative and General Literature* 48, pp. 95–106.
——. 2000a. "A Movement against a Structure: The Situation of Contemporary Arabic Literature in German-Speaking Countries Inside and Outside the Universities." *Awrāq: Estudios sobre el Mundo Arabe e Islámico Contemporáneo* 21, pp. 167–80.
Fakhreddine, Huda. 2015. *Metapoesis in the Arabic Tradition: From Modernists to Muḥdathūn*. Leiden: Brill.
——. 2017. "The Aesthetic Imperative: History Poeticized." In Lucian Stone and Jason Bahbak Mohaghegh (eds.). *Manifestos for World Thought*. London: Rowman & Littlefield, pp. 147–54.
——. *2021. The Arabic Prose Poem Poetic Theory and Practice*. Edinburgh: Edinburgh University Press.
Fanous, Mohamad Wajih Subhi. 1980. "Aspects of the Lebanese Contribution to Modern Arabic Literary Criticism." PhD thesis, University of Oxford.
Fanus, Wajih. 1986. "Sulaymān al-Bustānī and Comparative Literary Studies in Arabic." *Journal of Arabic Literature* 17, pp. 105–19.
Faraj, Nabīl. 1971. "Muqābala Adabiyya ma'a Yūsuf al-Shārūnī." *al-Ādāb*, January, pp. 50–2.
——. (ed.). 1995. *Yūsuf al-Shārūnī Mubdi'an wa-Nāqidan*. Cairo: al-Hay'a al-Miṣriyya al-'Āmma li-l-Kitāb.
Farānish (Faranesh), Alīf Yusūf. 2015. "al-Kitāba al-Būlīsiyya fī al-Adab al-'Arabī al-Ḥadīth." PhD thesis, Bar-Ilan University.
Fārūq, Nabīl. (n.d.1). *Milaff al-Mustaqbal (79): al-Taḥaddī*. Cairo: al-Mu'assasa al-'Arabiyya al-Ḥadītha.
——. (n.d.2). *Milaff al-Mustaqbal (97): Lahīb al-Kawākib*. Cairo: al-Mu'assasa al-'Arabiyya al-Ḥadītha.
——. (n.d.3). *Kūktīl 2000 (20): al-Ba'th wa-Qiṣaṣ Ukhrā*. Cairo: al-Mu'assasa al-'Arabiyya al-Ḥadītha.
——. (n.d.4). *Zūm (3): Lughz al-Kura al-Arḍiyya*. Cairo: al-Mu'assasa al-'Arabiyya al-Ḥadītha.
——. (n.d.5). *Zūm (6): Lughz al-Qiṭṭ al-Fiḍḍī*. Cairo: al-Mu'assasa al-'Arabiyya al-Ḥadītha.
Fatḥ al-Bāb, Ḥasan. 1992. "Andalus al-Shā'ir Samīḥ al-Qāsim." In Samīḥ al-Qāsim (ed.). *Samīḥ al-Qāsim fī Dā'irat al-Naqd*. Beirut: Dār al-Jīl, pp. 505–16.
al-Faytūrī, Muḥammad. 1979. *Dīwān*. Beirut: Dār al-'Awda.

Feodorov, Ioana. 2001. "Romanian Translations of Arabic Literature 1964–1994." *Romano-Arabica* 1, pp. 35–45.
——. 2001a. *The Arab World in Romanian Culture: 1957–2001*. Bucharest: Editura Biblioteca Bucureştilor.
Ferenczi, Sándor. 1924. "Stages in the Development of the Sense of Reality." In I. S. Van Teslaar (ed.). 1924. *An Outline of Psychoanalysis*. New York: The Modern Library, pp. 108–27.
Fernández-Parrilla, Gonzalo. 2013. "Translating Modern Arabic Literature into Spanish." *Middle Eastern Literatures* 16.1, pp. 88–101.
——. 2018. "Disoriented Postcolonialities: With Edward Said in (the Labyrinth of) Al-Andalus." *Interventions* 20.2, pp. 229–42.
Fernea, Elizabeth and Bezirgan, Basima Qattan (eds.). 1977. *Middle Eastern Muslim Women Speak*. Austin: University of Texas Press.
Festinger, Leon. 1957. *A Theory of Cognitive Dissonance*. Stanford, CA: Stanford University Press.
Filshtinsky, I. M. 1966. *Arabic Literature*, trans. Hilda Kasanina. Moscow: Nauka.
Fischel, W. J. 1938. "'Resh-Galuta' (*Ra's al-Jālūt*) in Arabic Literature." In F. I. Baer et al. (eds.). *Magnes Anniversary Book*. Jerusalem: Hebrew University Press, pp. 181–7.
Fitch, Brian T. 1982. *The Narcissistic Text: A Reading of Camus' Fiction*. Toronto: University of Toronto Press.
Flew, Antony. 1979. *A Dictionary of Philosophy*. London: Pan.
Flores, Angel. 1976. *A Kafka Bibliography 1908–1976*. New York: Gordian Press.
Forcione, Alban K. 1970. *Cervantes, Aristotle and the Persiles*. Princeton, NJ: Princeton University Press.
Foucault, Michel. 1966. *The Order of Things: An Archaeology of the Human Sciences*. Paris: Gallimard.
——. 1980 [1969]. "What Is an Author?" In Donald F. Bouchard (ed.). *Language, Counter-Memory, Practice: Selected Essays and Interviews by Michel Foucault*. Ithaca, NY: Cornell University Press, pp. 113–38.
France, Peter (ed.). 2000. *The Oxford Guide to Literature in English Translation*. Oxford: Oxford University Press.
Frolova, Olga. 1978. "Antifeodal'naya egipetskaya poėma 'Yasin i Bahiya' Nagiba Surura (An Anti-Feudal Poem 'Yāsin and Bahiya' of Nagīb Surūr)." *Palestinskiĭ Sbornik* 26 (89), pp. 22–7.
Gallagher, Nancy Elizabeth. 1994. *Approaches to the History of the Middle East: Interviews with Leading Middle East Historians*. Reading: Ithaca Press.
Gamal, Adel Suleiman. 1984. "Narrative Poetry in Classical Arabic Poetry." In A. H. Green (ed.). *In Quest of an Islamic Humanism: Arabic and Islamic Studies in Memory of Mohamed al-Nowaihi*. Cairo: American University in Cairo Press, pp. 25–38.
Ganguly, Debjani. 2015. "Polysystems Redux: The Unfinished Business of World Literature." *Cambridge Journal of Postcolonial Literary Inquiry* 2.2, pp. 272–81.
Gardet, L. 1971. "Ḥāl." *Encyclopaedia of Islam*, 2nd edn. III, pp. 83–5.
Gates, Henry Louis Jr., 1985. "Editor's Introduction: Writing 'Race' and the Difference It Makes." *Critical Inquiry* 12, pp. 1–20.
Geary, Grattan. 1878. *Through Asiatic Turkey: Narrative of a Journey from Bombay to the Bosphorus*. London: Sampson Low, Marston, Searle & Rivington.
Genette, Gérard. 1992. *The Architext: An Introduction*, trans. J. E. Lewin. Berkeley: University of California Press.
Gerber, Haim. 1999. *Islamic Law and Culture 1600–1840*. Leiden: Brill.
al-Ghamdi, Saleh. 1989. "Autobiography in Classical Arabic Literature." PhD thesis, Indiana University.
Ghanāyim, Maḥmūd. 1992. *Tayyār al-Wa'y fī al-Riwāya al-'Arabiyya al-Ḥadītha: Dirāsa Uslūbiyya*. Beirut: Dār al-Jīl.

Ghanāyim, Muḥammad Ḥamza. 1979. *Alif Lam Mīm*. Acre: Dār al-Aswār.
al-Ghazālī, Abū Ḥāmid. 1933. *Iḥyā' 'Ulūm al-Dīn*. Cairo: Maṭba'at 'Uthmān Khalīfa.
——. 1936. *Kīmyā' al-Sa'āda*. Cairo: n.p.
——. 1956. *al-Munqidh min al-Ḍalāl*, ed. Jamīl Ṣalība and Kāmil 'Ayyād. Damascus: Maṭba'at al-Taraqqī.
Ghazoul, Ferial J. 2006. "From the Spokesman of the Tribe to a Tribune of the Dispossessed." In Andreas Pflitsch and Barbara Winckler (eds.). *Poetry's Voice: Society's Norms: Forms of Interaction between Middle Eastern Writers and Their Societies*. Wiesbaden: Reichert Verlag, pp. 1–10.
al-Ghīṭānī, Jamāl. (ed.). 1980. *Najīb Maḥfūẓ Yatadhakkaru*. Beirut: Dār al-Masīra.
——. (ed.). 1981 [1980]. *Khiṭaṭ al-Ghīṭānī*. Beirut: Dār al-Masīra.
——. 1986. "al-Turāth al-Ṣūfī wa-l-Judhūr." *al-Akhbār*, May 28, p. 9.
——. 1986a. "al-Karāma al-Ṣūfiyya." *al-Akhbār*, June 16, p. 9.
——. 1986b. "Turāthunā al-Qaṣaṣī—1." *al-Akhbār*, July 16, p. 9.
——. 1986c. "Turāthunā al-Qaṣaṣī—3." *al-Akhbār*, August 6, p. 9.
——. 2006. *al-Majālis al-Maḥfūẓiyya*. Cairo: Dār al-Shurūq.
Ghosn, Katia and Tadié, Benoît (eds.). 2021. *Le récit criminel arabe / Arabic Crime Fiction*. Wiesbaden: Harrassowitz Verlag.
Ghurayyib, Ma'mūn. 1984. *Ma'a Mashāhīr al-Fikr wa-l-Fann*. Cairo: Dār al-Ma'ārif.
Giacconi, Marina. 2018. "Fantascienza e distopia in Tawfiq al-Ḥakīm. Fī sanat malyūn." *Occhialì: Laboratorio sul Mediterraneo islámico* 2, pp. 112–25.
Gibb, Hamilton A. R. 1962. *Studies on the Civilization of Islam*. London: Routledge.
——. 1962a. *Arabic Literature*. Oxford: Oxford University Press.
Gibb, Hamilton A. R. and Landau, Jacob. 1968. *Arabische Literaturgeschicte*. Zurich: Artemis Verlag.
——. and ——. 1970. *Arabic Literature: An Introduction* (in Hebrew). Tel Aviv: Am Oved.
Gibran, Kahlil. 1918. *The Madman*. New York: Alfred A. Knopf.
——. 1920. *The Forerunner*. New York: Alfred A. Knopf.
——. 1924. *The Prophet*. New York: Alfred A. Knopf.
——. 1926. *Sand and Foam*. New York: Alfred A. Knopf.
——. 1928. *Jesus, the Son of Man*. New York: Alfred A. Knopf.
——. 1931. *The Earth Gods*. New York: Alfred A. Knopf.
——. 1932. *The Wanderer: His Parables and His Sayings*. New York: Alfred A. Knopf.
——. 1933. *The Garden of the Prophet*. New York: Alfred A. Knopf.
——. 1957. *The Broken Wings*, trans. A. R. Ferris. New York: Citadel Press.
——. 1973. *Lazarus and His Beloved: A One Act Play*, ed. the author's cousin and namesake Kahlil Gibran and his wife Mary Gibran. Greenwich, CT: New York Philosophical Society.
——. 1982. *Dreams of Life* (*Lazarus and His Beloved* and *The Blind*), ed. the author's cousin and namesake Kahlil Gibran and his wife Mary Gibran. Philadelphia: Westminster.
Gill, R. B. 2013. "The Uses of Genre and the Classification of Speculative Fiction." *Mosaic: A Journal for the Interdisciplinary Study of Literature* 46.2, pp. 71–85.
Giovannucci, Perri. 2008. *Literature and Development in North Africa: The Modernizing Mission*. New York: Routledge.
Göçek, Fatma Müge and Balaghi, Shiva (eds.). 1994. *Reconstructing Gender in the Middle East*. New York: Columbia University Press.
Goethe, Johann Wolfgang von. 1964. *Iphigenia fī Tauris*, trans. Muḥammad 'Abd al-Ḥalīm Karāra. Alexandria: Munsha'at al-Ma'ārif.
——. 1966. *Nazwat al-'Āshiq wa-l-Shurakā'*, trans. Muṣṭafā Māhir. Cairo: al-Masraḥ al-'Ālamī.
——. 1967. *Tasso*, trans. 'Abd al-Ghaffār Makkāwī. Cairo: Dār al-Kātib al-'Arabī.
——. 1968. *Ālām Werther*, trans. Aḥmad Ḥasan al-Zayyāt. Beirut: Dār al-Kitāb al-'Arabī.

——. 1978. *Ālām Werther*, trans. Lānā Abū Muṣliḥ. Beirut: al-Maktaba al-Ḥadītha li-l-Ṭibā'a wa-l-Nashr.
——. 1980. *al-Dīwān al-Sharqī li-l-Mu'allif al-Gharbī*, trans. 'Abd al-Raḥmān Badāwī. Beirut: al-Mu'assasa al-'Arabiyya li-l-Dirāsāt wa-l-Nashr.
——. 1980a. *al-Ansāb al-Mukhtāra*, trans. 'Abd al-Raḥmān Badāwī. Beirut: Dār al-Andalus.
——. 1999. *Mukhtārāt Shi'riyya wa-Nathriyya*, trans. Abū al-'Īd Dūdū. Cologne: Manshūrāt al-Jamal.
——. 1999a. *Mukhtārāt Shi'riyya: Johann Wolfgang von Goethe fī al-Almāniyya wa-l'Arabiyya*, trans. Fu'ād Rifqa. Beirut: Dār al-Andalus.
Goldziher, Ignác. 1910. *Vorlesungen über den Islam*. Heidelberg: C. Winter.
——. 1966. *A Short History of Classical Arabic Literature*. Hildesheim: Georg Olms Verlag.
Golley, Nawar Al-Hasan. 2003. *Reading Arab Women's Autobiographies: Shahrazad Tells Her Story*. Austin: University of Texas Press.
Goodman, Dena. 1994. *The Republic of Letters: A Cultural History of the French Enlightenment*. Ithaca, NY: Cornell University Press.
Goodman, Lenn Evan (ed.). 1972. *Ibn Tufayl's Hayy Ibn Yaqzan*. New York: Twayne.
——. 1983. "The Greek Impact on Arabic Literature." In A. F. L. Beeston et al. (eds.). *Arabic Literature to the End of the Umayyad Period*. Cambridge: Cambridge University Press, pp. 460–82.
Gordon, Elizabeth Hope. 1917. *The Naming of Characters in the Works of Charles Dickens*. Lincoln: University of Nebraska Press.
Gordon, Haim. 1990. *Naguib Mahfouz's Egypt*. New York: Greenwood Press.
Gordon, Milton. 1964. *Assimilation in American Life*. New York: Oxford University Press.
Giorgio, Pasqualina. 2001. "Narrativa araba contemporanea: alcune problematiche di traduzione. (Abstract: Contemporary Arab Fiction: Some Translation Issues)." *Traduttore Nuovo* 56.1, pp. 23–8, 111–12.
Gorton, T. J. 1974. "Arabic Influence on the Troubadours: Documents and Directions." *Journal of Arabic Literature* 5, pp. 11–16.
Granara, William. 2005. "Nostalgia, Arab Nationalism, and the Andalusian Chronotope in the Evolution of the Modern Arabic Novel." *Journal of Arabic Literature* 36.1, pp. 57–73.
Grey, Jerry and Grey, Vivian (eds.). 1962. *Space Flight Report to the Nation*. New York: Basic Books.
Grey, Jerry and Grey, Vivian 1966. *Taqrīr 'an al-Faḍā' al-Yawm wa-Ghadan*, trans. Zakariyya al-Barāda'ī. Cairo: Dār al-Fikr al-'Arabī.
Günther, Sebastian. 1999. "Hostile Brothers in Transformation: An Archetypal Conflict in Classical and Modern Arabic Literature." In Angelika Neuwirth et al. (eds.). *Myths, Historical Archetypes and Symbolic Figures in Arabic Literature*. Beirut: Orient-Institut der DMG, pp. 309–36.
Günther, Sebastian and Milich Stephan (eds.). 2016. *Representations and Visions of Homeland in Modern Arabic Literature*. Hildesheim: Georg Olms Verlag.
Gutas, Dimitri. 1998. "Tardjama (Translations from Greek and Syriac)." *Encyclopaedia of Islam*, 2nd edn. X, pp. 225–31.
——. 1999. *Greek Thought, Arabic Culture: The Graeco-Arabic Translation Movement in Baghdad and Early 'Abbāsid Society (2nd–4th/8th–10th Centuries)*. London: Routledge.
——. 2000. *Greek Philosophers in the Arabic Tradition*. Aldershot: Ashgate.
Guth, Stephan (ed.). 2019. *Literary Visions of the Middle East: An Anthology of Canonical Masterpieces of Arabic, Persian, Turkish and Hebrew Fiction (Mid-19th to Early 21st Centuries)*. Wiesbaden: Harrassowitz Verlag.

Guth, Stephan and Pepe, Teresa (eds.). 2019. *Arabic Literature in a Posthuman World: Proceedings of the 12th Conference of the European Association for Modern Arabic Literature (EURAMAL), May 2016, Oslo.* Wiesbaden: Harrassowitz Verlag.
Guth, Stephan and Ramsay, Gail (eds.). 2011. *From New Values to New Aesthetics: Turning Points in Modern Arabic Literature (Proceedings of the 8th EURAMAL Conference, 11–14 June, 2008, Uppsala, Sweden). 2. Postmodernism and Thereafter.* Wiesbaden: Harrassowitz Verlag.
Guyer, Jonathan. 2014. "The Case of the Arabic Noirs." *Paris Review*, August 20, 2014, pp. 1–4.
Ḥabībī, Imīl (Habibi). 1974. *al-Waqā'i' al-Gharība fī Ikhtifā' Sa'īd Abī al-Naḥs al-Mutashā'il.* Haifa: Dār al-Ittiḥād.
——. 1985. *Sudāsiyyat al-Ayyām al-Sitta; al-Waqā'i' al-Gharība fī Ikhtifā' Sa'īd Abī al-Naḥs al-Mutashā'il wa-Qiṣas Ukhrā.* Haifa: Dār al-Ittiḥād.
——. 1985a. *Ikhtayya.* Nicosia: Bīsān.
Habiby, Emile. 1982. *The Secret Life of Saeed, the Ill-Fated Pessoptimist*, trans. Trevor Le Gassick. New York: Vintage Press.
——. 1985. *The Secret Life of Saeed the Pessoptimist*, trans. Salma Khadra Jayyusi and Trevor Le Gassick. London: Zed Books.
Ḥaddād, Mīshīl Iskandar. 1985. *Fī al-Nāḥiya al-Ukhrā.* Shfaram: Dār al-Mashriq.
Haddad, Robert M. 1970. *Syrian Christians in Muslim Society: An Interpretation.* Princeton, NJ: Princeton University Press.
Haddāra, Muḥammad Muṣṭafā. 1981. "al-Naz'a al-Ṣūfiyya fī al-Shi'r al-'Arabī al-Ḥadīth." *Fuṣūl* 1.4, pp. 107–22.
Hafez, Sabry. 1975. "Innovation in Egyptian Short Story." In R. C. Ostle (ed.). *Studies in Modern Arabic Literature.* Warminster: Aris & Phillips, pp. 99–112.
——. 2014. "World Literature after Orientalism: The Enduring Lure of the Occident." *Alif* 34, pp. 1–29.
——. 2017. "Cultural Journals and Modern Arabic Literature: A Historical Overview. " *Alif* 37, pp. 1–41.
Haggerty, James and Woodburn, John H. 1961. *Spacecraft.* New York: Scholastic Book Services.
——. 1964. *Spacecraft*, trans. Zakariyya al-Barāda'ī. Cairo: Maktabat al-Qāhira al-Ḥadītha.
Haikal, Mohammed Hussein. 1989. *Zainab*, trans. John Mohammed Grinted. London: Darf.
Haim, Sylvia G. 1962. *Arab Nationalism: An Anthology.* Berkeley: University of California Press.
al-Ḥājj, 'Azīz. 1983. *al-Ghazw al-Thaqāfī wa-Muqāwamatuhu.* Beirut: al-Mu'assasa al-'Arabiyya li-l-Dirāsāt wa-l-Nashr.
——. 1999. *Baghdad Dhālika al-Zamān.* Beirut: al-Mu'assasa al-'Arabiyya li-l-Dirāsāt wa-l-Nashr.
al-Ḥakīm, Su'ād. 1981. *al-Mu'jam al-Ṣūfī.* Beirut: Dār Nadra.
al-Ḥakīm, Tawfīq. 1986. "al-Riwāya Aṣīla fī al-Turāth al-'Arabī." *al-Akhbār*, August 6, p. 9.
——. 1990. *Return of the Spirit*, trans. William M. Hutchins. Washington, DC: Three Continents Press.
al-Ḥallāj, al-Ḥusayn ibn Manṣūr. 1974. *Dīwān*, ed. Kāmil Muṣṭafā al-Shaybī. Baghdad: Maṭba'at al-Ma'ārif.
Ḥamāda, Muḥammad Māhir. 1992. *Riḥlat al-Kitāb al-'Arabī ilā Diyār al-Gharb Fikran wa-Māddatan.* Beirut: Mu'assasat al-Risāla.
al-Hamadhānī, Abū al-Faḍl. 1973. *The Maqamat of Badi' al-Zaman al-Hamadhani*, trans. W. J. Prendergast. London: Curzon.
——. 1983. *Maqāmāt Abī al-Faḍl Badī' al-Zamān al-Hamādhānī.* Beirut: al-Dār al-Muttaḥida li-l-Nashr.

——. 2005. *Maqāmāt Abī al-Faḍl Badī' al-Zamān al-Hamādhānī*. Beirut: Dār al-Kutub al-'Ilmiyya.
Hamdouchi (al-Ḥamdūshī), Abdelilah ('Abd al-Ilāh). 2008. *The Final Bet*, trans. Jonathan Smolin. Cairo: American University in Cairo Press.
——. 2016. *White Fly*, trans. Jonathan Smolin. Cairo: Hoopoe.
al-Ḥamdūshī, 'Abd al-Ilāh. 2000. *al-Dhubāba al-Bayḍā'*. al-Muḥammadiyya, Morocco: Muttaqī.
——. 2001. *al-Rihān al-Akhīr*. al-Muḥammadiyya, Morocco: Muttaqī.
Hämeen-Anttila, Jaakko. 2002. *Maqama: A History of a Genre*. Wiesbaden: Harrassowitz Verlag.
——. 2008. "Building an Identity: Place as an Image of Self in Classical Arabic Literature." *Quaderni di Studi Arabi* 3, pp. 25–38.
Hamori, Andras. 1980. "Ilyādhat Hūmīrūs Bayna al-Ḥaqīqa wa-l-Taqlīd." In Sasson Somekh (ed.). *Abḥāth fi al-Lugha wa-l-Uslūb*. Tel Aviv: Tel Aviv University Press, pp. 15–22.
Handal, Nathalie (ed.). 2000. *The Poetry of Arab Women: A Contemporary Anthology*. New York: Interlink Books.
——. 2012. *Poet in Andalucía*. Pittsburgh: University of Pittsburgh Press.
——. 2019. *Shā'ira min al-Andalus*, trans. 'Ābid Ismā'īl. Damascus: al-Takwīn li-l-Ṭibā'a wa-l-Nashr wa-l-Tawzī'.
Hanssen, Jens. 2012. "Kafka and Arabs." *Critical Inquiry* 39.1, pp. 167–97.
Hanssen, Jens and Weiss, Max (eds.). 2016. *Arabic Thought beyond the Liberal Age: Towards an Intellectual History of the Nahda*. Cambridge: Cambridge University Press.
Haq, S. Nomanul. 2011. "Occult Sciences and Medicine." In Robert Irwin (ed.). *The New Cambridge History of Islam: Islamic Cultures and Societies to the End of the Eighteenth Century*, vol. 4. Cambridge: Cambridge University Press, pp. 640–67.
Harb, Lara. 2020. *Arabic Poetics: Aesthetic Experience in Classical Arabic Literature*. Princeton, NJ: Princeton University Press.
al-Ḥarīrī (al-Hariri), Abū Muḥammad. 1969 [1867]. *The Assemblies of al Hariri*, trans. Thomas Chenery. Farnborough: Gregg.
——. 1980. *The Assemblies of al-Hariri: Fifty Encounters with the Shaykh Abu Zayd of Seruj*, retold by Amina Shah from the Makamat of al-Hariri of Basra. London: Octagon.
——. 1985. *Maqāmāt al-Ḥarīrī*. Beirut: Dār Beirut.
Hartigan, Karelisa. 1979. *The Poets and the Cities: Selections from the Anthology about Greek Cities*. Meisenheim: Hain.
al-Hāshim, Jūzīf. 1960. *Sulaymān al-Bustānī wa-l-Ilyādha*. Beirut: Maktabat al-Madrasa wa-Dār al-Kitāb al-Lubnānī.
al-Hassan, Nawar. 1994. "A Feminist Reading of Arab Women's Autobiographies." PhD thesis, University of Nottingham.
Hatina, Meir. 2007. "Where East Meets West: Sufism, Cultural Rapprochement and Politics." *International Journal of Middle East Studies* 39, pp. 389–409.
——. 2011. "Arab Liberal Discourse: Old Dilemmas, New Visions." *Middle East Critique* 20, pp. 3–20.
Hatina, Meir and Sheffer, Yona (eds.). 2021. *Cultural Pearls from the East: In Memory of Shmuel Moreh, 1932–2017*. Leiden: Brill.
al-Ḥaydarī, Buland. 1990. *Abwāb ilā al-Bayt al-Ḍayyiq*. London: Riyāḍ al-Rayyis.
——. 1993. *al-A'māl al-Kāmila*. Kuwait City: Dār Su'ād al-Ṣabāḥ.
Haykal, Muḥammad Ḥusayn. 1968 [1913]. *Zaynab*. Cairo: Maktabat al-Nahḍa.
Haywood, John A. 1971. *Modern Arabic Literature 1800–1970*. London: Lund Humphries.
Hazo, Samuel. 1971. *The Blood of Adūnīs*. Pittsburgh: University of Pittsburgh Press.
Heiler, Friedrich. 1958. *Prayer*. New York: Oxford University Press.
Hejaiej, Monia. 1996. *Behind Closed Doors: Women's Oral Narratives in Tunis*. London: Quartet.

Helgesson, Stefan. 2015. "Tayeb Salih, Sol Plaatje, and the Trajectories of World Literature." *Cambridge Journal of Postcolonial Literary Inquiry* 2.2, pp. 253–60.
Herbert, Frank. 1965. *Dune*. Philadelphia and New York: Chilton.
Hermes, Nizar F. 2012. *The [European] Other in Medieval Arabic Literature and Culture*. New York: Palgrave Macmillan.
——. 2016. "Nostalgia for al-Andalus in Early Modern Moroccan *Voyages en Espagne*: al-Ghassānī's Riḥlat al-Wazīr Fī Iftikāk al-Asīr (1690–91) as a Case Study." *Journal of North African Studies* 21.3, pp. 433–52.
——. 2017. "'It Eclipsed Cairo and Outshone Baghdad!': Ibn Rashiq's Elegy for the City of Qayrawan." *Journal of Arabic Literature* 48.3, pp. 270–97.
Hever, Hannan. 1987. "Hebrew in an Israeli Arab Hand: Six Miniatures on Anton Shammas's *Arabesques*." *Cultural Critique* 7, pp. 47–76.
——. 1989. "Israeli Literature's Achilles's Heel." *Tikkun* 4.5, pp. 30–2.
——. 1991. "Minority Discourse of a National Majority; Israeli Fiction of the Early Sixties." *Prooftexts* 11, pp. 129–47.
Heym, Stefan. 1981. *Ahasver*. Munich: Bertelsmann.
al-Ḥifnī, ʿAbd al-Munʿim. 1980. *Muʿjam Muṣṭalaḥāt al-Ṣūfiyya*. Beirut: Dār al-Masīra.
Ḥijāzī, Aḥmad ʿAbd al-Muʿṭī. 1982. *Dīwān*. Beirut: Dār al-ʿAwda.
Hilāl, Muḥammad Ghunaymī. 1977. *al-Mawqif al-Adabī*. Beirut: Dār al-ʿAwda.
Hill, Christopher. 1971. *Antichrist in Seventeenth-Century England*. London: Oxford University Press.
Hill, Peter. 2015. "Translations of English Fiction into Arabic: *The Pilgrim's Progress* and *Robinson Crusoe*." *Journal of Semitic Studies* 60.1, pp. 177–212.
——. 2019. "Translation and the Globalisation of the Novel: Relevance and Limits of a Diffusionist Model." In Marilyn Booth (ed.). *Migrating Texts: Circulating Translations around the Ottoman Mediterranean*. Edinburgh: Edinburgh University Press, pp. 95–211.
——. 2020. *Utopia and Civilisation in the Arab Nahda*. Cambridge: Cambridge University Press.
Hilu, Virginia. 1976. *Beloved Prophet*. London: Quartet.
Hinchliffe, Arnold P. 1981. *The Absurd*. London: Methuen.
Hirsch, Lester M. (ed.). 1966. *Man and Space*. New York: Pitman.
——. (ed.). 1972. *al-Insān wa-l-Faḍā'*, trans. Ṣalāḥ Jalāl. Cairo: Maktabat al-Nahḍa al-Miṣriyya.
Hirschler, Konrad. 2012. *The Written Word in the Medieval Arabic Lands: A Social and Cultural History of Reading*. Edinburgh: Edinburgh University Press.
Hitti, Philip K. 1946. *History of the Arabs*. London: Macmillan.
——. 1962. *Islam and the West: A Historical Cultural Survey*. Princeton, NJ: Van Nostrand.
Hofstadter, Douglas R. 1979. *Godel, Escher, Bach*. New York: Vintage.
Høigilt, Jacob. 2019. *Comics in Contemporary Arab Culture*. London: I. B. Tauris.
Holmberg, Bo. 2006. "Transculturating the Epic: The Arabic Awakening and the Translation of the *Iliad*." In Margareta Petersson (ed.). *Literary Interactions in the Modern World*. Berlin: Mouton de Gruyter, pp. 141–65.
Homer. *The Odyssey*. 1984. Harmondsworth: Penguin.
Hopwood, Derek. 1999. *Sexual Encounters in the Middle East: The British, the French and the Arabs*. Reading: Ithaca Press.
Hottinger, Arnold. 1957. "Patriotismus und Nationalismus bei den Araben." *Neue Zurcher Zeitung*, May 12.
Hourani, Albert H. 1947. *Minorities in the Arab World*. London: Oxford University Press.
——. 1983. *Arabic Thought in the Liberal Age 1798–1939*. Cambridge: Cambridge University Press.
——. 1991. "Sulaiman al-Bustani and the *Iliad*." In *Islam in European Thought*. Cambridge: Cambridge University Press, pp. 174–87.

Hourani, Albert H. and Stern, S. M. (eds.). 1970. *The Islamic City: A Colloquium*, held at all Souls College, June 28–July 2, 1965. Oxford: Bruno Cassirer.
Howarth, Herbert and Shukrallah, Ibrahim. 1944. *Images from the Arab World: Fragments of Arab Literature Translated and Paraphrased with Variations and Comments*. London: Pilot Press.
Huart, Clément. 1966. *A History of Arabic Literature*. Beirut: Khayats.
Hujwīrī, Abū al-Ḥasan. 1926. *Kashf al-Maḥjūb* ed. V. A. Zukovski. Leningrad: n.p.
——. 1959. *The "Kashf al-Maḥjūb," the Oldest Persian Treatise on Sufism by al-Hujwīrī*, trans. R. A. Nicholson. London: Gibb Memorial Series.
——. 1999 [1926]. *Kashf al-Maḥjūb*, ed. V. A. Zukovski. Leningrad: Dār al-ʿUlūm.
al-Ḥumaydī, Abū ʿAbd Allāh. 1989. *Jadhwat al-Muqtabis fī Ta'rīkh ʿUlamā' al-Andalus*, ed. Ibrāhīm al-Abyārī. Cairo: Dār al-Kitāb al-Miṣrī and Beirut: Dār al-Kitāb al-Lubnānī.
Hunke, Sigrid. 1965. *Allahs Sonne über dem Abendlang*. Frankfurt and Hamburg: Fischer Bücherei.
——. 1979. *Shams al-ʿArab Tastaʿu ʿalā al-Gharb*, trans. Fārūq Bayḍūn and Kamāl Dasūqī. Beirut: al-Maktab al-Tijārī li-l-Ṭibāʿa wa-l-Tawzīʿ wa-l-Nashr.
Ḥusayn, ʿAbd al-Qādir. 1983. *Fann al-Badīʿ*. Beirut and Cairo: Dār al-Shurūq.
Ḥusayn, ʿAlī Ṣāfī. 1964. *al-Adab al-Ṣūfī fī Miṣr fī al-Qarn al-Sābiʿ*. Cairo: Dār al-Maʿārif.
Ḥusayn, Ṭāhā. n.d. [1929]. *al-Ayyām*. Cairo: Dār al-Maʿārif.
——. 1945. "al-Adab al-ʿArabī Bayna Amsihi wa-Ghadihi." *al-Kātib al-Miṣrī* I.1, pp. 4–27.
——. n.d. [1958]. *Alwān*. Cairo: Dār al-Maʿārif.
——. 1967 [1956]. *Naqd wa-Iṣlāḥ*. Beirut: Dār al-ʿIlm li-l-Malāyīn.
al-Ḥusaynī, ʿAlī. 1980. *Sifr ʿAbd al-Raḥmān al-Dākhil*. Baghdad: Dār al-Ḥurriyya.
al-Ḥusnī, ʿAbd al-Razzāq. 1974. *Ta'rīkh al-Ḥukūmāt al-ʿIrāqiyya*. Beirut: Maṭbaʿat Dār al-Kutub.
al-Ḥuṣrī, Abū Khaldūn Sāṭiʿ. 1965. *Yawm Maysalūn: Ṣafḥa min Ta'rīkh al-ʿArab al-Ḥadīth*. Beirut: Manshūrāt Dār al-Ittiḥād.
——. 1965 [1955]. *al-ʿUrūba Awwalan!* Beirut: Dār al-ʿIlm li-l-Malāyīn.
Ibn al-Akfānī. 1998. *Kitāb Irshād al-Qāṣid ilā Asnā al-Maqāṣid*, ed. Maḥmūd Fākhūrī et al. Beirut: Maktabat Lubnān.
Ibn ʿArabī, Muḥyī al-Dīn (Muhyiddin). 1938. *Iṣṭilāḥāt al-Ṣūfiyya*. Cairo: Maṭbaʿat al-Ḥalabī.
——. 1966. *Tarjumān al-Ashwāq*. Beirut: Dār Ṣādir.
——. 1978 [1911]. *The Tarjuman al-Ashwaq, by Ibn al-Arabi*, trans. Reynold A. Nicholson. London: Theosophical Publishing House.
——. 2021. *The Translator of Desires: Poems*, trans. Michael Sells. Princeton, NJ: Princeton University Press.
Ibn al-ʿArīf. 1933. *Maḥāsin al-Majālis*, ed. and trans. Miguel Asin Palacios. Paris: Librairie Orientaliste Paul Geuthner.
——. 1980. *Maḥāsin al-Majālis*, trans. William Elliott and Adnan K. Abdulla. Amersham: Avebury.
Ibn al-Athīr. 1987. *al-Kāmil fī Ta'rīkh*, ed. Muḥammad Yūsuf al-Daqqāq. Beirut: Dār al-Kutub al-ʿIlmiyya.
Ibn Bassām, Abū al-Ḥasan ʿAlī. 1979. *al-Dhākhīra fī Maḥāsin Ahl al-Jazīra*, ed. Iḥsān ʿAbbās. Beirut: Dār al-Thaqāfa.
Ibn al-Fuwaṭī, Kamāl al-Dīn. 2008. *Manāqib Baghdad*. Amman: Dār al-Fārūq.
Ibn al-Jahm, ʿAlī. n.d. *Dīwān*. Riyadh: Wizārat al-Maʿārif.
——. 1981. *Dīwān*, ed. Khalīl Mardam. Beirut: Dār al-Āfāq al-Jadīda.
Ibn Ḥanbal, Aḥmad. n.d. *Musnad*. Cairo: n.p.
——. 1969. *Musnad*. Beirut: al-Maktab al-Islāmī and Dār Ṣādir.
Ibn ʿImrān, al-Muʿāfā. n.d. *Kitāb al-Zuhd* (MS). Damascus: al-Ẓāhiriyya.
Ibn Kathīr. 1966. *al-Bidāya wa-l-Nihāya*. Beirut and Riyadh: Maktabat al-Maʿārif and Maktabat al-Naṣr.

Ibn al-Khaṭīb, Lisān al-Dīn. 1901. *al-Iḥāṭa fī Akhbār Ghranāṭa*. Cairo: Maṭbaʿat al-Mawsūʿāt.
Ibn Manẓūr. n.d. *Lisān al-ʿArab*. Beirut: Dār Ṣādir.
Ibn al-Mubārak, ʿAbd Allāh. 1966. *al-Zuhd wa-l-Raqaʾiq*, ed. Ḥabīb al-Raḥmān al-Aʿẓamī. Beirut: Dār al-Kutub al-ʿIlmiyya.
Ibn Munqidh, Usāma. 1930. *Kitāb al-Iʿtibār*, ed. Philip K. Hitti. Princeton, NJ: Princeton University Press.
——. 1987. *Memoirs of an Arab-Syrian Gentleman and Warrior in the Period of the Crusades*, trans. Philip K. Hitti. London: I. B. Tauris.
Ibn Qutayba, ʿAbd Allāh ibn Muslim. 1928. *ʿUyūn al-Akhbār*. Cairo: Maṭbaʿat Dār al-Kutub al-Miṣriyya.
Ibn Rashīq al-Qayrawānī. 1963. *al-ʿUmda*, ed. Muḥammad Muḥyī al-Dīn ʿAbd al-Ḥamīd. Cairo: al-Maktaba al-Tijāriyya al-Kubrā.
Ibn Ṭabāṭabā, Muḥammad ibn ʿAlī. 1966. *al-Fakhrī fī al-Ādāb al-Sulṭāniyya wa-l-Duwal al-Islāmiyya*. Beirut: Dār Ṣādir.
Ibn Taghribirdī, Jamāl al-Dīn. 1930. *al-Nujūm al-Zāhira fī Mulūk Miṣr wa-l-Qāhira*. Cairo: Maṭbaʿat Dār al-Kutub.
——. 1992. *al-Nujūm al-Zāhira fī Mulūk Miṣr wa-l-Qāhira*. Cairo: Maṭbaʿat Dār al-Kutub.
Ibn Ṭufayl. 1940. *Ḥayy ibn Yaqẓān*, ed. Jamīl Ṣalība and Kāmil ʿAyyād. Damascus: Maṭbaʿat al-Taraqqī.
Ibn Warraq. 2003. *Why I Am Not a Muslim*. Amherst, NY: Prometheus.
Ibn Zaydūn. 1958. *Dīwān Ibn Zaydūn wa-Rasāʾiluhu*, ed. ʿAlī ʿAbd al-ʿAẓīm. Cairo: Maktabat Nahḍat Miṣr.
Ibrāhīm, Ḥāfiẓ. n.d. [1937]. *Dīwān*, ed. Aḥmad Amīn et al. Beirut: Dār al-ʿAwda.
ʿĪd, Rajāʾ. 1993. *al-Madhhab al-Badīʿī fī al-Shiʿr al-ʿArabī*. Alexandria: Munshaʾat al-Maʿārif.
Idrīs, Suhayl. 1973. "Muʾtamar al-Udabāʾ wa-Ḥurriyyat al-Taʿbīr." *al-Ādāb* (April), pp. 2–7.
Idrīs, Yūsuf. 1988 [1971]. *al-Jins al-Thālith*. Cairo: Miṣr li-l-Ṭibāʿa.
Igbaria, Khaled. 2013. "Laylá Baʿalbakī and Feminism Throughout Her Fiction." PhD thesis, University of Edinburgh.
——. 2015. "Feminism throughout Laylá Baʿalbaki's Fiction." *International Journal of Gender and Women's Studies* 3.1, pp. 152–64.
Imruʾ al-Qays. 1964. *Dīwān*, ed. Muḥammad Abū al-Faḍl Ibrāhīm. Cairo: Dār al-Maʿārif.
ʿInāyāt, Rājī. 1980. *Sirr al-Aṭbāq al-Ṭāʾira*. Cairo: Dār al-Shurūq.
——. 1984. *Aḥlām al-Yawm Ḥaqāʾiq al-Ghad*. Cairo: Dār al-Shurūq.
——. 1993 [1983]. *Aghrab min al-Khayāl: Laʿnat al-Farāʿina: Wahm am Khayāl?* 5th edn. Cairo: Dār al-Shurūq.
——. 1995. *Aghrab min al-Khayāl: al-Ashbāḥ al-Mushāhgiba wa-Gharāʾib Ukhrā*. Cairo: Dār al-Shurūq.
Irwin, Robert. 2000. "Adonis in the Levant." *The Times Literary Supplement*, September 1, pp. 14–15.
——. (ed.). 2011. *The New Cambridge History of Islam: Islamic Cultures and Societies to the End of the Eighteenth Century*, vol. 4. Cambridge: Cambridge University Press.
ʿĪsā, Yūsuf ʿIzz al-Dīn. 1979. "Jules Verne wa-l-Adab al-ʿIlmī." *ʿĀlam al-Fikr*, April–June, pp. 199–232.
Ishtiaque Ullah, Sahar. 2016. "Postclassical Poetics: The Role of the Amatory Prelude for the Medieval Islamic Republic of Letters." *Cambridge Journal of Postcolonial Literary Inquiry* 3.2, pp. 203–25.
Iskandar, Makram Shākir. 1992. *Udabāʾ Muntaḥirūn*. Beirut: Dār al-Rātib al-Jāmiʿiyya.
al-Iskandarī, ʿAbd al-Muʿṭī al-Lakhmī. 1954. *Sharḥ Manāzil al-Sāʾirīn*, ed. Serge de Laugier de Beaurecueil. Cairo: Imprimerie de l'Institut Français d'Archéologie Orientale.

Iskander, Ghareeb. 2021. *English Poetry and Modern Arabic Verse Translation and Modernity*. London: I. B. Tauris.
Ismael, Jacqueline S. 1981. "The Alienation of Palestine in Palestinian Poetry." *Arab Studies Quarterly* 3.1, pp. 43–55.
Ismāʿīl, ʿIzz al-Dīn. 1978. *al-Shiʿr al-ʿArabī al-Muʿāṣir: Qaḍāyāhu wa-Ẓawāhiruhu al-Fanniyya wa-l-Maʿnawiyya*. Cairo: Dār al-Fikr al-ʿArabī.
al-Jābirī, Muḥammad ʿĀbid. 1982. *al-Khiṭāb al-ʿArabī al-Muʿāṣir: Dirāsa Taḥlīliyya Naqdiyya*. Beirut: Dār al-Ṭalīʿa and Casablanca: al-Markaz al-Thaqāfī al-ʿArabī.
Jabrā, Ibrāhīm Jabrā. 1968. "al-Tanāquḍāt fī al-Masraḥ wa-l-Marāya." *Shiʿr* 39, pp. 112–25.
——. 1989. *Taʾammulāt fī Bunyān Marmarī*. London: Riyāḍ al-Rayyis.
——. 1992. *Aqniʿat al-Ḥaqīqa wa-Aqniʿat al-Khayāl*. Beirut: al-Muʾassasa al-ʿArabiyya li-l-Dirāsāt wa-l-Nashr.
Jacquemond, Richard. 1992. "Translation and Cultural Hegemony: The Case of French–Arabic Translation." In Lawrence Venuti (ed.). *Rethinking Translation: Discourse, Subjectivity, Ideology*. New York: Routledge, pp. 139–58.
——. 1992a. "al-Tarjama wa-l-Haymana al-Thaqāfiyya: Ḥālat al-Tarjama al-Faransiyya/al-ʿArabiyya." *Fuṣūl* 11.2, pp. 43–57.
Jacquemond, Richard and Lagrange, Frédéric (eds.). 2020. *Culture pop en Égypte. Entre mainstream commercial et contestation*. Paris: Riveneuve
Jafri, Naqi Husain. 2004. "The Poetics and Politics of Troubadours: The Hispano-Arabic Connection." In Naqi Husain Jafri (ed.). *Critical Theory: Perspectives from Asia*. New Delhi: Jamia Millia Islamia, pp. 374–87.
al-Jāḥiẓ, Abū ʿUthmān. 1938. *al-Ḥayawān*. Cairo: al-Ḥalabī.
James, William. 1945. *The Varieties of Religious Experience*. New York: Mentor.
Jameson, Fredric. 1972. *The Prison-House of Language: A Critical Account of Structuralism and Russian Formalism*. Princeton, NJ: Princeton University Press.
al-Janābī, ʿAbd al-Qādir. 1994. *Risāla Maftūḥa ilā Adūnīs*. Paris: Manshūrāt Farādīs.
——. 2012. *Unḥutnī fī al-Ḍawʾ li-kay lā Tuṣāb Lughatī bi-l-Duwār*. Beirut: al-Ghāwūn.
al-Jarrāḥ, Nūrī. 2019. *Lā Ḥarba fī Ṭurwāda: Kalimāt Hūmīrūs al-Akhīra*. Milan: Manshūrāt al-Mutawassiṭ.
Jarrar, Maher. 2011. "'A Tent for Longing': Maḥmūd Darwīsh and al-Andalus." In Ramzi Baalbaki et al. (eds.). *Poetry and History: The Value of Poetry in Reconstructing Arab History*. Beirut: American University of Beirut Press, pp. 361–93.
al-Jawāhirī, Muḥammad Mahdī. 1982. *Dīwān al-Jawāhirī*. Beirut: Dār al-ʿAwda.
Jayyusi, Salma Khadra. 1977. *Trends and Movements in Modern Arabic Poetry*. Leiden: Brill.
——. (ed.). 1992. *Anthology of Modern Palestinian Literature*. New York: Columbia University Press.
——. 2008. "Response to Thomas Bauer." *Mamlūk Studies Review* 12.1, pp. 193–207.
al-Jazrāwī, Aḥmad. 2005. *Baghdād baʿḍ al-Gharīb wa-l-Ṭarīf min Maḍīha al-Ẓarīf*. Baghdad: Dār al-Shuʾūn al-Thaqāfiyya al-ʿĀmma.
al-Jīlānī, ʿAbd al-Qādir. 1331H. *al-Ghunya li-Ṭālibī al-Ḥaqq*. Cairo: Dār al-Kutub al-ʿArabīyya al-Kubrā.
Joad, C. E. M. 1948. *Guide to Modern Thought*. London: Pan.
Johnson, Rebecca Carol. 2017. "Archive of Errors: Aḥmad Fāris al-Shidyāq, Literature, and the World." *Middle Eastern Literatures* 20.1, pp. 31–50.
——. 2021. *Stranger Fictions: A History of the Novel in Arabic Translation*. Ithaca, NY: Cornell University Press.
Johnson-Davies, Denys. 1967. *Modern Arabic Short Stories*. London: Oxford University Press.
——. 1994. "On Translating Arabic Literature." In Ferial J. Ghazoul and Barbara Harlow (eds.). *The View from Within: Writers and Critics on Contemporary Arabic Literature*. Cairo: American University in Cairo Press, pp. 272–82.

Johnston, John H. 1984. *The Poet and the City: A Study in Urban Perspectives*. Athens: University of Georgia Press.

Jones, Alan. 1988. *Romance Kharjas in Andalusian Arabic Muwaššaḥ Poetry*. London: Ithaca Press.

Jones, Richard Glyn and Williams, Arlene (eds.). 1996. *The Penguin Book of Erotic Stories by Women*. Harmondsworth: Penguin.

Joyaux, Georges J. 1980. "Driss Chraïbi, Mohammed Dib, Kateb Yacine, and Indigenous North African Literature." In Issa J. Boullata (ed.). *Critical Perspectives on Modern Arabic Literature*. Washington, DC: Three Continents Press, pp. 117–27.

al-Ju'aydī, Muḥammad 'Abd Allāh. 1997. *Ḥuḍūr al-Andalus fī al-Adab al-Filasṭīnī al-Ḥadīth*. International Conference about Palestinian Literature, Birzeit University, May 17–19.

——. 2000. "Ḥuḍūr al-Andalus fī al-Adab al-Filasṭīnī al-Ḥadīth." *'Ālām al-Fikr* 28.4, pp. 7–52.

Jubrān, Jubrān Khalīl. n.d. [1912]. *al-Ajniḥa al-Mutakassira*. Beirut: n.p.

——. 1981. *al-Majmū'a al-Kāmila li-Mu'allafāt Jubrān Khalīl Jubrān al-Mu'arraba 'an al-Inklīziyyia*. Beirut: n.p.

——. 1985. *al-Majmū'a al-Kāmila li-Mu'allafāt Jubrān Khalīl Jubrān al-'Arabiyya*. Beirut: n.p.

Jubrān, Sulaymān. 1989. *al-Mabnā wa-l-Ṣūra fī Shi'r 'Abd al-Wahhāb al-Bayyātī*. Acre: Dār al-Aswār.

al-Jundī, Anwar. 1963. *al-Lugha al-'Arabiyya Bayna Ḥumātihā wa-Khuṣūmihā*. Cairo: Maktabat al-Anglo al-Miṣriyya.

Junge, Christian. 2021. "Affective Readings: Emotion and Society in/of Egyptian Literature, 1990 to 2020," TRAFO: Blog for Transregional Research, October 19 2021, available at: https://trafo.hypotheses.org/31191, last accessed October 21, 2021.

Jurji, Edward Jabra. 1938. *Illumination in Islamic Mysticism*. Princeton, NJ: Princeton University Press.

Kabbani, Rana. 1986. *Europe's Myths of Orient: Devise and Rule*. London: Macmillan.

Kadi, Joanna (ed.). 1994. *Food for Our Grandmothers: Writing by Arab-American and Arab-Canadian Feminists*. Boston, MA: South End Press.

Kafka, Franz. 1931. *Beim Bau der Chinesischen Mauer*. Berlin: Gustav Kiepenheuer.

——. 1946. *Beschreibung eines Kampfes*. New York: Schocken.

——. 1948. *The Penal Colony: Stories and Short Pieces*, trans. Willa and Edwin Muir. New York: Schocken.

——. 1953. *Hochzeitsvorbereitungen auf dem Lande*. New York: Schocken.

——. 1954. *Dearest Father*. New York: Schocken.

——. 1958. *Briefe 1902–1924*. New York: Schocken.

——. 1966. *Letter to His Father*. Bilingual edn. New York: Schocken.

——. 1971. *The Complete Stories*, ed. N. Glazer. New York: Schocken.

——. 1977. *Letters to Friends, Family, and Editors*, trans. Richard Winston and Clara Winston. New York: Schocken.

——. 2007. *Metamorphosis and Other Stories*, trans. Michael Hofmann. New York: Penguin.

——. 2014. *al-A'māl al-kāmila*, trans. Yusrī Khamīs. Cairo: al-'Arabī li-l-nashr wa-l-tawzī'.

al-Kalābādhī, Abū Bakr Muḥammad. 1980. *al-Ta'arruf li-Madhhab Ahl al-Taṣawwuf*, ed. Maḥmūd Amīn al-Nawawī. Cairo: Maktabat al-Kulliyyāt al-Azhariyya.

Kamal, Hala. 2021. "Virginia Woolf in Arabic: A Feminist Paratextual Reading of Translation Strategies." In Jeanne Dubino et al. (eds.). *The Edinburgh Companion to Virginia Woolf and Contemporary Global Literature*. Edinburgh: Edinburgh University Press, pp. 166–82.

Kashua, Sayed (Sayyid Qashshū'a). 2002. *Dancing Arabs* (in Hebrew). Ben-Shemen: Modan.

——. 2004. *Let It Be Morning* (in Hebrew). Jerusalem: Keter.

——. 2006. *Let It Be Morning*, trans. Miriam Shlesinger. New York: Black Cat.

——. 2010. *Second Person Singular* (in Hebrew). Jerusalem: Keter.

——. 2013. *Second Person Singular*, trans. Mitch Ginsburg. New York: Grove Press.

——. 2015. *Native* (in Hebrew). Jerusalem: Keter.

——. 2016. *Native: Dispatches from an Israeli-Palestinian Life*, trans. Ralph Mandel. New York: Grove Press.

——. 2017. *Follow the Changes* (in Hebrew). Shoham: Kinneret, Zmora, Dvir.

Kassem, Cez and Hashem, Malak (eds.). 1985. *Flights of Fantasy: Arabic Short Stories*. Cairo: Elias Modern Publishing House.

Kassem, Cez and Hashem, Malak (eds.). 1996. *Flights of Fantasy: Arabic Short Stories*, 2nd edn. Cairo: Elias Modern Publishing House.

Kattānī, Yāsīn. 2000–2001. "Qaṣṣ al-Ḥadātha: Dirāsa fī al-Tashkīl al-Fannī li-Riwāyat al-Kharrāṭ *Turābuhā Za'farān*." *al-Karmil: Studies in Arabic Language and Literature* 21/22, pp. 315–63.

Kawar, Irfan Arif. 1954. "Early Islam and Poetry." PhD thesis, Princeton University.

Kaylānī, Muḥammad Sayyid. 1962. *al-Adab al-Qubṭī Qadīman wa-Ḥadīthan*. Cairo: Dār al-Qawmiyya al-'Arabiyya li-l-Ṭibā'a.

Kayyal, Mahmoud. 2000. "Translational Norms in the Translations of Modern Hebrew Literature into Arabic Between 1948 and 1990." PhD thesis, Tel Aviv University.

——. 2006. *Translation in the Shadow of Confrontation: Norms in the Translations of Modern Hebrew Literature into Arabic between 1948 and 1990* (in Hebrew). Jerusalem: Magnes Press.

——. 2016. *Selected Issues in the Modern Intercultural Contacts between Arabic and Hebrew Cultures: Hebrew, Arabic, and Death*. Leiden: Brill.

Kazantzakis, Nikos. 1996 [1946]. *Zorba the Greek*, trans. Carl Wildman. New York: Simon & Schuster.

Kedourie, Elie. 1970. *The Chatham House Version and Other Middle Eastern Studies*. London: Weidenfeld & Nicolson.

——. 1971. "The Jews in Baghdad in 1910." *Middle Eastern Studies* 7.3, pp. 355–61.

——. 1974. *Arabic Political Memoirs and Other Studies*. London: Frank Cass.

——. 1989. "The Break between Muslims and Jews in Iraq." In Mark R. Cohen and Abraham L. Udovitch (eds.). *Jews among Arabs: Contacts and Boundaries*. Princeton, NJ: Darwin Press, pp. 21–63.

Kedourie, Sylvia (ed.). 1998. *Elie Kedourie CBE, FBA 1926–1992: History, Philosophy, Politics*. London: Frank Cass.

Kennedy, Philip F. 1991. "Thematic Relationships between the *Kharjas*, the Corpus of *Muwaššaḥāt* and Eastern Lyrical Poetry." In Alan Jones and Richard Hitchcock (eds.). *Studies on the Muwaššaḥ and the Kharja*. Reading: Ithaca Press, pp. 68–87.

Khaḍr, Mahā Maẓlūm. 2001. *Binā' Riwāyat al-Khayāl al-'Ilmī fī al-Adab al-Miṣrī al-Mu'āṣir*. Cairo: Maṭba'at al-Offset al-Ḥadītha.

al-Khāl, Yūsuf. 1979. *Dīwān*. Beirut: Dār al-'Awda.

Khalaf, Roseanne Saad. 2006. *Hikayat: Short Stories by Lebanese Women*. London: Telegram.

Khaldi, Boutheina. 2009. "Epistolarity in a *Nahḍah* Climate: The Role of Mayy Ziyādah's Letter Writing." *Journal of Arabic Literature* 40, pp. 1–36.

Khalifah, Omar. 2017. "Anthologizing Arabic Literature: The Longman Anthology and the Problems of World Literature." *Journal of World Literature* 2, pp. 512–26.

——. 2018. *Nasser in the Egyptian Imaginary*. Edinburgh: Edinburgh University Press.

Khalil, Iman. 1994. "Narrative Strategies as Cultural Vehicles: Rafik Schami's Novel *Erzahler der Nacht*." In Carol Aisha Blackshire-Belay (ed.). *The Germanic Mosaic: Cultural and Linguistic Diversity in Society*. New York: Greenwood Press, pp. 217–24.

——. 1995. "Arab-German Literature." *World Literature Today* 69, pp. 521–7.

Khalīl, Jūrj Najīb. 1967. *al-Shi'r al-'Arabī fī Khidmat al-Salām*. Tel Aviv: Dār al-Nashr al-'Arabī.

Khāliṣ, Walīd Maḥmūd. 2005. *Baghdād al-Ta'rīkh wa-l-Shi'r*. Beirut: al-Mu'assasa al-'Arabiyya li-l-Dirāsāt wa-l-Nashr.

Khan, Hasan-Uddin. 2008. "Identity, Globalization, and the Contemporary Islamic City." In Salma Khadra Jayyusi et al. (eds.). *The City in the Islamic World*. Leiden: Brill, pp. 1035–62.

al-Kharrāṭ, Idwār. 2005. *Mujāladat al-Mustaḥīl: Maqāṭi' min Sīra Dhātiyya li-l-Kitāba*. Cairo: Dār al-Bustānī li-l-Nashr wa-l-Tawzī'.

al-Khashin, Fu'ād. 1972. *Sanābil Ḥazīrān*. Cairo: Dār al-Ma'ārif.

al-Khaṭīb, Muḥammad Kāmil (ed.). 1994. *Naẓariyyat al-Masraḥ (al-Qism al-Thānī: Muqaddimāt wa-Bayānāt)*. Damascus: Manshūrāt Wizārat al-Thaqāfa.

——. 1995. *al-Riwāya wa-l- Yūtūbyā*. Damascus: Dār al-Madā li-l- Thaqāfa wa-l- Nashr.

al-Khaṭīb al-Baghdādī, Abū Bakr Aḥmad ibn 'Alī. 1931. *Ta'rīkh Baghdād*. Baghdad: Maṭba'at al-Sa'āda.

——. 1971. *Ta'rīkh Baghdād*. Beirut: Dār al-Kutub al-'Ilmiyya.

Khoury, Jeries. 2016. *The Impact of the Arabian Nights on Modern Arabic Poetry*. Wiesbaden: Harrassowitz Verlag.

Khūrī (Khoury), Ilyās (Elias). 1974. *Tajribat al-Baḥth 'an Ufq: Muqaddima li-Dirāsat al-Riwāya al-'Arabiyya Ba'da al-Hazīma*. Beirut: Markaz al-Abḥāth fī Munaẓẓamat al-Taḥrīr al-Filasṭīniyya.

——. (ed.). 1981. *al-Masīḥiyyūn al-'Arab: Dirāsāt wa-Munāqashāt*. Beirut: Mu'assasat al-Abḥāth al-'Arabiyya.

Kilito, Abdelfattah. 1983. *Les séances: récits et codes culturels chez Hamadhani et Hariri*. Paris: Sindbad.

——. 1993. *al-Maqāmāt: al-Sard wa-l-Ansāq al-Thaqāfiyya*, trans. 'Abd al-Kabīr al-Sharqāwī. Casablanca: Dār Tūbqāl li-l-Nashr.

——. 1999. *al-Ḥikāya wa-l-Ta'wīl: Dirāsāt fī al-Sard al-'Arabī*. Casablanca: Dār Tūbqāl li-l-Nashr.

——. 2001. *Lisān Ādam*, trans. 'Abd al-Kabīr al-Sharqāwī. Casablanca: Dār Tūbqāl li-l-Nashr.

——. 2002. *Lan Tatakallam Lughatī*. Beirut: Dār al-Ṭalī'a.

——. 2007. *al-Adab wa-l-Irtiyāb*. Casablanca: Dār Tūbqāl li-l-Nashr.

——. 2008. *Thou Shalt Not Speak My Language*, trans. Waïl S. Hassan. Syracuse, NY: Syracuse University Press.

——. 2020. *Fī Jaww min al-Nadam al-Fikrī*. Milan: Manshūrāt al-Mutawassaṭ.

Kilpatrick, Hilary. 1991. "Autobiography and Classical Arabic Literature." *Journal of Arabic Literature* 22, pp. 1–20.

——. 1998. "The 'Genuine' Ash'ab: The Relativity of Fact and Fiction in Early *Adab* Texts." In Stefan Leder (ed.) *Story-Telling in the Framework of Non-Fictional Arabic Literature*. Wiesbaden: Harrassowitz Verlag, pp. 94–117.

——. 2015. "Modern Arabic Literature as Seen in the Late 19th Century: Jurji Murqus's Contribution to Korsh and Kipichnikov's *Vseobshchaya Istoria Literatury*." In Roger Allen and Robin Ostle (eds.). *Studying Modern Arabic Literature: Mustafa Badawi, Scholar and Critic*. Edinburgh: Edinburgh University Press, pp. 83–101.

Kincaid, Paul. 2005. "On the Origins of Genre." In James Gunn and Matthew Candelaria Gunn (eds.). *Speculations on Speculation: Theories of Science Fiction*. Lanham, MD: Scarecrow Press, pp. 41–53.

Kirchner, Henner. 2001. "Internet in the Arab World: A Step Toward 'Information Society?'" In Kai Hafez (ed.). *Mass Media, Politics, and Society in the Middle East.* Cresskill, NJ: Hampton Press, pp. 137–58.

Kirkpatrick, Peter and Dixon, Robert (eds.). 2012. *Republics of Letters: Literary Communities in Australia.* Sydney: Sydney University Press.

Kishk, Muḥammad Jalāl. 1966. *al-Ghazw al-Fikrī.* Cairo: al-Dār al-Qawmiyya li-l-Ṭibā'a wa-l-Nashr.

Knight, Damon (ed.). 1977. *Turning Points: Essays on the Art of Science Fiction.* New York: Harper & Row.

Knipp, C. 1974. "The *Arabian Nights* in England: Galland's Translation and Its Successors." *Journal of Arabic Literature* 5, pp. 44–54.

Knox, Ronald A. 1951. *Enthusiasm.* Oxford: Clarendon Press.

Konerding, Peter et al. 2021. *Approaches to Arabic Popular Culture.* Bamberg: University of Bamberg Press.

König, Daniel G. 2016. "The Unkempt Heritage: On the Role of Latin in the Arabic-Islamic Sphere." *Arabica* 63, pp. 419–93.

Konstantinovic, Zoran. 1988. "Response to Claus Clüver's 'The Difference of Eight Decades: World Literature and the Demise of National Literatures.'" *Yearbook of Comparative and General Literature* 37, pp. 141–2.

Korteling, Jacomina. 1928. *Mysticism in Blake and Wordsworth.* Amsterdam: n.p.

Krachkovskii, I. J. 1927. "Die Literatur der arabischen Emigranten in Amerika (1895–1915)." *Monde Oriental* 21, pp. 193–213.

——. 1989. *al-Riwāya al-Ta'rīkhiyya fī al-Adab al-'Arabī al-Ḥadīth wa-Dirāsāt Ukhrā,* trans. 'Abd al-Raḥīm al-'Aṭāwī. Rabat: Dār al-Kalām li-l-Nashr wa-l-Tawzī'.

Kritzeck, James. 1964. *Anthology of Islamic Literature.* New York: Holt, Rinehart & Winston.

Krivoshein, Basil. 1938–1939. "The Ascetic and Theological Teaching of Gregory Palamas." *Eastern Churches Quarterly,* I, pp. 26–33, II, pp. 71–84, III, pp. 138–56, IV, pp. 193–214.

Kronholm, Tryggve. 1993. "Arab Culture—Reality or Fiction?" In Heikki Palva and Knut S. (eds.). *Papers from the Second Nordic Conference on Middle Eastern Studies, Copenhagen, 22–25 October 1992.* Copenhagen: Nordic Institute of Asian Studies, pp. 12–25.

Kropp, Manfred. 2004–2005. "The Office as a Universe—The Mystic Experience as the Initial Spark of a Civil Servant's Career: A New Reading into the Novel *ḥaḍrat al-muḥtaram* by Naguib Mahfouz." *Beiruter Blätter: Mitteilungen des Orient-Instituts Beirut* 12/13, pp. 61–9.

al-Kutubī, Ibn Shākir. 1951. *Fawāt al-Wafayāt,* ed. Muḥammad Muḥyī al-Dīn 'Abd al-Ḥamīd. Cairo: Maktabat al-Nahḍa al-Miṣriyya.

al-Lababīdī, Maḥmūd. 1943. "al-'Arab Bayna al-Falsafa al-Yūnāniyya wa-l-Adab al-Yūnānī." *al-Adīb,* May, pp. 29–35.

Labanieh, Aya. 2021. "Science Fiction, Rational Enchantment, and Arabic Literature." *Journal of Science Fiction* 4.2, pp. 8–12.

Lane, Edward William. 1859 [1839–1841]. *The Arabian Nights' Entertainments.* London: John Murray.

——. 1914 [1859]. *The Arabian Nights' Entertainments.* New York: Bigelow Brown.

——. 1968 [1863–1893]. *An Arabic–English Lexicon.* Beirut: Librairie du Liban.

Lapidus, Ira M. 1969. *Middle Eastern Cities.* Berkeley: University of California Press.

——. 2002. *A History of Islamic Societies.* Cambridge: Cambridge University Press.

Lassner, Jacob. 1970. "The Caliph's Personal Domain: The City Plan of Baghdad Re-Examined." In Albert H. Hourani and S. M. Stern (eds.). *The Islamic City: A Colloquium,* held at all Souls College, June 28–July 2, 1965. Oxford: Bruno Cassirer, pp. 103–18.

——. 1970a. *The Topography of Baghdad in the Early Middle Ages: Text and Studies.* Detroit: Wayne State University Press.

Lawall, Sarah. 1993. "Naguib Mahfouz and the Nobel Prize." In Michael Beard and Adnan Haydar (eds.). *Naguib Mahfouz: From Regional Fame to Global Recognition.* Syracuse, NY: Syracuse University Press, pp. 21–7.

Lawrence, Bruce B. 2011. "Sufism and Neo-Sufism." In Robert Hefner (ed.). *The New Cambridge History of Islam: Muslims and Modernity Culture and Society since 1800*, vol. 6. Cambridge: Cambridge University Press, pp. 355–84.

Lawrence, D. H. 2005 [1920]. *Women in Love.* New York: Barnes & Noble.

Lefevere, André. 1990. "Translation: Its Genealogy in the West." In Susan Bassnett and André Lefevere (eds.). *Translation, History and Culture.* London and New York: Pinter, pp. 14–28.

Le Gassick, Trevor. 1992. "The Arabic Novel in English Translation." *Mundus Arabicus* 5, pp. 47–60.

Lejeune, Philippe. 1975. *Le pacte autobiographique.* Paris: Éditions du Seuil.

——. 1982. "The Autobiographical Contact." In Tzvetan Todorov (ed.). *French Literary Theory Today: A Reader*, trans. R. Carter. Cambridge: Cambridge University Press, pp. 192–222.

——. 1989. *On Autobiography.* Minneapolis: University of Minnesota Press.

——. 1994. *al-Sīra al-Dhātiyya: al-Mīthāq wa-l-Ta'rīkh al-Adabī*, trans. 'Umar Ḥillī. Casablanca: al-Markaz al-Thaqāfī al-'Arabī.

Lenze, Nele. 2019. *Politics and Digital Literature in the Middle East: Perspectives on Online Text and Context.* New York: Palgrave Macmillan.

Leonard, Jonathan Norton. 1953. *Flight into Space.* New York: Random House.

——. 1957. *al-Safar ilā al-Kawākib*, trans. Ismā'īl Ḥaqqī. Cairo: Maktabat al-Nahḍa al-Miṣriyya.

Le Strange, Guy. 1900. *Baghdad during the Abbasid Caliphate: From Contemporary Arabic and Persian Sources.* Oxford: Clarendon.

Levine, Lawrence. 1988. *Highbrow/Lowbrow: The Emergence of Cultural Hierarchy in America.* Cambridge, MA: Harvard University Press.

Levy, Reuben. 1977 [1929]. *A Baghdad Chronicle.* Philadelphia: Porcupine Press.

Lewis, Bernard. 1968. *The Middle East and the West.* London: Weidenfeld & Nicolson.

——. 1970. *The Arabs in History.* London: Hutchinson.

——. 1973. *Islam in History: Ideas, Men and Events in the Middle East.* London: Alcove Press.

——. 1995. *Cultures in Conflict: Christians, Muslims, and Jews in the Age of Discovery.* New York and Oxford: Oxford University Press.

——. 2003. *What Went Wrong? The Clash between Islam and Modernity in the Middle East.* New York: Perennial.

Lichtenstadter, Ilse. 1976. *Introduction to Classical Arabic Literature.* New York: Schocken.

Livne-Kafri, Ofer. 2006. "Luka' B. Luka' in Muslim Apocalyptic Traditions." *Quaderni di Studi Arabi* 19, pp. 49–53.

Longrigg, Stephen Hemsley and Stoakes, Frank. 1958. *Iraq.* New York: Fredrick A. Praeger.

López, Silvia L. 2011. "Dialectical Criticism in the Provinces of the 'World Republic of Letters': The Primacy of the Object in the Work of Roberto Schwarz." *A Contracorriente* 9.1, pp. 69–88.

López-Baralt, Luce. 2006. "Islamic Influence on Spanish Literature: Benengeli's Pen in 'Don Quixote.'" *Islamic Studies* 45.4, pp. 579–93.

López-Calvo, Ignacio. 2019. "The Afterlife of al-Andalus: Muslim Iberia in Contemporary Arab and Hispanic Narratives." *Review: Literature and Arts of the Americas* 52.2, pp. 274–8.

Lorca, Federico García. 1940. *Poeta en Nueva York*. Mexico City: Séneca.
——. 1994–1996. *Obras completas*, ed. Miguel García-Posada. Barcelona: Círculo de Lectores/Galaxia Gutenberg.
——. 2008. *Poet in New York*, trans. Pablo Medina and Mark Statman. New York: Grove Press.
——. 2014. *Los mejores poemas para niños de Federico García Lorca*. Madrid: Editorial VERBUM.
Lowry, Joseph E. and Stewart, Devin J. (eds.). 2009. *Essays in Arabic Literary Biography 1350–1850*. Wiesbaden: Harrassowitz Verlag.
al-Lughawī, Abd al-Wāḥid Abū al-Ṭayyib. 1963. *Kitāb al-Aḍdād fī Kalām al-'Arab*, ed. 'Izzat Ḥasan. Damascus: al-Majma' al-'Ilmī al-'Arabī.
Lu'lu'a, 'Abd al-Wāḥid. 1989. "Ṣūrat Jabrā fī Shabābihi, Shi'r bi-l-Inklīziyya." *al-Nāqid* 10, pp. 26–31.
Lyall, Charles James (ed.). 1930. *Translation of Ancient Arabian Poetry*. London: Williams & Norgate.
Maalouf, Amin. 1989. *Samarkand*. Paris: Jean-Claude Lattèrs.
——. 1993. *Le rocher de Tanois*. Paris: Grasset.
——. 1994. *Samarkand*, trans. R. Harris. London: Abacus.
——. 1995. *The Rock of Tanios*, trans. D. S. Blair. London: Abacus.
al-Ma'arrī, Abū al-'Alā'. 1975. *Risālat al-Ghufrān*, ed. 'Alī Shalaq. Beirut: Dār al-Qalam.
Macaulay, Thomas Babington. 1972. *Selected Writings*, ed. J. Clive and T. Pinney. Chicago: University of Chicago Press.
MacDonald, Duncan Black. 1932. "A Bibliographical and Literary Study of the First Appearance of the Arabian Nights in Europe." *Library Quarterly* 2, pp. 387–420.
——. 1960 [1903]. *Muslim Theology, Jurisprudence and Constitutional Theory*. Lahore: Premier Book House.
Machado, Antonio. 1973. *Poesias completas*. Madrid: Espasa-Calpe.
Machut-Mendecka, Ewa. 1999. "The Individual and the Community in Arabic Literary Autobiography." *Arabica* 46.3/4, pp. 510–22.
Mack, Robert L. 2008. "Cultivating the Garden: Antoine Galland's *Arabian Nights* in the Traditions of English Literature." In Saree Makdisi and Felicity Nussbaum (eds.). *The Arabian Nights in Historical Context between East and West*. Oxford: Oxford University Press, pp. 51–81.
al-Māghūṭ, Muḥammad. 1981. *al-Āthār al-Kāmila*. Beirut: Dār al-'Awda.
Mahfouz, Naguib. 1969. "Under the Umbrella," trans. Nissim Rejwan. *New Outlook*, November–December, pp. 50–5.
——. 1973. *God's World*, trans. Akef Abadir and Roger Allen. Minneapolis: Bibliotheca Islamica.
——. 1981. *Children of Gebelawi*, trans. Philip Stewart. London: Heinemann.
——. 2001. *Naguib Mahfouz at Sidi Gaber: Reflections of a Nobel Laureate 1994–2001*. Cairo and New York: American University in Cairo Press.
Maḥfūẓ, Najīb. n.d. [1957]. *al-Sukkariyya*. Cairo: Dār Miṣr.
——. 1963. *Dunyā Allāh*. Cairo: Dār Miṣr.
——. 1967. *Awlād Ḥāratinā*. Beirut: Dār al-Ādāb.
——. n.d. [1967a]. *Mīrāmār*. Cairo: Dār Miṣr.
——. 1968. "al-Adab, al-Ḥurriyya, al-Thawra." *Mawāqif* I (October/November), pp. 85–6.
——. 1973 [1938]. *Hams al-Junūn*. Beirut: Dār al-Qalam.
——. n.d. [1974]. *al-Karnak*. Cairo: Dār Miṣr.
——. n.d. [1977]. *Malḥamat al-Ḥarāfīsh*. Cairo: Maktabat Miṣr.
——. 1977 [1973]. *al-Ḥubb Taḥt al-Maṭar*. Cairo: Dār Misr.
——. 1978 [1969]. *Taḥt al-Miẓalla*. Cairo: Dār Miṣr.
——. n.d. [1979]. *al-Shayṭān Ya'iẓu*. Cairo: Dār Miṣr.

——. n.d. [1982]. *Layālī Alf Layla*. Cairo: Maktabat Miṣr.
——. n.d. [1982a]. *al-Bāqī min al-Zaman Sā'a*. Cairo: Dār Miṣr.
——. n.d. [1983]. *Amāma al-'Arsh*. Cairo: Dār Miṣr.
——. 2006. *Awlād Ḥāratinā*. Cairo: Dār al-Shurūq.
Māhir, Muṣṭafā (ed.). 1970. *Ṣafaḥāt Khālida min al-Adab al-Almānī: Min al-Bidāya Ḥattā al-'Aṣr al-Ḥāḍir*. Beirut: Dār Ṣādir.
——. (ed.). 1974. *Alwān min al-Adab al-Almānī al-Ḥadīth: al-Qiṣṣa, al-Shi'r, al-Maqāl*. Beirut: Dār Ṣādir.
Mahmoud, Alaaeldin. 2019. "Glocalizing the (Arab) *Nahḍah*: An Investigation of the *Nahḍah*'s Literacies and Multimodalities." *Comparative Literature Studies* 56.3, pp. 557–72.
Maḥmūd, 'Alī 'Abd al-Ḥalīm. 1979. *al-Qiṣṣa al-'Arabiyya fī al-'Aṣr al-Jāhilī*. Cairo: Dār al-Ma'ārif.
Maḥmūd, Muṣṭafā. 1956. *Allāh wa-l-Insān*. Cairo: Dār al-Jumhūriyya.
——. 1959. *Lughz al-Mawt*. Cairo: Dār al-Nahḍa al-'Arabiyya.
——. 1960. *al-Mustaḥīl*. Cairo: Dār al-Nahḍa al-'Arabiyya.
——. 1961. *Einstein wa-l-Nisbiyya*. Cairo: Dār al-Nahḍa al-'Arabiyya.
——. 1961a. *al-Aḥlām*. Cairo: Dār al-Nahḍa al-'Arabiyya.
——. 1966. *Rajul Taḥt al-Ṣifr*. Cairo: Dār al-Ma'ārif.
——. 1972. *Rajul Taḥt al-Ṣifr*. Beirut: Dār al-'Awda.
——. 1985. *Rajul Taḥt al-Ṣifr*, 3rd edn. Cairo: Dār al-Ma'ārif.
——. 1996. *Ziyāra li-l-Janna wa-l-Nār*. Cairo: Dār Akhbār al-Yawm.
Majali, J. S. A. al-G. 1988. "Poetic Creativity in Arabic Literary Criticism: A Study of Arab Critical Views up to the End of the 5th/11th Century." PhD thesis, University of Manchester.
Makdisi, George. 1981. *The Rise of Colleges: Institutions of Learning in Islam and the West*. Edinburgh: Edinburgh University Press.
——. 1990. *The Rise of Humanism in Classical Islam and the Christian West*. Edinburgh: Edinburgh University Press.
Makiya, Kanan. 1993. *Cruelty and the Silence: War, Tyranny, Uprising, and the Arab World*. New York: W. W. Norton.
Al-Makkari. 1967. *Analectes sur l'histoire et la littérature des arabes d'Espagne*, ed. Reinhart Pieter Anne Dozy et al. Amsterdam: Oriental Press.
al-Malā'ika, Nāzik. 1981. *Dīwān*. Beirut: Dār al-'Awda.
——. 1983 [1962]. *Qaḍāyā al-Shi'r al-Mu'āṣir*. Beirut: Dār al-'Ilm li-l-Malāyīn.
Malti-Douglas, Fedwa. 1988. "Classical Arabic Crime Narratives: Thieves and Thievery in *Adab* Literature." *Journal of Arabic Literature* 19, pp. 108–27.
——. 1988a. "The Classical Arabic Detective." *Arabica* 35, pp. 59–91.
——. 1988b. *Blindness and Autobiography: Al-Ayyam of Taha Husayn*. Princeton, NJ: Princeton University Press.
——. 2001. *Medicines of the Soul: Female Bodies and Sacred Geographies in a Transnational Islam*. Berkeley: University of California Press.
Mandūr, Muḥammad. 1970. *A'lām al-Shi'r al-'Arabī al-Ḥadīth*. Beirut: al-Maktab al-Tijārī li-l-Ṭibā'a wa-l-Nashr wa-l-Tawzī'.
Mansour, Jacob. 1978. *Arabic and Islamic Studies* (in Hebrew). Ramat Gan: Bar-Ilan University.
al-Maqqarī, Aḥmad ibn Muḥammad. 1968. *Nafḥ al-Ṭīb fī Ghuṣn al-Andalus al-Raṭīb*, ed. Iḥsān 'Abbās. Beirut: Dār Ṣādir.
al-Marrākushī, 'Abd al-Wāḥid. 1963. *al-Mu'jib fī Talkhīṣ Akhbār al-Maghrib*, ed. Muḥammad Sa'īd al-'Iryān. Cairo: Lajnat Iḥyā' al-Turāth al-Islāmī.
Martínez Lillo, Rosa-Isabel. 2011. "Mixtificación de al-Andalus en la literatura árabe actual." *Awraq: Revista de Análisis y Pensamiento sobre el Mundo Árabe e Islámico Contemporáneo* 3 (Nueva época), pp. 57–86.

Massad, Joseph A. 2014. "Love, Fear, and the Arab Spring." *Public Culture* 26.1, pp. 129–54.
——. 2015. *Islam in Liberalism*. Chicago: University of Chicago Press.
Massignon, L. 1971. "al-Ḥallādj." In *Encyclopaedia of Islam*, 2nd edn. III, pp. 99–104.
——. 1982. *The Passion of al-Ḥallāj*, trans. H. Mason. Princeton, NJ: Princeton University Press.
Ma'tūq (Maatouk), Muḥammad. 1992. "A Critical Study of Anṭūn Sa'āda and His Impact on Politics: The History of Ideas and Literature in the Middle East." PhD thesis, University of London.
——. 2013. *Fa-l-Nujarrib Hādhā al-Rajul: Dirāsāt wa-Abḥāth fī Fikr Anṭūn Sa'āda*. Beirut: Dār al-Furāt.
Mavroudi, Maria. 2015. "Translations from Greek into Arabic and Latin during the Middle Ages: Searching for the Classical Tradition." *Speculum* 90.1 (January), pp. 28–59.
Mawāsī, Fārūq. 1989. *al-Khurūj min al-Nahr*. Kafr Qara': Dār al-Shafaq.
——. 2002. *Aqwās min Sīratī al-Dhātiyya*. Kafr Qara': Dār al-Hudā.
McAuley, Denis. 2012. *Ibn 'Arabī's Mystical Poetics*. Oxford: Oxford University Press.
McNelly, Willis E. (ed.). 1974. *Science Fiction: The Academic Awakening*. Shreveport, LA: College English Association.
Meisami, Julie Scott and Starkey, Paul (eds.). 1998. *Encyclopaedia of Arabic Literature*. London: Routledge.
Mendelson, David. 1986. *The Manifestos of Surrealism* (in Hebrew). Tel Aviv: Sifriyat Poalim.
Menocal, Maria Rosa. 1985. "Pride and Prejudice in Medieval Studies: European and Oriental." *Hispanic Review* 53, pp. 61–78.
——. 1987. *The Arabic Role in Medieval Literary History*. Philadelphia: University of Pennsylvania Press.
Messick, Brinkley Morris. 1993. *The Calligraphic State: Textual Domination and History in a Muslim Society*. Berkeley: University of California Press.
Mestyan, Adam. 2016. "Muḥammad Yūsuf Najm (1925–2009): A Maker of the *Nahḍa*." *Al-Abhath* 64, pp. 97–118.
Metlitzki, Dorothee. 1977. *The Matter of Araby in Medieval England*. New Haven, CT: Yale University Press.
M'henni, Mansour (ed.). 1993. *Tahar Ben Jelloun: Stratégies d'écriture*. Paris: Éditions L'Harmattan.
Michalak-Pikulska, Barbara. 1999. "Gibran Khalil Gibran's Significance and Role in Arabic and World Literature and His Creative Reception in the World." *Folia Orientalia* 35, pp. 93–100.
——. 2011. "The Beginning of Modern Prose Writing in Oman." In Frederek Musall and Abdulbary al-Mudarris (eds.). *Im Dialog bleiben: Sprache und Denken in den Kulturen des Vorderen Orients. Festchrift für Raif Georges Khoury*. Wiesbaden: Harrassowitz Verlag, pp. 281–91.
Micheau, Françoise. 2008. "Baghdad in the Abbasid Era: A Cosmopolitan and Multi-Confessional Capital." In Salma Khadra Jayyusi et al. (eds.). *The City in the Islamic World*. Leiden: Brill, pp. 221–45.
Micklethwait, Christopher Dwight. 2011. "Faits Divers: National Culture and Modernism in Third World Literary Magazines." PhD thesis, University of Texas at Austin.
Mīkhā'īl, Amāṭanyūs. 1968. *Dirāsāt fī al-Shi'r al-'Arabī al-Ḥadīth*. Sidon: al-Maktaba al-'Aṣriyya.
Mīkhā'īl, Murād. 1988. *al-A'māl al-Shi'riyya al-Kāmila*. Tel Aviv: Dār al-Sharq.
Miller, Judith. 1996. *God Has Ninety-Nine Names: Reporting from a Militant Middle East*. New York: Simon & Schuster.
Milson, Menahem. 1970. "Najīb Maḥfūẓ and the Quest for Meaning." *Arabica* 17, pp. 178–80.

——. 1976. "Reality, Allegory and Myth in the Work of Najīb Maḥfūẓ." *Asian and African Studies* 11, pp. 157–79.
——. 1977. "Religion and Revolution in an Allegory by Najīb Maḥfūẓ: A Study of *Rūḥ Ṭabīb al-Qulūb.*" In Myriam Rosen-Ayalon (ed.). *Studies in Memory of G. Wiet.* Jerusalem: Hebrew University Press, pp. 435–62.
——. 1989. "Najib Maḥfūẓ and Jamāl 'Abd al-Nāṣir: The Writer as Political Critic." *Asian and African Studies* 23, pp. 1–22.
Milstead, John et al. 1974. *Sociology through Science Fiction.* New York: St. Martin's Press.
al-Miṣrī, Ḥusayn Mujīb. 1994. *al-Andalus Bayna Shawqī wa-Iqbāl.* Aleppo: Dār al-Wa'y.
——. 1999. *al-Andalus Bayna Shawqī wa-Iqbāl.* Cairo: al-Dār al-Thaqāfiyya li-l-Nashr.
al-Miṣrī, Nash'at. 1983. *Ṣalāḥ 'Abd al-Ṣabūr—al-Insān wa-l-Shā'ir.* Cairo: al-Hay'a al-Miṣriyya al-'Āmma li-l-Kitāb.
Moch, Michal. 2017. *Naṣr Abū Zayd: A Critical Rereading of Islamic Thought.* Bydgoszcz: Kazimierz Wielki University Publishing Office.
Monroe, James T. 1974. *Hispano-Arabic Poetry.* Berkeley: University of California Press.
——. 1993. "*Zajal* and *Muwashshaḥa.*" In Salma Khadra Jayyusi (ed.). *Islamic Spain.* Leiden: Brill, pp. 398–419.
Montávez, Pedro Martínez. 1992. *Al-Andalus, España, en la literatura árabe contemporánea.* Madrid: MAPFRE.
Montgomery, James E. 2013. *Al-Jāḥiẓ: In Praise of Books.* Edinburgh: Edinburgh University Press.
Moreh, Shmuel. 1969. "The Influence of Western Poetry and Particularly T. S. Eliot on Modern Arabic Poetry (1947–1964)." *Asian and African Studies* 5, pp. 1–50.
——. 1973. "The Neoclassical *Qaṣīda*: Modern Poets and Critics." In Gustave E. Von Grunebaum (ed.). *Arabic Poetry Theory and Development.* Wiesbaden: Harrassowitz Verlag, pp. 155–79.
——. 1976. *Modern Arabic Poetry 1800–1970.* Leiden: Brill.
——. 1984. "Town and Country in Modern Arabic Poetry from Shawqī to al-Sayyāb." *Asian and African Studies* 18, pp. 161–85.
——. 1988. *Studies in Modern Arabic Prose and Poetry.* Leiden: Brill.
——. 1992. *Live Theatre and Dramatic Literature in the Medieval Arabic World.* Edinburgh: Edinburgh University Press.
Moreh, Shmuel and Maḥmūd 'Abbāsī. 1987. *Tarājim wa-Āthār fī al-Adab al-'Arabī fī Isrā'īl 1948-1986.* Shfaram: Dār al-Mashriq.
Moretti, Franco. 1996. *The Modern Epic: The World-System from Goethe to García Márquez,* trans. Quintin Hoare. London: Verso.
——. 2000. "Conjectures on World Literature." *New Left Review* 1, pp. 54–68.
al-Mousa, Nedal. 1998. "The Fortunes of Faust in Arabic Literature: A Comparative Study." *New Comparison: A Journal of Comparative and General Literary Studies* 26, pp. 103–17.
Mowafy, Waheed Mohamed Awad. 1999. "Modern Arabic Literary Biography: A Study of Character Portrayal in the Works of Egyptian Biographers of the First Half of the Twentieth Century, with Special Reference to Literary Biography." PhD thesis, University of Leeds.
al-Mozany, Hussain. 2010. "The Last Trip to Baghdad." *Banipal* 37, pp. 6–19.
Mubārak, 'Alī. 1882. *'Alam al-Dīn.* Alexandria: Maṭba'at Jarīdat al-Maḥrūsa.
Mubārak, Zaki. n.d. *al-Taṣawwuf al-Islāmī fī al-Adab wa-l-Akhlāq.* Beirut and Sidon: al-Maktaba al-'Aṣriyya.
——. 1935. *al-Madā'iḥ al-Nabawiyya fī al-Adab al-'Arabī.* Cairo: Dār al-Kātib al-'Arabī.
Mughulṭāy, Abū 'Abd Allāh. 1997. *al-Wāḍiḥ al-Mubīn fī Dhikr Man Ustushhida min al-Muḥibbīn.* Beirut: Dār al-Intishār al-'Arabī.
Muḥammad, Muḥammad Sayyid. 1994. *al-Ghazw al-Thaqāfī wa-l-Mujtama' al-'Arabī al-Mu'āṣir.* Cairo: Dār al-Fikr al-'Arabī.

Muhanna, Elias. 2017. *The World in a Book: Al-Nuwayri and the Islamic Encyclopedic Tradition*. Princeton, NJ: Princeton University Press.
al-Muḥāsibī, al-Ḥārith. 1964. *Risālat al-Mustarshidīn*, ed. ʿAbd al-Fattāḥ Abū Ghudda. Halab: al-Maṭbūʿāt al-Islāmīyya.
Muir, William. 1924. *The Caliphate: Its Rise, Decline, and Fall*. Edinburgh: John Grant.
al-Munāwī, ʿAbd al-Ra'ūf. 1321H. *Kunūz al-Ḥaqā'iq fī Ḥadīth Khayr al-Khalā'iq*. Cairo: n.p.
Mūsā, Ṣabrī. 1987. *al-Sayyid min Ḥaql al-Sabānik*. Cairo: al-Hay'a al-Miṣriyya al-ʿĀmma li-l-Kitāb.
Mūsā, Salāma. 1945. *al-Balāgha al-ʿAṣriyya wa-l-Lugha al-ʿArabiyya*. Cairo: al-Maṭbaʿa al-ʿAṣriyya.
——. 1947. *al-Tathqīf al-Dhātī aw Kayfa Nurabbī Anfusanā*. Cairo: Maṭbaʿat Lajnat al-Ta'līf wa-l-Tarjama wa-l-Nashr.
——. 1962. *Mā Hiya al-Nahḍa*. Beirut: Manshūrāt Maktabat al-Maʿārif.
al-Mūsawī (= al-Musawi), Muḥsin Jāsim. 1973. *al-Nafṭ al-ʿIrāqī: Dirāsa Wathā'iqiyya min Manḥ al-Imtiyāz ḥattā al-Ta'mīm*. Baghdad: Dār al-Ḥurriyya li-l-Ṭibāʿa.
——. 1973a. *al-Thawra al-Jadīda: Dirāsāt Taḥlīliyya fī al-Siyāsa wa-l-Iqtiṣād wa-l-Fikr*. Beirut: al-Mu'assasa al-ʿArabiyya li-l-Dirāsāt wa-l-Nashr.
——. 1981. *Scheherazade in England*. Washington, DC: Three Continents Press.
——. 1986. *Alf Layla wa-Laylā fī Naẓariyyat al-Adab al-Inklīzī*. Beirut: Manshūrāt Markaz al-Inmā' al-Qawmī.
——. 1993. *al-Istishrāq fī al-Fikr al-ʿArabī*. Beirut: al-Mu'assasa al-ʿArabiyya li-l-Dirāsāt wa-l-Nashr.
——. 2000. *Mujtamaʿ Alf Layla wa-Laylā*. Tunis: Markaz al-Nashr al-Jāmiʿī.
——. 2001. *al-Nukhba al-Fikriyya wa-l-Inshiqāq: Qirā'a fī Taḥawwulāt al-Ṣafwa al-ʿĀrifa fī al-Mujtamaʿ al-ʿArabī al-Ḥadīth*. Beirut: Dār al-Ādāb.
——. 2003. *The Postcolonial Arabic Novel: Debating Ambivalence*. Leiden: Brill.
——. 2005. *al-Naẓariyya wa-l-Naqd al-Thaqāfī: al-Kitāba al-ʿĀrabiyya fī ʿĀlam Muthaghyyir, Wāqiʿuhā, Siyāqātuhā wa-Bunāhā al-Shuʿūriyya*. Beirut: al-Mu'assasa al-ʿArabiyya li-l-Dirāsāt wa-l-Nashr.
——. 2006. "Pre-Modern Belletristic Prose." In: Allen and Richards 2006, pp. 101–33.
——. 2006a. *Arabic Poetry: Trajectories of Modernity and Tradition*. London: Routledge.
——. 2006b. *Reading Iraq: Culture and Power in Conflict*. London: I. B. Tauris.
——. (ed.). 2009. *Arabic Literary Thresholds: Sites of Rhetorical Turn in Contemporary Scholarship*. Leiden: Brill.
——. 2009a. *Islam in the Street: The Dynamics of Arabic Literary Production*. Lanham, MD: Rowman & Littlefield.
——. 2009b. *The Islamic Context of the Thousand and One Nights*. New York: Columbia University Press.
——. 2013. "The Medieval Islamic Literary World-System: The Lexicographic Turn." *Mamlūk Studies Review* 17, pp. 43–71.
——. 2014. "The Republic of Letters: Arab Modernity? (Part1)." *Cambridge Journal of Postcolonial Literary Inquiry* 1.2, pp. 265–80.
——. 2015. "The Republic of Letters: Arab Modernity? (Part 2)." *Cambridge Journal of Postcolonial Literary Inquiry* 2.1, pp. 115–30.
——. 2015a. "The Medieval Islamic Republic of Letters as World Model." *Cambridge Journal of Postcolonial Literary Inquiry* 2.2, pp. 281–6.
——. 2015b. *The Medieval Islamic Republic of Letters: Arabic Knowledge Construction*. Notre Dame, IN: University of Notre Dame Press.
——. 2016. *al-Dhākira al-Shaʿbiyya li-Mujtamaʿāt Alf Layla wa-Layla: al-Sard wa-Marjaʿiyyatuhu al-Ta'rīkhiyya wa-Āliyyatuhu*. Beirut: al-Markaz al-Thaqāfī al-ʿArabī.

——. 2018. "Postcolonial Theory in the Arab World: Belated Engagements and Limits." *Interventions: International Journal of Postcolonial Studies* 20.2, pp. 174–91.

——. 2020. *Jumhūriyyat al-Ādāb fī al-ʿAṣr al-Islāmī al-Wasīṭ: al-Bunya al-ʿArabiyya li-l-Maʿrifa*, trans. Ḥabība Ḥasan. Beirut: al-Shabaka al-ʿArabiyya li-l-Abḥāth wa-l-Nashr.

——. 2020a. "Canons, Thefts, and Palimpsests in the Arabic Literary Tradition." *Journal of Arabic Literature* 51, pp. 165–88.

——. 2021. *The Arabian Nights in Contemporary World Cultures Global Commodification, Translation, and the Culture Industry*. Cambridge: Cambridge University Press.

——. 2022. *Arabic Disclosures: The Postcolonial Autobiographical Atlas*. Notre Dame, IN: University of Notre Dame Press.

Musʿid, Aḥlām Wāsif. 2006. *Marāyā al-Ab wa-l-Sulṭa—Qirāʾa Sūsyū-Thaqāfiyya fī al-Sīra al-Dhātiyya al-ʿArabiyya al-Muʿāṣira*. Amman: Dār Azmina.

Myers, Richard K. 1986. "The Problem of Authority: Franz Kafka and Najīb Maḥfūẓ." *Journal of Arabic Literature* 17, pp. 82–96.

Na'āmneh, Maḥmūd. 2022. "Ṣūfī Language and the Opening of Signification: al-Ḥallāj as an Example Maḥmūd Na'āmneh." *International Journal of Literature and Arts* 10.1, pp. 59–67.

al-Nabhānī, Yūsuf ibn Ismāʿīl. 1984. *Jāmiʿ Karāmāt al-Awliyāʾ*, ed. Ibrāhīm ʿUṭwa ʿAwaḍ. Cairo: Ḥalabī.

Naddaff, Sandra. 2014. "The Thousand and One Nights as World Literature." In Theo D'haen (ed.). *The Routledge Companion to World Literature*. London: Routledge, pp. 487–96.

Naff, Thomas. 1993. *Paths to the Middle East: Ten Scholars Look Back*. Albany: State University of New York Press.

al-Nafzāwī, Muḥammad ibn Muḥammad. 1983. *Shahādāt wa-Mukhtārāt min al-Rawḍ al-ʿĀṭir fī Nuzhat al-Khāṭir*, ed. Hānī al-Khayyir. Damascus: Maktabat Usāma.

Nahas, Michael. 1985. "A Translation of *Ḥayy b. Yaqẓān* by the Elder Edward Pococke (1604–1691)." *Journal of Arabic Literature* 16, pp. 88–90.

Naimy, Mikhail. 1950. *Kahlil Gibran: A Biography*. New York: Philosophical Library.

Najm, Muḥammad Yūsuf. 1956. *al-Masraḥiyya fī al-Adab al-ʿArabī al-Ḥadīth*. Beirut: Dār Bayrūt li-l-Ṭibāʿa wa-l-Nashr.

Naqqāsh, Samīr. 1995. *Nubūʾāt Rajul Majnūn fī Madīna Malʿūna*. Jerusalem: Rābiṭat al-Jāmiʿiyyīn al-Yahūd al-Nāziḥīn min al-ʿIrāq.

——. 2004. *Shlūmū al-Kurdī wa-Anā wa-Zaman*. Cologne: Manshūrāt al-Jamal.

al-Nāshif, Zakī. 1989. "Shakespeare am al-Shaykh Zubayr." *al-Mawākib*, September/October, pp. 36–41.

Natour, Hanan. 2019. "Language Contacts in Arabic Poetry: Patterns of Merging Languages in the Poetry of Adonis and Fuad Rifka." *META: Middle East Topics & Arguments* 13, pp. 77–87.

Navarrete, Ignacio. 1986. "A Polysystemic Approach to Literary Theory: In Response to Barry Jordan." *Yearbook of Comparative and General Literature* 35, pp. 122–6.

al-Nawas, Ahmed. 2018. "View of the Conditions of Arabic Literature in the Nordic Region." *International Journal of Art, Humanities and Social Sciences* 11.1, pp. 160–83.

Nawfal, Muḥammad. 1983. *Taʾrīkh al-Muʿāraḍāt fī al-Shiʿr al-ʿArabī*. Beirut: Mu'ssasat al-Risāla and Dār al-Furqān.

al-Nawrasī, Rūnāk Tawfīq ʿAlī. 2009. *Baghdād fī al-Shiʿr al-ʿAbbāsī: Dirāsa fī Shiʿr al-Madīna: al-Ruʾyā wa-l-Fann*. Beirut: al-Dār al-ʿArabiyya li-l-Mawsūʿāt.

Neuwirth, Angelika. 1999. "Maḥmūd Darwīsh's Re-staging of the Mystic Lover's Relation Towards a Superhuman Beloved." In Stephan Guth et al. (eds.). *Conscious Voices: Concepts of Writing in the Middle East*. Beirut: Orient-Institut der DMG, pp. 153–78.

——. et al. (eds.). 2010. *Arabic Literature: Postmodern Perspectives*. London: Saqi.

Nicholson, Linda. 1995. "Introduction." In Seyla Benhabib et al. (eds.). *Feminist Contentions: A Philosophical Exchange*. New York: Routledge, pp. 1–16.

Nicholson, Reynold A. 1956. *A Literary History of the Arabs*. Cambridge: Cambridge University Press.
——. 1969 [1907]. *A Literary History of the Arabs*. Cambridge: Cambridge University Press.
——. 1975. *The Mystics of Islam*. London: Routledge.
Nieten, Ulrike-Rebekka. 2006. "Arabic Poetry and the Songs of the Troubadours: A Cross-Cultural Approach." In Angelika Neuwirth and Andreas Christian Islebe (eds.). *Reflections on Reflections: Near Eastern Writers Reading Literature. Dedicated to Renate Jacobi*. Wiesbaden: Reichert Verlag, pp. 253–61.
Nietzsche, Friedrich W. 1941. *The Antichrist*, trans. Henry Louis Mencken. New York: Alfred A. Knopf.
——. 1955. *Die Geburt der Tragödie*. Stuttgart: Alfred Kröner.
——. 1967. *The Birth of Tragedy and the Case of Wagner*, trans. W. Kaufmann. New York: Vintage.
Nigg, Joe. 2016. *The Phoenix: An Unnatural Biography of a Mythical Beast*. Chicago: University of Chicago Press.
Noack, Rick and Gamio, Lazaro. 2015. "The World's Languages, in 7 Maps and Charts." *Washingtonpost.com*, April 23, 2015, available at: https://www.washingtonpost.com/news/worldviews/wp/2015/04/23/the-worlds-languages-in-7-maps-and-charts, last accessed on March 6, 2021.
Nocke, Alexandra. 2006. "Rewriting Israeliness: Arabs Writing in Hebrew and Jews Writing in Arabic." In Andreas Pflitsch and Barbara Winckler (eds.). *Poetry's Voice: Society's Norms: Forms of Interaction between Middle Eastern Writers and Their Societies*. Wiesbaden: Reichert Verlag, pp. 173–85.
Noorani, Yaseen. 1999. "The Lost Garden of al-Andalus: Islamic Spain and the Poetic Inversion of Colonialism." *International Journal of Middle East Studies* 31, pp. 237–54.
——. 2016. "Estrangement and Selfhood in the Classical Concept of Waṭan." *Journal of Arabic Literature* 47.1/2, pp. 16–42.
——. 2019. "Translating World Literature into Arabic and Arabic into World Literature: Sulayman al-Bustani's al-Ilyadha and Ruhi al-Khalidi's Arabic Rendition of Victor Hugo." In Marilyn Booth (ed.). *Migrating Texts: Circulating Translations around the Ottoman Mediterranean*. Edinburgh: Edinburgh University Press, pp. 236–65.
Nsiri, Imed. 2020. "The Question of Tradition between Eliot and Adūnīs." *Journal of Arabic Literature* 51, pp. 215–37.
Nūr, ʿAdlī Ṭāhir. 1973. *al-Mustashriq al-Kabīr Edward William Lane*. Cairo: Dār al-Nashr li-l-Jāmiʿāt al-Miṣriyya.
Nuṣayr, ʿĀyida. 1992. "Qanāt al-Tarjama Bayna al-Thaqāfatayn al-ʿArabiyya wa-l-Faransiyya fī Qarnayn." *ʿĀlam al-Kitāb*, April/June, pp. 43–7.
Nuʿayma, Mīkhāʾīl. 1934. *Jubrān Khalīl Jubrān: Ḥayātuhu, Mawtuhu, Adabuhu, Fannuhu*. Beirut: Maṭbaʿat Lisān al-Ḥāl.
——. 1951 [1923]. *al-Ghirbāl*. Cairo: Muʾassasat Nawfal.
——. 1964 [1923]. *al-Ghirbāl*. Beirut: Dār Ṣādir and Dār Bayrūt.
——. 1989 [1917]. *al-Ābāʾ wa-l-Banūn*. Beirut: Muʾassasat Nawfal.
Nykl, A. R. 1946. *Hispano-Arabic Poetry and Its Relations with the Old Provençal Troubadours*. Baltimore: J. H. Furst.
Obadyā, Ibrāhīm. 2003. *60 ʿĀman: Anā wa-l-Shiʿr*. n.p.: n.p.
O'Fahey, Rex Séan and Radtke, Bernd. 1993. "Neo-Sufism Reconsidered, with Special Reference to Aḥmad ibn Idris." *Der Islam* 70, pp. 52–87.
Ogunnaike, Oludamini. 2020. *Poetry in Praise of Prophetic Perfection: A Study of West African Arabic Madīḥ Poetry and Its Precedents*. Cambridge: Islamic Texts Society.
Olša Jr., Jaroslav. 1995. "Arabic SF." In John Clute and Peter Nicholls (eds.). *The Encyclopedia of Science Fiction*. New York: St. Martin's Griffin, p. 49.

Omri, Mohamed-Saleh. 1998. "'Gulf Laughter Break': Cartoons in Tunisia during the Gulf Conflict." In Fatma Müge Göçek (ed.). *Political Cartoons in the Middle East*. Princeton, NJ: Markus Wiener, pp. 133–54.

——. 2000. "*Adab* in the Seventeenth Century: Narrative and Parody in al-Shirbīnī's *Hazz al-Quḥūf*." *Edebiyât* 11.2, pp. 169–96.

——. 2011. "Notes on the Traffic between Theory and Arabic Literature." *International Journal of Middle East Studies* 43.4, pp. 731–3.

Orfali, Bilal. 2012. "A Sketch Map of Arabic Poetry Anthologies up to the Fall of Baghdad." *Journal of Arabic Literature* 43, pp. 29–59.

——. 2017. "Mystical Poetics: Courtly Themes in Early Sufi Akhbār." In Maurice Pomerantz and Evelyn Birge Vitz (eds.). *In the Presence of Power Court and Performance in the Pre-Modern Middle East*. New York: New York University Press, pp. 196–214.

Orfali, Bilal and Baalbaki, Ramzi. 2015. *The Book of Noble Character: Critical Edition of Makārim al-akhlāq wa-maḥāsin al-ādāb wa-badā'i' al-awṣāf wa-gharā'ib al-tashbīhāt, Attributed to Abū Manṣūr al-Tha'ālibī (d. 429/1039)*. Leiden: Brill.

Orsini, Francesca. 2015. "Whose Amnesia? Literary Modernity in Multilingual South Asia." *Cambridge Journal of Postcolonial Literary Inquiry* 2.2, pp. 266–72.

Ostle, R. C. (ed.). 1991. *Modern Literature in the Near and Middle East 1850–1970*. London: Routledge.

——. et al. (eds.). 1998. *Writing the Self: Autobiographical Writing in Modern Arabic Literature*. London: Saqi.

Otterbeck, Jonas. 2021. *The Awakening of Islamic Pop Music*. Edinburgh: Edinburgh University Press.

Otto, Annie S. 1970. *The Letters of Kahlil Gibran and Mary Haskell*. Houston: A. S. Otto.

Ouyang, Wen-chin. 1997. *Literary Criticism in Medieval Arabic-Islamic Culture: The Making of a Tradition*. Edinburgh: Edinburgh University Press.

——. 2012. *Poetics of Love in the Arabic Novel: Nation-State, Modernity and Tradition*. Edinburgh: Edinburgh University Press.

——. 2013. *Poetics of Nostalgia in the Arabic Novel: Nation-State, Modernity and Tradition*. Edinburgh: Edinburgh University Press.

——. 2018. "Orientalism and World Literature: A Re-reading of Cosmopolitanism in Ṭāhā Ḥusayn's Literary World." *Journal of Arabic Literature* 49.1/2, pp. 125–52.

Pacha, S. E. Yacoub Artin (ed. and trans.). 1968. *Contes populaires inédis de la Vallée du Nil*. Paris: Maisonneuve et Larose.

Palgrave, Turner Francis. 1906 [1861]. *The Golden Treasury*. London: Dent.

Pamuk, Orhan. 2006. *Istanbul—Memories and the City*, trans. Maureen Freely. New York: Vintage.

——. 2009. *The Museum of Innocence*, trans. Maureen Freely. New York: Alfred A. Knopf.

Parr, Nora. 2021. "Ghetto, Nakba, Holocaust: New Terms (of Relationship) in Elias Khoury's *Awlad al-Ghitu*." In Jane Hiddleston and Wen-cin Ouyang (eds.). *Multilingual Literature as World Literature*. London: Bloomsbury, pp. 167–83.

Patel, Abdulrazzak. 2013. *The Arab Nahḍah: The Making of the Intellectual and Humanist Movement*. Edinburgh: Edinburgh University Press.

Peled, Mattityahu. 1979. "Creative Translation." *Journal of Arabic Literature* 10, pp. 128–50.

——. 1983. *Religion, My Own: The Literary Works of Najīb Maḥfūẓ*. New Brunswick, NJ: Transaction Books.

——. 1986. "Nodding the Necks: A Literary Study of Shirbīnī's *Hazz al-Quḥūf*." *Die Welt des Islams* 26, pp. 57–75.

Peled, Mattityahu and Shamir, Shimon (eds.). 1978. *Egyptian Intellectuals on National Priorities* (in Hebrew). Jerusalem: Hebrew University of Jerusalem.

Pepe, Teresa. 2012. "Improper Narratives: Egyptian Personal Blogs and the Arabic Notion of Adab." *LEA: Lingue e Letterature d'Oriente e d'Occidente* 1, pp. 547–62.

——. 2015. "When Writers Activate Readers: How the Autofictional Blog Transforms Arabic Literature." *Journal of Arabic and Islamic Studies* 15, pp. 73–91.

——. 2019. *Blogging in Egypt: Digital Literature, 2005–2016*. Edinburgh: Edinburgh University Press.

Perrin, Valérie. 2018. *Changer l'eau des fleurs*. Paris: Albin Michel.

———. 2020. *Fresh Water for Flowers*, trans. Hildegarde Serle. New York: Europa Editions.

Philipp, Thomas. 1993. "The Autobiography in Modern Arab Literature and Culture." *Poetics Today* 14.3, pp. 573–604.

Phillips, Christina. 2008. "An Attempt to Apply Gérard Genette's Model of Hypertextuality to Najīb Maḥfūẓ's *Malḥamat al-Ḥarāfish*." *Middle Eastern Literatures* 11.3, pp. 283–300.

Plato. 1937 [1892]. *The Dialogues of Plato*, trans. B. Jowett. New York: Random House.

Plotinus. 1956 [1917–1930]. *The Enneads*, trans. S. Mackenna. London: Faber & Faber.

Preminger, Alex (ed.). 1974. *Princeton Encyclopedia of Poetics and Poetry*. Princeton, NJ: Princeton University Press.

Prendergast, Christopher. 2001. "Negotiating World Literature." *New Left Review* 8, pp. 100–21.

——. (ed.). 2004. *Debating World Literature*. New York: Verso.

Puccetti, Roland. 1956. "Lorca and Arab Andalusia." *Middle East Forum* 31 (July), pp. 22–5.

Qabbānī, Nizār. 1974. *al-A'māl al-Siyāsiyya*. Beirut: Manshūrāt Nizār Qabbānī.

Qabbish, Aḥmad. 1970. *Ta'rīkh al-Shi'r al-'Arabī al-Ḥadīth*. Damascus: n.p.

Qaddafi, Muammar. 1998. *Escape to Hell and Other Stories*. Montreal: Stanké.

al-Qāḍī, Muḥammad. 1993. "al-Ẓāhir wa-l-Bāṭin fī Kitāb *al-Ayyām*: Baḥth fī al-Tab'īr." In *Mā'wiyyt Ṭāhā Ḥusayn: Waqā'i' Nadwat Bayt al-Ḥikma bi-Qarṭāj 27 wa–28 June 1990*. al-Majma' al-Tunisī li-l-'Ulūm wa-l-Ādāb wa-l-Funūn: Bayt al-Ḥikma, pp. 207–32.

al-Qāḍī, Wadād. 2009. "In the Footsteps of Arabic Biographical Literature: A Journey, Unfinished, in the Company of Knowledge." *Journal of Near Eastern Studies* 68.4, pp. 241–52.

al-Qalamāwī, Suhayr. 1966. *Alf Layla wa-Layla*. Cairo: Dār al-Ma'ārif.

al-Qashṭīnī, Khālid. 2004. *Ayyām Fātat: Ḥikāyāt wa-Khāṭirāt*. London: Dār al-Ḥikma.

Qāsim, Maḥmūd. 1990. "Adab al-Khayāl al-Siyāsī." *al-Karmil* 36/37, pp. 285–301.

——. 1993. *al-Khayāl al-'Ilmī fī Adab al-Qarn al-'Ishrīn*. Cairo: al-Hay'a al-Miṣriyya al-'Āmma li-l-Kitāb.

——. 1996. *al-Adab al-'Arabī al-Maktūb bi-l-Faransiyya*. Cairo: al-Hay'a al-Miṣriyya al-'Āmma li-l-Kitāb.

——. 2002. *Dalīl al-Aflām fī al-Qarn al-'Ishrīn fī Miṣr wa-l-'Ālam al-'Arabī*. Cairo: Maktabat Madbūlī.

Qasim, Qasim. 1991. *al-Riḥla*. Beirut: Dār al-Ḥamrā'.

——. 1993. *La'nat al-Ghuyūm*. Beirut: Dār al-Wurūd.

——. 1995. *Ḥadatha An Ra'ā*. Beirut: Dār Amwāj.

——. 2001. *Lamsat al-Ḍaw'*. Beirut: Dār Amwāj.

——. 2004. *Jasad Ḥarr*. Beirut: Bīsān li-l-Nashr wa-l-Tawzī' wa-l-I'lām.

al-Qāsim, Samīḥ. 1986. *Persona Non Grata*. Dālyat al-Karmil: al-'Imād.

——. 1987. *Dīwān*. Beirut: Dār al-'Awda.

——. 1992. *A'māl Samīḥ al-Qāsim al-Kāmila*. Beirut: Dār al-Jīl.

Qa'wār, Jamāl. 1988. *Zaynab*. Nazareth: al-Mawākib.

al-Qazwīnī, Zakariyyā ibn Muḥammad. 1849. *Kitāb 'Ajā'ib al-Makhlūqāt—Die Wunder der Schöpfung*, ed. Ferdinand Wüstenfeld. Göttingen: im Veralg der dietrichschen Buchhandlung.

——. 1960. *Āthār al-Bilād wa-Akhbār al-'Ibād*. Beirut: Dār Ṣādir and Dār Bayrūt.
Qilāda, Wilyam Sulaymān. 1993. *al-Masīḥiyya wa-l-Islām fī Miṣr wa-Dirāsāt Ukhrā*. Cairo: Sīnā li-l-Nashr.
al-Qushayrī (al-Qushayri), Abū al-Qāsim. n.d. *al-Risāla fī 'Ilm al-Taṣawwuf*. Cairo: Maṭba'at Ṣabīḥ.
——. 1940. *al-Risāla fī 'Ilm al-Taṣawwuf*. Cairo: Ḥalabī.
——. 1990. *Principles of Sufism*, trans. B. R. von Schlegell. Berkeley, CA: Mizan Press.
al-Quwayrī, Yūsuf. 1997. *Min Mufakkirat Rajul lam Yulad*. Beirut: Dār al-Jīl.
Rabinowitz, Dan and Mansour, Johnny. 2011. "Historicizing Climate: *Hayfawis* and *Haifo'im* Remembering the Winter of 1950." In Mahmoud Yazbak and Yfaat Weiss (eds.). *Haifa Before and After 1948: Narratives of a Mixed City*. Dordrecht: Institute for Historical Justice and Reconciliation, pp. 119–48.
Radtke, Bernd. 1996. "Sufism in the 18th Century: An Attempt at a Provisional Appraisal." *Die Welt des Islams* 36, pp. 326–64.
Rāghib, Nabīl. 1981. *Dalīl al-Nāqid al-Adabī*. Cairo: Maktabat Gharīb.
Rā'if, Aḥmad. 1972. *al-Bu'd al-Khāmis*. Kuwait: Dār al-Buḥūth al-'Ilmiyya.
——. 1987. *al-Bu'd al-Khāmis*. Cairo: al-Zahrā' li-l-I'lām al-'Arabī.
al-Ramlī, Līnīn. 1992. *Sa'dūn al-Majnūn*. Kuwait City: Dār Su'ād al-Ṣabāḥ.
Ramsay, Gail. 2017. *Blogs and Literature and Activism: Popular Egyptian Blogs and Literature in Touch*. Wiesbaden: Harrassowitz Verlag.
Rastegar, Kamran. 2005. "The Changing Value of *Alf Laylah wa Laylah* for Nineteenth-Century Arabic, Persian, and English Readerships." *Journal of Arabic Literature* 36.3, pp. 269–87.
Raven, John. 2010. "Using Digital Storytelling to Build a Sense of National Identity amongst Emirati Students." *Education, Business and Society: Contemporary Middle Eastern Issues* 3.3, pp. 201–17.
al-Rāwī, Muḥammad (ed.). 1982. *Udabā' al-Jīl Yataḥaddathūna*. Suez: Maṭbū'āt al-Kalima al-Jadīda.
Raymond, André. 1994. "Islamic City, Arab City: Orientalist Myths and Recent Views." *British Journal of Middle Eastern Studies* 21, pp. 3–18.
——. 2002. *Arab Cities in the Ottoman Period: Cairo, Syria and the Maghreb*. Aldershot: Ashgate.
Recapito, Joseph. 1998. "Al-Andalus and the Origin of the Renaissance in Europe." *Indiana Journal of Hispanic Literatures* 8, pp. 55–74.
Reeves, Minou. 2000. *Muhammad in Europe*. New York: New York University Press.
Reid, J. M. 1976. *The Concise Oxford Dictionary of French Literature*. Oxford: Oxford University Press.
Rejwan, Nissim. 1985. *The Jews of Iraq: 3000 Years of History and Culture*. London: Weidenfeld & Nicolson.
——. 2004. *The Last Jews in Baghdad: Remembering a Lost Homeland*. Austin: University of Texas Press.
Retsö, Jan. 2003. *The Arabs in Antiquity: Their History from the Assyrians to the Umayyads*. Abingdon: RoutledgeCurzon.
——. 2010. "Arabs and Arabic in the Age of the Prophet." In Angelika Neuwirth et al. (eds.). *The Qur'ān in Context: Historical and Literary Investigations into the Qur'ānic Milieu*. Leiden: Brill, pp. 281–92.
——. 2013. "What Is Arabic?" In Jonathan Owens (ed.). *The Oxford Handbook of Arabic Linguistics*. Oxford: Oxford University Press, pp. 433–50.
Reynolds, Dwight Fletcher. 1995. *Heroic Poets, Poetic Heroes: The Ethnography of Performance in an Arabic Oral Epic Tradition*. Ithaca, NY: Cornell University Press.
——. 1997. "Shā'ir (E. The Folk Poet in Arab Society)." *The Encyclopaedia of Islam*, IX, pp. 233–6.

——. (ed.). 2001. *Interpreting the Self: Autobiography in the Arabic Literary Tradition.* Berkeley: University of California Press.
——. (ed.). 2005. "Symbolic Narratives of Self: Dreams in Medieval Arabic Autobiographies." In Philip F. Kennedy (ed.). *On the Fiction and Adab in Medieval Arabic Literature.* Wiesbaden: Harrassowitz Verlag, pp. 261–84.
——. (ed.). 2015. *The Cambridge Companion to Modern Arab Culture.* Cambridge: Cambridge University Press.
——. 2020. *The Musical Heritage of Al-Andalus.* London: Routledge.
——. 2021. *Medieval Arab Music and Musicians: Three Translated Texts.* Leiden: Brill.
Riad, Mustafa. 2000. "The 'Absurd' in Naguib Mahfouz's Plays." Sixth International Symposium on Comparative Literature: Modernism and Postmodernism East and West, available at: http://greatliteraryworks.blogspot.com/2007/11/absurd-in-naguib-mahfouzs-plays.html, last accessed April 15, 2021.
Ricci, Ronit. 2011. *Islam Translated: Literature, Conversion, and the Arabic Cosmopolis of South and Southeast Asia.* Chicago: University of Chicago Press.
——. 2014. "World Literature and Muslim Southeast Asia." In Theo D'haen (ed.). *The Routledge Companion to World Literature.* London: Routledge, pp. 497–506.
Rice, Laura Hamdy and Hamdy, Karim. 2008. "Said's Impact on Arab Intellectuals: Reverberations of Said's Thought in the Current Debates over Islam, and U.S.–Muslim/Arab Relations." In Silvia Nagy-Zekmi (ed.). *Paradoxical Citizenship: Essays on Edward Said.* Lanham, MD: Lexington Books, pp. 15–23.
Riedel, Dagmar Anne. 1998. "Medieval Arabic Literature between History and Psychology: Gustave von Grunebaum's Approach to Literary Criticism within the Western Orientalist Tradition." *Arabist: Budapest Studies in Arabic* 19/20, pp. 111–22.
Rifāʿī, Maḥmūd Muḥammad Aḥmad. 1990. *Safīnat al-Faḍāʾ al-Ghāmiḍa.* Cairo: al-Hayʾa al-Miṣriyya al-ʿĀmma li-l-Kitāb.
al-Rīḥānī, Amīn Fāris. 1955. *Hutāf al-Awdiya: Shiʿr Manthūr.* Beirut: Dār Rīḥānī li-l-Ṭibāʿa wa-l-Nashr.
——. 1968. *al-Rīḥāniyāt.* Beirut: Dār Rīḥānī li-l-Ṭibāʿa wa-l-Nashr.
Ron-Gilboa, Guy. 2021. "'Anqāʾ Mughrib: The Poetics of a Mythical Creature." *Journal of Abbasid Studies* 8.1, pp. 75–103.
Ronnow, Gretchen. 1984. "The Oral vs. the Written: A Dialectic of Worldviews in Najib Maḥfūẓ's *Children of Our Alley.*" *Al-ʿArabiyya* 17, pp. 87–118.
Rooke, Tetz. 1997. *In My Childhood: A Study of Arabic Autobiography.* Stockholm: Almquist & Wiksell.
——. 1997a. "Moroccan Autobiography as National Allegory." *Oriente Moderno* 17.2, pp. 289–305.
——. 2000. "The Influence of *Adab* on the Muslim Intellectuals of the *Nahda* as Reflected in the Memoirs of Muhammad Kurd Ali (1876–1953)." In Bjørn Utvik and Knut Vikør Utvik (eds.). *The Middle East in a Globalized World.* Bergen: Nordic Society for Middle Eastern Studies, pp. 193–219.
——. 2001. "From Self-Made Man to Man-Made Self: A Story about Changing Identities," available at: http://rooke.se/rooketime21e.html, last accessed Septemeber 17, 2021.
——. 2002. *Fī al-Ṭufūla, Dirāsa fī al-Sīra al-Dhātiyya al-ʿArabiyya,* trans. Ṭalʿat al-Shāyib. Cairo: al-Majlis al-Aʿlā li-l-Thaqāfa (2nd edn 2009, Cairo: al-Markaz al-Qawmī lil-Tarjama).
——. 2006. "Translation of Arabic Literature: A Mission Impossible?" In Lutz Edzard and Jan Retsö (eds.). 2006. *Current Issues in the Analysis of Semitic Grammar and Lexicon II, Oslo-Göteborg Cooperation, 4th–5th November 2005, Abhandlung für die Kunde des Morgenlandes (Band LIX).* Wiesbaden: Harrassowitz Verlag, pp. 214–25.
——. 2008. "*In the Presence of Absence*: Mahmoud Darwish's Testament." *Journal of Arabic and Islamic Studies* 8.2, pp. 11–25.

——. 2011. "The Emergence of the Arabic Bestseller: Arabic Fiction and World Literature." In Stephan Guth and Gail Ramsay (eds.). *From New Values to New Aesthetics: Turning Points in Modern Arabic Literature (Proceedings of the 8th EURAMAL Conference, 11–14 June, 2008, Uppsala, Sweden). 2. Postmodernism and Thereafter*. Wiesbaden: Harrassowitz Verlag, pp. 201–13.
——. 2011a. "Arabic World Literature: New Names, Old Games?" In Kerstin Eksell and Stephan Guth (eds.). *Borders and Beyond Crossings and Transitions in Modern Arabic Literature*. Wiesbaden: Harrassowitz Verlag, pp. 127–46.
——. 2017. "The Slippers That Keep Coming Back: Gender and Race in Two Swedish Theatre Adaptations, *Abu Kasems Slippers* (1908) and *The Weaver of Baghdad* (1923)," paper presented in the Conference *One Thousand and One Nights*: Comparative Perspectives on Adaptation and Appropriation, University of St. Andrews, August 31–September 1, 2017.
Rosenthal, Franz. 1979. "Literature." In Joseph Schacht and C. B. Bosworth (eds.). *The Legacy of Islam*. Oxford: Oxford University Press, pp. 321–49.
Roskies, David G. 1984. *Against the Apocalypse: Responses to Catastrophe in Modern Jewish Culture*. Cambridge, MA: Harvard University Press.
Rossetti, John Joseph Henry. 2017. "A Shared Imaginary City: The Role of the Reader in the Fiction of Muḥammad Khuḍayyir." PhD thesis, University of Pennsylvania.
Roth, Joseph. 1934. *Der Antichrist*. Amsterdam: A. De Lang.
Rothstein, Edward. 2005. "Regarding Cervantes, Multicultural Dreamer." *New York Times*, June 13, available at: https://www.nytimes.com/2005/06/13/arts/regarding-cervantes-multicultural-dreamer.html, last accessed August 22, 2021.
al-Rouayheb. 2005. *Before Homosexuality in the Arabic-Islamic World 1500–1800*. Chicago: University of Chicago Press.
Royer, Diana. 2001. *A Critical Study of the Works of Nawal El Saadawi, Egyptian Writer and Activist*. Lewiston, NY: Edwin Mellen Press.
Rudnyckyj, J. B. 1959. "Functions of Proper Names in the Literary Work." In Paul Böckmann (ed.). *Stil und Formprobleme in der Literatur: Vortäge des VII. Kongresses der Internationalen Vereinigung für Moderne Sprachen und Literaturen in Heidelberg*. Heidelberg: Carl Winter, pp. 378–83.
Rūmī, Ǧalāl ud-dīn Muḥammad. 1925. *Maṯnawī-i Ma'nawī*, ed. and trans. R. A. Nicholson. London: Gibb Memorial Series.
——. 1968. *Maṯnawī-i Ma'nawī*, ed. and trans. R. A. Nicholson. London: Gibb Memorial Series.
Ruocco, Monica. 2000. "A Survey of Translation and Studies on Arabic Literature Published in Italy (1987–1997)." *Arabic and Middle Eastern Literatures* 3.1, pp. 63–73.
——. 2001. "La traduzione della terminologia teatrale in lingua araba (Abstract: The Translation of Arabic Theatre Terminology)." *Traduttore Nuovo* 56.1, pp. 29–37, 112.
al-Ruṣāfī, Ma'rūf. 1986. *Dīwān*. Beirut: Dār al-'Awda.
Ryding, Karin Christina. 2021. "The Arabic of *Dune*: Language and Landscape." In Daniela Francesca Virdis et al. (eds.). *Language in Place: Stylistic Perspectives on Landscape, Place and Environment*. Amsterdam: John Benjamins, pp. 106–23.
Saad el Din, Mursi and Cromer, John. 1991. *Under Egypt's Spell: The Influence of Egypt on Writers in English from the Eighteenth Century*. London: Bellew.
Ṣābir, Majdī. 1991. *Discovery: al-Qamar al-Mal'ūn*. London: Mid-Light.
Sabra, Martina. 2010. "The Poem of the Day Direct to Your Smartphone? Modern Arabic Literature on the Worldwide Web." *Fikrun wa Fann* 93, pp. 32–35.
Sacks, Jeffrey. 2015. *Iterations of Loss: Mutilation and Aesthetic Form, Al-Shidyaq to Darwish*. New York: Fordham Universiy Press.
Sa'dāwī, Aḥmad. 2013. *Frankenstein fī Baghdād*. Baghdad: Manshūrāt al-Jamal.
Sadeh, Pinḥas. 1974 [1958]. *Life as a Parable* (in Hebrew). Tel Aviv: Schocken.

Sáenz-Badilios, A. 1997. "Philologians and Poets in Search of the Hebrew Language." In Ross Brann (ed.). *Languages of Power in Islamic Spain*. Bethesda, MD: CDL Press, pp. 49–75.
al-Ṣafadī, Ṣalāḥ al-Dīn. 2000. *Kitāb al-Wāfī bi-l-Wafayāt*. Beirut: Dār Iḥyā' al-Turāth al-'Arabī.
Said, Edward W. 1985 [1978]. *Orientalism*. London: Penguin.
Sa'īd, Fatḥī. 1994. *Andalusiyyāt Miṣriyya*. Cairo: al-Hay'a al-Miṣriyya al-'Āmma li-l-Kitāb.
Sakkout, Ḥamdī. 1975. "Najīb Maḥfūẓ's Short Stories." In R. C. Ostle (ed.). 1975. *Studies in Modern Arabic Literature*. Warminster: Aris & Phillips, pp. 114–25.
Sakr, Naomi (ed.). 2007. *Arab Media and Political Renewal*. London: I. B. Tauris.
Salem, Elise. 2003. *Constructing Lebanon: A Century of Literary Narratives*. Gainesville: University Press of Florida.
Ṣāliḥ, Fakhrī (ed.). 1995. *al-Mu'aththirāt al-Ajnabiyya fī al-Shi'r al-'Arabī al-Mu'āṣir*. Beirut: al-Mu'assasa al-'Arabiyya li-l-Dirāsāt wa-l-Nashr.
Ṣāliḥ, Rushdī (ed.). 1982. *Bayram al-Tūnisī: Bayram wa-l-'Arab wa-l-'Ālam*. Cairo: al-Hay'a al-Miṣriyya al-'Āmma li-l-Kitāb.
Sanaullah, Muhammad. 2010. "Symbolic Islamo-European Encounter in Prosody: *Muwashshaḥāt, Azjāl* and the Catalan Troubadours." *Islamic Studies* 49.3, pp. 357–400.
Sarḥān, Hāla. 1990. "Sirr al-Markabāt al-Faḍā'iyya fī Ḥuqūl al-Qamḥ al-Barīṭāniyya." *Kull al-Nās*, August, pp. 20–3.
Sartre, Jean-Paul. 1964. *Les Mots*. Paris: Gallimard.
——. 1983. *Sīratī al-Dhātiyya: al-Kalimāt*, trans. Suhayl Idrīs. Beirut: Dār al-Ādāb.
Ṣawāyā, Mīkhā'īl. 1960. *Sulaymān al-Bustānī Rā'id al-Baḥth al-Adabī wa-l-Naqd al-Ḥadīth*. Beirut: Manshūrāt Dār al-Sharq al-Jadīd.
al-Sayyāb, Badr Shākir. 1971. *Dīwān*. Beirut: Dār al-'Awda.
——. 2007. *Kuntu Shuyū'iyyan*. Cologne: Manshūrāt al-Jamal.
Schachtel, E. G. 1963. *Metamorphosis*. London: Routledge.
Schami, Rafik. 1987. *Erzähler der Nacht*. Weinheim: Beltz.
——. 1989. *Eine Hand Voller Sterne*. Weinheim: Beltz.
——. 1993. *Damascus Nights*, trans. Philip Boehm. New York: Farrar, Straus & Giroux.
——. 1995. *Reise zwischen Nacht und Morgen*. Munich: Carl Hanser Verlag.
——. 1996. *A Hand Full of Stars* (in Hebrew), trans. Daphna Amit. Tel Aviv: Schocken.
——. 2004. *Die dunkle Seite der Liebe*. Munich: Carl Hanser Verlag.
——. 2009. *The Dark Side of Love*, trans. Anthea Bell. Northampton, MA: Interlink Books.
——. 2010. *The Calligrapher's Secret*, trans. Anthea Bell. London: Arabia.
Scharfstein, Ben-Ami. 1973. *Mystical Experience*. Oxford: Blackwell.
——. 1993. *Ineffability: The Failure of Words in Philosophy and Religion*. Albany: State University of New York Press.
Schildgen, Deen et al. (eds.). 2007. *Other Renaissances: A New Approach to World Literature*. New York: Palgrave Macmillan.
Schimmel, Annemarie. 1975. *Zeitgenössische Arabische Lyrik*. Tübingen: Horst Erdmann Verlag.
——. 1982. *As Through a Veil: Mystical Poetry in Islam*. New York: Columbia University Press.
——. 1983. *Mystical Dimensions of Islam*. Chapel Hill: University of North Carolina Press.
Scholem, Gershom G. 1954. *Major Trends in Jewish Mysticism*. New York: Schocken.
——. 1972. *On the Kabbalah and Its Symbolism*. New York: Schocken.
——. 1974. *The Messianic Idea in Judaism*. New York: Schocken.
Schuman, L. O. 1965. *Een Moderne Arabische Vertelling: Nagib Mahfuz, Awlad Haritna*. Leiden: Brill.
Sebeok, Thomas A. (ed.). 1986. *Encyclopedic Dictionary of Semiotics*. Berlin: Mouton de Gruyter.
Sedillot, L. A. 1877. *Histoire Generale des Arabes*. Paris: Maisonneuve.

Selim, Samah. 2004. *The Novel and the Rural Imaginary in Egypt, 1880–1985*. London: RoutledgeCurzon.

——. 2004a. "The Nahda, Popular Fiction and the Politics of Translations," *The MIT Electronic Journal of Middle East Studies* 4, pp. 75–89.

——. 2011. "Roundtable: Theory and Arabic Literature in the United States." *International Journal of Middle East Studies* 43.4, p. 721.

——. 2011a. "Toward a New Literary History." *International Journal of Middle East Studies* 43.4 (2011), pp. 734–736.

——. 2019. *Popular Fiction, Translation and the Nahda in Egypt*. New York: Palgrave Macmillan.

Sells, Michael A. "Longing, Belonging, and Pilgrimage in Ibn al-'Arabī's Interpreter of Desires (*Tarjumān al-Ashwāq*)." In Ross Brann (ed.). *Languages of Power in Islamic Spain*. Bethesda, MD: CDL Press, pp. 188–96.

Semaan, Khalil I. 1969. "T. S. Eliot's Influence on Arabic Poetry and Drama." *Comparative Literature Studies* 5.4, pp. 472–89.

——. 1979. "Islamic Mysticism in Modern Arabic Poetry and Drama." *International Journal of Middle East Studies* 10, pp. 517–31.

Semah, David. 1974. *Four Egyptian Literary Critics*. Leiden: Brill.

Serjeant, R. B. (ed.). 1980. *The Islamic City*, selected papers from the Colloquium Held at the Middle East Centre, Faculty of Oriental Studies, Cambridge, United Kingdom, from 19 to 23 July 1976. Paris: UNESCO.

Sha'bān, Buthayna. 1986. "Bayna al-Adab al-Nisā'ī al-'Arabī wa-l-Adab al-Nisā'ī al-Inglīzī: Ghāda al-Sammān wa-Virginia Woolf." *al-Mawqif al-Adabī* 16.186, pp. 64–89.

——. 1999. *100 'Āmm min al-Riwāya al-Nisā'iyya al-'Arabiyya (1899–1999)*. Beirut: Dār al-Ādāb.

Sha'bān, Sa'd. 1993. *Nāfidha 'alā al-Faḍā'*. Cairo: al-Hay'a al-Miṣriyya al-'Āmma li-l-Kitāb.

Shafik, Viola. 1998. *Arab Cinema: History and Cultural Identity*. Cairo: American University in Cairo Press.

Shahīd, Irfan. 1965. "A Contribution to Koranic Exegesis." In George Makdisi (ed.). *Arabic and Islamic Studies in Honor of Hamilton A. R. Gibb*. Cambridge, MA: Harvard University Press, pp. 563–80.

——. 1983. "Another Contribution to Koranic Exegesis: The Sūra of the Poets (xxvi)." *Journal of Arabic Literature* 14, pp. 1–21.

——. 2000. "Gibran and the American Literary Canon: The Problem of *The Prophet*." In Kamal Abdel-Malek and Wael Hallaq (eds.). *Tradition, Modernity, and Postmodernity in Arabic Literature: Essays in Honor of Professor Issa J. Boullata*. Leiden: Brill, pp. 321–34.

——. 2004. "The Sūra of the Poets, Qur'ān xxvi: Final Conclusions." *Journal of Arabic Literature* 35, pp. 175–220.

Shakespeare, William. n.d. *The Complete Works*. London: Spring Books.

——. 1964. *The Merchant of Venice*. London: Methuen.

——. 1971. *Julius Caesar*. London: Longman.

Shākir, Tahānī 'Abd al-Fattāḥ. 2002. *al-Sīra al-Dhātiyya fī al-Adab al-'Arabī: Fadwā Ṭūqān wa-Jabrā Ibrāhīm Jabrā wa-Iḥsān 'Abbās Namūdhajan*. Beirut: al-Mu'assasa al-'Arabiyya li-l-Dirāsāt wa-l-Nashr.

Sha'lān, Ibrāhīm Aḥmad. 1993. *al-Nawādir al-Sha'biyya al-Miṣriyya: Dirāsa Ta'rīkhiyya Ijtimā'iyya*. Cairo: Madbūlī.

Shalaq, 'Alī. 1979. *Najīb Maḥfūẓ fī Majhūlihi al-Ma'lūm*. Beirut: Dār al-Masīra.

Shalash, 'Alī. 1966. "Virginia Woolf wa-Qiṣṣat Tayyār al-Wa'y." *al-Fikr al-Mu'āṣir* 15, pp. 50–9.

Shalḥat, Anṭwān. 1989. *Samīḥ al-Qāsim min al-Ghaḍab al-Thawrī ilā al-Nubu'a al-Thawriyya*. Acre: Dār al-Aswār.

Shāmī, Rafīq. 1997. *Yad Mil'uhā al-Nujūm*, trans. from English by Marsel Sagiv. Tel Aviv: Schocken.

Shannon, Jonathan. 2007. "Performing al-Andalus, Remembering al-Andalus: Mediterranean Soundings from Mashriq to Maghrib." *Journal of American Folklore* 120.477, pp. 308–44.

Sharaf, 'Abd al-'Azīz. 1992. *Adab al-Sīra al-Dhātiyya*. Cairo: al-Sharika al-Miṣriyya al-'Ālamiyya li-l-Nashr—Longman.

Sharbal, Mūrīs Ḥannā. 1996. *Mawsū'at al-Shu'arā' wa-l-Udabā' al-Ajānib*. Tripoli: Jarrūs Press.

Sharfuddin, Mohammed. 1994. *Islam and Romantic Orientalism*. London: I. B. Tauris.

Sharīf, Nihād. 1981. *Alladhī Taḥaddā al-I'ṣār*. Cairo: al-Hay'a al-Miṣriyya al-'Āmma li-l-Kitāb.

——. 1989. *al-Shay'*. Cairo: al-Hay'a al-Miṣriyya al-'Āmma li-l-Kitāb.

——. 1994. *Mu'allafāt Nihād Sharīf*. Cairo: al-Hay'a al-Miṣriyya al-'Āmma li-l-Kitāb.

al-Shārūnī, Yūsuf. 1971. "Muqaddima fī Adabinā al-Riwā'ī al-Mu'āṣir 1952–1971." *al-Majalla*, October, pp. 8–14.

——. 1980. "al-Khayāl al-'Ilmī fī al-Adab al-'Arabī." *'Ālam al-Fikr*, October/December, pp. 243–76.

Sha'shū'a, Salīm. 1979. *al-'Aṣr al-Dhahabī: Ṣafaḥāt min al-Ta'āwun al-Yahūdī al-'Arabī fī al-Andalus*. Tel Aviv: Dār al-Mashriq.

Shā'ul, Anwar. 1980. *Qiṣṣat Ḥayātī fī Wādī al-Rāfidayn*. Jerusalem: Rābiṭat al-Jāmi'iyyīn al-Yahūd al-Nāziḥīn min al-'Irāq.

——. 1983. *Wa-Bazagha Fajr Jadīd*. Jerusalem: Rābiṭat al-Jāmi'iyyīn al-Yahūd al-Nāziḥīn min al-'Irāq.

Shawqī, Aḥmad. 1932. *Amīrat al-Andalus*. Cairo: Dār al-Kutub al-Miṣriyya.

——. 1964. *al-Shawqiyyāt*. Cairo: al-Maktaba al-Tijāriyya al-Kubrā.

Shawqī, Sharīf. n.d. *Idārat al-'Amaliyyāt al-Khāṣṣa—al-Maktab Raqam 19 (51): al-Tāj al-Dhahabī*. Cairo: al-Mu'assasa al-'Arabiyya al-Ḥadītha.

al-Shayyāl, Jamāl al-Dīn. 1950. *Ta'rīkh al-Tarjama fī Miṣr fī 'Ahd al-Ḥamla al-Faransiyya*. Cairo: Dār al-Fikr al-'Arabī.

——. 1951. *Ta'rīkh al-Tarjama wa-l-Ḥaraka al-Thaqāfiyya fī Miṣr fī 'Aṣr Muḥammad 'Alī*. Cairo: Dār al-Fikr al-'Arabī.

Sheehi, Stephen. 2004. *Foundations of Modern Arab Identity*. Gainesville: University Press of Florida.

Sheeler, Charles. 1939. *Paintings, Drawings, Photographs*, with an Introduction by William Carlos Williams. New York: Museum of Modern Art.

Sheetrit, Ariel M. 2012. "The Poetics of the Poet's Autobiography: Voicings and Mutings in Fadwā Ṭūqān's Narrative Journey." *Journal of Arabic Literature* 43.1, pp. 102–31.

Shenberg, Galia. 1998. "Diglossia and Bilingualism: Storytelling by Druze Women" (in Hebrew). *'Iyyun ve-Mehkar be-Hachsharat Morim* (Gordon College, Haifa) 21, pp. 21–9.

al-Shīdī, Fāṭima. 2021. "Ṣalāḥ Fā'iq al-Siryālī al-Akhīr." *Jarīdat 'Umān*, available at: https://www.facebook.com/fatma.sheedi/posts/10222562225056613, last accessed September 5, 2021.

Shih, Shu-Mei. 2004. "Global Literature and the Technologies of Recognition." *PMLA* 119.1, pp. 16–30.

——. 2013. "Global Literature and the Technologies of Recognition." In Theo D'haen et al. (eds.). *World Literature: A Reader*. London: Routledge, pp. 259–74.

Shiloah, Amnon. 1995. *Music in the World of Islam: A Socio-Cultural Study*. Aldershot: Scolar Press.

Shimon, Samuel (ed.). 2018. *Baghdad Noir*. New York: Akashic Noir.

Shipley, Joseph. 1972. *Dictionary of World Literature*. Totowa, NJ: Littlefield, Adams.

al-Shirbīnī, Yūsuf. 2005. *Kitāb Hazz al-Quḥūf bi-Sharḥ Qaṣīd Abī Shādūf* (*Brains Confounded by the Ode of Abū Shādūf Expounded*), vol. 1, ed. Humphrey Davies. Dudley, MA: Peeters.

——. 2007. *Yusuf al-Shirbini's Brains Confounded by the Ode of Abū Shādūf Expounded* (*Kitāb Hazz al-Quḥūf bi-Sharḥ Qaṣīd Abī Shādūf*), vol. 2, trans. Humphrey Davies. Dudley, MA: Peeters.

Shīrīzī, Marsīl. 2002. *Awrāq Munāḍil Īṭālī fī Miṣr*. Cairo: Dār al-ʿĀlam al-Thālith.

Shoair, Mohamed. 2022. *The Story of the Banned Book: Naguib Mahfouz's Children of the Alley*, trans. Humphrey Davies. Cairo: American University in Cairo Press.

Shoham, S. Giora. 1980. *Salvation through the Gutters* (in Hebrew). Tel Aviv: Cherikover.

Shoshan, Boaz. 1991. "High Culture and Popular Culture in Medieval Islam." *Studia Islamica* 73, pp. 67–107.

Shuʿayr, Muḥammad. 2018. *Awlād Ḥāratinā: Sīrat al-Riwāya al-Muḥarrama*. Cairo: Dār al-ʿAyn.

Shuiskii, Sergei A. 1982. "Some Observations on Modern Arabic Autobiography." *Journal of Arabic Literature* 13, pp. 111–23.

Shukrī, Ghālī. 1978. *Shiʿrunā al-Ḥadīth ... Ilā Ayna?* Beirut: Dār al-Āfāq al-Jadīda.

——. 1982. *al-Muntamī*. Beirut: Dār al-Āfāq al-Jadīda.

Shulman, David. 1984. "Muslim Popular Literature in Tamil: The Tamīmancāri Mālai." In Yohanan Friedman (ed.). *Islam in Asia*. Jerusalem: Magnes Press, I, pp. 174–207.

Shūmān, Muḥammad Zīnū. 1994. "Amīn Maʿlūf wa-l-Kūmīdyā al-Ilāhiyya." *al-Bilād*, March 26, p. 41.

Shūsha, Fārūq. 1980. *Fī Intiẓār Mā Lā Yajī'*. Cairo: Madbūlī.

Shusterman, Richard. 1993. "Too Legit to Quit? Popular Art and Legitimation." *Iyyun, The Jerusalem Philosophical Quarterly* 42 (January), pp. 215–24.

Silverberg, Robert (ed.). 1983. *The Nebula Awards Stories Eighteen*. Enfield, CT: Science Fiction Writers of America.

——. (ed.). 1986. *Qiṣaṣ min al-Khayāl al-ʿIlmī*, trans. Fatḥī ʿAbd al-Fattāḥ. Cairo: Maktabat Gharīb.

Simon, Reeva S. 1986. *Iraq between the Two World Wars: The Creation and Implementation of a Nationalist Ideology*. New York: Columbia University Press.

Smith, Anthony D. 1991. *National Identity*. Harmondsworth: Penguin.

Smith, Wilfred Cantwell. 1963. *Islam in Modern History*. New York: Mentor.

Smolin, Jonathan. 2013. "Didactic Entertainment: The Moroccan *Police Journal* and the Origins of the Arabic Police Procedural." *International Journal of Middle East Studies* 45, pp. 695–714.

——. 2013a. *Moroccan Noir: Police, Crime, and Politics in Popular Culture*. Bloomington: Indiana University Press.

Snir, Reuven. 1982. "Kitāb al-Zuhd by al-Muʿāfā ibn ʿImrān." MA thesis, Hebrew University of Jerusalem.

——. 1984. "Sufi Elements in Modern Arabic Poetry and the Role of the Egyptian Poet Ṣalāḥ ʿAbd al-Ṣabūr." *Bulletin of the Israeli Academic Center in Cairo* 5, pp. 12–13.

——. 1985. "Ṣūfiyya bi-lā Taṣawwuf Islāmī: Qirā'a Jadīda fī Qaṣīdat Ṣalāḥ ʿAbd al-Ṣabūr ʿal-Ilāh al-Ṣaghīr.'" *al-Karmil: Studies in Arabic Language and Literature* 6, pp. 129–46.

——. 1986. "Sufi Elements in Modern Arabic Poetry 1940–1980" (in Hebrew). PhD thesis, Hebrew University of Jerusalem.

——. 1986a. *Anthology of Ascetic, Mystic and Metaphysical Arabic Poetry From the 8th Century to Our Days*. Jerusalem: Academon.

——. 1988. "The Books: Blessing or Curse—A Study of 'The Books' by Mīshīl Ḥaddād" (in Hebrew). *Journal of the Teachers of Arabic Language* 4, pp. 9–16.

——. 1988a. "From War to Peace." *Middle East Focus* 10, pp. 2, 11.

——. 1988–1989. "Two Egyptian Writers in the Service of Peace." *Middle East Review* 21, pp. 41–5.

——. 1989. "The Arab–Israeli Conflict as Reflected in the Writing of Najīb Maḥfūẓ." *Abr-Nahrain* 27, pp. 120–53.
——. 1989a. "Human Existence According to Kafka and Ṣalāḥ 'Abd al-Ṣabūr." *Jusūr* 5, pp. 31–43.
——. 1990. "'A Wound Out of His Wounds': Palestinian Arabic Literature in Israel" (in Hebrew). *Alpayim* 2, pp. 244–68.
——. 1991a. "Figliastri pieni d'amore: Scrittori arabi in lingua ebraica." *La Rassegna Mensile di Israel* 57.1/2 (June/August), pp. 245–53.
——. 1991b. "*Mundus Inversus* in Arabic Literature in the Twentieth Century" (in Hebrew). In H. Z. Levy (ed.). *Fathers and Sons: Myth, Theme and Literary Topos*. Jerusalem: Magnes Press, pp. 88–107.
——. 1992. "Step-Sons and Lovers" (in Hebrew). *Moznaim*, May, pp. 6–9.
——. 1992a. "'al-Zayt fī al-Miṣbāḥ Lan Yajiffa'—Jadaliyyat al-Burj al-'Ājī' / al-Manāra fī Mir'āt al-Shi'r al-Multazim." *al-Karmil: Studies in Arabic Language and Literature* 13, pp. 7–54.
——. 1992b. "Neo-Sufism in the Writing of the Egyptian Poet Ṣalāḥ 'Abd al-Ṣabūr." *Sufi: A Journal of Sufism* 13, pp. 24–6.
——. 1992c. "Arabic Literature in Syria between Distinctiveness and Unity" (in Hebrew). *Moznaim*, December, pp. 61–4.
——. 1993. "Al-'Anāṣir al-Masraḥiyya fī al-Turāth al-Sha'bī al-'Arabī al-Qadīm" (review article of Moreh 1992). *al-Karmil: Studies in Arabic Language and Literature* 14, pp. 149–70.
——. 1993a. "The Inscription of 'En 'Abdat: An Early Evolutionary Stage of Ancient Arabic Poetry." *Abr Nahrain* 31, pp. 110–25.
——. 1993b. "'Limādhā Tunfā al-Kalimāt?'—al-Shā'ir wa-Ṣakhratuhu fī Mir'āt al-Shi'r al-Multazim." *al-Karmil: Studies in Arabic Language and Literature* 14, pp. 49–93.
——. 1994. "Adab, Ta'rīkh, wa-Ta'rīkh al-Adab." *al-Karmil: Studies in Arabic Language and Literature* 15, pp. 61–85.
——. 1994a. "The 'World Upsidedown' in Modern Arabic Literature: New Literary Renditions of an Antique Religious Topos." *Edebiyât* 5.1, pp. 51–75.
——. 1994b. "'Under the Patronage of Muḥammad': Islamic Motifs in the Poetry of Jewish Writers from Iraq" (in Hebrew). In Tamar Alexander et al. (eds.). *History and Creativity in the Sephardi and Oriental Jewish Communities* (in Hebrew). Jerusalem: Misgav Yerushalayim, pp. 161–93.
——. 1994c. "Arabic Literature in the 20th Century: An Historical Dynamic Functional Model" (Hebrew), *HaMizrah HeHadash* 36, pp. 49–80.
——. 1994d. "A Study of *Elegy for al-Ḥallāj* by Adūnīs." *Journal of Arabic Literature* 25.2, pp. 245–56.
——. 1994–1995. "Mysticism and Poetry in Arabic Literature." *Orientalia Suecana* 43/44, pp. 165–75.
——. 1995. "'Hebrew as the Language of Grace': Arab-Palestinian Writers in Hebrew." *Prooftexts* 15, pp. 163–83.
——. 1995a. "Qirā'a fī Qaṣīdat 'Abārīq Muhashshama' li-'Abd al-Wahhāb al-Bayyātī." *al-Karmil: Studies in Arabic Language and Literature* 16, pp. 7–53.
——. 1996. "'Armed with Roses and Sweet Basil': The Emergence of Feminist Culture in the Arab World" (Hebrew). *Motar: Journal of the Yolanada and David Katz Faculty of the Arts, Tel Aviv University* 4, pp. 65–72.
——. 1997. "'And I Hallucinate in No-Man's Land': Arab-Palestinian Writers in Hebrew" (in Hebrew). *Hebrew Linguistics* 41/42, pp. 141–53.
——. 1998. "Synchronic and Diachronic Dynamics in Modern Arabic Literature." In Shimon Ballas and Reuven Snir (eds.). *Studies in Canonical and Popular Arabic Literature*. Toronto: York Press, pp. 87–121.

——. 1998a. "The Palestinian al-Ḥakawati Theater: A Brief History." *Arab Studies Journal* 6.2/7.1, pp. 57–71.
——. 1999. "Virginia Woolf in Arabic Literature: Translations, Influence, and Reception." *Virginia Woolf Miscellany* 54, pp. 6–7.
——. 2000. "'Al-Andalus Arising from Damascus': Al-Andalus in Modern Arabic Poetry." *Hispanic Issues* 21, pp. 263–93.
——. 2000a. "Modern Arabic Literature and the West: Self-Image, Interference, and Reception." *Yearbook of Comparative and General Literature* 48, pp. 53–71.
——. 2000b. "The Emergence of Science Fiction in Arabic Literature." *Der Islam* 77.2, pp. 263–85.
——. 2000c. "'Poète des secrets et des racines': L'Adonis hallajien" In Adūnīs, *Adonis: un poète dans le monde d'aujourd'hui 1950–2000*. Paris: Institut du monde arabe, pp. 171–2.
——. 2001. *Modern Arabic Literature: A Functional Dynamic Historical Model*. Toronto: York Press.
——. 2001a. "'Postcards in the Morning': Palestinians Writing in Hebrew." *Hebrew Studies* 42, pp. 197–224.
——. 2002. *Rak'atān fī al-'Ishq: Dirāsa fī Shi'r 'Abd al-Wahhāb al-Bayyātī*. Beirut: Dār al-Sāqī.
——. 2002a. "Science Fiction in Arabic Literature: Translation, Adaptation, Original Writing and Canonization." *Arabic Language and Literature* (Seoul) 2, pp. 209–29.
——. 2004. "Shā'ir al-Asrār wa-l-Judhūr, Adūnīs al-Ḥallājī." In Adūnīs. *al-Ḍaw' al-Mashriqī: Adūnis ka-mā Yarāhu Mufakkirūn wa-Shu'arā' 'Ālamiyūn*. Damascus: Dār al-Ṭalī'a, pp. 177–9.
——. 2004–2005. "'Will Homer Be Born after Us?': Intertextuality and Myth in Maḥmūd Darwīsh's Poetry in the 1980s." *al-Karmil: Studies in Arabic Language and Literature* 25/26, pp. 17–85.
——. 2005. *Arabness, Jewishness, Zionism: A Clash of Identities in the Literature of Iraqi Jews* (in Hebrew). Jerusalem: Ben-Zvi Institute for the Study of Jewish Communities in the East.
——. 2005a. "'When the Time Stopped': Ishaq Bār-Moshe as Arab-Jewish Writer in Israel." *Jewish Social Studies* 11.2, pp. 102–35.
——. 2006. *Religion, Mysticism and Modern Arabic Literature*. Wiesbaden: Harrassowitz Verlag.
——. 2007. "'The Tail above the Head': Literary Representations of 'Abd al-Nāṣir's Regime as a World Upside Down." *Quaderni di Studi Arabi* n.s. 2, pp. 181–208.
——. 2008. "'Other Barbarians Will Come': Intertextuality, Meta-Poetry, and Meta-Myth in Maḥmūd Darwīsh's Poetry." In Hala Khamis Nassar and Najat Rahman (eds.). *Mahmoud Darwish, Exile's Poet: Critical Essays*. Northampton, MA: Interlink Books, pp. 123–66.
——. 2011. "'The More the Vision Increases, the More the Expression Decreases': Muslim Mysticism between Experience, Language and Translation" (in Hebrew). *Jama'a: Interdisciplinary Journal of Middle East Studies*19, pp. 83–133.
——. 2012. *Adonis—Index of the Acts of the Wind* (in Hebrew). Tel Aviv: Keshev.
——. 2013. *Baghdad: The City in Verse*. Cambridge, MA: Harvard University Press.
——. 2013a. "'I Saw My God in the Eye of My Heart': Mysticism, Poetry, and the Creative Process in Modern Secular Arabic Literary Culture." In Ali Hussein (ed.). *Branches of the Goodly Tree: Studies in Honor of George Kanazi*. Wiesbaden: Harrassowitz Verlag, pp. 194–229.
——. 2015. *Who Needs Arab-Jewish Identity? Interpellation, Exclusion, and Inessential Solidarities*. Leiden: Brill.
——. 2017. *Modern Arabic Literature: A Theoretical Framework*. Edinburgh: Edinburgh University Press.

——. 2019. "World Literature, Republics of Letters, and the Arabic Literary System: The 'Modernists' in the Defendants' Bench: A Review Article." *Mamlūk Studies Review* 22, pp. 137–92.
——. 2019a. *Arab-Jewish Literature: The Birth and Demise of the Arabic Short Story* (With an Anthology of 16 Translated Short Stories by Arabized Jews). Leiden: Brill.
——. 2021. "'The Eye's Delight': Baghdad in Arabic Poetry." *Orientalia Suecana* 70, pp. 4–40.
——. 2021a. "Kafka's 'Frightened Mouse': Existentialist vis-a-vis Mystical Concepts in Ṣalāḥ 'Abd al-Ṣabūr's Poetry." *Quaderni di Studi Arabi* 16, pp. 1–24.
Sobolev, Dennis. 2017. "The Concept of 'World Literature' and Its Problems" (in Russian). In Olga Polovinkina (ed.). *Noscere est comparare: Komparativistika v kontekste isotricheskoi poetiki* (*Comparative Literature in the Context of Historical Poetics*). Moscow: RGGU, pp. 20–53.
Somekh, Sasson. 1970. "Za'balāwī: Author, Theme and Technique." *Journal of Arabic Literature* 1, pp. 24–35.
——. 1971. "The Sad Millennarian: An Examination of *Awlād Ḥāratinā*." *Middle Eastern Studies* 7.1, pp. 49–61.
——. 1973. "Arabic Literature and Hebrew Translation" (in Hebrew). In Jacob Mansour (ed.). *Arabic and Islamic Studies* (in Hebrew). Ramat Gan: Bar-Ilan University, pp. 141–52.
——. 1973a. *The Changing Rhythm*. Leiden: Brill.
——. 1982. "Bidāyāt al-Tarjama al-Adabiyya fī al-Qarn al-Tāsi' 'Ashar wa-Mushkilat al-Uslūb al-Qaṣaṣī." *al-Karmil: Studies in Arabic Language and Literature* 3, pp. 45–59.
——. 1983. "A Literature in Search of Language." Inaugural Lecture, Irene Halmos Chair of Arabic Literature, Tel Aviv University, October 23 (reprint).
——. 1987–1988. "A Minute to Midnight: War and Peace in the Novels of Naguib Maḥfūẓ." *Middle East Review* 20, pp. 7–13.
——. 1991. *Genre and Language in Modern Arabic Literature*. Wiesbaden: Harrassowitz Verlag.
——. 1992. "The Neoclassical Arab Poets." In M. M. Badawi (ed.). *Modern Arabic Literature*. Cambridge: Cambridge University Press, pp. 36–81, 491–4.
——. (ed.). 1993. *Translation as a Challenge: Papers on Translation of Arabic Literature into Hebrew* (in Hebrew). Tel Aviv: Tel Aviv University Press.
Soons, C. A. 1959. "Cide Hamete Benengeli: His Significance for 'Don Quijote.'" *Modern Language Review* 54.3, pp. 351–7.
Sophocles. 2007. *Sophocles: Oedipus the King*, ed. Ian Johnston. Arlington, VA: Richer Resources.
——. 2018. *Sophocles: Oedipus the King*, ed. P. J. Finglass. Cambridge: Cambridge University Press.
Southern, R. W. 1962. *Western Views of Islam in the Middle Ages*. Cambridge, MA: Harvard University Press.
Spencer, Robert. 2013. "The 'War on Terror' and the Backlash against Orientalism." In Ziad Elmarsafy et al. (eds.). *Debating Orientalism*. New York: Palgrave Macmillan, pp. 155–74.
Sperl, Stefan and Shackle, Christopher (eds.). 1996. *Qasida Poetry in Islamic Africa and Asia: Classical Traditions and Modern Meanings*. Leiden: Brill.
——. and ——. (eds.). 1996a. *Qasida Poetry in Islamic Africa and Asia: Eulogy's Bounty, Meaning's Abundance: An Anthology*. Leiden: Brill.
Stagh, Marina. 1992. "A Critical Review of a Contemporary Work on the Literary History of Egypt." In Bo Utas and Knut S. Vikør (eds.). *Papers from the First Nordic Conference on Middle Eastern Studies, Uppsala 26–29 January 1989*. Bergen, Norway: Nordic Society for Middle Eastern Studies, pp. 63–72.

——. 1993. *The Limits of Freedom of Speech: Prose Literature and Prose Writers in Egypt under Nasser and Sadat*. Stockholm: Almqvist & Wiksell.
——. 1999. "The Translation of Arabic Literature into Swedish." *Cuadernos (Escuela de Traductores de Toledo)* 2, pp. 41–6.
——. 2000. "The Translation of Arabic Literature into Swedish." *Yearbook of Comparative and General* Literature 48, pp. 107–14.
Stanton, Anna Ziajka. 2019. Review of *Modern Arabic Literature: A Theoretical Framework,* by Reuven Snir. *Modernism/Modernity* 26.3, pp. 681–3, available at: muse.jhu.edu/article/733199, last accessed September 17, 2021.
——. 2021. "Vulgar Pleasures: The Scandalous Worldliness of Burton's 'Arabian Nights.'" *Journal of World Literature* 6.1, pp. 45–64.
Starkey, Paul. 2006. *Modern Arabic Literature*. Edinburgh: Edinburgh University Press.
Starkey, Paul and Starkey, Janet (eds.). 1998. *Travellers in Egypt*. London: I. B. Tauris.
Stapleton, Michael. 1985. *The Cambridge Guide to English Literature*. Cambridge: Cambridge University Press.
Stearns, Justin. 2009. "Representing and Remembering al-Andalus: Some Historical Considerations Regarding the End of Time and the Making of Nostalgia." *Medieval Encounters* 15, pp. 355–74.
Steiner, Peter. 1984. *Russian Formalism: A Metapoetics*. Ithaca, NY: Cornell University Press.
Steinmetz, Horst. 1988. "Response to Claus Clüver's 'The Difference of Eight Decades: World Literature and the Demise of National Literatures.'" *Yearbook of Comparative and General Literature* 37, pp. 131–3.
Stern, Samuel Miklos. 1974. *Hispano-Arabic Poetry*. Oxford: Clarendon Press.
Stetkevych, Jaroslav. 1969. "Arabism and Arabic Literature: Self-View of a Profession." *Journal of Near Eastern Studies* 28.3, pp. 145–56.
——. 1993. *The Zephyrs of Najd: The Poetics of Nostalgia in the Classical Arabic Nasib*. Chicago: University of Chicago Press.
Stetkevych, Suzanne Pinckney. 2017. "Abbasid Panegyric: *Badīʿ* Poetry and the Invention of the Arab Golden Age." *British Journal of Middle Eastern Studies* 44.1, pp. 48–72.
Stewart, Devin J. 1997. "Cide Hamete Benengeli, Narrator of *Don Quijote*." *Medieval Encounters* 3.2, pp. 111–27.
Stoddart, William. 1976. *Sufism*. Wellingborough: Thorsons.
Stoll, Georg. 1998. "Immigrant Muslim Writers in Germany." In John C. Hawley (ed.). *Postcolonial Crescent: Islam's Impact on Contemporary Literature*. New York: Peter Lang, pp. 266–83.
al-Suhrawardī, Shihāb al-Dīn. 1957. *Hayākil al-Nūr*. Cairo: al-Maktaba al-Tijāriyya al-Kubrā.
——. 1993. *Maqāmāt al-Ṣūfiyya*, ed. Emile Maalouf. Beirut: Dar el-Machreq Sarl Éditeurs.
al-Sulamī, Abū ʿAbd al-Raḥmān. 1953. *Ṭabaqāt al-Ṣūfiyya*, ed. Nūr al-Dīn Sharība. Cairo: Dār al-Kitāb al-ʿArabī.
al-Sulṭānī, Fāḍil. 2021. *al-Arḍ al-Yabāb wa-Tanāṣṣuhā maʿa al-Turāth al-Insānī*. Baghdad: Dār al-Madā.
Ṣunʿ Allāh, Ibrāhīm. 1981. *al-Lajna*. Beirut: Dāa al-Kalima.
Surūr, Ṭāhā ʿAbd al-Bāqī. 1957. *Rābiʿa al-ʿAdawiyya wa-l-Ḥayāt al-Rūḥiyya fī al-Islām*. Cairo: Dār al-Fikr al-ʿArabī.
al-Suyūṭī, Jalāl al-Dīn. n.d. *al-Muzhir fī ʿUlūm al-Lugha wa-Anwāʿihā*. Cairo: Dār Iḥyāʾ al-Kutub al-ʿArabiyya.
——. n.d.I. *Nuzhat al-Julasāʾ fī Ashʿār al-Nisāʾ,* Cairo: Maktabat al-Qurʾān.
Swanson, Maria and Gould, Rebecca Ruth. 2021. "The Poetics of *Nahḍah* Multilingualism: Recovering the Lost Russian Poetry of Mikhail Naimy." *Journal of Arabic Literature* 52, pp. 170–201.

Szyska, Christian. 1995. "On Utopian Writings in Nasserist Prison and Laicist Turkey." *Die Welt des Islams* 35.1, pp. 95–125.

——. 1997. "Rewriting the European Canon: 'Alī Aḥmad Bākathīr's 'New Faust.'" In Lutz Edzard and Christian Szyska (eds.). *Encounter of Words and Texts: Interculture Studies in Honor of Stefan Wild on the Occasion of his 60th Birthday*. Hildesheim: Georg Olms Verlag, pp. 131–45.

——. 1997–1998. "Ḥawla al-Kitāba al-Ṭūbāwiyya fī Sujūn Jamāl 'Abd al-Nāṣir." *al-Karmil: Studies in Arabic Language and Literature* 18/19, pp. 115–42.

Tabur, Merve. 2019. "A View from the Moon: Allegories of Representation in Tawfiq al-Ḥakīm and H. G. Wells." *Alif: Journal of Comparative Poetics* 39, pp. 63–90.

Tageldin, Shaden M. 2011. "The Returns of Theory." *International Journal of Middle East Studies* 43.4, pp. 728–30.

Ṭāhā (Taha), Ibrāhīm. 1990. *al-Bu'd al-Ākhar*. Nazareth: Rābiṭat al-Kuttāb al-Filasṭīniyyīn.

——. 1997. "Duality and Acceptance: The Image of the Outsider in the Literary Work of Shimon Ballas." *Hebrew Studies* 38, pp. 63–87.

——. 2000. "The Palestinians in Israel: Towards a Minority Literature." *Arabic and Middle Eastern Literatures* 3.2, pp. 219–34.

——. 2000a. "Text–Genre Interrelations: A Topographical Chart of Generic Activity." *Semiotica* 132.1/2, pp. 101–9.

——. 2002. *The Palestinian Novel: A Communication Study*. London: RoutledgeCurzon.

——. 2008. "'Swimming against the Current': Toward an Arab Feminist Poetic Strategy." *Orientalia Suecana* 56, pp. 193–222.

——. 2009. *Arabic Minimalist Story: Genre, Politics and Poetics in the Self-Colonial Era*. Wiesbaden: Reichert Verlag.

——. 2017. "Palestine." In Waïl S. Hassan (ed.). *The Oxford Handbook of Arab Novelistic Traditions*. Oxford: Oxford University Press, pp. 371–82.

Ṭāhā, Maḥmūd Ṭāhā. 1965. "A'lām al-Qiṣṣa fī al-Adab al-Inglīzī al-Ḥadīth: Virginia Woolf." *al-Qiṣṣa* 2.13, pp. 23–42.

——. 1966. *Dirāsāt li-A'lām al-Qiṣṣa fī al-Adab al-Inglīzī al-Ḥadīth*. Cairo: 'Ālam al-Kutub.

——. 1975. "Sīrat Ḥayāt Woolf." *'Ālam al-Fikr* 5.4, pp. 249–72.

——. 1979. "Virginia wa-Leonard Woolf." *'Ālam al-Fikr* 9.4, pp. 225–6.

Ṭāhir, Bahā'. 2006. *Fī Madīḥ al-Riwāya*. Amman: Azmina li-l-Nashr wa-l-Tawzī'.

——. 2007. *Wāḥat al-Ghurūb*. Beirut: Dār al-Ādāb.

Taji-Farouki, Suha. 2007. *Beshara and Ibn 'Arabi: A Movement of Sufi Spirituality in the Modern World*. Oxford: Anqa Publishing.

Tājir, Jāk. 1945. *Ḥarakat al-Tarjama bi-Miṣr Khilāla al-Qarn al-Tāsi' 'Ashar*. Cairo: Dār al-Ma'ārif.

——. 2014. *Ḥarakat al-Tarjama bi-Miṣr Khilāla al-Qarn al-Tāsi' 'Ashar*. Cairo: Hindāwī.

Tal, David (ed.). 2013. *Israeli Identity between Orient and Occident*. London: Routledge.

——. 2017. "Jacqueline Kahanoff and the Demise of the Levantine." *Mediterranean Historical Review* 32, pp. 237–54.

Talmud Bavli, Sotah (Jerusalem, 1981) (photostat of the 1884 edition of Vilnius).

al-Tami, Ahmed. 1993. "Arabic 'Free Verse': The Problem of Terminology." *Journal of Arabic Literature* 24, pp. 185–98.

Ṭāqa, Shādhil. 1969. *al-A'war al-Dajjāl wa-l-Ghurabā'*. Beirut: Dār Maktabat al-Ḥayāt.

Ṭarābīshī, George. 1972. "Waqā'i' al-Mu'tamar al-Thāmin li-l-Udabā' al-'Arab." *al-Ādāb* (January), p. 91.

Ṭarrāzī, Philip de. 1913 (vol. I–II); 1914 (vol. III); 1933 (vol. IV). *Ta'rīkh al-Ṣiḥāfa al-'Arabiyya*. Beirut: al-Maṭba'a al-Adabiyya.

Tart, Charles T. (ed.). 1969. *Altered States of Consciousness*. New York: Wiley.

al-Ṭawīl, Tawfīq. 1990. *al-Ḥaḍāra al-Islāmiyya wa-l-Ḥaḍāra al-Ūrubiyya*. Cairo: Maktabat al-Turāth l-Islāmī.

Tayan, E. 1965. "Djihād." In *The Encyclopaedia of Islam*, 2nd edn. II, pp. 538–40.

Taylor, John Russell. 1984. *The Penguin Dictionary of the Theatre*. Harmondsworth: Penguin.

Teggart, Hope. 2019. "Frankenstein in Baghdad: A Novel Way of Understanding the Iraq War and Its Aftermath." *International ResearchScape Journal* 6, pp. 1–30.

al-Tha'ālibī, Abū Manṣūr 'Abd al-Malik. 1983. *Tatimmat Yatīmat al-Dahr fī Maḥāsin Ahl al-'Aṣr*, ed. Mufīd Muḥammad Qumayḥa. Beirut: Dār al-Kutub al-'Ilmiyya.

The Arab World: A Catalogue of Doctoral Dissertations, 1938–1984. University Microfilms International, February 1985.

The Talmud of Babylonia, XVII, Tractate Sotah. 1984, trans. Jacob Neusner. Chico, CA: Scholars Press.

Thiher, Allen. 1984. *Words in Reflection: Modern Language Theory and Post Modern Fiction*. Chicago: University of Chicago Press.

Thompson, Thomas Levi. 2017. "Speaking Laterally: Transnational Poetics and the Rise of Modern Arabic and Persian Poetry in Iraq and Iran." PhD thesis, University of California, Los Angeles.

Tibawi, Abd al-Latif. 1972. *Islamic Education: Its Traditions and Modernization into the Arab National Systems*. London: Luzac.

al-Tirmidhī, al-Ḥakīm. 1947. *Adab al-Nafs*, ed. A. J. Arberry and 'Alī Ḥasan 'Abd al-Qādir. Cairo: Maṭba'at al-Ḥalabī.

——. 1947a. *al-Riyāḍa*, ed. A. J. Arberry and 'Alī Ḥasan 'Abd al-Qādir. Cairo: Dār al-Fikr al-'Arabī.

Tobi, Yosef. (ed.). 1995. "The Reaction of Rav Sa'adia Gaon to Arabic Poetry and Poetics." *Hebrew Studies* 36, pp. 35–53.

——. (ed.). 2004. *Contacts between Arabic Literature and Jewish Literature in the Middle Ages and Modern Times*, vol. III (in Hebrew). Tel Aviv: Afikim.

Tomiche, Nada. 1993. *La littérature arabe contemporaine*. Paris: Éditions Maisonneuve et Larose.

Toorawa, Shawkat M. 2005. *Ibn Abi Tahir Tayfur and Arabic Writerly Culture: A Ninth-Century Bookman in Baghdad*. London: RoutledgeCurzon.

——. 2006. "Modern Arabic Literature and the Qur'an." In Glenda Abramson and Hilary Kilpatrick (eds.). *Religious Perspectives in Modern Muslim and Jewish Literatures*. London: Routledge, pp. 239–57.

Toral-Niehoff, Isabel. 2015. "History in Adab Context: 'The Book on Caliphal Histories' by Ibn 'Abd Rabbih (246/860–328/940)." *Journal of Abbasid Studies* 2, pp. 61–85.

Tresilian, David. 2008. *A Brief Introduction to Modern Arabic Literature*. London: Saqi.

Trimingham, J. Spencer. 1971. *The Sufi Orders in Islam*. Oxford: Clarendon Press.

Trudewind, Stephan. 2000. "al-Adab al-'Arabī al-Mu'āṣir al-Mutarjam ilā al-Almāniyya." *Fikr wa-Fann* 72, pp. 49–51.

al-Tūnisī, Bayram. 1976. *al-Maqāmāt*. Cairo: al-Hay'a al-Miṣriyya al-'Āmma li-l-Kitāb.

Turgenev, Ivan Sergeyevich. 1951 [1917]. *A House of Gentlefolk*, trans. Constance Garnett. New York: Macmillan.

al-Ṭūsī, Abū Naṣr al-Sarrāj. 1960. *al-Luma'*, ed. 'Abd al-Ḥalīm Maḥmūd and Ṭāhā 'Abd al-Bāqī Surūr. Cairo: Dār al-Kutub al-Ḥadītha.

al-Udhari, Abdullah (ed. and trans.). 1984. *Mahmud Darwish, Samih al-Qasim, Adonis*. London: Saqi.

al-'Umarī, Ibn Faḍl Allāh. 2010. *Masālik al-Abṣār fī Mamālik al-Amṣār*, ed. Kāmil Salmān al-Jubbūrī. Beirut: Dār al-Kutub al-'Ilmiyya.

Underhill, Evelyn. 1961. *Mysticism*. New York: E. P. Dutton.

al-'Urayyiḍ, Ibrāhīm. 1958. *Min al-Shi'r al-Ḥadīth 1900–1950*. Beirut: Dār al-'Ilm li-li-Malāyin.

Urmson, J. O. and Rée, Jonathan (eds.). 1989. *The Concise Encyclopaedia of Western Philosophy and Philosophers*. London: Unwin Hyman.

'Uthmān, I'tidāl. 1981. "Ṣalāḥ 'Abd al-Ṣabūr wa-Binā' al-Thaqāfa." *Fuṣūl* II.1, pp. 193–8.

——. 1988. *Iḍā'at al-Naṣṣ*. Beirut: Dār al-Ḥadātha.

Van Gelder, Geert Jan. 2017. "Foul Whisperings: Madness and Poetry in Arabic Literary History." In Joseph E. Lowry and Shawkat Toorawa (eds.). *Arabic Humanities, Islamic Thought: Essays in Honor of Everett K. Rowson*. Leiden: Brill, pp. 150–75.

Van Leeuwen, Richard. 1999. "The Poet and His Mission: Text and Space in the Prose Works of Maḥmūd Darwīsh." In Stephan Guth et al. (eds.). 1999. *Conscious Voices: Concepts of Writing in the Middle East*. Beirut: Orient-Institut der DMG, pp. 265–6.

Vatikiotis, P. J. 1971. "The Corruption of *Futuwwa*: A Consideration of Despair in Najīb Maḥfūẓ's *Awlad Haritina*." *Middle Eastern Studies* 7.2, pp. 169–84.

Venuti, Lawrence (ed.). 1992. *Rethinking Translation: Discourse, Subjectivity, Ideology*. New York: Routledge.

Vial, Ch. 1986. "Ḳiṣṣa." *The Encyclopaedia of Islam*, 2nd edn. V, pp. 187–93.

Viteri Marquez, Elisa Andrea. 2020. "Literary Masculinities in Contemporary Egyptian Dystopian Fiction: Local, Regional and Global Masculinities as Social Criticism in *Utopia* and *The Queue*." MA thesis, Stockholm University.

Viviani, Paola. 2012. "'Acting Like a Thief': Fatimah Na'ut Translates Virginia Woolf in Egypt." In Oriana Palusci (ed.). *Translating Virginia Woolf*. Bern: Peter Lang, pp. 145–55.

von Grunebaum, Gustave E. 1953. *Medieval Islam*. Chicago: University of Chicago Press.

——. 1962. *Modern Islam: The Search for Cultural Identity*. Berkeley: University of California Press.

——. 1967. "Literature in the Context of Islamic Civilization." *Oriens* 20, pp. 1–14.

Wādī, Ṭāhā. 2001. *al-Qiṣṣa Dīwān al-'Arab: Qaḍāyā wa-Namādhij*. Cairo: al-Sharika al-Miṣriyya al-'Ālamiyya li-l-Nahsr—Longman.

Wahba, Magdi. 1974. *A Dictionary of Literary Terms*. Beirut: Librairie du Liban.

Wajdī, Wafā'. 1980. *al-Ḥubb fī Zamāninā*. Cairo: al-Hay'a al-Miṣriyya al-'Āmma li-l-Kitāb.

——. 1985. *al-Ḥarth fī al-Baḥr*. Cairo: Madbūlī.

Walder, Dennis. 1998. *Post Colonial Literatures in English: History, Language, Theory*. Oxford: Blackwell.

Wallace, David Foster. 2006. *Consider the Lobster and Other Essays*. New York: Little, Brown.

Walters, Keith. 2021. "Introduction: The Arabic Language and Identity." In Reem Bassiouney and Keith Walters (eds.). *The Routledge Handbook of Arabic and Identity*. New York: Routledge, pp. 3–10.

al-Wardī, 'Alī. 1971. *Lamaḥat Ijtimā'iyya min Ta'rīkh al-'Irāq al-Ḥadīth*. Baghdad: Maṭba'at al-Irshād.

al-Washshā', Abū al-Ṭayyib Muḥammad ibn Isḥāq. 1965. *al-Muwashshā*. Beirut: Dār Ṣādir.

al-Waṣīfī, 'Abd al-Raḥmān Muḥammad. 2002. *Nizār Qabbānī Shā'iran Siyāsiyan*. Cairo: Dār al-Fikr al-Ḥadith li-l-Ṭibā'a wa-l-Nashr.

Wasserstrom, Steven M. 1995. *Between Muslim and Jew: The Problem of Symbiosis under Early Islam*. Princeton, NJ: Princeton University Press.

Watson, Helen. 1992. *Women in the City of the Dead*. London: Hurst.

Watt, Montgomery W. 1963. *The Faith and Practice of al-Ghazali*. London: George Allen & Unwin.

——. 1972. *The Influence of Islam on Medieval Europe*. Edinburgh: Edinburgh University Press.

Waṭṭār, al-Ṭāhir. 1977. *al-Zilzāl*. Acre: Dār al-Aswār.

——. 2000. *The Earthquake*, trans. William Granara. London: Saqi Books.

Waugh, Earle H. 1989. *The Munshidīn* (sic!) *of Egypt: Their World and Their Song*. Columbia: University of South Carolina Press.

Wehr, Hans. 1976. *A Dictionary of Modern Written Arabic*. Ithaca, NY: Spoken Language Services.

Weidner, Stefan. 2012. "Exile that Enriches: The Cultural Achievements of Iranian and Arab Authors in Germany." *Fikrun wa Fann* 97, pp. 68–74.

Wensinck, A. J. and Mensing, J. P. (eds.). 1936–1969. *Concordance et Indices de la Tradition Musulmane*. Leiden: Brill.

Wheeler, Deborah L. 2017. *Digital Resistance in the Middle East: New Media Activism in Everyday Life*. Edinburgh: Edinburgh University Press.

White, Hayden. 2008. "'With No Particular Place to Go': Literary History in the Age of the Global Picture." *New Literary History* 39.3 (Summer), pp. 727–45.

Wien, Peter. 2017. *Arab Nationalism : The Politics of History and Culture in the Modern Middle East*. London: Routledge.

Wiet, Gaston. 1966. *Introduction à la littérature arabe*. Paris: Maisonneuve et Larose.

Wild, Stefan. 1996. "Islamic Enlightenment and the Paradox of Averroes." *Die Welt des Islams* 36.3, pp. 379–90.

——. 1999. "A Tale of Two Redemptions: A Comparative Analysis of Ṭāhā Ḥusayn's *The Days* and Muḥammad Shukrī's *For Bread Alone*." In Angelika Neuwirth et al. (eds.). *Myths, Historical Archetypes and Symbolic Figures in Arabic Literature*. Beirut: Orient-Institut der DMG, pp. 349–61.

Wilpert, Gero von. 1964. *Sachwörterbuch der Literatur*. Stuttgart: Kröner.

Wilson, Edmund. 1941. *The Wound and the Bow: Seven Studies in Literature*. Cambridge, MA: Houghton Mifflin.

Wimbush, Andy. 2016. "The Pretty Quietist Pater: Samuel Beckett's Molloy and the Aesthetics of Quietism." *Literature and Theology* 30.4, pp. 439–55.

Winckler, Barbara. 2018. "'New Media' and the Transformation of the Public Sphere in the *Nahḍa* Period and Today: How the Advent of the Periodical Press and the Internet Have Affected the Arabic Literary Field—Analogies and Differences." In Roger Allen et al. (eds.). *New Geographies: Texts and Contexts in Modern Arabic Literature*. Madrid: Ediciones Universidad Autónoma de Madrid, pp. 27–64.

Woolf, Virginia. n.d. *al-Amwāj*, trans. Murād al-Zumar; rev. Aḥmad Khākī. Cairo: Dār al-Kātib al-ʿArabī.

——. 1925. *Mrs. Dalloway*. New York: Harcourt, Brace.

——. 1963. *The Waves*. London: Hogarth Press.

——. 1968. *al-Amwāj*, trans. Murād al-Zumar. Cairo: Dār al-Maʿārif.

——. 1968a. *The Common Reader—First Series*. London: Hogarth Press.

——. 1968b. *al-Manār*, trans. Jurjis Mansī. Cairo: al-Hilāl.

——. 1971. *al-Qāri' al-ʿĀdī: Maqālāt fī al-Naqd al-Adabī*, trans. ʿAqīla Ramaḍān. Cairo: al-Hay'a al-Miṣriyya al-ʿĀmma li-l-Ta'līf.

——. 1974. *Mrs. Dalloway* (in Hebrew), trans. Rina Litwin. Tel Aviv: Machbarot Lesifrut.

——. 1992. *Flāsh*, trans. ʿAṭā ʿAbd al-Wahhāb. Baghdad: Dār Shamas.

——. 1994. *al-Sayyida Dalloway*, trans. ʿAbd al-Karīm Maḥfūḍ. Homs: Dār Jafrā li-l-Nashr.

——. 1998. *al-Sayyida Dalloway*, trans. ʿAṭā ʿAbd al-Wahhāb. Beirut: al-Mu'assasa al-ʿArabiyya li-l-Dirāsāt wa-l-Nashr.

——. 2008. *Yawm al-Ithnayn aw al-Thulāthā' (wa-Qiṣaṣ Ukhrā)*, trans. Laylā Muḥammad ʿUthmān Najātī. Cairo: al-Markaz al-Qawmī li-l-Tarjama.

——. 2009. *Athar ʿalā al-Ḥā'iṭ (Qiṣaṣ)*, trans. Fāṭima Nāʿūt. Cairo: al-Markaz al-Qawmī li-l-Tarjama.

——. 2009a. *Ghurfa Takhuṣṣu al-Mar' Waḥdahu*, trans. Sumayya Ramaḍān. Cairo: Madbūlī.

——. 2009b. *Juyūb Muthqala bi-l-Ḥijāra wa-"Riwāya lam Tuktab Baʿd"*, trans. Fāṭima Nāʿūt. Cairo: al-Markaz al-Qawmī li-l-Tarjama.

——. 2015. *Ilā al-Fanār*, trans. Isabel Kamāl. Cairo: al-Hay'a al-ʿĀmma l-Quṣūr al-Thaqāfa.

——. 2016. *Orlando*, trans. Tawfīq al-Asadī. Baghdad: Dār al-Madā.

——. 2017. *Ghurfa Takhuṣṣu al-Mar' Waḥdahu*, trans. 'Ahd Ṣabīḥa. Damascus: Dār Nīnwā.
Wordsworth, William. 1965. *Selected Poems and Prefaces*, ed. Jack Stillinger. Boston, MA: Houghton Mifflin.
al-Yāfi'ī, Abū Muḥammad. 1961. *Nashr al-Maḥāsin al-Ghāliya fī Faḍl al-Mashāyikh al-Ṣūfiyya Aṣḥāb al-Maqāmāt al-'Āliya*, ed. Ibrāhīm 'Aṭiyya 'Awaḍ. Cairo: Maṭba'at al-Ḥalabī.
Yāghī, 'Abd al-Raḥmān. 1980. *Fī al-Juhūd al-Masraḥiyya al-Ighrīqiyya al-Ūrūbiyya al-'Arabiyya (min al-Naqqāsh ilā al-Ḥakīm)*. Beirut: al-Mu'assasa al-'Arabiyya li-l-Dirāsāt wa-l-Nashr.
Yaḥyāwī, Rashīd. 2015. *al-Kalām 'alā al-Kalām fī al-Turāth: Madākhil li-Maqāṣid al-Ta'rīb wa-l-Tadyīn*. Amman: Dār Kunūz al-Ma'rifa.
Yanat, Kamel. 1985. "Note sur Dib et la science fiction: l'exemple de Cours sur la rive sauvage." *Kalim, Langues et littératures* (Algiers) 6, pp. 197–203.
Yāqūt. 1990. *Mu'jam al-Buldān*, ed. Farīd 'Abd al-'Azīz al-Jundī. Beirut: Dār al-Kutub al-'Ilmiyya.
——. 1991. *Mu'jam al-Udabā'*. Beirut: Dār al-Kutub al-'Ilmiyya.
Yazbak, Mahmoud. 1998. *Haifa in the Late Ottoman Period, 1864–1914: A Muslim Town in Transition*. Leiden: Brill.
Yosefi, Maksim. 2017. "The Attitude of the Religious Establishment towards Poets and Poetry in the First Centuries of Islam: A Textual Discussion." *Jama'a* 23, pp. 49–82.
Young, George. 1927. *Egypt*. London: Ernest Benn.
Younis, Eman. 2021. "Contemporary Arabic Literature and Its Obsession with the Internet." In Meir Hatina and Yona Sheffer (eds.) *Cultural Pearls from the East: In Memory of Shmuel Moreh, 1932–2017*. Leiden: Brill, pp. 224–43.
Zach, Natan. 1983. *All the Milk and Honey* (in Hebrew). Tel Aviv: Am Oved.
Zachs, Fruma. 2005. *The Making of a Syrian Identity: Intellectuals and Merchants in 19th-Century Beirut*. Leiden: Brill.
Zachs, Fruma and Halevi, Sharon. 2015. *Gendering Culture in Greater Syria: Intellectuals and Ideology in the Late Ottoman Period*. New York: I. B. Tauris.
——. 2018. "al-Bustānī family." In *Encyclopaedia of Islam*, 3rd edn. Edited by Kate Fleet, Gudrun Krämer, Denis Matringe, John Nawas, Everett Rowson. Available at: http://dx.doi.org/10.1163/1573-3912_ei3_COM_25436.
Zachs, Fruma and Bawardi, Basilius 2019. "Arab Nation-building through Detective Stories in al-Ḍiyā': The Cultural Translations of Nasīb al-Mash'alānī." *Die Welt des Islams* 60.1, pp. 1–23.
Zadādiqa, Sufyān. 2008. *al-Ḥaqīqa wa-l-Sarāb: Qirā'a fī al-Bu'd al-Ṣūfī fī Shi'r Adūnīs Marji'an wa-Mumārasatan*. Beirut: al-Dār al-'Arabiyya li-l-'Ulūm Nāshrūn and Manshūrāt al-Ikhtilāf.
Zaydān, Joseph. 1986. *Maṣādir al-Adab al-Nisā'ī fī al-'Ālam al-'Arabī al-Ḥadīth*. Jidda: al-Nādī al-Adabī al-Thaqāfī.
Zaydān, Jurjī. 1905. *Fatḥ al-Andalus aw Ṭāriq ibn Ziyād*. Cairo: al-Hilāl.
——. 1910–1911. *'Abd al-Raḥmān al-Nāṣir*. Cairo: al-Hilāl.
——. 1913. *Ta'rīkh Adab al-Lugha al-'Arabīyya*. Cairo: Maṭba'at al-Fajjāla.
——. 1960. *Ta'rīkh al-Adab al-'Arabī*. Cairo: Maktabat Nahḍat Miṣr.
——. 1992. "Al-Qiṣṣa 'Inda al-Ṣūfiyya." *al-Hilāl*, May, pp. 48–55.
al-Zayyāt, Aḥmad Ḥasan. n.d. *Ta'rīkh al-Adab al-'Arabī*. Cairo: Maktabat Nahḍat Miṣr.
Zeidan, Joseph T. 1979. "Myth and Symbol in the Poetry of Adūnīs and Yūsuf al-Khāl." *Journal of Arabic Literature* 10, pp. 71–94.
Zekavat, Massih. 2015. "A Comparative Study of the Poetics of Plato and the *Qur'ān*." *Primerjalna književnost* (Ljubljana) 38.3, pp. 39–58.

Zipin, Amnon. 1980. *Bibliography of Modern Hebrew Literature in Arabic Translation, 1948–1979*. Tel Aviv: Institute for the Translation of Hebrew Literature.
Ziter, Edward. 2015. *Political Performance in Syria From the Six-Day War to the Syrian Uprising*. New York: Palgrave Macmillan.
——. 2021. "Repurposing Romantic Drama in Late-Nineteenth-Century Egypt: Najīb al-Ḥaddād's Arabizations of Victor Hugo." *Journal of Arabic Literature* 52, pp. 394–424.
Zurayk, Constantine K. 1956. *The Meaning of the Disaster*. Beirut: Khayat.
Zwettler, Michael N. 1978. *The Oral Tradition of Classical Arabic Poetry: Its Character and Implications*. Columbus: Ohio State University Press.
——. 1990. "A Mantic Manifesto: The Sūra of 'The Poets' and the Qur'ānic Foundations of Prophetic Authority." In James L. Kugel (ed.). *Poetry and Prophecy: The Beginnings of a Literary Tradition*. Ithaca, NY: Cornell University Press, pp. 75–119, 205–31.
——. 2007. "The Sura of the Poets: 'Final Conclusions'?" *Journal of Arabic Literature* 38, pp. 111–66.

Index

Note: The definite article *al* is not taken into consideration in the alphabetical order. It appears in this form throughout the entire book before solar and lunar letters. The following terms and their derivatives do not appear in the Index as independent entries or appear only partly: Arab, Arabic, Baghdad, culture, Egypt, Iraq, Islam, language, literature, modern, poetry, popular, reading, religion, system, text, translation, West.